HOCKEN

Exegi monumentum aere perennius
(I have reared a monument more lasting than bronze.)
Odes of Horace, Book III

Collectors appear to non-collectors as selfish, rapacious, and half-mad, which is what collectors frequently are, but they may also be enlightened, generous, and benefactors of society, which is the way they like to see themselves. Mad or sane, they salvage civilization.
Wilmarth Lewis, collector of Walpoliana, 1952

The book-collector is in fact one of the assault troops in literature's and history's battle against the inequity of oblivion.
John Carter, 1979

We in New Zealand owe an inestimable debt to the private book collectors of the past ... Without them the resources for scholarship and research in our libraries would be pitifully weak and our ability to understand our distinctively New Zealand experience would be greatly hindered.
*J.E. Traue,'For the ultimate good of the nation'
in Committed to Print, 1991*

I have visited many of these old stations, now deserted or desolate spots, or else converted to purposes of a far different character. Nothing brought back to me so vividly the bygone past of old New Zealand as wandering through these ruined remains ... Such scenes I have more than once seen, and very sad they are – food for much painful thought and retrospect. Of scenes like these are the antiquities of New Zealand; and they indeed deserve the name. Surely people unthinkingly say that New Zealand is too new a country, that it has as yet little or no historical interest and no antiquities. To my mind associations make antiquities, rather than great lapse of time.
T.M. Hocken, 'The early history of New Zealand', 18 September 1880

Omit no detail.
Elsdon Best, citing Hocken, 1901

HOCKEN

Prince *of* Collectors

Donald Jackson Kerr

Published by Otago University Press
Level 1, 398 Cumberland Street
Dunedin, New Zealand
university.press@otago.ac.nz
www.otago.ac.nz/press

First published 2015
Copyright © Donald Jackson Kerr

The moral rights of the author have been asserted.
ISBN 978-1-877578-66-3

A catalogue record for this book is available from the National Library of New Zealand. This book is copyright. Except for the purpose of fair review, no part may be stored or transmitted in any form or by any means, electronic or mechanical, including recording or storage in any information retrieval system, without permission in writing from the publishers. No reproduction may be made, whether by photocopying or by any other means, unless a licence has been obtained from the publisher.

Publisher: Rachel Scott
Editor: Anna Rogers
Design concept and jacket design: Ralph Lawrence
Index: Diane Lowther

Front cover: Hocken on the deck of the Japanese steamer *Yawata Maru*, on which the family sailed from Sydney on 9 August 1901 on a long overseas trip to England via Japan and the East. SO9-393a, Hocken Collections, Uare Toaka o Hakena, University of Otago.
Back cover: Robley's personalised book label for Hocken, c. 1900.
Ref: A-080-006, Alexander Turnbull Library, Wellington

Printed in China through Asia Pacific Offset Ltd

This book is dedicated to collectors everywhere.

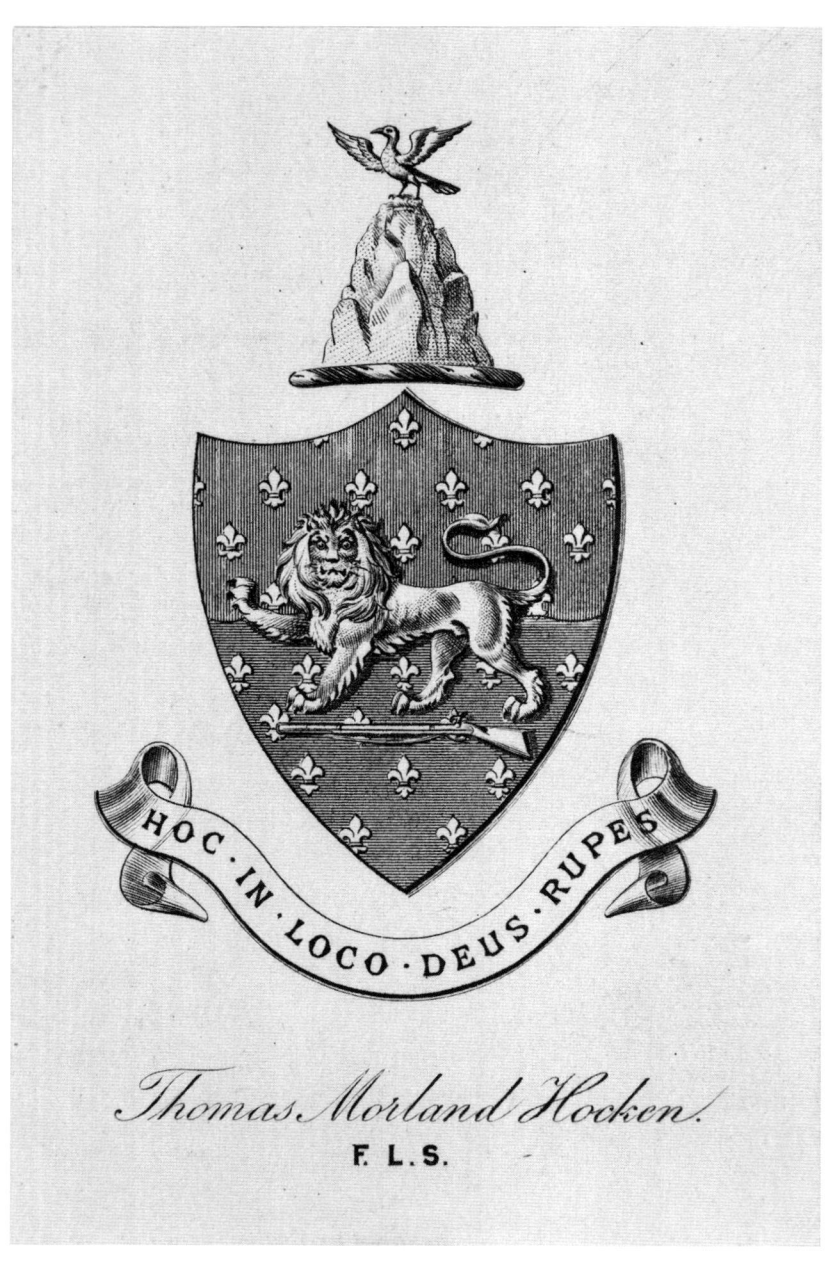

Hocken's 'F.L.S.' bookplate. The Latin motto translates as 'In this place God is a rock.'
S14-078i, Hocken Collections, Uare Taoka o Hakena, University of Otago

Contents

Foreword by Sharon Dell 9
Acknowledgements 11
Timeline 14
Introduction 17

1. Childhood and Schooling 24
2. Surgeon and Sailor 34
3. Early Beginnings in Dunedin 52
4. Home and Garden 66
5. A Fondness for Anything New Zealand 76
6. Cultivating Contacts 90
7. Good Fortune, Dr Hocken, FLS 104
8. In Her Own Right 114
9. A Reputation Established 126
10. 'A Very Big Affair Indeed' 144
11. Bibliographic Connections 157
12. The Fieldwork Continues 175
13. A Gift, a 'Literary Venture' and the South Seas 188
14. 'For a Boxful of Such *Rubbish* I Should be Infinitely Obliged' 200
15. A Welcome Break 211
16. The CMS, the Colonial Office and Home 220
17. 'Marsden or Some Other Old Historical Subject' 229
18. The Pinnacle 237
19. An Act of Patriotism 258
20. The Hocken Legacy 279

Appendices
  I. T.M. Hocken's Letter to his Friend George Fenwick 301
  II. T.M. Hocken's Last Will and Testament 304
  III. Selected Book-collecting Letters 309

Notes 319
Bibliography 374
Index 394

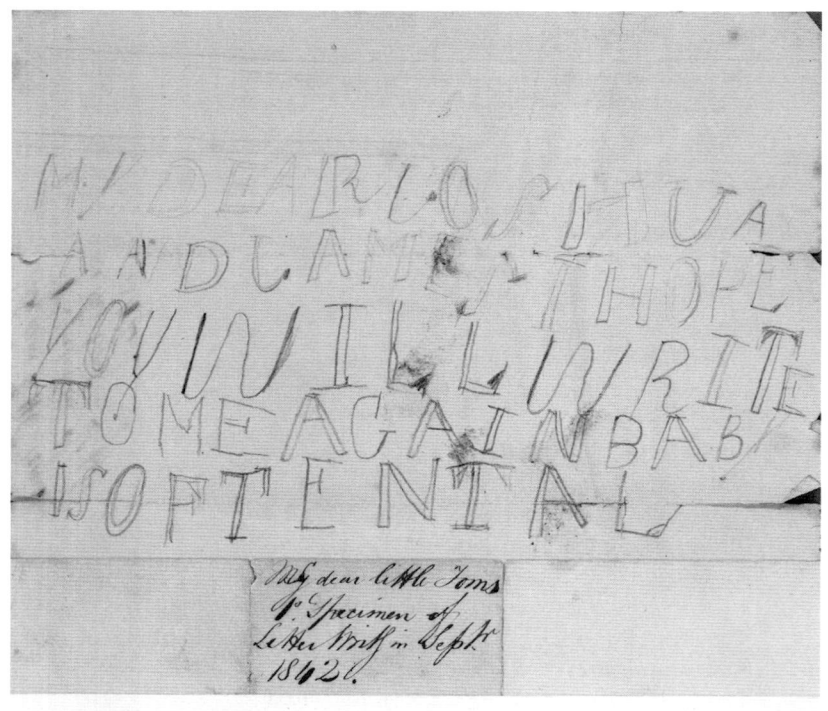

Life comes full circle: Thomas Morland Hocken's first (1842) and last (1910) writings. S14-078h, Hocken Collections, Uare Taoka o Hakena, University of Otago

Foreword

Ka Taoka Hakena: Treasures of the Hocken Collections was published in 2007 to mark the centenary of the signing of the deed of trust that transferred the collection of Thomas Morland Hocken to the University of Otago. In the preface to that volume, then Vice-Chancellor Professor Sir David Skegg wrote that many great universities had a great research library donated by a private collector or benefactor but, unlike most of those libraries, Hocken has the words 'open to the public' inscribed on its walls.

Many of the treasures highlighted in that book were part of Hocken's original collection, a testament to the quality of the founding collection and also to the growth that has occurred in the years that have followed Hocken's gift to the university.

Hocken: Prince of Collectors will be of great value to researchers in book history, book collecting, and the development of libraries in New Zealand. It will certainly increase understanding and appreciation of Hocken's legacy to New Zealand.

As Special Collections Librarian at the University of Otago Library Dr Donald Kerr was well placed to undertake this task, and the University Library was pleased to support his research. His familiarity with the two other great New Zealand collectors, Sir George Grey and Alexander Turnbull, has also allowed him to place Hocken in the wider context of New Zealand and Australian book collectors.

Donald has searched out and examined every volume in the original Hocken collection. He has pored over correspondence in libraries and archives and, following Hocken's own principles, has visited significant locations across the world in the course of his research. He has thus been able to create a detailed picture of Hocken's collecting methods. We also now know more about his motivation and his use of the material he gathered in lectures and publications.

We can read about Hocken's many connections and networks among sources, fellow collectors and experts in various fields. We gain insights into the loving father and family man and see how his wife Bessie was drawn into his enterprise: drawing, translating and copying for him.

I have worked in both the Alexander Turnbull Library and the Hocken Collections and it is interesting to note the differences in the collections as a reflection of the characters of two founders.

Bibliophile Alexander Turnbull was interested in books as objects. He had them bound and embellished in London by the superstar craftsmen of the day, and built a collection about the history of the book and book arts around them.

Hocken had a far more practical approach, developing his collection primarily as a database to use in his own historical research. He bound pamphlets and manuscripts into serviceable volumes that he would take with him to his public lectures; he would annotate them, index them and provide keys to features in works of art.

Hocken was also a bibliographer, and this book details his relationships with Australian counterparts and places his work in the context of other attempts at compiling comprehensive records. Hocken's *A Bibliography of the Literature Relating to New Zealand* was published in July 1909, and endured for 60 years as the principal record of New Zealand publications.

As a researcher Hocken knew the value of even the most seemingly trivial material. 'My own extensive experience in these matters leads me to say that no letter or document should be cast aside as too trivial for the purpose in view. It may contain but a grain of information, may supply a missing date, or may throw some light on something obscure.'[1]

The value of documenting New Zealand's founding collections is nowhere more evident than in the case of Hocken's enthusiasm for Samuel Marsden and the Church Missionary Society. This book tells the full story of Hocken's acquisition of material from CMS offices in London and his pursuit of relatives of the early missionary settlers. He travelled several times to the Bay of Islands to see for himself the site of their endeavours and interviewed many people associated with the mission. He felt deep regret that his own publication on Marsden and the mission would remain incomplete at his death, although his work formed the basis of J.R. Elder's two volumes published in the 1930s.

In late 2014 Hocken's CMS records were inscribed on the New Zealand Register of the UNESCO Memory of the World programme. November 2014 also saw the launch of the Marsden Online Archive containing 3700 pages of 600 of the manuscript letters and journals in Hocken's collection, along with transcripts and sophisticated online research tools.

Some 110 years after their acquisition and 200 years after the events they describe, these records of the foundation of New Zealand are now accessible anywhere in the world. The project is one of many giving a contemporary twist to words 'open to the public', as more and more of the collections that Hocken created and inspired become accessible online.

For Thomas Morland Hocken – collector, bibliographer, communicator and benefactor – his work was a labour of love. For those of us who continue to build and care for his collection and the great research library that has developed from it, this book is a valuable resource as we gain inspiration from our founder, understanding of his methods and motivations, and deeper knowledge of the origins of the collection with which we work.

Sharon Dell, Hocken Librarian, February 2015

Acknowledgements

It is a pleasure to acknowledge the many debts accumulated during the years in which this work has been written. As Special Collections Librarian at the University of Otago, I have had valuable access to the Hocken Library, a mere seven minutes' walk away. In my quick jaunts back and forth, and via telephone and email, I have received support and encouragement from the staff at the Hocken. It is therefore to my colleagues there that I offer first thanks: Sharon Dell (Hocken Librarian), Anna Blackman, Ali Clarke, Natalie Poland, Katherine Milburn, Mark Quarrie, Lucy Clark, Mary Lewis, Anna Petersen, Karen Craw, Alexander Ritchie, Iain Chambers and Anne Jackman, now Director, Presbyterian Research Centre, Knox College.

In March 2007 I received a Ministry for Heritage and Culture New Zealand History Research Trust Fund Award, which facilitated my research, especially at libraries and research institutions throughout New Zealand and Australia. To the ministry I offer sincere thanks for the opportunity to work in the State Library of Victoria, the State Library of New South Wales, the State Library of Tasmania, the University of Tasmania Library, the Alexander Turnbull Library, Canterbury Museum and the Sir George Grey Special Collections at Auckland Libraries. In 2010 I received a Winston Churchill Memorial Award that enabled five weeks' research in Britain, following the 'Hocken Trail'. I am grateful not only to this agency, but to all those fine libraries and institutions that held materials pertinent to my work on Hocken.

Of course the institutions are nothing without the people within them, and encouragement from colleagues concerning one's project is always gratifying. Personal thanks must go to: John Cardwell and Sarah Preston (Royal Commonwealth Collection and Cambridge University Library), James Stevenson and Carol Tasker (Lincoln Archives, Lincoln), Jennie Mooney (Grimsby Public Library), Beverley Osborne, Hugh Knowles and Jackie Balaam (Woodhouse Grove School, North Yorkshire), Kath Cassidy and Derek Tree (Newcastle Public Library), Melanie Wood and Allan Callender (Robinson Library, University of Newcastle), Joseph Marshall (Special Collections, University of Edinburgh), Mary O'Doherty (Mercer Library, Royal College of Surgeons in Ireland, Dublin), Brid O'Sullivan (National Library of Ireland), Beata Bradford (SS Great Britain Archive, Bristol), Colin Harris (Bodleian Library, Oxford), Nicholas Martland and John Goldfinch (British Library), Lynda Brooks (Linnean Society, London), Sarah Walpole (Royal Anthropological Institute, London) and Heidi Potter (Japan Society, London). In Australia I thank Des Cowley (State Library of Victoria, Melbourne), Paul Brunton and Jim Andrighetti (Mitchell Library, State Library of New South Wales), Mark Hildebrand (Dixson Librarian, State Library of New South

Wales), Emilia Ward, Juanita Wertepny and Gill Ward (University of Tasmania, Hobart) and Ian Morrison (State Library of Tasmania, Hobart).

In the search for relevant material on Hocken, I have been helped by many people, and their responses, in person, by letter or email, have greatly refined my research and assisted my work. My thanks to: John Adams, Robin Adams, Charles Benson and Eileen O'Flaherty (Trinity College Library, Dublin), Captain Masaharu Akamine (NYK Maritime Museum, Yokohama, Japan), Wyn Beasley, James Beattie, Simon Beattie (ex-Quaritch), David Bell, Roger Blackley, Simon Blundell (Reform Club, London), Robert Booth, Kate Boyes (Capetown), Tom Brooking, Eileen Chanin, Rosemary Clarkson, Ruth Long and Adam Perkins (Darwin Archive, Cambridge Library), Neil Clayton, Roger Collins, Richard Dingwall, John Eggling, Simon Eliot (University of London), Ian Farquhar, Jan Flood, Colin Franklin (Oxford), Lydia Fraser (Textile Museum, Washington, DC), David Galloway, Rowan Gibbs, Peter Griffiths, Robert Hannah, Michael Harlow, Gordon Haws, John Holmes, Susan Irvine, Michael Jeans (Cambridge Museum, New Zealand), Edmund King, Michael Laird, Helen Leach, Gregor Macaulay, Johanna Massey, John Montgomery (Royal United Services Institute Librarian, London), Jerry Morris, Peter Nockles, Suzanne Fagan and Dominic Whitehead (John Rylands Library, University of Manchester), Geraldine O'Driscoll (Royal College of Surgeons of England, London), Erik Olssen, Richard Overell (Monash Library), Phil Parkinson, Lachy Paterson, Richard Reeves, Michael Reilly, James Ritchie, Shef Rogers, Peter Skegg, John Stenhouse, Lucy Sussex, Garry Tee, Philip Temple, Linda Tyler, David Verran, John and Michele Walker (Calverley Vicarage, Calverley, Pudsey, West Yorkshire), Ian Wards, Jane Stemp Wickenden (Institute of Naval Medicine), John Wilson (North East Lincolnshire Archives) and Kathy Young.

New Zealand libraries and institutions, and their personnel, also deserve gratitude for their support and encouragement. Thanks to Martin Collett and Elizabeth Lorimer (Auckland Institute and Museum Library), Bruce Ralston (ex-manager, Library and Information Service, Auckland War Memorial Museum), Lorraine Johnston (Heritage Collection Librarian, Dunedin Public Library), Jean Strachan and Anthony Tedeschi (both ex-Dunedin Public Library), Alison Breese and Chris Scott (Dunedin City Archives), Scott Reeves and Dimitri Anson (Otago Museum), Jennifer Twist and John Yaldwyn (Museum of New Zealand Te Papa Tongarewa Archives), Jocelyn Chambers (Alexander Turnbull Library), Joanna Condon (ex-Canterbury Museum) and my former colleagues at the Sir George Grey Special Collections, Auckland Libraries, especially Georgia Prince, Iain Sharp, Keith Giles and Kate de Courcy.

The University of Otago Library has been exceedingly supportive in this project and I offer thanks to the Executive Management Group who, in 2007, approved a six-month secondment that allowed time to examine Hocken's collection. For this initiative I have to thank Stuart Strachan, ex-Hocken Librarian, who not only read parts of the original draft but has been extremely supportive of my work. I would also like to thank Dr A.G. Hocken (no relation), who not only read a few draft chapters, but also kindly supplied a copy of the diary of Gladys Hocken from the Fish Hoek Archives, Cape Town, South Africa. Others who have assisted, apart from the Hocken colleagues listed above, and who deserve thanks, include John Hughes and Richard Munro (University of Otago Library) and Rosalind Andrews and Pam Treanor, now ex-University of Otago Library.

A number of individuals require special mention. Sincere thanks must go to Christopher de Hamel, Nicolas and Joanna Barker, David and Rosalind McKitterick, and Christopher and Ros Buckland Wright. Their friendship and encouragement helped me enormously while I was visiting Britain. Ralph Lawrence has not only provided encouragement in this project but, being a designer, has worked his magic on the design of the book and jacket. For this I thank him heartily. And special gratitude to David Elliot and his wife Gillian, a colleague at the University of Otago. David accompanied me on my trip to England, and I would not have accomplished so much if I had not been able to share the costs of a car while chasing Dr Hocken. David also embarked on 'a little research', for which I will be forever grateful. To Gillian I still relate fond memories of this 'boys' trip' and our experiences on the road.

For permission to use and quote from unpublished manuscripts in their care or ownership I thank the following: the Hocken Collections, especially the Fish Hoek Archives, Cape Town; Mrs D.E. Hotmoller (Johannesburg; MS-3741); the Alexander Turnbull Library; the Sir George Grey Special Collections at Auckland Libraries; the Auckland Institute and Museum Library; the British Library; and Lincoln Archives. Permission to reproduce photographs was granted by Hocken Collections, the Alexander Turnbull Library and the State Library of New South Wales.

A book like this is not done alone. At various stages, a number of people have read the typescript and provided invaluable suggestions for its improvement. For their time and energy I am grateful to Tony Ballantyne, David Murray, Gordon Parsonson, David Skegg and Stuart Strachan, who applied the red pen to passages, phrases and grammatical errors I have taken on board their suggestions. Nevertheless, all mistakes and misconceptions are mine alone. I would also like to thank the publisher and the team at Otago University Press for their efforts to transform the manuscript to book form.

And finally, warm and sincere thanks to Jude and Sam for their patience and tolerance. Without their support, the completion of this book would not have been possible.

Donald Kerr, Dunedin, 2015

Timeline

Dr Thomas Morland Hocken 1836–1910

14 January 1836	Born Stamford, Lincolnshire
1844–50	Attends Woodhouse Grove School
1851	Apprenticed to Robert McNichol, apothecary, St Helens, Lancashire
1853–58	Assistant to Dr Septimus William Rayne, Newcastle upon Tyne
1854–58	Attends medical courses at the Practical School of Science, Newcastle
1858–59	Medical student, Original Theatre of Anatomy and School of Medicine and Surgery, Dublin
May 1859	Admitted to the Royal College of Surgeons of England
October 1859	Secures post of surgeon-superintendent on *White Star*
January 1861	Secures post of surgeon-superintendent on SS *Great Britain*
October 1861	First appearance in print: 'Treatment of sea-sickness', *The Lancet*
1861	Salvages shipboard newspapers
February 1862	Arrives in Dunedin from Melbourne
December 1862	Delivers a talk on botany to Dunedin citizens
January 1863	Appointed coroner, Dunedin district
July 1867	Marries Julia Anne Dakyne Simpson, Waikouaiti
1869	Foundation member of the Otago Institute
June 1871	Moves into Atahapara, Moray Place
December 1881	Julia Hocken dies

March 1882	Leaves for England
December 1882	Returns from England
March 1883	Accepted as a Fellow of the Linnean Society, London
July 1883	Marries Elizabeth Mary Buckland, Invercargill
1884	Gladys Hocken, only daughter, born
1885	Gazetted out of coronership
March 1897	Announces 'gift' to the Dominion
March 1898	*Contributions* published
April 1898	Visits Samoa and Fiji
August 1901	Leaves for England via Japan
June 1902	Accepted as a Non-Resident Fellow of the Royal Colonial Institute, London
June 1902	Accepted as a corresponding member of the Japan Society, London
July 1903	Granted permission to examine Colonial Office Records
November 1903	Secures Church Missionary Society manuscripts
November 1903	Accepted as an Ordinary Fellow of the Royal Anthropological Institute, London
July 1904	Returns from England via Japan
2 September 1907	Deed of trust signed
July 1909	*Bibliography* published
March 1910	Appointed Vice-Chancellor, University of Otago
31 March 1910	Opening of the Hocken Wing
17 May 1910	Dies of cancer, Dunedin

Introduction

Dr Thomas Morland Hocken (1836–1910) is one of the Holy Trinity of first book collectors in New Zealand, alongside Governor Sir George Grey in Auckland and Wellington's Alexander Horsburgh Turnbull. Throughout his busy life as a medical practitioner in Dunedin he collected books, manuscripts, sketches, maps and photographs pertinent to the history and development of early New Zealand. Much of the driving force for his collecting was based around James Cook and early discovery narratives, the Rev. Samuel Marsden and his contemporaries, Edward Gibbon Wakefield and the New Zealand Company, Maori, and early settlement and colonisation, especially in the south. In March 1910 his extensive collection was gifted to New Zealand and eventually passed over to the University of Otago for full stewardship. Still one of the country's best repositories of New Zealand and Pacific materials, it continues to attract scholars both local and international.

Apart from Eric McCormick's essay on Hocken in his *Fascinating Folly* (1961), A.G. Hocken's lecture, *Dr T.M. Hocken 1836–1910: A gentleman of his time* (1986), and his more recent *Dr Hocken of Dunedin: A life* (2008), John Ross's article on Hocken in the *Dictionary of Literary Biography* (Volume 184; 1997) and an earlier thesis study by Olga Fitchett (1928), little systematic and specific work has been done on Hocken as a collector. A comprehensive study of him in this guise is long overdue.

This book is the first to provide a full account of Hocken's collecting and the development of his library. I have used a bio-bibliographical approach, which allows for coverage of five important aspects. First, there are the types and categories of materials he collected. Apart from the occasional foray into more traditional areas of book collecting – that is, rare books – his collecting was focused on the above-mentioned subjects. It was confined, specific collecting at its best.

Second, there is the collecting process and how Hocken acquired his material. His arrival in Dunedin in February 1862 signalled the beginning of his collecting in New Zealand, his adopted home. Both opportunistic and visionary, he recognised that there were things about his newly adopted country that were worth saving. He began collecting at the right time, when those individuals who had played such a significant role in the early development of the country were old, or had just died, and their close family members were keen to talk about the past and perpetuate the memory of those stored experiences. Many were increasingly concerned about what to do with family papers, books and newspapers. Hocken would have agreed wholeheartedly with Turnbull, his fellow collector, who wrote that: 'The present day New Zealand public is apt to forget those who bore the heat & burden of the troublous times the colony passed through in the sixties and that is one reason why I strive to make my collection of New Zealand literature as complete as I can.'[1] Hocken made every effort to obtain such documents and attempted to ground his collection and subsequent publications on the efforts of others. His frequent pilgrimages north, the networking that evolved from these trips, the friendships and relationships that resulted, his use of events such as the New Zealand and South Seas Exhibition and organisations such as the Otago Institute, and his sheer persistence in hunting down books and manuscripts, form integral components of his activities as a collector. He obtained much material from individuals throughout the country, and almost every outgoing letter in his voluminous correspondence contained a plea for historical matter that he was willing to take in and save. He was forever asking, and his requests bore fruit.

He bought from book dealers such as Chapman in Auckland, Angus & Robertson in Sydney and Bernard Quaritch in London, but little evidence of such transactions survives. He certainly obtained books over the counter while visiting England during his two trips there and secured important caches of manuscript materials. Yet again, for the books at least, few invoices remain. Book collectors like Grey and Turnbull purchased from antiquarian dealer catalogues and these remain in their collections, enabling trends of purchase to be established and estimates of how much was paid for an item and when. There are too few catalogues in Hocken's collection to draw any such conclusions.

Third, there is the development of his library within New Zealand and, to a certain extent, Australia. Because much of his collecting focused on the local, he did not have to worry too much about the supply or availability of books. Although many of the publications he acquired had London imprints, many were available in selected bookshops throughout New Zealand and Australia. As time went on, increasing numbers of books, pamphlets, maps and broadsheets were published locally for a growing local market. Hocken took advantage of this trend. His acquisition of primary materials such as manuscripts and maps was often serendipitous, aided by his growing reputation as an authority on New Zealand history and as a collector. Indeed, documents and books were generously given to him, usually without any conditions attached. He also had contact with the four major book collectors in Australia and New Zealand: Sir George Grey, Alexander Turnbull, David Scott Mitchell and Sir William Dixson.

Fourth, there are his publications, his *Contributions to the Early History of New Zealand (Settlement of Otago)* (1898), *Bibliography* (1909) and the posthumous *The Early History of New Zealand* (1914), all of which are tangible results of his collecting. Integral to these works are the lectures he delivered, which were first published in local newspapers. Hocken was above all an educator. In 1908, for example, he offered the Polynesian Society £100 towards publishing manuscripts submitted to the society, if the 200 or so other members could raise a further £400 for that purpose. He wanted materials such as Elsdon Best's Urewera history (over 700 foolscap pages), various collections of Rarotongan and Marquesan traditions and other papers on better-known Maori subjects to be published and gain wider readership. In conveying this generous offer by 'one of our original members', Stephenson Percy Smith appealed to society members in words that could have been penned by Hocken:

> Here is a chance for many of our New Zealand Colonists, who are well able to afford it, to assist in the National work of preserving the old records of a race that is rapidly passing away – at any rate those who are able to supply information so often required when the details of these manuscripts come to be studied. The liberal offer now made is one that, on no account should be allowed to fall through, for a similar one may never be repeated.

A circular was posted out to all members.[2] Unfortunately, by 7 August 1908, only £30 10s had been collected.[3] Hocken had experienced poor responses and inertia from others before, and had predicted a similar outcome. He stoically continued regardless.

Last, further light is cast on Dr Thomas Morland Hocken or, as he was occasionally called, Dr Horching, Hockin, Hawkins, Hocking, Hocklen and Hocker. Indeed, one citizen gave him a wooden leg.[4] True, there is much known and written about the 'wee doctor', but it is hoped that new and relatively unknown facts pertinent to his collecting will form a better and more rounded picture and understanding of him. His relationship with and reliance on his second wife Bessie is of particular importance.

Hocken's collection itself is a source of much of this light. Since the advent of the handpress and the printing of books, bookplates or ex libris (from the books) have been used by book collectors to denote ownership. The pasting of a bookplate (armorial, pictorial or an amalgam of these) into a book is an integral part of a good collector's notion of forming a collection. It is the ideal opportunity for the collector to handle the book and examine its condition and contents. It also offers aesthetic decision-making about where to place the bookplate: on the front pastedown endpaper? Over an existing bookplate? Beside an existing one? This process also presupposes having a bookplate, either designed by the owner or commissioned, as in some cases, from an artist. Of course, pasting it in is never a quick process. It can be done at the time of acquisition; often it is done later, when there is more time available. Every good collector recognises the validity of this experience. It says, 'This book is mine.' It represents order, control, ownership verification and immortality. It is the same with the signing of one's books.

As Hocken's collection took shape, he made its contents his own. He had an armorial bookplate made, which he placed in most of his books and manuscript volumes. Though he could not bear arms by right, he appropriated them for his bibliophilic purpose. Tradition has it that John Hockin, Vicar of Oakhampton and Rector of Lydford, county Devon, and chaplain to the Rt Hon. George, Lord Lyttelton, obtained a grant from the College of Arms that commemorated an incident in the time of Queen Anne. The tale goes that one Thomas Hockin single-handedly drove off a landing party from a French privateer in the Bristol Channel that was intent on raiding Godrevey, the family estate. The privateers were forced to withdraw after Hockin, from behind a rock, vigorously fired back at them. The 'spade' shield on the College of Arms grant shows the English lion and Hockin's gun on the red top half, with a wavy shoreline separating the blue (sea) in the bottom strewn with French fleur-de-lys in disarray. The crest depicts a rock with a seagull rising, all proper, on a wreath. Hocken's amended bookplate has the lion and gun central and the fleur-de-lys over the whole shield and in neat array. The motto *Hoc in loco Deus rupes* (In this place God is a rock) backs up the original story and confirms the spelling 'Hockin'.[5]

He had two bookplates: one printed with 'F.L.S.' (Fellow of the Linnean Society, London) and one without. The latter was the first produced and almost always has a scripted ink version of 'F.L.S.' added to it. The printed 'F.L.S.' bookplate was certainly produced after 1 March 1883, the day he officially became a Fellow of the Linnean Society. There is no definite date when the first was created, although a small embossed stamp of 'his' coat-of-arms may offer a clue. Some books, but not all of them, have an embossed stamp on page 35.[6] Although the reason why Hocken chose this page number is not known, a reasonable suggestion is that it was in 1871, when he was 35 and had moved into his home, Atahapara. The collector had a firm base; why not a bookplate, which he surely designed himself?

A 'Hocken' book or manuscript is easily distinguishable. His bookplate and embossed arms aside, he was a prolific signer, signing many of his books three times: on a preliminary page, on the title page and on the first part of the text proper. In addition to this, he had a hei tiki stamp and a hei tiki label, each containing the Maori version of his name, 'Hakena'. These two items were created by his friend, General Horatio Gordon Robley, about 1899. The green tiki label read 'NGA TE HAKENA TENEI TIKI' – 'this tiki belongs to Hocken'. It should have read 'na', so Hocken cancelled the 'g' with a pen. Using green ink, Hocken stamped only some of his books. The label was pasted in, and was also seldom used. And as with so many provenance markers, endless variations are found in his books.

Occasionally dates are given that help us to determine when he acquired a book. Early acquisitions include W.C. Wentworth's *A Statistical, Historical, and Political Description of the Colony of New South Wales* (1819), which has all of Hocken's accoutrements ('F.L.S.' bookplate, signature, etc), and the date '1871'. Another book is the second edition of William Eden's *The History of New*

Holland, from its First Discovery in 1616, to the Present Time (1787), which has his provenance markers, but also 'T.M. Hocken 1872' on the title page. Hocken was inordinately proud of his collection.

There are three general caveats. First, this work is not about Hocken and his career as coroner and surgeon. True, his medical profession helped to establish his standing and credentials in Dunedin (and the wider community); it gave him entrée to various levels of society; it enabled him to foster useful networks; and it gave him the wherewithal to build a large house to accommodate his collection, to travel and to buy books and manuscripts. Acknowledging that it was an integral part of his being, I mention it in passing, preferring to give greater prominence to the activity of collecting. For those interested in his medical career, I recommend A.G. Hocken's biography.

Second, Hocken collected hundreds of Maori and Pacific Island artefacts, many of which are now housed at the Otago Museum. Some are mentioned, but this work does not cover the more specialised area of artefacts, their provenance and ethnographic importance.

Third, Hocken was a small man, possibly 4 ft 8 in (142 cm), and certainly not 5 ft. Throughout his collecting career there is evidence that he was pushy, persistent, dogged (as every collector must be) and sometimes irritating. The small-man syndrome comes to mind: perhaps he did overcompensate for his size. Despite his stature, he was certainly noticed and had a presence. His extremely scrupulous determination to assert ownership – bookplate, signature, hei tiki stamp – reflects much of how he saw himself, his collection and the future. The psychology of collecting I leave to others.

Collecting has been defined by Werner Muensterberger in his *Collecting: An unruly passion* (1994), as 'the selecting, gathering, and keeping of objects of subjective value'.[7] Collecting is a highly individualistic activity, and Hocken was engaged in it for a good 50 years. Fortunately, his collection is extant: 5200 books, hundreds of manuscripts, 34 volumes of 'Variae' (some 650 disparate manuscripts and ephemeral printed materials bound together), 17 volumes of 'Flotsam and Jetsam' (hereafter F&J), 2800 pamphlets in 210 volumes, maps, sketches, paintings and photographs. This book is not only about patient assembly, it is also biographical, teasing out aspects that promote greater understanding of his life and activities as a collector.

In 1517 the Dukes of Bavaria appointed Johannes Avetinus their historiographer and commissioned him to prepare an official history of their realm. 'Day and night without rest,' Avetinus reported, he went 'across the entire land of Bavaria, pounding at the door of every convent and monastery, sifting every box of papers, perusing and copying word for word every pertinent manuscript, charter, privilege, letter, chronicle, verse, saying, adventure story, missal, prayer book, inventory, calendar, obituary, saint's life …' in fulfilment of his ducal commission 'to discover, inspect, and transcribe the old documents, antiquities, and records stored in our Bavarian monasteries'.[8] A growing sense of national pride led to the collection and compilation of historical records. Hocken was such an historiographer.

In this role he was very fortunate. He was likeable, methodical, persistent and an excellent field worker, willing to get his hands dirty as he trawled through mountains of documents and printed books. In fact, by this manner he 'rescued' the Treaty of Waitangi from the basement of Wellington's Government Buildings in 1908. Although facsimiles had been made as early as 1877, he discovered the nation's prime document 'damaged' and 'rat eaten' amid a heap of old papers. As J.H. Aumblin wrote of Hocken: 'I can fancy you poking about in all sorts of curious & queer old shops for New Zealand things. Don't forget envelopes or letters with old N.Z. stamps.'[9] Hocken was also lucky to meet people who were history-makers in New Zealand, or their kith and kin. His enthusiasm was infectious, especially when he appealed to their good nature in preserving materials for the future. Without doubt, Hocken was not only the right collector at the right time, but also truly visionary. Although penned by his friend Augustus Hamilton, the following sentiments could well apply to him:

> Even the things that seem most common, least worthy, when in use, all gain some being as time passes. Each little thing that carelessly we value not at first, grows rich with store of years. Still more do places gain their hold upon us unheeded at the time. A store of memories of days spent amidst strong associations that stirred and built the mind are the truest riches in all after-life ... The man who knows and dwells in history adds a new dimension of his existence: he no longer lives in the one plane of present ways and thoughts; he lives in the whole space of life — past, present, and dimly future ... He values the present as the most complete age of history for study, as explaining the past. He values the past as the long continuity that has brought about the result of the present, in which he happens to breathe. He lives in all time; the ages are his; all live alive, to him ...[10]

In September 1901 Hocken advised Elsdon Best to 'omit no detail'.[11] I have not been able to follow that dictum. I physically examined Hocken's entire collection, and though this was an enjoyable exercise, it produced more data: provenance details, bibliographical nuances to certain volumes, and numerous notations and marginalia. By necessity, I have had to be selective. I have used what correspondence there is, but much of it is incomplete, allowing only part of his story to be told. I have, however, quoted generously from the many incoming and outgoing letters because they give authority to the factual record upon which his life and activities as a collector stand. Any faults or omissions are mine alone.

On two separate occasions the Nelson-based Francis Arnot Blackader Bett, fellow medico and corresponding member of Pat Lawlor's 'bookmen', called Hocken 'the perfect collector' and 'the Prince of Collectors', acknowledging that he was one of that rare breed of individuals who amass their collections in their chosen fields and then selflessly give them away for the benefits of others.[12] As an avid collector himself, Bett had the right credentials to make this claim. This, then, is Hocken's story.

1
Childhood and Schooling

The picturesque Lincolnshire town of Stamford, Hocken's birthplace, is located in the southern part of Kesteven on the River Welland, 80 km from Lincoln and approximately 160 km north of London (just off the A1). Because it was an old thoroughfare to and from the capital, several parliaments were held there in the Middle Ages. Initially a pottery centre, it became recognised as a wool and cloth production centre. Stamford has always been a town of churches, spires dominating its skyline. Five medieval churches are still in use, and three non-conformist chapels. A number of other fine buildings, such as the medieval Browne's Hospital and Burghley House, built by William Cecil, secretary of state to Elizabeth I, are among the town's 600 listed buildings and have won it conservation area status. Because of this, Stamford has been used as the setting for a number of television shows and films.[1]

Thomas Morland Hocken was born here on 14 January 1836, though his exact place of birth remains unknown. His father, Joshua, an itinerant Methodist preacher, was in the third year of his Stamford circuit, which took in some 24 local towns and villages.[2] He shared his duties with James Cook Jr and Martin Tubb, and looked to Methodist church members to raise funds to meet the costs of family, servants, washing, coals and candles, letter charges and medicines.[3]

Amid anxious moments on 14 January, Joshua Hocken noted in his diary: 'This evening at 7 o'clock my dear Anne was safely delivered of a fine and lovely boy; prayer was answered in the event, and we now have additional cause for praise and devotedness to God. Oh that my insensible heart *felt* more.'[4] By March 1836, the £2 fee for Anne Hocken's confinement was duly noted in the circuit accounts. The boy's second name was most favoured: a letter written by Joshua in May 1853 is addressed to 'My dear James and Joshua and Morland'. Hocken himself preferred and always used his middle name.

Joshua Hocken, born one of four brothers at Bodmin, Cornwall, in 1798, joined the Wesleyan Methodists in 1815, where 'he obtained the blessedness of "those whose iniquities are forgiven, and whose sin is covered"'.[5] After diligent service as a local minister, he entered the Methodist Society ministry in 1824. Thus began his 29-year career as an itinerant Methodist preacher. His preaching was described as 'plain, evangelical, practical and earnest and blessed with the conversion of many souls'.[6] Through what he called 'the revolvings of the mysterious wheel of divine providence', Joshua met Anne, daughter of John and Jane Richardson of Richmond, Yorkshire.[7] On 19 August 1828 they were married in Manchester by the Rev. William Marsden.[8] The licence indicates that they were both 21, but in fact they were 30. A small 1829 oil portrait of Anne Hocken shows a kindly but determined woman, her dark hair hidden by a white bonnet.⁹ Little is known of her except that she had one sister, Mary, and six brothers. Anne died on 22 November 1887 and was interred in St Giles Church Yard, Durham.¹⁰

Anne and Joshua had five children, and their birthplaces give an excellent indication of the transient life of a nineteenth-century circuit preacher. Morland's oldest brother, James Richardson, was born at Abergavenny, Monmouthshire, Wales, in 1829; Joshua was born in Hampshire, Winchester, in 1831; younger brother William Henry was born in Caistor, Lincolnshire in 1838; and his only sister, Eliza Anne, was born in 1840 at Shardlow, near Derby. Two other children died in infancy: John Wesley (1833) and Andorania (1834).¹¹

Circuit tenure was usually for three years, followed by a move to another designated area. Itinerant preaching was often arduous and demanded strength of character, not to mention fitness. Some 10 years before Joshua began his work, 62-year-old Joseph Taylor, based in Derby 'in the 38th year of my itinerant labours', described the life: 'We are only two Preachers, and one horse, and are 2 weeks in and 2 weeks out. In the time we are in we walk to 5 places in the country, the most distant of which is about 4 miles.'¹² Horses played an important part in the rise and progress of Methodism. At one conference when a circuit clamoured for another minister, the Rev. Jabez Bunting suggested, 'Send them a horse! … The beast would help the existing ministers to do double the work.'¹³

Bunting was important to Joshua Hocken: he sanctioned his appointment. The conscientious custodian of John Wesley's system, Bunting was ordained in 1803, made secretary of the Wesleyan Conference in 1814 and served as president in 1820 and 1828. The vigorous and rigorous Bunting, known not so affectionately as the 'Methodist Pope', described the circuit from London via Manchester to Hull: 'But you will remember that to travel 800 miles, attend some nine or ten public meetings, and preach once at all of the places, or nearly all, in the space of sixteen days, is rather trying to one's strength.'¹⁴ Bunting was a good man to know and Joshua no doubt exhibited the right credentials.

Joshua was in Aberdeen in 1824 and 1825, and then from 1831 to 1833 in Jersey on the Guernsey district.¹⁵ The family returned there later: the 1861 census places Anne and her daughter Eliza at 17 Alley Street, St Peter Port.¹⁶ In September 1836 Joshua received £19 10s 1d from the Methodist Council as his last pay installment for duties completed on the Stamford circuit. By October 1836 the family had moved to Grimsby, on the Humber Estuary in northeast Lincolnshire, where young Morland Hocken spent his formative years. His father was often absent. For example, from May to July 1837 Joshua covered the towns of Grimsby, Caistor, Cleethorpes, Waltham, Limber, Keelby and Laceby.¹⁷ It was a well-defined and demanding schedule, involving many kilometres and a number of services every Sunday – and this was outside the usual weekday service and administrative obligations. Amid all this continuous activity Morland was baptised, somewhat belatedly, on 25 February 1837 at the Wesleyan Chapel in Grimsby.[18] John Jones, who shared Joshua's circuit duties, was the presiding minister.

For the Hocken family the Methodist circuit life provided a livelihood, a firm religious base, a sense of community and a strong culture of achievement. These were earnest, simple, pious lives removed from worldly pleasures and centred on home, chapel and business, a sense of duty, hard work, foresight and thrift, moderation and self-discipline. And Joshua was the prime driver: the zealous preacher, full of optimism, preaching and singing with fervour, and no doubt setting villages ablaze with his religious enthusiasm and gospel of forgiveness.[19] It is no wonder that Edward Gibbon Wakefield termed Methodists full of 'a desperate conscientiousness', while Thomas Carlyle disliked their preoccupation with themselves: 'Methodism with its eye forever turned on its own navel; asking itself with torturing anxiety of Hope and Fear, "Am I right? Am I wrong? Shall I be saved? Shall I not be damned?"'[20]

With her husband so often absent, Anne Hocken was the chief caregiver, comforter and the cornerstone of family stability. She saved the scrap of paper, still in his collection (see frontispiece), that showed Morland's first attempts at writing: 'My dear Joshua and James I hope you will write to me again. Baby is often tal –'. This specimen, all in capital letters, was written when he was six, and was verified by his mother's note: 'My dear little Toms 1st specimen of letter writing in Septr 1842'.[21] Although there is no evidence of his early schooling, it is presumed that he attended a Methodist day school. Sunday school was also compulsory, and the discipline was uncompromising, as just the first four of the 1836 'Rules to be observed in the Sunday School, Great Coates' indicate:

> Rule 1: Parents are to send their Children regularly to School, when Divine Service is in the Morning, at the hours of Nine and Two during the Summer months – at Half-past Nine and Two during the Winter months. When Service is in the Evening, the School will meet at Ten and Two, throughout the year.
>
> Rule 2: The Children are to come perfectly neat and clean, or a mark of disgrace will be entered in the book for each offence: – if often repeated, it will lead to expulsion.
>
> Rule 3: The Parents are never to keep their Children from School, except in case of sickness, or by especial leave of the Teachers. In all cases they must obtain a Leave Ticket.
>
> Rule 4: Any Child who shall be absent Three Sundays, without leave, will be expelled.[22]

Joshua Hocken was also an author, carefully following the rule that works emanating from the society were to 'contain no news, no politics, no personal invectives, nothing offensive either to religion, decency, good nature, or good manners'.²³ In 1839 he wrote *A Brief History of the Wesleyan Methodism, in the Grimsby Circuit*. This 66-page document, with its 'Grimsby Wesleyan Methodistic Tree' frontispiece, was printed and sold by W. Skelton in Grimsby and by John Mason in London. The preface reveals a possible influence on his son's later devotion to collecting and rescuing historical material:

> As the writer of the following pages believes the system of Wesleyan Methodism to be the work of God, and an important section of His church, he deems every thing illustrative of its history, valuable and interesting; and as this cause has existed in the Town of Grimsby, and in many other places on the Eastern side of Lincolnshire, for nearly a century, and no written document directly bearing on its history, has yet appeared; he, in accordance with his own feelings, and the wishes of numerous friends, has made an effort to rescue from oblivion, many facts which perhaps in a few years, would have been for ever lost.²⁴

Joshua also relied on the *Journals* of the Wesley brothers, various issues of the Wesleyan Methodist magazines and circuit documents. Here he set an example that was followed by Hocken, most notably in his later publications, which all relied strongly on documentary sources. As befits an earnest Methodist preacher, there are few light moments in Joshua Hocken's book. His son adopted a similar style: strongly informational, fact-based historical narrative, with little comic relief.

By late 1839 and 1840 the Hockens were in North Yorkshire, where Joshua was employed on the Stokesley circuit and struggling to do his work. In August 1840 from Castle Donington, a small town in the district of Shardlow where Eliza was born, he wrote to his mentor, Bunting, explaining that although he was still happy to undertake ministerial duties, he could not walk the circuit. He had a rupture – probably a hernia – which had developed when he was on the Stamford circuit. It was '*difficult* and *dangerous* to walk the distances that I am obliged to in this' and he was no longer able to do the '*long* walks', even though a horse was available.²⁵ Another practical reason for the plea was 'the long and expensive journey of about 130 miles [209 km] with a Family of three small children, one of which is at the breast, and my wife's health delicate'.²⁶ Not one to shirk his responsibilities, he offered his services to 'the Melton Mowbray Circuit, only 20 miles away', adding that with a horse, which was available, he could 'promote the cause efficiently'.²⁷ The following year Joshua was 'so fully occupied' that he scarcely had time to see his wife and children.²⁸ By 1844 he had moved south to the Norwich circuit, where he took on additional responsibilities as financial secretary and was the promoter of 'the general objects of our Educat'l movement' on the

Bungay–North Walsham–Yarmouth–Bury St Edmunds circuit.[29] That year, too, young Morland enrolled at Woodhouse Grove, a boarding school for the sons of Methodist preachers at Apperley Bridge, Yorkshire.

In 1845 Joshua put pen to paper again. His *Hints and Helps to Local Preachers*, a smaller pamphlet of 14 pages, proved so popular that no known copy of the first edition exists. A 'Second Thousand' copy has survived, with the prefatory note: 'The rapid sale of the following Hints has induced the Author to issue another edition of them, in their present form.' It is dated 19 April 1845. John Wesley had maintained that 'the work of grace would die out in one generation if the Methodists were not a reading people'.[30] Literature was 'a weapon, a tool' and preachers like Joshua were expected to be disseminators of literature, taking it all with great seriousness. Accordingly his hints included advice on book-related topics. Number 5, for example, noted, in part: 'in reading, comprehend the meaning of the page you are upon, before you turn to another. One book well digested is more useful than twenty read in the usual cursory manner.' Number 6 stated: 'If you buy only one work in a year, let it be the best of the kind extant, if your means will allow. A standard work is prized more than gold by a man of mind.' He also covered how best to speak to an audience, something his son would later do frequently in Dunedin: 'Always aim at simplicity, unction, and ease … Avoid bombast and jocularity. It is better to be pious without eloquence than eloquent without piety.' A '*short* introduction' was advisable.

Back in 1820, Jabez Bunting had produced his own 'Best means of preparing missionaries for their work', which also dealt with education and books. Missionary candidates should write themes and remarks on the books they read, especially books of missionary biography; have a 'General knowledge of natural history, astronomy, geography'; and prepare their minds for '*patient* labour'.[31] Joshua had wanted to include a brief catalogue of the most suitable books to read, but realised this was not possible. In another time and place his son would be free to create much more substantial book lists, particularly his *Bibliography* (1909). Hocken never owned copies of his father's works but he did have in his collection such publications as John Pearson's *The Life of William Hey* (1823), the biography of a distinguished provincial surgeon who had been a friend of Wesley, and the *Arminian Magazine* (later the *Methodist Magazine*), which had been established by Wesley in 1778 and which only ceased publication in 1969.[32] But all this lay far in the future. First young Morland had to be formally educated.

Woodhouse Grove School

At Apperley Bridge, 6.5 km across the fields and open moorland from Bradford and 13 km from Leeds, sits Woodhouse Grove School. It was here, between 1844 and 1850, that Morland was a pupil. The school, which sits on a sloping hill overlooking the valley of the River Aire, was founded by the

Methodist Conference in 1811 and opened on 8 January 1812. It not only provided a balance to Kingswood School, established in the south by Wesley, but also provided another outlet to train and educate boys for the ministry.[33]

The school started small with nine founding pupils. By the end of the first year there were 70 boys, all of them boarders. Pupils entered at the age of eight and left at 14.[34] There was no entry examination or selection policy and, before 1829, no fees, with the education of the boys being maintained by the Methodist Conference, which ruled the school.

The main school building ran from south to north with a corridor from the front door through the original Tudor building. There were three dormitories, the remnants of which remain: the top bedroom housed 45 boys, the bottom another 45, and the crib, next to the governor's bedroom, accommodated 10. To the west of the main building was the schoolroom. The school was served by one water pump and the boys washed in large troughs of cold water. In 1828 each boy was given his own towel, brush and comb. Sometime after 1836 'play and promenade cloisters' were constructed, a huge concession considering Wesley's dictum: 'He that plays when he is a child will play when he is a man.'[35] The pupils' activities tended to focus on the useful: gardening, chopping wood and felling trees, assisting with the hay-making or at the Sunday school services at the local village. All were considered admirable diversions from the days devoted to schoolwork. Much of the surrounding wood was out of bounds to the boys.

After 1833, when the school chapel was built, the boys were marched there on Sundays at 10.30 am, 3 pm and 6 pm to learn catechisms by heart, while the older boys were drilled in the Greek Testament. On the front of the pulpit, *inside*, was printed in ink in well-formed Roman letters, the phrase: 'Be short and lively'.[36]

In 1838 William Grear began his stint as headmaster. A lay teacher, he had worked as a classics master at Kingswood and then ran a school in Liverpool. In 1843 the Rev. William Lord began 15 years as governor. In this role he was the school representative, the go-between with the Methodist Conference, and acted *in loco parentis*, leading and maintaining the boys' spiritual and moral welfare.[37] Unlike his predecessors, Grear favoured competition. In 1840 he introduced reports and records of pupil progress in class and in subjects studied. This innovative programme was designed to encourage the pupils to excel. In 1842 a new external examiner, C. Duncan, was appointed. He made suggestions to broaden the scope of the examination to include reading, spelling, English grammar and geography; there was also the introduction of singing to the curriculum and the use of staff as supervisors in all examinations. Many of these ideas were implemented.

To combat outbreaks of influenza, measles and cholera and improve the general health of the boys, gymnastics was introduced in 1842. However, even this activity was not without its hazards. In 1848 a boy called Tindall fell on his head from the trapeze and died. According to reports, his death affected the school greatly.

Morland left 'the Grove' before a new west wing was built with money offered in compensation for school land required by the Leeds to Bradford line of the Midland Railway Company. He and other keen readers may, however, have enjoyed the introduction in 1849 of gas lighting, which replaced candles and oil lamps.[38]

When Morland entered the school in 1844 he donned the school uniform of a dark blue jacket, corduroy trousers and a large flat cap of red and yellow with a slanting peak.[39] Affectionately known as the 'Grove Costume', it made the Grovians easily recognisable in the wider community. He was also expected to bring two suits, two pairs of shoes, six linen shirts and six pairs of stockings. The first day at a new school is often an intimidating experience, but Morland had brothers there: James was in his last year and Joshua had one more year to go. Younger brother William arrived in 1846. Parents paid four guineas towards the upkeep of the uniform, and the inevitable 'hand-me-downs' may have reduced the Hockens' costs.

To modern eyes the education system at the Grove seems gruelling, but that was the nineteenth-century Methodist way. As the school's biographer and former teacher Josiah Thomas Slugg wrote in 1885:

> A boy had nothing to do but yield to obedience, and learn the lesson set before him, which all the other boys of the same standing in the school were learning at the same time. The consequence was that discipline was maintained and progress was made. No time was wasted. The only days on which there was no teaching were Christmas Day and Good Friday. We knew nothing practically of either Easter or Whitsuntide.[40]

And so it began. Each morning at 5.45 in summer, 6.45 in winter, the most junior master would ring the rising bell. The master of the day would then enter the bedroom and shout 'All rise!' The boys would get out of their wooden cribs (iron beds were not introduced until 1866) and five minutes later, it was 'All kneel down' for a brief reflective prayer, then 'Rise' again, with sleepy-eyed charges marched off to the lavatories. Morning school from 6 to 8 am would follow. With the exceptions of Saturday afternoon and evening and Sunday, the rest of the day ran as follows:

8 am	Family prayers
8.30 am	Breakfast
9 am–12 noon	School (with a 10-minute break for airing room)
12.30 pm	Dinner
1–2 pm	Playground (schoolroom or playshed in wet weather)
2–5 pm	School (with ventilation break)

5.30 pm	Supper
6.30 pm	Night school (from 1835 'prep' for the next day's lessons)
8 pm	Bed (irrespective of age)

The Sabbath was full of prayers, reading and preaching, but William H. Shaw, a pupil between 1827 and 1833 and later a minister, thought well of Sunday, which 'instead of being a day of gloom, was the happiest day in the week, when the boys, instead of being schooled, cabined, and confined, unnaturally "bunged up" with religion, walked arm in arm, and took sweet counsel together as friends'.[41]

The food was less than appetising. Breakfast consisted of dry bread and milk on five days, with porridge, treacle and water providing a change on the other two. Dinner, the main meal, was Spartan, with portions of meat and potatoes ranging from 'small', 'common' and 'small common' to 'large' and 'very large'. Only 'Gobbles' (gluttonous boys), who were frowned upon, ate very large portions. Monday's dinner was suet pudding, served with melted butter. Dinner was eaten in silence, although reading was permitted. Supper, the last meal of the day, was dry bread and milk drunk from tin mugs.

As a new boy beginning in the minor classes, Morland's week was broken up into classics (22 hours) and reading, writing and accounts (26½ hours). In all this, he would have encountered Virgil, Horace, Caesar's *Commentaries*, Ovid's *Metamorphoses*, Cicero's *Orationes*, Xenophon, Homer and the Greek Testament. The Eton Latin Grammar predominated. Attendance at evening lectures on geography, geometry, philosophy and English grammar was also expected. The subjects taught at the school in 1846, Morland's third year, were English grammar, English composition or dictation, spelling, Latin, Greek, French, history, geography, arithmetic, algebra, mensuration (geometry), bookkeeping, writing, Scripture reading, Conference Catechism, Evidences of Christianity and Scripture Antiquities.[42]

Aside from class routines there were legitimate diversions. The playground offered a break from classes, as did traditional schoolyard games such as marbles, fives, peg-top and conkers. There were the usual rough and tough games such as pegging, which involved the hitting, punching, kicking and thumping of a luckless boy on a given day, usually the eighteenth before a vacation. There was also a game called 'slavery', in which small boys were captured by larger boys and sold to others for money, represented by paper or tin discs. The authorities frowned on this as 'fostering too favourable an idea of slavery in the Institution'.[43] Cricket and football were forbidden because these games were too hard on the boys' clothing.

The boys were provided with pocket money during their six years at school. On the Saturday half-holiday, a later introduction, 1½d from the school and 1d from parents were distributed. In Hocken's day a ha'penny was allocated to the Methodist Overseas Mission Fund, leaving 2d minus any fines to spend. Outlets were limited, but the 'spice man', an outdoor vendor who sold treats to the boys outside the school gates, was popular. Occasionally the boys were allowed out of the school, to bathe in the nearby Aire River, to walk in the neighbourhood, to enjoy a picnic in Bolton Woods or to tramp to The Chevin, a ridge overlooking the nearby market town of Otley. These activities always depended on the availability, inclination and generosity of the master.

There were transgressions. Clandestine food cooking is recorded, particularly potatoes obtained from a nearby field over a climbable wall. There was no allowance for youthful enterprise and high-jinks. Boys caught were punished – the cane, fines or solitary confinement – and sometimes expelled. There were monitors for almost every aspect of school life – bell, book, bedroom and so on – who formed part of the disciplinary team and helped to regulate, perhaps unwittingly, their unruly contemporaries.

Two aspects of life at Woodhouse Grove are interesting when considering Hocken's future profession as a practising surgeon and his future interest in books and bibliography. Science was little taught there when he was a pupil. Samuel Ebenezer Parker, the headmaster from 1817 to 1832, developed a science programme, but it lapsed after his departure.[44] Any science teaching was completely dependent on the strengths of a particular master; in reality it received scant attention until about the 1870s.[45] The formation of a proper school library was slow at Woodhouse Grove. From the beginning an appeal was made for suitable books and they trickled in, by donation and gift, and the occasional purchase. In 1825 'a select Juvenile Library for the use of the school' was proposed and a list of required books drawn up, but no one was given responsibility for forming the library. Governor Lord was so despondent over the lack of a library that in 1843 he asked parents to subscribe 1s per quarter for each boy. The following year he obtained a £25 grant for book purchases. When Peter McOwan took over the library in the mid-1850s, he introduced historical novels to balance the then staple diet of old issues of the *Methodist Magazine*. Yet even so E.G. Sugden's 1883 ground plan of the school has no library room.[46]

According to his good friend George Fenwick, Hocken 'always entertained for this old school a great affection and pride, and was never tired of describing the strenuous school discipline and Spartan diet … or of relating anecdotes of schoolboy pranks and all the little great events which go to make up a schoolboy's life'.[47] In 1902 Hocken visited Woodhouse Grove and, after discussion with the head, he was able to secure a half-day holiday for the boys as well as a gift of 6d each all round. Those present did not get off scot-free; they had to listen to a brief address by this 'old' Grovian. Hocken also donated £5 towards the school's Coronation Clock, which celebrated the accession of Edward VII in 1901. Shortly after this he attended an anniversary dinner for old Grovians in London, where he discovered he was one of two survivors of his year; the other was a celebrated London barrister, who may have been Henry Priestley.[48]

There had been another connection with Woodhouse Grove some years earlier. In 1887 Hocken purchased a 'splendid picture' of a group of Maori chiefs and their wives, the interpreter, the Rev. and Mrs Jobson and Mrs Brames Hall assembled in a room in John Wesley's London house. It was painted by the minor pre-Raphaelite artist James Smetham, later friend to Ruskin and Rossetti. While Smetham was attending the Grove as an 11-year-old in 1832, he is said to have 'copied Raphael's cartoons from the *Penny Magazine*. What time was not consumed in drawing was spent prowling about the Grove, and slipping away to Calverley Wood, and inventing ghost-stories to fit old Calverley Hall.'[49] Hocken also collected books on Smetham and corresponded with his widow, Sarah.

2
Surgeon and Sailor

In 1851 the Great Exhibition, a celebration of scientific and technological advancements instigated by Prince Albert, the Queen's consort, was opened at the Crystal Palace in London's Hyde Park. By this time the Hockens – Joshua, Anne, James (now an accountant), Eliza and Morland, registered in the census as a 'medical student' – were living in Windle, St Helens, in Lancashire. Sometime late in 1845 the family had moved to the Leeds area, specifically Cleckheaton south of Bradford, and by June 1847 they were living in Stanningley.[1] Hocken was indentured to 30-year-old Robert McNichol, a member of the Royal College of Surgeons of England, and in general practice as an apothecary.[2] McNichol, who lived with his wife Elizabeth and his mother in nearby New Market Street, would later become president of the North West Association of Medical Officers of Health.

The Hockens were a self-improving, ambitious family, yet educating four boys was by no means cheap. The decision for Morland to follow the medical line may have been an economic one, although evidence on the cost of the profession is at best contradictory. M. Jeanne Peterson cites figures such as £500, £600 and £1000, including educational fees and living expenses.[3] She also cites Jukes de Styrap, who claimed that 'medicine was a cheap profession' and suggested that, for most, the annual cost would be nearer to £100.[4] There were three 'medical' orders: physicians, surgeons and apothecaries. The apothecaries were an ancient society, once part of the Grocers' Company of the City of London, and then defined by royal charter in 1617. With the passing of the Apothecaries Act of 1815, members could fulfil their traditional role of druggists – supplying, compounding and selling – and the new practice of prescribing medicines. They could also perform minor surgical operations such as dental extractions and bleeding. Like surgeons, apothecaries were trained through apprenticeships.

All apothecary students had to sit a 'Latin Examination at any time after their first registration', and Hocken presumably sat some sort of preliminary entrance examination and impressed McNichol enough to take him on. The apprenticeship term lasted five years, with formal courses in chemistry, anatomy and physiology, *materia medica* (the body of knowledge about the properties of medicines) and therapeutics, botany and vegetable physiology, forensic medicine and the theory and practice of medicine. Practical sessions – anatomical demonstrations and dissections – were held in recognised hospitals or dispensaries. Rules on attendance, the fitness of instructors and examinations are outlined in *Regulations to be Observed by Students Intending to Qualify Themselves to Practice as Apothecaries in England and Wales 1843* which Hocken secured second hand.[5] Although he was required to attend the formal lectures, much of Hocken's education and learning came from his master, who imparted his own knowledge and skills.

Hocken did not, however, complete the five-year term with McNichol. In 1853, after only two years, he transferred his apprenticeship (or assistantship) to Dr Septimus William Rayne of Newcastle upon Tyne. Rayne was surgeon to the police for almost 40 years, surgeon to Trinity House (home to a seafarers' charitable guild), tutor in operative surgery in the town, surgeon to the North-Eastern Railway and medical referee for the Eagle Insurance Company. He was described as 'kindly and genial', and 'considerate and sympathetic' to the poor.[6] As both pupil and surgeon assistant to this experienced, well-connected, urbane man, Hocken lived with him in Newcastle for six years: at 18 and 19 Blackett Street, and then at 61 Westgate Street.

It is uncertain why Hocken moved to Newcastle. McNichol was born there and he may have recognised his pupil's potential and used home-town contacts. Indeed he may have recommended Hocken to Rayne. Newcastle did, of course, boast a reputable medical school. Another factor may have been his father's death. Joshua had been ill for some four years. On 10 May 1853 he wrote to a colleague in Leeds:

> My dear Bro, I am sorry that severe affliction prevents me from going *out* and making any effort to accomplish your benevolent wishes. I have not been able to preach since 1st March, and I have abandoned the idea of ever taking another circuit ... Within the last two months my recovery has been very doubtful, but I *think* I am now a little better. An affection in the chest – threatening consumption.

In true evangelical spirit he looked forward to a meeting at Manchester and hoped it would be a success.[7] But 16 days later Joshua died, aged 54, at Friar Street in Lancaster.[8] According to his obituary, during his final illness he repeated: 'Heaven is my home. For me to live is Christ, and to die is gain.'[9]

Newcastle was a bustling industrial town with a population of 87,784 in 1851.[10] The Tyne generated a busy river life with industries such as coal, textiles and ship-building providing employment. The railway connected Newcastle to other parts of England and Scotland, and amenities such as the Royal Arcade and Grainger Market attracted buyers to the town, which was also home to some 198 Methodist chapels.[11] The Methodists, along with the Quakers, the Baptists and the Independents, formed an influential contingent in civic life. By 1851 Joshua Hocken's mentor, Jabez Bunting, was living in Newcastle, as was a Miss Richardson, a possible relative on Hocken's maternal side. She had the future distinction, or not, of marrying the prolific and garrulous Dunedin writer J.G.S. Grant, whose works Hocken would later collect.[12]

The position of surgeon to which Hocken aspired was a step up from that of an apothecary. A surgeon could perform operations, set broken bones (manipulation), treat accident cases and skin disorders, and minister to some gynaecological ailments. The surgeon's skill or 'craft' 'demanded speed, dexterity, and physical strength, as well as expertise'.[13] Like an apothecary, a surgeon was also permitted to dispense drugs.

In 1854 Hocken attended a 'course of lectures and practical tuition in medical and pre-medical sciences' at the Newcastle upon Tyne College of Practical Science. The courses offered were taught in the Barber Surgeons' Hall in Victoria Street and had to conform to regulations laid down by the University of London, the Royal College of Surgeons of England and the Worshipful Company of Apothecaries.[14] The school had a dissecting room, a library, a students' waiting room on the ground floor and a large museum above. According to a local newspaper, 'no similar institution in the kingdom is provided with equal facilities so far as it respects building accommodation'.[15]

Among the subjects Hocken studied, in a busy schedule of classes, were anatomy and physiology, the 'principles and practice of physic, and of surgery', chemistry, midwifery, medical jurisprudence and botany (for which he won a silver medal in 1855). Also on offer was hospital practice through the Newcastle Infirmary. If Hocken had attended every class it would have cost him and his parents more than 31 guineas, not including living expenses. He may, however, have availed himself of a 'Perpetual Ticket to all the Lectures', which cost 40 guineas.

Dublin Bound

In 1858 Hocken moved again, this time to Dublin, where he enrolled at the Original Theatre of Anatomy and School of Medicine and Surgery, attending courses during the winter and summer terms of 1858 and 1859. Beginning lectures on 1 November 1858, he was one of 154 students. Although the Original's building was deemed inadequate, there was a relatively new laboratory built in 1856 and a museum. There were courses similar to those in Newcastle and daily demonstrations, aided by the fact that the school was within five minutes' walk of two medical and surgery hospitals and the adjoining Anglesey Lying in Hospital and Dispensary.

As well as paying his fees – the cost for attendance was 26 guineas – Hocken had the expense of equipping himself with the correct surgical instruments, such as a dissecting case (8s 6d), a pocket case containing 13 instruments (£1 5s), a case of 'tooth instruments' (1 guinea) and a midwifery case (£1 10s).[16]

Again his days were full. At 1 o'clock each week day he faced anatomy, physiology and surgery; at 12 o'clock on Tuesday, Thursday, Friday and Saturday he had theory and practice of surgery; at 3 o'clock on Monday, Wednesday and Friday he had theory and practice of medicine; at 2 o'clock on Monday, Wednesday and Friday he had *materia medica* and therapeutics; at 4 o'clock on Monday and Wednesday he had forensic medicine and hygiene; and at 2 o'clock on Tuesday, Thursday and Saturday he had theory of chemistry, practical chemistry and natural philosophy. He also attended courses on midwifery and diseases of women and children.[17] There is no glimpse of Hocken as a student apart from one brief mention in Lambert Hepenstal Ormsby's *Medical History of the Meath Hospital and County Dublin Infirmary*, where T. Morland Hocken is listed as one of 21 'Former Pupils of the Meath Hospital' session of 1858–59.[18]

Of course the end result of attendance and study was to qualify as a fellow or licentiate of the Royal College and be issued with letters and testimonials that enabled one to 'exercise and enjoy all rights of practice in the art or science of surgery'.[19] On 28 April 1859 Hocken, along with 16 other students, received his certificate to practise. In *The Lancet* of 7 May 1859 his name was listed under the Apothecaries' Hall entry as having passed his 'examination in the science and practice of medicine',[20] and on 21 May his name was among 25 others in both *The Lancet* and the *British Medical Journal* as 'gentlemen' admitted to the Royal College of Surgeons of England.[21] He could now put after his name the initials MRCS (Member of the Royal College of Surgeons) and LSA (Licentiate of the Society of Apothecaries).

Surgeon-Superintendent

Hocken had stayed in touch with Rayne in Newcastle, of whom he was very fond: '[Hocken] always spoke with the greatest reverence and affection of his old master, and often lamented that the good old custom of articling a young inexperienced and simply theoretical doctor to some older practitioner who acted as mentor and guide in practical work, should have fallen into disuse.'[22] Rayne had offered Hocken a partnership, which must have been tempting for a young man faced with the difficulties of establishing a private practice in England in the mid-nineteenth century. Hocken, however, replied that for health reasons he had decided to seek his fortune in the Antipodes. As he later noted on the back of the testimonial he received from fellow passengers in 1861, 'my health had not been good for two or three years & I thought it on the whole better to cast in my lot with those who were seeking fortune in so new & so fine a country as New Zealand. This step I never regretted.'[23]

Health was often a factor in the decision to emigrate. Thomas Naghten FitzGerald, a near contemporary of Hocken's at the Original, had been advised to escape the English winters. He emigrated to Melbourne in 1858 and became one of Australia's most influential surgeons.[24] Hocken, by nature conservative, came to the idea of emigration slowly. About July 1859 he began applying for a position as a surgeon-superintendent on board one of the many emigrant ships; FitzGerald had gone to Australia in this way.

The role of surgeon–superintendent was an important one. Disease and sickness were prevalent on board crowded vessels, and the cramped conditions on a two- to three-month sea journey could exacerbate and escalate any illness on board. A good doctor could bolster morale and keep sickness and disease at bay; a bad one could do much damage. There were also a number of non-medical duties. An 1841 copy of *Instructions to the Surgeons-Superintendent Appointed by the Court of Directors to Board the Emigrant Ships of the New Zealand Company* in Hocken's collection lists 37 duties, which include the following: 'You are not in any way to interfere with the navigation of the ship; but you are to the best of your ability, to preserve order among the Emigrants on board'; 'You are to take care that the Emigrants' berths are kept clean, and as airy as possible'; and 'You are, every Sunday, to read Prayers and a Sermon, to such Emigrants as shall voluntarily attend you for that purpose.'[25] After a pre-embarkation examination of the emigrants, the surgeon-superintendent was required to keep 'a Journal, or daily register, of the number of sick, their names, ages, nature and character of disease, symptoms, termination and treatment, and to lose no opportunity of making a post mortem examination, should the disease terminate fatally, and to insert the result carefully in the register'.[26] As one writer has suggested, the surgeon-superintendent was 'a sanitary inspector, a medical officer, an emigration official, and a moral guardian'.[27]

The requirements for such a post were specific. The applicant must include 'the usual certificates of medical education from the teachers of the several branches of medicine, as also his diplomas in Physic, Surgery, and Midwifery'. He would 'also be subject to an examination as to his practical knowledge in these three branches'.[28] In order to satisfy these requirements, Hocken began compiling a dossier. He approached those he knew best and finally obtained 10 professional endorsements to his personal character and skill as a medical man. These were full of praise: several mentioned his manner – 'extremely amiable and courteous' and 'gentlemanly and retiring' – as well as endorsing his surgical and medical skills.[29] William Stokes, Regius Professor of Medicine in the University of Dublin, wrote: 'I think him a gentleman of great natural ability, an excellent observer, and a most sound practitioner.'[30] Despite the formulaic phrases, these testimonials provide a glimpse of a young man who, at 23, was ready to step out into the world.[31] They helped him to secure his first post as surgeon-superintendent on board the *White Star* in October 1859.[32]

Part of the White Star Shipping Line, the *White Star* was a Yankee hard-pine ship built specifically for passage to Australia. Once gold was discovered there in 1851, the rush of emigrants clamouring for a new life had obliged British shipowners to ask American builders for suitably large and swift vessels.[33] The *White Star*'s maiden passage to Melbourne in April 1855 took 79 days. On her return voyage she carried 80,000 ounces of gold. In 1858 she reached Australia in 72 days, the best passage of the year. When Hocken sailed on her, she left Liverpool on 9 November 1859 and reached Melbourne on 19 January 1860 (72 days). Her captain, Ayrshire Scot John Kerr, was not reckless but 'liked to keep his ship going under as much canvas' as possible.[34]

On board were 13 saloon passengers, travelling in comfortable cabins and paying for the privilege, and 294 steerage passengers carried in much less salubrious conditions between decks.³⁵ Just before the ship docked, as was customary when a journey had been satisfactory, the saloon passengers gave a sum of money to the captain and the doctor: Hocken's came in a velvet purse. An accompanying letter, signed by 10 grateful passengers, acknowledged his 'decided ability', 'general kindness of heart' and 'most untiring assiduity'. Hocken received another glowing testimonial when the *White Star* arrived back in Liverpool on 12 May 1860, having left Melbourne on 18 February.

Little is known of what occupied Hocken over the next eight months, but sometime over the winter of 1860 he secured a post on the SS *Great Britain*, described by one marine historian as 'the most famous ship which ever floated, excepting Noah's ark'.³⁶ She was the world's first ocean-going propeller-driven iron ship, an engineering triumph designed by Isambard Kingdom Brunel. Capable of carrying 1000 tonnes of cargo, she could accommodate 600 passengers and boasted a saloon, a surgery, a mess room, a pantry, a bar, three kitchens, a carpenters' and joiners' workshop, a butcher's shop, a cow house and space for 160 sheep, 40 pigs and 100 dozen poultry.³⁷

The SS *Great Britain* was the only steam vessel designed for passengers on the Australian route until 1875. During her remarkable career she made 32 trips to Australia between 1852 and 1876; she was the oldest emigration vessel to reach the colony. Hocken travelled on her twentieth voyage, her tenth to Australia under Captain John Gray, a Shetland Islander who once told a passenger that he loved 'every plank' of the *Great Britain*.³⁸ Hocken's daughter Gladys recalled the 'thrilling tales' her father used to tell, and was quoted saying: 'He became great friends with the *Great Britain*'s famous master, Captain Grey [sic] ...'³⁹ When the ship sailed from Liverpool to Melbourne on 17 February 1861 there were 136 crew on board, including Hocken, and 406 passengers.⁴⁰ Hocken had no assistants, and may have relied on help from the stewards or pursers. It was not a propitious beginning: the ship's departure was delayed and there was also a furious gale, which caused some damage. She first steamed to Cork, and then the voyage proper began.

Rachel Henning, one of the first-class passengers, hinted at how busy Hocken must have been, since 'so many people were unwell at various times'. She, however, was determined not to need his services. Before the ship left Liverpool, Henning sat in the saloon and wrote a letter to her sister Etta: 'The doctor appeared at breakfast today, a droll little man ... and covered with yellow buttons to express his being an officer. I hope I shall never want him, and it is most unlikely.'⁴¹

For amusement on the long voyage, there were the usual board games such as chess, draughts, whist and backgammon, along with piano playing, songs and dancing, and reading. One morale booster actively encouraged by the captain was the ship's newspaper, the *Great Britain Magazine and Weekly Screw*, which was produced from 16 March to 27 April 1861. An extracted version of 200 copies was reprinted by Mason & Firth in Melbourne later that year. This newspaper is significant in that it contains Hocken's first writings. The copy that survives in the SS *Great Britain* Archives in Bristol was the first printed item he salvaged. His note on the title page reads: 'T.M. Hocken, Surgeon S.S. *Great Britain*, 1860 & 1861.' It was kept as a treasured family item by Hocken's daughter until she gave it to the archive.[42]

The contents page has his pencilled initials beside his contributions: 'The *Great Britain* steamship and her inhabitants', 'Sea-sickness', 'Our sanitary condition', 'The island of Martin Vaz', 'The infernal regions of the *Great Britain*', 'Eyes', 'The world we inhabit and its continuation', 'Lost', 'Consolation', 'A story of *un*-true love' and 'Our last'. Two articles – 'Our sanitary condition', stressing cleanliness, dryness and ventilation, and 'Our last', an advertising and subscription 'pump' for the proposed printing of the newspaper – have his initials printed at the end. 'Sea-sickness', both sections of 'The world we inhabit' and 'Our last' are unsigned but he added his name on his copy. The remainder carry Hocken's initials or nom-de-plumes: 'W.E.' for 'The island of Martin Vaz', 'Aleu' for 'Eyes', 'Francis Forlorn' for 'Lost' and 'Tabitha Green' for 'Consolation'. 'A story of *un*-true love' is missing from the 1861 reprint, and one can only speculate about its content: a shipboard romance? A tale of unrequited love, disappointment and rejection? Perhaps Hocken also signed it 'Francis Forlorn'.

His first contribution, 'The *Great Britain* steamship and her inhabitants', begins with a rhetorical flourish:

> We have left our dear old native land, we have lost sight of those white cliffs which but lately were so familiar to our view, and are ploughing the great ocean, to reach another distant shore to form a new home, and perchance return no more. We don't mean to say it will be so, for every Briton loves his country, loves all corners, and counts the days he will be absent. But in the chapter of accidents, we say it may be so.
>
> With what different plans we are skimming over the blue sea were a difficult task to enumerate, but let us halt awhile, and look on the heterogeneous mass of human beings studding the decks of the *Great Britain*.

He could be describing himself when he writes of the 'gay gentleman' who is 'boldly launching on to the waves of life, buoyantly hoping that they will cast him on some friendly shore, where he may earn an honourable independence, and perchance, as time rolls on, enable him by honest labours to provide for those aged parents to whom he owes everything in this life'.

But, he asks, how many emigrants will 'run their course unchequered? How many more will have to encounter bitter disappointment at the non-fulfilment of those overexalted ideas with which they are going to Australia?' And how many will 'manfully battle against the strong reverses which will cross them at every step, till Dame Fortune shall smile upon them'? He discusses the realities of a new life in a new country, and the anticipated opportunities – a new beginning, new love, riches. His Methodist upbringing surfaces with the admonition that 'it is only by steady labour and attention to our vocations that we may expect success to our undertakings'. There is a positive ending: 'everyone will have cause to rejoice at the step they are now taking, and in so doing, we beg to conclude by offering them sincere good wishes for their welfare, and bidding them God speed.'[43]

Hocken's literary debut was not without controversy. A passenger named Walker took exception to his reference to the 'less fortunate older maids ... whose matrimonial chances are gradually lowering in the horizon' but who may experience the 'capricious shaft from Cupid's quiver'. He called it a 'spiteful allusion'. His retort culminated in the stanza: 'There never was a goose so grey,/ But some day soon or late;/ An honest gander came that way,/ And took her for his mate.'[44] One 'Tabitha Scroggins' was harsher. She not only called Hocken 'some idiot Jackanapes, whose schoolboy scribbling you have thought fit to publish' but also a 'silly Correspondent'. It would not be the last time that his writing was criticised.

As *The Lancet* had noted on 4 December 1858, seasickness, which usually affected most passengers in the first few weeks of a voyage, was 'a malady so provoking and hitherto so invincible, that every man may claim a fair hearing if he promises a cure'.[45] Self-assured, and ever ready to enhance his name and reputation, Hocken penned his own two-page article on the subject. He suggested a formula 'of the greatest use, though by no means a certain cure': '3 drachms Nitro Hydrochloric Acid (dilute); 16 drops Hydrocyanic Acid; ½ grain of Muriate of Morphia; and eight ounces of water. Take two tablespoonfuls every three or four hours.' The article, which ends, 'Many sea sick folk assure me that they will never, never again trust the treacherous sea', contains a bastardised Latin quote by Horace: 'Nauta infelix immemor praeteritum,/ Moc reficit navim ac reccnsendrit navem.'[46] 'Treatment of sea-sickness' became Hocken's first real appearance in print when he submitted it to the editor of *The Lancet* in September 1861. It appeared on 5 October that year, by which time Hocken was a veteran of four sea voyages. He made small amendments to the formula, included far more medical details and, perhaps not wanting to risk criticism from a larger, more informed audience, deleted the Horace quotation. The ending now read: 'All persons about to undertake a voyage – especially a protracted one – should take, two days before going on board, a sound purgative, followed up by the medicines just named. When on board they should resolutely refuse to yield to the temptations of sea-sickness, constantly pacing the upper deck, and so becoming accustomed to the vessel's disagreeable roll.' A subdued sense of humour is evident in the final sentence: 'Otherwise Neptune is pretty certain to demand payment of the customary impost.'[47]

Other articles in the *Great Britain Magazine and Weekly Screw* reflect Hocken's liking for descriptive history, but one item stands out. It is 'The mythology of the Maori' which, although not indicated as being by him, carries the initials 'T.M.'.[48] It is a marvellously prescient piece, given his future in New Zealand and his interest in and collecting of things Maori. Arthur Thomson's recently published *The Story of New Zealand: Past and present – savage and civilized* (1859) was the basis for Hocken's brief examination of the Maori religion, which 'will prove instructive to the readers of the *Great Britain Magazine*'. He then outlines the Creation process, the Maui myth, including Hawaiki as the name of Maui's home, and the tale of the maiden from heaven and the father of the child who eventually ascended to heaven on a spider's web. Rather than continue with more 'remarkable fictions', he writes, 'what a strange mixture of truth and error there is in all this', and then explains how easy it would be to trace the origins of these legends through the Mosaic account of creation and flood. The last paragraph provides the first tangible evidence of his interest in missionaries and conveys the prevailing contemporary view that assimilation of the Maori was a desirable outcome of European 'civilisation':

> It is, however, gratifying to know that the labours of the missionary, education, intercourse with the whites, and a written language, which the Maori now possess, are gradually inducing them to the relinquishment of their ancient beliefs, and to the adoption of a purer faith of the Gospel. The races are besides amalgamating. The Anglo-Saxon blood already flows in the veins of at least 1000 natives, and thus, if the Maori did not ultimately become one with the whites, enough of the Saxon blood shall have been infused into the race as will preserve it from the fate of all aborigines – extinction. We have no fears of the future of New Zealand. The most distant of England's colonies will ere long become the brightest gem in her diadem of glory, and the Maori will contribute their full share to the zeal, energy, and the intelligence which will secure to New Zealand the honorable appellation of the Queen of the South.

Crossing the line on 17 March meant that Hocken, by now an experienced hand, faced the customary rituals. When the ship passed the volcanic island of Martin Vaz, about 1190 km east of Vitória in the southern Atlantic Ocean, the crew and passengers enacted a repossession of the island that reads like a *Swallows and Amazons* escapade. Hocken, as chief reporter, seems to have enjoyed himself. As a step towards improving the islanders, who were nowhere to be seen, he and his 'gang' left behind relics of English civilisation: copies of the ship's magazine, an old brown wide-awake (hat), two pocket handkerchiefs, five empty bottles, a toothpick and a dozen cigars.

Good Friday, 29 March, brought fine weather, moderate winds and sightings of albatrosses and Cape hens. Deaths – from measles, croup and consumption – kept Hocken busy on the professional front. There were also happier medical events: when a boy was born on board, his proud parents wanted to name him 'Thomas Gray Morland Hocken Great Britain Magazine'.[49]

The SS *Great Britain* arrived in Melbourne on 2 May 1861. During the voyage the boilers had been lit 24 times and, out of a total 71 days at sea, 732 hours or nearly 31 days had been spent under steam. A day before the ship docked 37 passengers had a 'whip-round' for Hocken and presented this to him with a testimonial, which he kept.[50]

The Second Run

The SS *Great Britain* was re-equipped and ready to leave Melbourne on 30 May 1861. The passage back, with the same captain and officers, took 64 days, ending at Liverpool on 4 August.[51] On board were 682 people: 542 passengers and a crew of 140.[52] Spotting icebergs – those 'most sublime of Nature's masterpieces' – near Cape Horn provided a treat for passengers.[53] These also became suitable subjects for amateur and professional sketchers alike, including young Charles Chomley from Ireland, who kept a diary on the voyage.[54] So too did Clara Aspinall, another saloon passenger, who was returning to England. As she recorded, her fellow travellers included Antonia Jones, an American tragedian, G.V. Brooke, famous for playing Othello,[55] and Australian politician and statesman Henry (later Sir Henry) Parkes. Also a journalist and a poet, Parkes told Aspinall that he owned '500 volumes of modern poets, and the works of every person who had written on Australia'.[56] To any prospective collector, a boast such as this could well have been a challenge.

Aspinall's *Three Years in Melbourne* (1862), based on her diary, provides an early glimpse of Hocken's personality and professionalism: 'All ships have a doctor, but they have not all one like ours, who combined so many qualities desirable in a ship-surgeon. He was generally called "the little doctor", partly because he was a favourite – for the best things are supposed to be wrapped up in the smallest compass – and partly because he was very small in stature.'[57] Later she refers to him as an 'angel of goodness'. He was 'excessively kind and untiringly energetic in his attention to his patients of all classes'.[58] Hocken owned a copy of Aspinall's book and acknowledged her on the title page as 'sister of the well-known Melbourne barrister'. He also added a note: 'Dr T.M. Hocken, S.S. Great Britain', and later, at the beginning of Chapter 15, '*Great Britain, Cap. John Gray. I was surgeon of the vessel.' Hocken also, as some ship's surgeons did, took on the role of chaplain, reading the morning and evening services on Sundays and taking funeral services.

The attraction was not one-sided, as Aspinall records in her diary: 'I went into luncheon & found the good little doctor had reserved me one of the best seats. It was next to Capt. Palsey, opposite C. Chomley, Capt Lyteleton [sic] & Mr Wildash.' When she was 'horribly' seasick he attended her in her cabin and on Sunday 2 June, 'The doctor read the prayers, which I could follow throughout whilst lying in my berth.' She writes of Hocken's diminutive height, noticing that he overcame his pique at this physical characteristic by making a point of offering his arm to the tallest women on the ship. With full confidence in himself, he would then promenade around the deck. Aspinall was not initially one of those he escorted. As her entry for Saturday 15 June reads, 'The little doctor wanted me to take his arm but I always get off as it would look so truly ridiculous. He then went to Mrs [indecipherable]; Dr Hunter who stooped down & tried to lean upon him. I would have given anything for a photograph of them.' The very next day, however, she writes:

> The little doctor has won the respect of every body by the way in which he conducts his services & the energy he had displayed in getting up an evening service though some few objected. Besides having won mine he has won a large amount of gratitude from me for having cured my sickness or at all events stopped it for a time. He offered his arm again to me on deck & I took it for the first time as there were few people about, still I think I saw some of them looking amused at seeing me stooping down & trying to accommodate myself to his height.

On a more gossipy note Aspinall records, on 11 July, hearing that 'the Doctor had proposed to Miss Sampson & been refused'.[59] Hocken was a young, single, healthy male. Although possibly breaching professional etiquette, his offer of marriage was understandable. Chomley, who may have heard about Hocken's plight, summed up the dangers on board: 'for be it known that a marine residence is just the most dreadful place for scandal that can exist, for instance a gentleman sleeps on deck & the report goes that he's drunk & cannot go to bed. I walk with one young lady more than another simply because she can talk sence [sic] & make herself agreeable and it is reported that we are engaged.'[60] One wonders what Clara Aspinall thought of Hocken trying his luck.

The usual on-board amusements were organised, and once again there was a newspaper, the *Great Britain Gazette*, in which Hocken was involved. Four issues, each four pages long, were produced on 6, 20 and 27 July and 3 August. (There was a single sheet supplement to the 20 July issue.) Hocken's reports on the 'Health of the ship' and his advocacy for pure air in 'Keep on deck' are easily recognisable. The former indicates what he had to deal with and his approach to health:

> The general Sanitary Condition of the Ship, I am happy to say, continues good. We have now no infectious disease on board, though it is very probable that Measles will re-appear as we enter warm latitudes. Dysentery and Bronchitis are the prevailing complaints; besides which there is a fair amount of general sickness. Our Little Stranger – puny and sickly from the first – paid us but a short visit, – dying within a fortnight of his birth. The other death, a female Infant, was exceedingly sudden, – the patient dying

within nine hours after being first visited. The causes of death in this case were Convulsions and Infantile Pneumonia.

The necessity of *Cleanliness* and *Ventilation*, both in berth and person, cannot be too strongly insisted upon. Moisture and Dampness of Berths should be *carefully avoided*, as they form a powerful *incubator* of disease, and doubly so when associated with dirt and insufficient ventilation.[61]

In this instance other contributions by him are not easily distinguished, but there is certainty about the historical overview of the SS *Great Britain*, titled 'The history of our ship', in the last issue. This long article is unsigned, yet has a distinctive, fact-based tone that could come only from Hocken's pen. His authorship is verified by the existence of a typed version of the article in his collection, along with a poster advertising the ship and two newspaper engravings depicting her in full sail.[62]

Clara Aspinall was disappointed with the newspaper. Although a contributor herself writing under the name 'Cecelia', she felt most contributors were 'positively too indolent'.[63] She was also displeased with the ship's library, claiming that only the works of Channing (either William Ellery or his brother, Edward Tyrrel), a few guidebooks to the colonies and some fiction, including John Bunyan's *Pilgrim's Progress*, were available. There was plenty of literary talk. Aspinall mentions discussions on, among others, Thackeray, Oliver Wendell Holmes's *Elsie Venner*, Richard Alfred Millikin's *The Groves of Blarney*, Elizabeth Gaskell's *Cranford*, Byron and Shakespeare. Other entertainments for 'raising our sinking spirits', in Charles Chomley's words, included the reading of selections from British poets, reciting Irish songs and Negro melodies, and the playing of overtures on the flute and violin.[64]

When available, Hocken was part of such occasions. In fact he tended to parade his knowledge a little, often to his cost. On 26 July Aspinall recorded that Captain Palsey asked Antonia Jones, who was reading *Cranford*, how she liked 'Folfoody's Poems'. He then enquired if Hocken had read them. At his reply, 'Ye—es oh yes, very fine, very fine indeed', Palsey 'shrieked with laughter & warned me [Aspinall] against ever pretending to know more than I really did'.

With actors on board, there was opportunity for numerous theatrical performances. On the evening of 15 June, as Aspinall records, *The Serious Family* was performed, with Hocken taking the tiny role of Vincent. 'The little Doctor too did his part to perfection dressed in his best coat & buttons. We were so amused at him running onto the stage & instead of saying Lady Chomley he exclaimed: "Save us all, here comes Lady Chomley."'[65] Nine days later, on 24 June, he appeared in *The Loan of a Lover*: 'The little doctor looked intensely amusing dressed in wide breeches shoes & buckles – a pumper & belt like Dickeys & a knitted cap with tassel at the top of it. Though he did not know his part perfectly, he carried it off remarkably well, smiling & looking easy & natural.' On 2 July in *O'Callaghan on his Last Leg*s, 'the little Doctor as Dr Banks amused us as much as he did in "The Loan of a Lover"'. On 17 July in *The Invincible Prince*, a burlesque set on the Spanish Main, Hocken gets character mention only: he played 'Don Moustachey (de Haroy), Barbos of the Guard'.

Aspinall describes Hocken's enthusiasm for these activities: 'He was always ready to do anything towards promoting amusement, and would take any part that was assigned to him in the amateur performances; and, if he had not time to learn his part thoroughly (for sometimes very short notice was given), he bowed, and smiled, and conducted himself with so much ease, and was always so picturesquely attired, that by his manner he quite made up for the matter.'[66] In one of her 'Cecelia' pieces, concerning the lack of male singers on board, Aspinall also mentions Hocken by his nickname, the rather apt 'Professor Swyzel': 'Then there is the young and gifted Professor Swyzel, so mellifluous in common parlance, what would he not be in song, breathing out, "Queen of My Soul", or "I Love Her, How I Love Her".'[67]

At one point in the voyage, Hocken and Captain Gray attended a birthday party given by Miss Maggie Smith in the saloon quarters. Among dishes of dried fruits and cakes and pink, white and azure bonbons, the two men uncorked the champagne and lemonade bottles. Clara Aspinall notes that 'Professor' Hocken's favourite topics for discussion were 'Science and Love'. According to her, he delighted in talking to the most scientifically inclined passengers on board and enjoying, to quote him, 'an intellectual feast'. He had, she writes, 'just a *soupçon* of romance about him which is useful on board ship, and which helped to give a poetic flavour to his physic'. From her observations, especially when discussing such cerebral topics, he would launch into 'the realms of Love', seemingly oblivious to the growing discomfort of his listeners. Despite his size, he carried his authority well: 'they always listened deferentially to "the little doctor"'.[68] Aspinall also records that his

> physical courage was very great; indeed, he had told me before we sailed that he had 'a morbid love of danger'. I was therefore not much alarmed, when one day, just as he was prescribing for me in my worst stage of *mal de mer*, and I had said, 'Oh, doctor! Is there any fear of our running into an iceberg?' he exclaimed, in a deep, tragical voice, 'Only let us touch an iceberg, and we shall not be three minutes above water!'[69]

Hocken was kept busy until the end of the voyage. Just before the ship docked, a steerage passenger, who had been assisting the sailors on the ropes, had a major seizure. He and Dr Hunter tried to revive the man, but he died and was buried at sea, like the two children who had died earlier on board. The ship sailed past Cork and Anglesey and into the Mersey. Hocken was home again. He would have three months before his next marine obligation.

The Last Run

Hocken embarked on his last voyage on the SS *Great Britain*, now part of the Black Ball Line, on 20 October 1861, reaching Melbourne on Christmas Eve that year. A quarter of the crew had been on the February voyage and Captain Gray was once again in command. Among the 687 people on board – 143 crew members, 456 adults, 80 children, 8 infants[70] – were the 'All England Eleven' cricketers, the first such team to travel to Australia.

Hocken performed his usual pre-departure medical checks but, as reported by an unknown writer in the *Cabinet*, the ship's newspaper, it 'was merely a nominal examination, and was more for the inspection of tickets, than to inquire into any of the physical defects of the passengers'.[71] The 65-day non-stop trip was fairly smooth, alternating engine power and sail, as verified by the diary of first class passenger Helen Roland.[72] Hocken was kept busy. Two Cornishmen died soon after crossing the equator, a child in steerage died and there was almost a fourth fatality when a young man from steerage was flung six metres from the royal mast during a gale, sustaining only severe sprains to his feet. In another serious incident, cricketer George 'Farmer' Bennett lost his grip on the belaying pin he was using as a bat in a game on deck. The pin smashed into the face of a saloon passenger, breaking his nose and lacerating his cheek. He was treated by Hocken and recovered slowly.[73] Another member of the team, William 'Terrible Billy' Caffyn, faced his own ordeal. As he recorded in his memoir *Seventy-One Not Out* (1889), the mosquitoes 'tormented the life out of me' and he was forced to see Hocken, who prescribed swathing his head in muslin and covering his arms with stockings. As can be imagined, he received a fair amount of ribbing from his team mates.[74] Other cricketers, such as Tom Sewell and Tom Hearne, suffered from bouts of seasickness and were no doubt ministered to by Hocken. After the Bay of Biscay, however, it was reported that 'the little cricketers were beginning to chirp again'.[75]

Despite noting, on 24 October 1861, that 'More than two-thirds of the passengers have been very sick' and describing how Jane Mack had 'been ill all Saturday and yesterday violent headache and pains in her limbs', Helen Roland wrote that Hocken 'has not had very much to do':

> He is a very little man and he is not very prepossessing in his manner I think. He was telling Miss Felkin the other day that Miss Ronald was the only lady on board with whom he had not spoken, and that he felt afraid of taking the liberty: Miss Felkin having told me, it has made me feel extremely foolish whenever I see him, and when the introduction will take place I know not. As usual with the Ronald family, I have got up a reputation, without at all wishing it, of being a bit of a blue stocking.

She also testified to Hocken's liking for 'intellectual feasting':

The other night the doctor actually came up and spoke to me; Jane Mack and I were sitting together, he came with the ostensible object of asking how she felt, but took the opportunity of asking me how I liked 'Darwin' and other questions of that kind. I am rather pleased I have spoken to him at last, as it seemed strange I should be the only one on board that had not done so.

Roland recorded finishing Charles Lyell's *Principles of Geology*, published between 1830 and 1833, with which she was 'much pleased, edified as well'. She noted that 'The doctor has lent me a review which appeared in the *Edinburgh Review* in 1845, on the 'Vestiges of Creation', a book of which you have perhaps heard.'[76]

Hocken may have read *Vestiges of Creation*, published anonymously in 1844, and Darwin's *On the Origin of Species*, published in 1859. It is interesting that he had with him on board the review he lent Roland, in which Cambridge Professor of Geology Adam Sedgwick famously railed against *Vestiges*. In fact, Sedgwick once wrote to Charles Lyell about the book's conclusions: 'If the book be true, the labours of sober induction are in vain; religion is a lie; human law is a mass of folly, and a base injustice; morality is moonshine; our labours for the black people of Africa were works of madmen; and man and woman are only better beasts!'[77] Hocken's Christian faith was strong and perhaps by lending the article out he was ensuring that his fellow passenger, a woman no less, would have the intellectual resources to counter the book's 'false philosophy'.

As usual, Hocken fulfilled his religious duties: 'We had service both morning and evening, and through the help of a melodeon we manage both chants and hymns. The purser and the doctor read in the morning, the doctor conducts the evening service.' At one stage Hocken was very ill with a sore throat and 'the fourth officer assisted the purser'.[78] Once again, there was a ship's newspaper, now recognised as 'an institution of the passage to and from Australia'.[79] The *Cabinet* was issued four times during the voyage: on 9 November (up to crossing the line), on 8 December (reaching the longitude of the Cape) and twice more during the remainder of the voyage.[80] Much of the *Cabinet*, in an edited version, was reset and printed with the sub-title *A repository of facts, figures, and fancies relating to the voyage of the 'Great Britain' S.S. from Liverpool to Melbourne with the Eleven of All England, and other distinguished passengers*, by J. Reid in Melbourne, 1862.

Captain Gray welcomed the newspaper. It broke the monotony of the voyage, and it enabled him to tell of the ship's progress: 'within these last few days Fortune has favoured us with a strong steady breeze … and I have every hope that we shall enjoy our Christmas dinner in Australia'. Gray could also happily state that 'the health of the ship continues perfectly satisfactory, which is a boon, considering how liable we are to retain any kind of sickness that may be infectious'.[81] The doctor's medical report, signed 'Morland Hocken', backs this up: 'I am happy to say that the general health continues excellent – attributable to the fine weather we have enjoyed since leaving England, and also to the great attention paid to cleanliness by our passengers. The cold weather has brought its usual amount of colds and coughs, and two or three cases of very severe bronchitis. The necessity of warm clothing need hardly be insisted upon.'[82]

Perhaps the food on board, at least in the saloon, contributed to the healthiness of the passengers. While steerage passengers faced preserved meat and plum pudding, the first-class passengers could dine on vermicelli soup, mutton, pork, geese, veal, duck, chicken, turkey, lamb, beef, ham, tongue, vegetables, rice, batter or custard pudding, gooseberry or blackcurrant tart, jam tart, omelette or macaroni, cheese, oranges, ginger, raisins, almonds, walnuts and Barcelona nuts.[83] Indigestion was surely one complaint that Hocken had to deal with.

Some *Cabinet* articles carry initials and pseudonyms, but most are unsigned making it difficult to identify Hocken's contributions. However, the tone and content of the two-part 'Natural history of the voyage' and the now familiar 'The world we inhabit' are surely his. In the former he displays knowledge of George Bennett's *Wandering in New South Wales* (1834), a book he would eventually own, and in the latter repeats from the *Great Britain Gazette and Weekly Screw* much about the ship, its physical dimensions, history and personnel. He even pretends to quote himself: 'In an interesting paper on this subject, Dr Hocken, our medical officer, gives us the benefit of his botanical knowledge. "We have," he says, "as all know, three lofty trees springing from the deck, their roots of course being deep below. Their names and characteristics are not to be found in any botanist's flora, but in *our* world they are termed fore, main, and mizzen masts ..."'. And so on until, under the paragraph 'Its Government', Hocken terms himself 'The Secretary of State – or the gentleman whom we imagine to be in the secret of the state of the health of each of us'.[84] Mr Meadon, chief engineer, is Cyclops, Mr Beckett the Chancellor of the Exchequer.

There are otherwise only a few glimpses of Hocken in the *Cabinet*, and those are mostly connected with bad Victorian humour. With jokes such as 'When is the "Great Britain" most like a bugler? When she gets a blow at the Horn' and 'Why is the "Great Britain" like an old lady wearing false hair? Because her head is grey (Gray)', Hocken did not escape notice. Under 'Puns professionals' readers are asked: 'At what time does the respected surgeon of the "Great Britain" S.S. appear most unprofessional? When he has no patience (patients).' His possible retort was under 'Advertisements': 'Found, at the surgery, by Dr Hocken, a large quantity of sham-pain.'[85]

The *Cabinet* was not the only magazine produced on this voyage. Three weeks after the ship left England, G.H. Wayte (later editor), F.E. Stewart, L.P. Traherne, W.V. Robinson and Hocken met in the saloon to establish a weekly periodical called the *'Great Britain' Miscellany*. They decided that 'all subjects, whether of a local or a generally literary character' would be admitted into its columns 'with the exception of political and religious topics and personalities'.⁸⁶

The tone of the *Miscellany* is more informal than that of the *Cabinet*. The bad jokes are still there, as are Captain Gray's enthusiastic reports. Reference is made to dancing and music every evening, backgammon in the saloon and a dog called Fury. Articles not printed in the *Cabinet* include 'Stray thoughts on smoking and smokers', 'The England Eleven', 'Hunting reminiscences', 'Our cricketers', 'Sporting in NZ', 'Remedies for sea-sickness', information on the poisonous herb tutu, and 'Gold in New Zealand'. Although the writers of these pieces are unidentified, the ones on smoking and seasickness are surely by Hocken. The appearance of tutu is of particular interest, especially in light of Hocken's later examination of this plant in Dunedin. There are three brief references to Hocken. The first is in a letter that suggests he could help the ladies 'put their hands to the good work and establish a "Great Britain Dorcas Society"' to sew clothing for the steerage passengers. The second reports his treatment of Heathfield Stephenson, captain of the cricket team, for a small injury caused by the rough weather: according to Hocken, the damage was 'only *local*'.⁸⁷ And finally, an article called 'Our microcosm', which contains an amusing medical anecdote noting that those on the voyage were 'a jolly community; when we are well, we have everything about us calculated to keep us so, and preserve our cheerfulness; when we are ill, we have the best of little doctors to apply to'.⁸⁸

Cape Otway and its lighthouse, on the coast of Victoria, came into view on 23 December 1861 and the ship soon nosed into Hobsons Bay and anchored off Sandridge Pier, within sight of the city of Melbourne.⁸⁹ Once again Gray and Hocken received testimonials: 82 and 50 sovereigns respectively. However, not everyone was appreciative, as Helen Roland noted:

> A testimonial is being got up for the doctor, or more properly those who have required his services are joining together in giving him something; the Lorimers do not give anything, nor do Kate and I and many others. We have not required him, and as I do not like him personally, I should not think of giving. Mrs Grey has required him a great deal, she was confined to her cabin for some weeks with bronchitis, she gives him fifteen guineas.⁹⁰

Nothing is known of Hocken's activities in Melbourne, although it is easy to guess that he was involved in producing the edited version of the *Cabinet* and the 172-page *'Great Britain' Miscellany* printed by Mason & Firth, who had earlier issued the *Weekly Screw*. As with the earlier *Great Britain Magazine*, he saw it as 'a thousand pities' to allow the pleasant memories of the voyage to dissipate.⁹¹ Printing such edited versions of the shipboard magazines, paid for by subscriptions, meant that passengers had copies that they could send home to friends or keep as souvenirs. The writing, editing and publishing experience would stand Hocken in good stead in the future.

After a full month in Melbourne, on 29 January 1862 Hocken 'left the old "Great Britain" at Melbourne … having permission from Messr Gibbs, Bright &c [steamship and general agents] to do so, in order to go down to Dunedin'. He sailed on the *Chariot of Fame*, along with some of the 'thousands of diggers [who] were making their way to the newly discovered Otago gold-fields'.[92] It was the beginning of an important chapter in his life.

3
Early Beginnings in Dunedin

Hocken arrived in Dunedin on 22 February 1862 after a 23-day passage out of Melbourne. The town was in the throes of gold fever. Gold had been discovered in the area in the 1850s, all to little stir, but in May 1861 Gabriel Read, a miner from Tasmania, found a rich mine at what became Gabriel's Gully at Tuapeka, and then another strike followed at nearby Waitahuna. The rush was on: 'Every able bodied man in town or village threw down his tools and was off to the diggings.' Ships poured in full of miners who had already tried their luck in California and across the Tasman; 69 docked in 1860, 256 in the following year.[1] By December 1861, 14,000 men had pitched their tents in the area.[2] Local poet John Blair captured the spirit:

> Gold! Gold! Is all the cry!
> Picks and shovels, blankets, buy!
> Off to Gabriel's Gully hie.
> Off to the Diggings! ...
> Where are all the hangers on
> Who Dunedin streets did throng?
> Gold! Gold! Off they're gone,
> Off to the Diggings ... [3]

As Hocken himself later wrote, 'Dunedin followed the lead; morning after morning fresh parties left the town, master and man on equal terms; clerks and mechanics, the better class, and the shopkeepers, all travelling to the same goal.'[4]

Otago's population had ballooned. In 1848 the province contained 350 males and 270 females; in 1860 the population had risen to 12,691; a year later the 1861 census revealed that the area contained 27,242 souls, excluding some 3000 miners and local Maori. Over 15 religious denominations were represented, with 10,596 Presbyterians pipping the Anglicans by about 1000, followed by 3160 'unknowns' and 2745 Roman Catholics. Other, smaller groups included Lutherans, Jews, Freethinkers, Mormons and Universalists.[5] Dunedin was the new El Dorado. Hocken was but one of hordes of eager, mostly single men, and some women, to try their luck at the diggings. He was not, however, set on gaining riches by the shovel and pan. Like Julius Vogel, founding editor of the *Otago Daily Times* and future politician, he envisaged other opportunities.[6]

From Port Chalmers Hocken would have caught one of the 'greasy, dirty little boats' that transported arrivals to the colour and confusion of the Dunedin jetty.[7] There were, in A.H. McLintock's words, 'diggers in every variety of costume, with the dandy or "flash" man resplendent in scarlet shirt, white moleskin trousers, cabbage-tree hat with long black ribbons, and crimson silk scarf set off by a fringe of tassels dangling from the waist. Also part of the crowd were 'smart young clerks, custom-house officers, soldiers ... in their bright scarlet tunics, policemen in blue with peaked leather hats', not to mention sailors and wharfies.[8] As Hocken walked through the town, treading a mixture of asphalt and mud, he would have seen a circular open space from which five streets opened up: the principal Princes Street, south and north, Stafford, Manse and Jetty streets. As well as shops he would have passed the post office, customs house, treasury, gold office and government offices (called the 'shabbiest').[9] The smell would have been memorable: animal and vegetable remains, fish, and moist, untreated and disease-producing sewage. There was no water supply: water for domestic purposes ran off shingle or iron roofs into old barrels and was then transported into houses in buckets. The cost of meat was high, from 1s 6d to 2s per pound (453g), and a loaf of bread cost anywhere between 10d and 1s. Many poorer people consumed low- or bad-quality goods. There had been cases of typhoid fever, dysentery, worms (especially in children), rheumatic fever, pneumonia, bronchitis, diphtheria, boils and erysipelas, particularly among the elderly. The need for town cleanliness and a proper sewage disposal system was a common cry in the newspapers, as was the real possibility of deaths: 'the Black Horses are harnessed, and every moment may be at the door.'[10] As a medical man, Hocken would not have been impressed. His thorough microscopic examination of the local spring and well-water in October 1862, tellingly mentioned in the report of the Dunedin Sanitary Commission of 1865, was but one example of his zealous professionalism in this area.[11]

Another glance would have revealed wooded gullies strewn with more mud, and cottages, calico huts and buildings of all shapes and sizes. Indeed, one resident maintained 'she went to sleep having seen Bell Hill covered with manuka and a few small houses, and woke to find the place white with tents'.[12] Rents were high: for some of the cottages between 25s and 40s per week. Manuka firewood, which was plentiful, could cost between 30s and 35s a load.[13] Landslips and stone avalanches were a common occurrence.

It is not known where Hocken first stayed in town — perhaps it was at Alexander Miller's 'comfortable board and lodging' at Moray House in Stuart Street or the Albion on Great King Street, 'combining the freedom of a Hotel, with the comforts of an English House'[14] — or how he found his business premises. Nevertheless, he was quick to make a good start. After submitting his credentials to A.C. Strode, the resident magistrate, he walked to the offices of the newly established *Otago Daily Times* and paid 3d for a business notice in the next issue on Monday, 24 February 1862.[15] It appeared on page three under 'Miscellaneous', between an advertisement for the Royal Princess Theatre and a notice issued by a disgruntled Port Chalmers resident: 'Dr Morland Hocken, late Surgeon of the steam-ship "Great Britain" has commenced practice in Princes-street, a few doors above Bank of New South Wales, Dunedin.'[16] Later, more successfully placed advertisements were expanded to: 'Dr Hocken, late Surgeon of the S.S. *Great Britain*, Princes-street Chambers, opposite the Exchange Hotel, and a few doors above the Bank of New South Wales. Hours of Consultation: 9 to 11 a.m., 2 to 4 p.m., and afterwards through the evening.'[17]

There is a paucity of information about Hocken's movements during his first year in Dunedin, but there is a hint of what was to come. On 17 December 1862 he gave a lecture on botany at Knox Church; it was the sixth in a series organised by the Dunedin Young Men's Christian Association. He followed J.L.C. Richardson, the provincial superintendent, and preceded local politician John McGlashan and William Lauder Lindsay, the Edinburgh-educated botanist who, because he had been so unwell, had his lecture, 'The place and power of natural history in colonization', read out to a packed audience on 22 November.[18] Hocken did not hear Lindsay's lecture but owned two written versions – a YMCA pamphlet of 1862 and an 1863 printing from Edinburgh. He later bound them up with Lindsay's *Observations on New Zealand Lichens* (1866) and *Contributions to New Zealand Botany* (1868), and inside made a typically long, factual annotation on the Scotsman:

> Dr Lindsay was a medical officer of the Perthshire County Lunatic Asylum & was also an accomplished botanist & geologist. Compelled by delicate health he visited NZ in 1861 returning in January 1862. During this time he made many observations & contributions to these sciences as they relate to NZ of which this volume forms part. He also wrote a paper 'On the Geology of the Gold Fields of Otago, N.Z.' in the Brit. Assoc Reports of Oct. 1862; 'On the Toot Plant & Poison of N.Z.' in No. 61 of the 'Westminster Review'; & a lecture on 'The Place & Power of Natural History in Colonization' delivered to the Young Mens' Xtian Assoc, reprinted & altered in the Edinburgh 'New Philosophical Journal' for April & July 1863. Dr Lindsay's head quarters when in Otago were with Mr Wm Martin, gardener of Fairfield. Dr L. was a poitinere [potinière – chatterbox, one who talks incessantly] & died.[19]

Hocken's talk was general in scope and his audience was, to quote the *Otago Daily Times*, 'more select than numerous' owing to the 'very unpropitious state of the weather'.[20] He used diagrams and his faithful microscope to inform his listeners about plants, floral systems, fungi and a particular local occurrence, fermenting cesspools. He also touched on New Zealand plants such as manuka, cabbage trees and ferns (which he later called 'beautiful waving'),[21] as well as tutu (*Coriaria arborea*), with its highly toxic green fruit and flowering racemes.[22] While in Otago, Lindsay was asked by the provincial council to examine 'toot', as it was known. Stock poisoning was common and occasionally humans died.[23] In fact, a few days before Hocken arrived in

Dunedin, a Frenchman named Rigan had died near Maungatua after eating tutu.[24] In his lecture Hocken offered his listeners a recipe for an antidote: 'first an emetic, to be followed by a breakfast cup of strong coffee, mixed with a teaspoonful of hartshorn, and a table spoonful of charcoal'.[25] As a young man eager to establish a reputation in his adopted country, Hocken deserves credit for familiarising himself so quickly with New Zealand plants and for appearing before an audience. At the end of his talk, he offered his services to anyone who was interested in botanical studies, adding that he would assist to the best of his ability. And all the while he was establishing a busy medical practice.

Hocken as Coroner

The resignation of the town's coroner, Henry Howorth, in late December 1862 provided Hocken with an excellent opportunity for social and professional advancement. He applied for the vacancy and secured his warrant of appointment, dated 12 January 1863, on 6 February.[26] Thus began a busy and productive 22-year colonial career. Robert Valpy Fulton, in his *Medical Practice in Otago and Southland in the Early Days* (1922), deemed it 'astonishing' that Hocken was not only able to establish and maintain a general practice but also to take on the office of coroner.[27]

His medical work was, in his own words, 'very hard, but I was young and strong, and the pay was very good'.[28] For several years he rarely took less than £10 a day in actual cash, gold, notes and gold dust, paid to him largely by an itinerant population coming and going from the diggings. Accidents were common: scalp wounds, eye injuries from explosions, broken bones from falls, gunshot and knife wounds. And then there were the 'house calls', often to outlying, desolate areas. He would either walk or ride, or, later when the tracks were laid, travel by train.

As coroner, his role was to enquire into the manner of deaths, especially those that were deemed violent and unnatural, or had no known cause. An inquest not only helped to determine how or why the person died but also to establish their identity. Hocken dealt with suicides, accidental deaths – especially by drowning – fatal injuries through fighting and gunshot wounds and loss of life through fires. It was a job that covered a wide territory, from Blueskin Bay (Waiputai) to the Taieri and inland to Outram and Hindon, as well as Port Chalmers, though the last named was removed from Hocken's jurisdiction in late 1866.[29] Each inquest demanded consummate skill, social sensitivity and sound judgement. Hocken was good at the job.

His duties began almost immediately. Much of his activity in this role – reporting on health, hospital administration and sanitary conditions in Dunedin, and later securing the positions of surgeon of the Dunedin Volunteer Naval Brigade (1865) and the Defence Forces (1885), and president of the Otago Medical Association – is ably covered in A.G. Hocken's biography.[30] Two incidents, however, are worth mentioning.

One was the Jarvey case of March 1865, which was a notable forensic first.[31] Captain William Andrew Jarvey, master of a small vessel trading between New Zealand and Australia, was charged with poisoning his wife Catherine, who had died the previous September. In a hand-written note saved by Hocken, Jarvey made special appeal for a trial by 'common jury'.[32] The first trial was presided over by Justice Henry Chapman. Unfortunately, no verdict was delivered, owing to what Hocken described as 'the ignorant stupidity of one of the jury – Schlesinger'.[33] Jarvey was tried again in September before Justice Christopher Richmond. As coroner, Hocken had Catherine Jarvey's body exhumed and tested for the organic poison strychnine. According to Hocken, the accused remained confident throughout the proceedings, under the illusion that the poison would have decomposed with the body and would leave no trace. When its presence was indisputably shown by a Melbourne-based expert, Jarvey fainted in the dock. A guilty verdict was eventually delivered. Jarvey was hanged in the Dunedin gaol on 24 October 1865.

Hocken not only saved the coarse cloth-bound pamphlet, *Trial of Captain Jarvey on a Charge of Poisoning his Wife* (1865), but also made extensive notes on the trial that reveal a characteristic often forgotten when it comes to the 'gentlemanly' doctor: he was capable of speaking plainly.

> Jarvey was a most atrocious criminal. Without doubt he had secretly murdered several of his illegitimate children in Tasmania & had this trial failed he would have been charged with these crimes. At the time that one of his daughters was lying dead of scarlet fever he was discovered by his wife in the attempt to have sexual connexions with her. The horrified mother threatened disclosure & to secure her silence Jarvey poisoned her. This – the real motive – did not appear in the trial.

There had initially been no reason to be suspicious, going by the statement of Dr Charles Hardy and the Jarvey daughter, Elizabeth Ann, who was the sole witness to her mother's death. Three months later, however, 'the terrible secret proved more than she could bear' and she told the police what had really happened. As Hocken recorded, 'On the night of the murder he [Jarvey] broke into his daughter's bedroom & attempted to ravish her. This she also concealed … Considerable interest was taken in his children who assumed different names, but in a few years they were entirely lost sight of.'[34]

The second incident occurred after Hocken's coronership had ended. He owned a copy of the *Full Report of the Trial of Thomas Hall for the Murder of Captain Henry Cain*, a notorious Timaru poisoning case that was tried in the Dunedin Supreme Court in January 1887.[35] Hocken's note on his copy, a reprint from one included in the *Otago Daily Times*, reveals that he was privy to information not readily available: 'There is little doubt but that Margaret Houston [Cain's live-in carer] was an accomplice in the attempt to murder, or at least that there was knowledge of what was going on. When Hall's goods were sold there were found amongst his photographic slides, many pictures of Miss Houston, taken in various attitudes and quite naked.'[36] Hall's death sentence was later quashed by the Court of Appeal.

Clubs and Associations in Dunedin

Hocken was a devout Christian, but in New Zealand he left his Methodist background behind and joined the Church of England. He became a pew holder at St Paul's Cathedral in 1862 and was later a churchwarden and lay canon. On 16 December 1862, the day before he gave his botany lecture, a bazaar and 'Industrial Exhibition' was opened to raise funds for a new Anglican church. The hastily organised exhibition featured a variety of natural and manufactured products from around the southern region and was 'as far as possible, an exposition of the products of the colony': it extended to areas such as Nelson and Wellington and was advertised in the *Lyttelton Times*. The exhibitor response was so good that there was too much to display. Hocken was mentioned in newspaper reports for his contribution of 'a number of specimens of dried ferns, prettily displayed on a large board'.[37] He was, as always, willing to be involved; he enjoyed such occasions.

As a young professional keen to make his mark, he joined organisations in Dunedin that would lead to further contacts. One that had personal and professional benefits was the Masonic Lodge, established in Otago on 8 August 1860.[38] On 7 January 1863 Hocken was initiated into the Lodge of Otago, No. 1146 EC (soon to be No. 844), along with accountant Hector Baxter, auctioneer John Daniels, tobacconist Philip Strelitz and storekeeper John Frederick Wilson.[39] He was listed as a surgeon, living and working at 128 Princes Street.[40] By the end of May that year Hocken had moved to a house in Rattray Street, 'a little above the Shamrock Hotel and formerly occupied by Dr Nelson'. His hours of consultation were 'during the forenoon and evening'.[41] This address was very handy for lodge meetings, which were held at the Shamrock, now the site occupied by Speight's Brewery.[42] Hocken's fellow members included his friend, artist William Mathew Hodgkins, former coroner Henry Howorth, local customs collector William Mills, secretary of the Goldfields Department Vincent Pyke, Otago superintendent John Hyde Harris, and William Lloyd of Lloyd, Taggart & Co., agents for New Zealand Steam Navigation. Hocken resigned from the Masons in 1883.

Hocken also joined the Dunedin (Otago) Club, which was established in 1858 and whose members included prominent runholders, merchants, judges, magistrates, barristers, surgeons and architects. His name appears on the first membership list of September 1863, alongside 80 other men.[43] Like them, he paid the annual subscription of eight guineas with the additional entrance fee of one guinea. And although his attendance at meetings is not well documented, he no doubt enjoyed the dinners, the social chat, the garden parties and the occasions held in honour of a visiting celebrity or a departing member.[44] When he died, the annual report described Hocken as 'one of the oldest members, his connection with the Club dating practically from its foundation'.[45] Over the years the social and political contacts he made here and at the lodge afforded him excellent connections when it came to expanding his collecting networks.

In 1864 Hocken joined the Benevolent Institute, paying the necessary two guinea membership fee. He was a committed member, listed on the committee of management with such people as Otago Police Commissioner St John Branigan, Julius Vogel and John Hyde Harris. He was nominated honorary surgeon, submitting the society's annual reports until 1889 when he was replaced by Dr William Stenhouse. He regularly visited the Dunedin Lunatic Asylum (52 visits in 1868) and attended a number of sick people at their homes.[46] His efforts were noticed: the Rev. Donald Stuart reported in 1871 that 'the health of the institution during the past year said a great deal in favour of Dr Hocken, who he also knew to be very attentive to the out-door patients'.[47] Hocken owned some 33 reports and pamphlets on the Benevolent Institute dated between 1864 and 1896, making brief notes on some about their printing.[48] He joined the Otago Acclimatisation Society in 1865 and continued to be involved and to collect the society's reports until 1886, when his membership lapsed.[49]

Lighter Moments

Public meetings and social occasions also provided ideal opportunities to become known. As a new arrival keen to understand the Dunedin community, Hocken may well have attended the public meeting held on 10 May 1862 and attended by some 1000 citizens to discuss the separation of the North and Middle Islands, as they were then known, so that the south could have its own government. He was certainly present at a later meeting in Riverton in March 1869, where an interested party formed a group to initiate the re-annexation of Southland to the province of Otago. Hocken kept the proposal and filed it in his second F&J volume.[50] On 12 December 1862 he was present at a party at the Provincial Hotel after a farewell benefit performance for Sandford Fawcett who, with his brother Tom, managed the Royal Princess Theatre, which had been opened in February that year. (The Theatre Royal had opened in July.) The Fawcetts ran their own company and imported visiting performers. One of the other party guests was actor Madame Marie Duret, whose benefit was to be held the following night. A toast was given to 'The Ladies', to which Hocken and Tom Fawcett responded.[51]

Hocken's interest in thespian matters was not confined to being an audience member. On 9 January 1864 George Fawcett produced a burlesque called *The Chamber of Horrors: A tale of wax and mystery* at the Princess Theatre. It included 'three caricatures of well known individuals', one of which was an impersonation of a character called Little May, 'a well-known member of the medical fraternity'.[52] This was, of course, Hocken: the newspaper advertisement listed 'Dr H–n ... Little May'.[53] On hearing of this proposed performance, Hocken went to the actress's 'dressing room' and said to her: 'Well Miss Holt, I understand you wish to burlesque me; may I sit down? I have come to give you as much assistance as I can. Now will you endeavour to make yourself up as carefully as possible, and if there are any clothes or properties I can lend you, pray mention them, and we will send round at once to my rooms for them.' On the night, when 'Little May' walked towards the footlights, schooled in walk, mannerisms and movement by Hocken, the packed house 'fairly rocked with laughter'. When Hocken acknowledged his counterpart from his box seat, 'the roof fairly came off'.[54] Hocken had the courage, spirit and sense of humour to allow a laugh at his own expense, especially when it involved his size. Such 'fun and gaiety' won him acceptance and provided much-needed relief from the harsh daily realities of his profession.[55]

Even in his job there were light moments. One day in June 1864 a number of men spied blood oozing from under the door of a former ham and beef shop in Manse Street. There was talk of murder but Hocken, who was passing, obtained some samples of the blood and determined that it was 'from a poor porker'.[56]

Hocken not only enjoyed entertaining – conversation, a round of cards and wine or coffee – but was fond of humorous stories and had a great store of 'side-splitting yarns' gained from his experiences out in the field. As Robert Fulton put it: 'An hour with Dr Hocken when in a reminiscent mood was worth more than a seven shilling novel.'[57]

The Collection Begins

Establishing his medical practice was of paramount importance to Hocken, but even in these early years his interest in New Zealand history and ethnography began to take shape. And, occasionally, professional life coincided with personal interests. On 17 November 1865 Hocken held an inquest at the Taieri River Hotel into the death of Charles Davis, a five-year-old Maori boy who had died of a lung infection while under the care of a man named Piripi who claimed to be a Hauhau prophet from the North Island.[58] While noting that part of Piripi's treatment included 'rasping the boy's chest with the serrated leaf of the toetoe grass', Hocken also took the time to record the prescription for the homeopathic infusion used, which involved leaves from the kowhai, ngaio and karamu trees. Above his translation, 'To make known the medicinal properties of certain trees', is the original Maori, but no mention of who first provided it.[59] Perhaps it was German missionary Johann Freidrich Riemenschneider, who was the interpreter at the inquest. Some months earlier Hocken had received visits from Riemenschneider, who had arrived in Nelson in 1843. On the same immigrant ship, the *St Pauli*, had been Johann Friedrich Heinrich Wohlers, the Lutheran missionary who lived among the Maori at Ruapuke Island in Foveaux Strait for 40 years, and with whom Hocken would eventually correspond. Riemenschneider, who was, in Hocken's words, 'the German missionary & schoolmaster at the Otago heads', also knew Nelson (and later Otago) surveyor Frederick Tuckett and many prominent Maori chiefs. It is not clear who initiated the first meeting, but the men discussed Maori health and disease before and after colonisation. Given Riemenschneider's rich experiences in New Zealand, Hocken would have learnt much from this 'very intelligent & observant man' who 'had had some medical training'.[60]

Happily, these meetings bore fruit. On 9 November 1864 the missionary wrote to say that he was sending through his 'On Maori habits of life', a closely packed essay of 33 leaves covering such subjects as venereal diseases, measles, tobacco use, diseases of the skin and asthma. Since Hocken's time was 'much occupied', Riemenschneider suggested he 'begin at the 12th or 13th page in looking over them':

> I commenced some time ago to write when I thought there was ample time for me to go into the subject, but I have found myself interrupted with other work, journeying, &c, & so it has been all along. From the same causes the whole from beginning to end was ill arranged, & I have found no time & leisure for either copying or revising it & must therefore read it just as it is with all its imperfections & which I trust you will kindly excuse. I do very much regret indeed that I should have had to wait this long & I do so sincerely apologise.

Riemenschneider also stressed that he had expressed his 'own private views & opinions', and left it to Hocken's 'professional knowledge & better judgement, to form your own opinion, & to decide for yourself as to what those remarks of mine are worth & may be relied on for correctness'.[61]

The manuscript has particular significance. It is the first recorded item Hocken accepted into his collection and, more importantly, the first result of his many requests for material on early New Zealand history. It also acknowledges a fact noted elsewhere, by many people – that Hocken was a busy man. He also had presence. Although 20 years older, Riemenschneider was obviously impressed by the young doctor. The annotation Hocken added to the missionary's material also establishes an important precedent: he was an inveterate scribbler on his materials, whether they were books, manuscripts or maps. His notes were almost always factual, with a strong focus on dates, historical events, places and people. As he once wrote, 'Dates are dry, but imperative.'[62]

The New Zealand Exhibition, 1865

Despite its short duration and the somewhat chaotic arrangements, the 1862 industrial exhibition was such a success in trumpeting the progress of the province that in August 1863 the provincial council voted £4000 towards the general expenses of a group of commissioners to plan a larger, grander event. This became the New Zealand Exhibition, held in Dunedin in 1865.[63] Governor Sir George Grey, advocate of scientific and technological advancements, had the exhibition noted in the *New Zealand Gazette* on 12 September 1863.[64]

The 14 commissioners appointed were 'old' community faces: James Hector (director of the Geological Survey of Otago and later director of the Geological Survey and Colonial Museum in Wellington), Thomas Dick (future Otago superintendent), T.B. Gillies (local lawyer and politician), James Paterson (local MP), E.B Cargill (prominent businessman and future castle builder) and his politician brother John Cargill, well-known merchants R.B. Martin and James Rattray, Alfred Eccles, Henry Clapcott (provincial treasurer), R.S. Cantrell (politician), W.H. Reynolds (businessman and politician), Julius Vogel and architect William Mason. Public endorsement was encouraged and, to that end, on 14 February 1864 a public holiday was given to celebrate the laying of the foundation stone of the exhibition building, designed by Mason and W.H. Clayton. The commissioners' enthusiasm for the scheme was infectious despite the inevitable budget blow-out, which rocketed the cost to £18,000. Hector undertook a whirlwind tour of the country and reported back on the developments. By the end of October 1864 he had a commitment from Hocken to provide copy on 'the analysis of the vital statistics of New Zealand'; another local, Vincent Pyke, would contribute gold mining statistics. From Wellington, politician Francis Dillon Bell was to cover the 'Native Races'. Hector himself, along with scientist and former explorer James Coutts Crawford and geologist and future Canterbury Museum director Julius Haast, would cover geology and mineralogy.[65] These writings were to form part of the catalogue.

On 12 January 1865 the exhibition opened in a newly erected Italianate brick building on Great King Street. It was an impressive structure with four square loggia-topped towers and a huge central hall with upper and lower galleries on all four sides. The show-stoppers were the Cape Saunders 'lighthouse' and the 6.4 m gilded obelisk strategically placed at the entrance, which represented the gold exported from New Zealand during the rush years.[66] Over 102 days some 29,000 visitors saw hundreds of exhibits from the provinces of Otago, Canterbury, Auckland and Nelson, from the Australian colonies, and from Britain, Canada, France, Germany and the Netherlands. Just a few of the many items on display were a Venetian bookcase, soap and candle goods, a moa egg, specimens of alpine flora, numerous stuffed birds, sketch maps and plans, samples of fencing and telegraphic wiring, early New Zealand printed books (from William Colenso), a model railway, a model of artificial salmon-breeding ponds, a sundial made of Oamaru stone, a locally built wooden boat, photographs by Joseph Perry and chromo-lithographs of ferns and flowering plants, castings and ornamental railings, Indian textiles, fleeces, bottled wine, Hector's botanical collection and a model of the bridge over the Clutha River. The Maori section, of particular interest to Hocken, included mats, flax (*Phormium tenax*), canoes and carved paddles, fish-hooks, mere, adzes, combs and greenstone pendants. There was also a Fine Arts Room containing 406 works (412 in the second and third printing of the catalogue) by New Zealand artists such as Charles Barraud, Henry Coote, John Gully and George O'Brien and, from abroad, *A. Bacchante* by the great Sir Joshua Reynolds.[67] According to one local reporter, this was 'the most delightful, and one of the most creditable, departments of the Exhibition'.[68]

Hocken owned a copy of Gully's *New Zealand Scenery* (1877), deemed an 'excellent' copy and purchased for 17s. He claimed that the artist's name and fame were established at this exhibition with works such as *The Peak of Mount Cook*, *Wairau Gorge* and *Lake Arthur, Rotoiti, Nelson* attracting purchasers such as Commissioners Eccles and Martin, who each paid £10 for a piece.[69] Later Hocken himself was able to secure 'The Peak of Mount Cook' from John Douglas, manager of the Bank of New South Wales, for an undisclosed sum. As Hocken noted in *New Zealand Scenery*, in 1899,

> I knew Mr John Gully well. He was an occasional visitor at my house on his trips from home at Nelson. Though not a professional artist he easily stands first amongst our N.Z. painters ... Gully thought highly of [*The Peak of Mount Cook*] which he always called to see when in Dunedin. On one occasion, after gazing at it a long time he said: 'Ah! I shall never paint like that again' ... He was a cheerful, merry fellow, & travelled much with his fellow artist Richmond.

The book, which originally cost £5, did not sell well because, in Hocken's words, of the 'dreadful renderings of [Gully's] beautiful originals' and because 'sheets were sold loose for framing. So little was the book prized that copies were tossed about in all the dust of auction rooms, & it is now [1899] beginning to be rare ...'[70]

The written material that accompanied the exhibits was exactly what Hocken liked to collect. Volume 11 of his F&J collection contains numerous documents pertaining to the exhibition. Some are substantial publications; others are single sheets, such as 'Notes on what sort of exhibits are required for New Zealand Exhibition' (1865), 'Decisions on points relating to the New Zealand Exhibition' (1865), an announcement of the decision not to award prizes in the Fine Arts Section, New Zealand Exhibition Certificate forms and the *Otago Daily Times* coverage of the opening.[71]

Hocken had, of course, been involved in mounting the exhibition. He prepared a cabinet of moa bones for display.[72] He also organised an exhibition of 'South Sea Island costumes',[73] and – along with naturalist, missionary and printer William Colenso, local businesswoman Amelia Muir and William

Jeffreys, son of the strongly evangelical independent minister the Rev. Charles Jeffreys – he exhibited specimens of tapa cloth and 'a numerous variety of Fiji clubs and other curiosities'.[74] Already Maori and Pacific Island materials were a focus for Hocken's collecting. Also evident is his self-assurance and his confidence in what he said and wrote. He had sufficient social skill and tact to collaborate with others, especially the strong-minded and irascible Colenso. The two men enjoyed a long friendship.

Hocken also, it would seem, had fun at the exhibition. He joined Vogel and eccentric demagogue and journalist J.G.S. Grant in some spoof lectures. A ditty in Charles Thatcher's *Otago Songster* (1865) reveals that Hocken's lecture (No. 16) was amusingly titled 'On Tectile [sic] Covering, from the days of Wat Tyler down to Thatcher, with a treatise on cocked hats'.[75] Hocken's small stature and his predilection for wearing hats to compensate for his lack of height made him ripe for lampooning. Years later, F.A. Bett recalled that one of the sights of Dunedin was 'the spectacle of Dr. H. walking with Dr [F.C.] Batchelor, both wearing silk hats, Dr B. must have been 6 ft. 6 inches high. It certainly was ridiculous to see the one peering down & the other peeping up as they engaged in conversation.'[76]

Hocken also featured in Thomas Redmayne's cartoon, 'Otago and her new doctors: A speedy cure anticipated', in *Dunedin Punch* of 9 September 1865. A bearded Hocken holding a glass or flask sits on a chair beside Dr Alexander Hunter. Both men are peering over at their young female patient, a youthful 'Otago' (a 'Britannia' lookalike), who is holding up a bowl marked 'Delicate Financial Soup'. A walking stick lies casually on the floor beside Hocken, and his legs – nowhere near the ground – dangle under the chair.[77] When the New Zealand Exhibition closed on 5 May 1865, the building was turned into a hospital.[78] It would become familiar territory as Hocken returned to the rigours of his professional duties.

New Zealand History

In the main, Hocken's historical interest lay in the period spanning the pre-history of New Zealand, including the early Maori, through to the New Zealand Company's emigration plans, and ending (generally) with the establishment of Christchurch, the last settlement in which the company was involved. Although much of his collecting encompassed the period up to 1850, Hocken did make comment on his own times. Found in his 'New Zealand Notes', his books, and on his paintings and sketches, are rare insights that not only reflect his responses to his environment, which he was still discovering, but also provide a modicum of gossip about others.

He had some fondness for 1862, calling the year 'those stirring times'. He pinpointed the town's somewhat notorious Vauxhall Pleasure Gardens, created by colourful promoter and 'little man' Shadrach Edward Robert Jones, 'as one of the excitements of an exciting time'.[79] Jones, a fellow medic, hotel owner and impresario was, in Hocken's view, 'a smart rogue & bankrupt'.[80] (He did in fact run into considerable financial trouble.) One particular event stuck in Hocken's mind:

> I remember the celebration at Vauxhall after the termination of the N.Z. Wars in 1865 at which Sir George Grey & the Maori chiefs (whom he was organizing at his best efforts to show the grandeur of the British Empire) were present. A lovely day, games, tent pegging, &c, a large tent in which was the banquet, & at every toast the chiefs filling their glasses with anything which was near & would point them to the Governor calling out 'Kawene, Kawene, Kawene'. Fine fellows they were too, but apparently without the least idea of a toast contained beyond liquor.[81]

He described, too, some of the physical changes in the city, for example at Andersons Bay:

> Nightly boats plied there & also occasionally a small steamer. The place was well lighted, there was provision for entertainment, walks out through the bush, fireworks one special feature of one being called the Siege of [Duppel]. On holidays, which were not infrequent, there was an incessant running to & fro through the day, tents, refreshments, games &c. It is impossible now to believe that all this wild & continuous excitement ever existed on what is now a quiet & unfrequented spot. But then the Australasian gold fever had not ceased & it was readily fanned into fresh flames.[82]

He also remembered the old farmhouse of Otago's religious leader, the Rev. Thomas Burns, at Grants Braes (now Waverley) – 'When I came to Dunedin this house was in ruins …' [83] – and detailed the changing (and fickle) fortunes of land speculation. Shortly after 'a great advertisement of the sale [of St Kilda sections in 1862] & a still greater champagne lunch which at first fell flat', Hocken treated George Scott, on Forbury Road, who had broken his leg. Scott, unable to pay anything for 'a long & troublesome attendance', made over a land order for some St Kilda sections instead, but these were of so little value that Hocken 'took no further trouble about them'. About 1869 Scott transferred his interest to John Reid, who put the sections on the market again. 'As there was a slight spurt – I applied to Mr Reid who generously (for I had never had any name or legal title to the sections) made over the property to me.' Then the Catholic Bishop of Dunedin, Patrick Moran, always keen to acquire real estate for church building, 'purchased sections everywhere, & amongst them mine, which fortunately adjoined. I got nearly £100 for them. Today [1894] I doubt whether I should get £25 …'[84]

This was the sort of historical minutiae that attracted Hocken, especially if such facts were in danger of disappearing or being forgotten. For example, on his copy of Redmayne's *Royal Hotel, Dunedin*, drawn in 1876 and taken from a photograph in 1858, he writes:

> The Royal Hotel, Princes St, Dunedin, now the site of the Bank of N.Z. Originally the house of Mr David Garrick who came out in the John Wickliffe in 1848. Leaving shortly he sold the section to a McDonald the first landlord for £100, afterwards sold to George Smith for £300, to W.C.Young & Ed. McGlashan for £1600 & then in 1863 to the Bank for £9000. For long it was the southernmost hotel in her Majesty's Dominions. To the right is just visible the Provincial Council Chambers where is now the Cargill monument.[85]

And finally, on William Handcock's 'very accurate' *City of Dunedin* (1864), he noted something of the artist, who was the 'first drawing master of the Boys' High School', and the changing cityscape:

> By the old cemetery is the junction of York Place, Rattray St, Arthur St & Half Way Bush Road lost under the hill. At the corners are the Robin Hood & the Salutation hotels. The Middle District School is at the top and left of Dowling St. A little below & on the right is the original Roman Catholic Church. Still lower on the right is the High School. To the left of the picture on the flat is the just erected N.Z. Exhibition, now part of the hospital. Knox Church is also seen. St. Paul's Church with its two gables marks Stewart [sic] St & the jetty below, with Bell Hill to the right.

4
Home and Garden

On 3 July 1867 Hocken married Julia Anne Dakyne Simpson at St John's Church, Waikouaiti. Sara Jones, C.F. Black and Henry Howorth, the retired coroner, were witnesses, and the Rev. Alexander Desant officiated.[1] Nothing is known of how 31-year-old Hocken and his 25-year-old wife met. According to her death certificate, she was born in Edinburgh. Her father, James Simpson, was a lace manufacturer; her mother's classification was 'not known'.[2] Julia lived in Sydney for a short period, and A.G. Hocken speculates that they may have met on the *White Star* or the SS *Great Britain*. She was certainly not on the *Chariot of Fame* when Hocken arrived in New Zealand. Tradition records that she was an alcoholic and caused Hocken much grief during their 14-year marriage, which was childless. Indeed, it is claimed that she tied up the night service bell so that it would not ring, thus forcing patients to go elsewhere. She also did not deliver messages, with the same result.[3] There is little information about her, but she was a good friend of Eliza Larnach, first wife of William Larnach. In April 1880 Eliza made one brief reference to the Hockens, suggesting that Julia may have been a similar height to her husband: 'Dunedin has become quite lively with all the weddings. Ruth Edwards married a Mr Hall, I am informed they are smaller than Dr and Mrs Hocken!'[4] When Eliza Larnach died suddenly of an apoplectic fit on 8 November 1880, it was Hocken's task to inform Larnach by telegram as the latter was on business in Melbourne. On 4 December 1880 Julia wrote a consoling letter to Eliza's son Donald, at Oxford.

> My dear Donny,
> I was at your Father's house today, and as he was writing to you, I asked him to give you my love and sympathy. He begged me to write to you myself. He is dreadfully distressed. He thought as I knew your dear Mother so well, and we were such friends, that it would please you to have a separate letter from me. Your Mother often spoke of you to me, and relied upon you and loved you very much, but I think since her return from England we have been more thrown together, and you were constantly spoken of. The day she died, she was to have dined and gone to the theatre afterwards. My maid saw her just twenty minutes before she was attacked. I tell you this to show you had you been in Dunedin you could not have seen her conscious ...[5]

Julia herself died just over a year later, on 7 December 1881, after suffering from jaundice for 10 days. She was 40 years old.[6]

Atahapara

On 28 July 1869 Hocken took out a lease on a large section of land on the corner of Moray Place and MacAndrew (now Burlington) Street. He then commissioned his friend Henry Frederick Hardy, who had a wealth of local experience, to design and build a large two-storey house.[7] It was a sensible move and may have been precipitated by what most collectors dread, a fire, even though in Hocken's case it was only a chimney fire at his Rattray Street house in May that year. For this 'minor offence' he was fined 5s.[8] A new home would help to consolidate Hocken's social and professional status, and he would be close to the centre of Dunedin's business and social activities. A larger house would also allow him space for his growing collection of books and paintings and, as an enthusiastic botanist, he would be able to have a garden and greenhouse filled with both imported and native plants. Its commanding position gave the house an attractive view down the harbour. He called it Atahapara ('time of the dawn'). Ready for occupation in June 1871, by 1875 it was described as 'brick with shop [Hocken's consulting room] adjoining house and premises, valued £110'.[9] By 1881 the house was valued at £150, and the following year the property was freehold.

Although Atahapara no longer exists, photographs and written evidence remain to tell us something of how it looked. On Moray Place a double iron gate set into a picket fence opened to a drive and a diagonal path leading up to a small verandah and the front door, which had a large bay window to its left. On the right-hand side of the house a path led to Hocken's surgery, which Fulton later described as a 'curious little glass windowed side entrance for patients'. At the back were sheds and stables; the latter, built about 1887 or 1888, housed Hocken's ponies, Tommy and Jack. Fulton also remembered 'a little greenhouse, a cherry tree, a very old pear tree with fruit in later years only to be described as stones, a karaka, a kowhai, a fine grass tree, and a cabbage tree'.[10] In 1891 Hocken proudly announced to Thomas Cheeseman, director of the Auckland Institute and Museum: 'I am growing many N.Z. plants in my garden' and 'I have a Meryta [puka] in my greenhouse – doing well. I think of planting it outside now that the Spring has come. What do you think?'[11]

A recently discovered interior plan of the house is headed 'Alterations to Residence in Moray Place Converting it into "The Soldiers' Club House"', which, by 1920, was designated as 469 Moray Place.[12] The alterations made by the Anzac Club owners were minor, involving a change to the bay window, a new door on the right side of the house and a sliding door between two rooms upstairs. The total cost was £70. Given these small alterations, it is safe to conclude that the interior structure remained much as it was in Hocken's day. The plan shows the position of the kitchen and pantry and storerooms at the back of the ground floor. At the front with the large bay window, porch and side entrance is the 'Billiard Room', which was once Hocken's consulting and surgery room. On the other front side of the hallway is the 'Reading

Room', a large room with a fireplace, which may have been a formal lounge. Next to it is the 'Library' which, given that Hocken had fixed shelves built to house his collection, was certainly retained for that purpose. The room has a double-backed fireplace. Atahapara was demolished in 1920, making way for a Returned Services Association hostel.

Surviving photographs hint at the interior. One taken by Hocken's friend, ethnologist and future Otago Museum director Augustus Hamilton, shows a partial view of an internal door. To the right is an imposing floor-to-ceiling Maori carving, and running parallel to this are three pictures of Maori, unmistakably by the artist Joseph Jenner Merrett (Hocken owned 16 of his works).[13] Another photograph taken in 1893 by Hocken's second wife shows the 57-year-old doctor sitting at a table in his library, poised to examine a botanical specimen with his microscope. At the back, striped curtains protect the books from sun and dust, and the table has a carpet covering.[14]

Mary Isabella Lee, who was the mother of Labour politician John A. Lee and employed by the Hockens as a seamstress, also noticed the carvings in Atahapara. As she noted in her journal, 'They had a lovely home – all the Door frames of drawing & Dineing rooms & The Drs Surgery & the Bannisters & Newel Posts – were all Maori Carveing & the Dr had a Small room of his own full of Maori Carveings – they are In the Museum now [the Hocken Wing].' The doctor himself she described as 'a funny little chap'.[15]

Another to report on the house was the American novelist and humourist Mark Twain, who was in Dunedin from 6 to 8 November 1895 during his world tour and was entertained by Hocken on the 6th. Twain's attention was taken by a fossilised caterpillar, which he proclaimed a 'ghastly curiosity', but he did notice other aspects of 'the residence of Dr. Hockin':

> He has a fine collection of books relating to New Zealand; and his house is a museum of Maori art and antiquities. He has pictures and prints in color of many native chiefs of the past – some of them of note in history. There is nothing of the savage in the faces; nothing could be finer than these men's features, nothing more intellectual than these faces, nothing more masculine, nothing nobler than their aspect. The aboriginals of Australia and Tasmania looked the savage, but these chiefs looked like Roman patricians. The tattooing in these portraits ought to suggest the savage, of course, but it does not. The designs are so flowing and graceful and beautiful that they are a most satisfactory decoration. It takes but fifteen minutes to get reconciled to the tattooing, and but fifteen more to perceive that it is just the thing. After that, the undecorated European face is unpleasant and ignoble.[16]

In January 1908 Anna (Annie) Trimble, second wife of bookseller William Heywood Trimble who later became the first Hocken Librarian, interviewed the doctor for the *Evening Star*.[17] This chatty piece published on

1 February offers a small glimpse of the layout of the house and Hocken's collection. Annie Trimble was shown into the large library. Instead of a conventional mantel over the fireplace, there was a large carving – the gable end of a Maori house. She spied one cabinet dedicated to some of Hocken's collection of early printed books in Maori, which included a facsimile transcription of the Auckland Institute and Museum Library's copy of Thomas Kendall's *A Korao no New Zealand* (1815) and one of Hocken's two copies of Kendall and Samuel Lee's *A Grammar and Vocabulary of the Language of New Zealand* (1820). There was shelving allocated for large folios such as Cook's navigational charts and maps. After being shown numerous treasures, which included Samuel Marsden's letters and journals, Sir William Fox's journal and Colonel Charles Stapp's journal about the expedition to Opotiki to avenge the 1865 murders of missionary Carl Sylvius Völkner and interpreter James Falloon, Trimble noted: 'the papers were all very beautifully mounted and arranged, and were bound in rich and durable bindings'. Various cupboards and 'dim recesses' held charts and plans of pa, including sketches by Charles Heaphy, one of Hocken's correspondents. The passage leading to and from this room was covered with pictures. Trimble was obviously taken with this section, as she asked if she could return at another time to view them.

Botanical Beginnings

Hocken's enthusiasm for botanical collecting was part of a long-established New Zealand tradition, which began with Captain James Cook, the irrepressible Sir Joseph Banks and Daniel Solander, a Swedish naturalist and pupil of Linnaeus. On Cook's second voyage Johann Reinhold Forster, his son Georg and Anders Sparrman, who was another pupil of Linnaeus, continued the collection of flora from the New World. One who was heavily influenced by the Forsters' work was the French explorer, Jules Dumont d'Urville, whose dedication to collecting was unflagging. As Hocken wrote, 'His name remains with us, not only attached to important surveys, but also to many of our New Zealand plants.'[18] Also important was Allan Cunningham, who worked mostly in Australia but spent two periods of some six months in New Zealand in 1827–28 and 1838, and William Colenso, who arrived in 1834 as a missionary and was prompted to continue his botanical collecting by Charles Darwin, whom he met briefly in December 1835. John Carne Bidwill began his botanising in 1839, as did explorer and naturalist Ernst Dieffenbach, who came to New Zealand as ship's surgeon on the *Tory*. Others who made botany their interest included doctor and politician David Monro, the three Hs (Ferdinand von Hochstetter, Julius von Haast and James Hector), Charles Knight, Thomas Gillies, Walter Mantell, the Rev. Richard Taylor, William Travers, George Malcolm Thomson, botanist Thomas Kirk, Cheeseman and the young Leonard Cockayne.[19] All added to the store of knowledge on New Zealand's botany, discovering, recording, sharing finds and disappointments. Hocken was part of this legacy, not only collecting in the field but also gathering the various publications that many of these men produced. He also corresponded with several of them. And although he increasingly turned to ethnography and matters historical, his enthusiasm for botany persisted.

In Trimble's *Catalogue of the Hocken Library* (1912) there are five pages dedicated to botanical books, with the last two listing publications on flax.[20] The oldest book in Hocken's collection is doctor and naturalist Pietro Andrea Mattioli's *Discorsi*, an encyclopedia of Renaissance pharmacology commenting on the work of first-century physician Pedanius Dioscorides and containing descriptions of many new medicinal plants. First published in 1554, it was exceedingly popular, and ran through a number of revised and corrected editions. Hocken's copy, printed in Venice in 1621 by Marco Ginami, is missing pages 781–816. Twenty-five late eighteenth- and early nineteenth-century publications are registered in the catalogue. They include works by the Scottish botanist Robert Brown, naturalist on Matthew Flinders's Australian expeditions and librarian to the Linnean Society; works by both Johann and Georg Forster, including *Characteres Generum Plantarum quas in initinere ad Insulas Maris Australis* (1776), *Beschreibungen der Gattungen von Pflanzen auf einer Reise Nach den Inseln der Süd-See* (1779), *Florulae Insularum Australium Prodromus* (1786) and *Dissertatio Inauguralis Botanico-Medica de Plantis Esculentis Insularum Oceani Australis* (1786); works by English botanist Sir William Jackson Hooker, including *Directions for Collecting and Preserving Plants in Foreign Countries* (1834) and *Companion to the Botanical Magazine* (1835) and *Icones Plantarum* (1837); and J.D. Hooker's *Flora Antarctica* (1847), *Flora Novae-Zelandiae* (1855) and *Florae Tasmaniae* (1860). Other nineteenth-century works include Allan Cunningham's *Florae Insularum Novae Zealandiae Precursor; or, A Specimen of the Botany of the Islands of New Zealand* (1836), Karl Alexander von Huegel's *Enumeratio Plantarum Quas in Novae Hollandiae* (1837), William Colenso's *Classification and Description of Some Newly-Discovered Ferns, Collected in the Northern Island of New Zealand in 1841–42* (1845) and *Choix de plantes de la Nouvelle Zélande* (1846) by Etienne Raoul, who was the surgeon and naturalist on the French ship *l'Aube*, sent to Akaroa in 1840. Other titles include British doctor, botanist and naturalist William Griffith's *Development of Organs in Phanoerogamous Plants* (1847), William Henry Harvey's *Phycologia Australica; or A History of Australian Seaweeds* (1858) and Mrs Stanley Jones's Auckland-printed *Handbook to the Ferns of New Zealand*, chiefly compiled from J.D. Hooker's *Flora Novae-Zealandiae* and W.J. Hooker's *Species Filicum, &c.* (1861).

The Otago Institute was central to Hocken's collecting life, especially with regard to natural history. Established under the auspices of the larger New Zealand Institute in 1869, the society had the broad objectives of encouraging art, science, literature and philosophy. Founding members of the Dunedin chapter included Justice Dudley Ward, Alfred Eccles, mathematician and scientist Arthur Beverly, and land agent and provincial councillor Robert Gillies. At the first meeting, held on 24 August in the upper room in the old Provincial Council Chambers (afterwards the Supreme Court), the first president, Justice Ward, spoke of the 'power of every man of average ability to leave behind him some "footprints on the sands of time" pointing in the onward direction' and the immediate need for 'the compilation of a complete Natural History of the colony', to which Otago could certainly contribute. And following the Baconian precept that knowledge is power, Ward continued: 'we should constantly keep in mind that there is not a rock on the mountain, a stratum of soil in the plain, a tree in the forest, or a herb in the pasture that has not its use – what that use is, it is for science and experience to discover; and every new discovery adds a new source of wealth to the colony, and a fresh incentive to immigration.'[21]

Such sentiments would have struck a chord with Hocken, but part of the address delivered by Vice-President Alfred Eccles on 2 November 1869 would have captured his full attention: 'Here will be a great and almost virgin field for the members of this Institute – to collect a really good library of works of reference, a want that is continually being felt, notwithstanding that many useful works are already found scattered amongst local libraries.'[22] Hocken needed no prompting: he had already begun collecting. Nevertheless, the institute was vital to him: as a vehicle for his burgeoning interest in early New Zealand history (some of his lectures were eventually published in the *Transactions and Proceedings of the New Zealand Institute*); as a focus for his collection and the preservation of sources of colonial history; as a social and intellectual outlet where he could compete and rub shoulders with kindred spirits; and as an opportunity to be part of a wider movement dedicated to social, scientific and historical advancements.[23]

At the first annual meeting of the institute on Monday, 11 July 1870, after a busy first year of 10 council and 10 general meetings, Hocken was appointed honorary secretary. By 1871 he was a vice-president, along with Gillies; he would later become president three times and remain on the executive board for 36 years. Initially the institute lacked a dedicated building in which to hold regular meetings, but on 16 September 1871 the botanical room at the Otago Museum was secured and then used for most of the gatherings. (In later years Atahapara was used.) The predominant subject discussed on that occasion was moa remains, resulting from James Hector's and W.D. Murison's work in the field. Two months later, Arthur T. Thomson wrote Hocken a letter detailing moa bones and remains found in a cave at the foot of the Obelisk mountains, near Alexandra.[24] This was the sort of exchange that greatly pleased Hocken, and just the kind of information that he was happy to convey to listeners. Indeed, he had initiated the correspondence with Thomson, pressing the historian, who was writing from Clyde, to become a member of the institute.

※ ※ ※

The 8 March 1870 meeting of the Otago Institute included what the *Otago Daily Times* described as a 'long discussion … on the important subject of flax culture'.[25] The growing and preparation of flax as a useful and valuable commodity was particularly important in colonial New Zealand. In his new role as honorary secretary, Hocken received publications from individuals and reciprocating institutions on a variety of subjects, including flax. Some of these works, especially the more ephemeral ones, were bound up in his pamphlet collection. Volume 20 is a prime example. Titled 'Industries', it contains numerous pamphlets about flax, from M.J.J. Donlan's *Phormium Tenax, or Neptune New-Rigged* (1833) to a first and second edition of James Hector's *Phormium Tenax as a Fibrous Plant* (1872; 1889). Other pamphlet volumes contain flax-related material, while some individual manuscript sheets, such as the convict Robert Williams's description of dressing flax and the Admiralty's tests on flax rope (April 1819), are embedded in Hocken's collection of Samuel Marsden's papers.[26]

The benefit of corresponding with like-minded individuals was self-evident. On 5 August 1870 Thomas Kirk sent Hocken a copy of F.W. Hutton's *New Zealand Flax. A Lecture on the Manufacture of New Zealand Flax* (1870) – geologist Hutton had worked as a flax-miller when he first came to New Zealand in 1866 – while the above-mentioned second edition of *Phormium Tenax as a Fibrous Plant* arrived as a presentation copy signed 'with best regards from his old friend J. Hector'. Some sources were more local. Edward McGlashan, a local runholder, merchant and fellow Mason, owned a number of flax-mills in the Otago area. In December 1866 he experimented with flax as a paper substitute. One of the sheets he produced is in Hocken's collection, given to him by the maker on 20 March 1867. A comment on it reads: 'a good specimen … for books & shows how well it takes ink'.[27]

Documentation on when and from whom a collector obtains his or her books is not often present. Occasionally, however, the book historian is thrown a morsel. From 19 October 1885, Hocken took advantage of a cheap return fare of 80s to visit the New Zealand Industrial Exhibition in Wellington.[28] During the journey he met Thomas Shearman Ralph, illustrator of the Maori language versions of *Robinson Crusoe* and *Pilgrim's Progress* and an accomplished medico, who established the Microscopical Society of Victoria.[29] On 29 December that year Ralph wrote to Hocken from Melbourne: 'When we were together on board the P & O steamer we had some talk on the subject of books; & now I am breaking up my library I shall be glad to find purchases for some portions, chiefly Botanical. I herewith send you a list.'[30] Ralph could not recall what he paid for the 24 books, but he did send some estimates. The titles on offer included Swiss botanist Augustin de Candolle's *Prodromus Systematis Regni Vegetabilis* (6 volumes only, £4), William Griffith's *Development of Organs in Phanerogamous Plants*; his *Posthumous Papers*, which contained *Icones Plantarum Asiaticarum* (1847–54); his *On the Higher Cryptogamous Plants* and

Monocotyledonous Plants (called 'rare & expensive'); Emmanuel Le Maout's *Atlas élémentaire de botanique* (1846, 5s); Robert Brown's *Prodromus Florae Novae Hollandiae* (1827) and his *Supplementum* (1830); Huegel's *Enumeratio*; botanist P.W. Watson's *Corpologie* (1825), deemed 'scarce' and which may have been his *Dendrologia Britannica*; J.D. Hooker's *Flora Antarctica* and *Flora Novae Zelandiae* (£5); an incomplete copy of Stephan Endlicher's *Genera Plantarum* (£1); a copy of *Lichenographia Universalis* (1810), a 600-page work by the Swedish 'father of lichenology' Erik Acherius (10s); C.M. Gottsche, J.B.G. Lindenberg and C.G. Nees ab Esenbeck's *Synopsis Hepaticarum* (1844, 5s); French scientist Benjamin Delessert's *Musée botanique* (1845); Swede J.G. Agardh's *Species, Genera et Ordines Algarum* (1853, 7s); W.J. Hooker's *Musci Exotici* (1818–20, 7s); Karl Müller's *Synopsis Muscorum frondosorum* (1 volume, facsimile, 5s); English botanist George Bentham's *Leguminosae* (2s 6d); *Systema Mycologicum* (1821–[32], 15s) by Elias Fries, the Swedish mycologist who first classified fungi; Acharius's *Methodus qua Omnes Detectos Lichenes* (1803, 7s), W.A. Leighton's *Angiospermus Lichens* (no doubt his *The British Species of Angiocarpous Lichens, elucidated by their Sporida* (1851, 3s 6d); and German botanist and pharmacist Adalbert Schnizlein's *Iconographia Familiarum Naturalium regni Vegetabilis* (£4 4s).

Throughout this transaction, Ralph was extremely accommodating. On planning a visit to Wellington, he not only offered to deliver the books to Hocken in Dunedin, but noted: 'If the whole number be taken I will add to these any more I have … if all are taken you had better telegram to me.'[31]

Thirteen of these titles have been identified and are now spread throughout the University of Otago system at the Hocken Library, Special Collections and Science Storage. These include titles such as Griffith's *Icones Plantarum Asiaticarum*, *On the Higher Cryptogamous Plants* and *Monocotyledonous Plants*, which were once presented to the Otago Museum by Hocken in 1900, but were subsequently transferred.[32] About two titles there is some doubt and 14 books have not been accounted for, perhaps because Hocken simply did not buy them. Whatever the reason, the purchase from Ralph highlights Hocken's continued interest in botany and provides evidence of a local supply of early botanical works.

Hocken's botanical interest remained active and undiminished throughout his life and although he was not systematic in collecting books on the topic, he used every opportunity to secure items that attracted his eye, mind and imagination.[33] In Athens during his world tour of 1901-04 he purchased a copy of Theodor von Heldreich's *Die Nutzpflanzen Griechenlands* (Athens, 1862); in Naples he acquired an Italian reprint edition of Ottaviano Targioni Tozzetti's *Dizionario botanico Italiano* (Firenzi, Guglielmo Piatti, 1825); and in Geneva during February 1903 he obtained Louis Bouvier's *Flore des Alpes, de la Suisse et de la Savoie, comprenant* (1882) and Auguste Gremli's *Flore analytique de la Suisse* (1886). Sometimes a purchase went astray. While in Switzerland, he ordered a copy of Giovanni Arcangeli's *Compendio della flora Italiana* (Turin, 1894). The bookseller posted the desired item to Athens, where it was then forwarded to Rome. A map of Switzerland, an alphabetical listing of plants in Hocken's handwriting and a postcard from T. Paleros, Athens, 12 January 1903, are tipped inside the book, which is now in his collection. The postcard reads: 'Mr Hocken: Your parcel has been lying in the Post Office, and it has been forwarded to your address today …'

Hocken also made botanical notes in his books. In his copy of Hooker's *Handbook of New Zealand Flora* (1864–67), there is a loosely tipped sheet between pages xx and xi (Fruit and Seed) headed 'Zoopsis, then Corpites' followed by Latin terms. Between pages 32 and 33 lies a pressed leaf specimen and a note in his hand that reads: 'Supposed Veronica from Longwood Range S.W. Otago Alt. 2000 ft, from P. Thomson.' (Peter Thomson was the founder of the Dunedin Naturalists' Field Club.) On pages 44 to 45 is a note dated 17 November 1894: 'Dodonote sepals 4 or 5 more or less copresent. Within them are (8 or 9) minute somethings, glands and stamens? Pistil something often frigid, semi-contorted …' John White's complete lecture edition of *Maori Customs and Superstitions* (1861) also received attention.[34]

Sometime after 14 February 1907 Hocken obtained a manuscript copy of Bishop Leonard Williams's 'Maori names of plants', which had been copied and collated by his son, the Maori language bibliographer Herbert Williams.[35] The changing nature of this document must have whetted Hocken's botanical appetite. A few years earlier, on 17 October 1904, the bishop had written:

> With regard to the Maori plant names I may tell you that I had in my hands a short time ago a list compiled by Cheeseman, who had been preparing the new Handbook which includes my list, and a good many others, – some of doubtful character. I have added my list since you copied it, but I do not know exactly where to lay my hand on the list as you saw it, so I do not know what the added names are. You are welcome to use what you got from me in any way you may wish.[36]

Hocken added to the 109-page list and made notes of a botanical nature, although wider ethnographic ones do exist. He added, for example, 'Akarewa – a variety of taro (purple)' and 'Piwai – small kumara overlooked when lifting the crop'.[37] Although seemingly insignificant these examples, taken together with others, form a larger store of botanical (and ethnographic) details. For Hocken, such notes merited his precious time and energy. He liked attending to such details and his comments stand as fine examples of his desire to set the record straight.

✳   ✳   ✳

Sometimes Hocken's botanical interests took on a more personal note. During 1874 and 1875 the Swedish botanist and explorer Sven Berggren (1837–1917) was in New Zealand on a botanising expedition to collect lichens, mosses, seaweeds and higher plants.[38] Berggren's enthusiasm for New Zealand was fuelled by William Lauder Lindsay, who had supplied him with a list of men in New Zealand who had scientific leanings. Among them was Hocken. Berggren reached Port Chalmers on 1 April 1874 and after 10 days, which included a preliminary excursion, he 'moved to Dr Hocken's'.[39] (His carte de visite is in Hocken's collection.) 'Dr Berggren,' Hocken noted, 'made my house his headquarters & during the winter we went through all the NZ. Musei. He sent home … a large collection of N Z. Algae specimens of which I have. He was a capital linguist & soon spoke Maori whilst in the North Island.' Typically, Hocken repeated part of this information elsewhere, in a note on page 46 of Berggren's *On New Zealand Hepaticæ* (1898): 'My house was Berggren's head quarters during his visit to New Zealand. A clever cryptogamic botanist. During the winter of 1874 we went through the whole of his collection of N.Z. Musei with microscope & dissections.'

While in Dunedin Berggren made several profitable excursions, attended a meeting of the Otago Institute[40] and named a liverwort after his host – *Balantiopsis Hockeni Berggr.*, as depicted in Hocken's copy of Berggren's *On New Zealand Hepaticæ* (1898).[41] After Berggren left Dunedin on 8 June 1874 the two men kept in touch. Sometime after June Hocken forwarded a letter addressed to Berggren and noted: 'Since your departure I have continued to be very busy & have had no leisure time. I have heard of you from two or three persons … I suppose you have found the locality of the Waikato to be all I described it in a colonial point of view. I shall be glad to have a few lines from you.'[42]

By December 1874 Berggren was in Auckland preparing for another North Island trip. On 5 February 1875, when near Oropi, he wrote to Hocken about his recent 'botanising trip' in the mountains (National Park) and the North (Hokianga and Bay of Islands), noting that 'as soon as my collections have been properly prepared and sent home I leave for South Otago'.[43] Berggren then added a plea for Hocken to 'collect some flowering specimens of *Viscum Lindsaye* in alcohol' and concluded: 'I hope you have made a very fine and large collection of mosses since I left Dunedin.'[44] The return to the south was wishful thinking. In April 1875 Berggren left Christchurch for Fiji, Hawaii and San Francisco, and by February 1876 he was home at Lund.

Distance did not deter contact. In 1888 Berggren sent Hocken a presentation copy of *Fresh-water Algae collected by Dr S. Berggren in New Zealand and Australia*, which had been published in Stockholm that year. Like most collectors, Hocken liked presentation copies and his collection is filled with many from a wide variety of individuals. This particular gift dealt with a subject in which he had a strong interest, and it undoubtedly conjured up pleasant memories of a shared experience.

5
A Fondness for Anything New Zealand

'There is an everlasting hope in [hero-worship] for the management of the world. Had all traditions, arrangements, creeds, societies that men ever instituted, sunk away, this would remain. The certainty of Heroes being sent us; our faculty, our necessity, to reverence Heroes when sent: it shines like a polestar through smoke-clouds, dust-clouds, and all manner of down-rushing and conflagration.' So wrote Thomas Carlyle, the influential nineteenth-century essayist.[1] Hocken had his own heroic polestars and he fortuitously discovered these collecting fields relatively early. The first was Captain James Cook, navigator and explorer; the second was the Rev. Samuel Marsden, missionary in Australia and New Zealand; and the third, Edward Gibbon Wakefield, political theorist, colonial reformer and founder of the New Zealand Company. In the first paragraph of his *Contributions* (1898), he encapsulates his field of concentration and announces his devotion to the focal points of his collection:

> The early history of the Australian Colonies is deeply interesting, and that of New Zealand especially so. The circumstances of its descry by Tasman and of its discovery by Cook, the study of its aboriginal inhabitants – foremost among the savage races of mankind – the introduction of Christianity and missionary labour by the venerated Samuel Marsden, and the story of its colonization under the scheme of that gifted man, Edward Gibbon Wakefield, form a fascinating study for the too few students, of whom the author enrols himself as one.[2]

His interest in Cook, Marsden and Wakefield was also evident in his views on the four great historical subjects worthy of depiction on canvas: 'the landing of Captain Cook at Poverty Bay, the first preaching of the Gospel at Rangihona [Rangihoua] by Samuel Marsden, the signing of the Treaty of Waitangi, and the arrival of the first immigrants at Port Nicholson [Wellington] in 1840'.[3] The Otago Institute, its parent organisation the New Zealand Institute and local newspapers became the perfect vehicles to promote his interest in these 'polestars', and the all-encompassing history, development and 'antiquities' of early New Zealand.

Stuart Strachan, former Hocken Librarian, is correct in noting that Hocken was initially interested in New Zealand's natural environment, but later turned his attention to local and national history, with its wider ethnographic implications.[4] This change was apparent in the subjects of the lectures he gave to the Otago Institute over the years. His first paper, delivered on 11 July 1870, was entitled 'Decrease in the number of whales'.[5] Because of his professional commitments – in 1869 he had been appointed the province's medical assessor and a member of the Otago Medical Board – the paper boasted little original research.[6] It was an amalgam of his conversations with a number of old whalers and information from his prime source, Walter Pearson, the Commissioner of Crown Lands. Extracting and synthesising this sort of information was a skill that Hocken would hone to perfection. Although a small beginning, the paper generated feedback from a most interesting quarter. After reading it, Frederick John Knox, who is credited with starting New Zealand's first public library in Port Nicholson in July 1840, wrote to Hocken on 25 November 1870 enclosing a note titled 'Whales and their capture'. Knox had other interesting connections. While in Edinburgh during the 1820s he was hired as an assistant to his older brother, Robert Knox, the anatomist who had purchased bodies from body-snatchers William Burke and William Hare. Hocken thought enough of Knox's note to file it away for safekeeping and made his own small annotation: 'The autograph of one who purchased bodies from the resurrectionists, & had to fly from the country in 1839 or 1840. He taught anatomy at Edinburgh.'[7]

During his years as an institute member, Hocken presented at least 20 lectures on topics relating to early New Zealand settlement history and the Maori and Polynesian peoples. As was the practice of the time, such addresses soon appeared in print in the *Otago Daily Times*, the *Otago Witness* or the *Saturday Advertiser*. As a fervent educationalist, Hocken was pleased to see them made available to a wider section of the community. Altruism apart, their appearance bolstered his reputation as a local expert on early New Zealand historical matters. Typically, he collected and compiled all these newspaper appearances and assorted articles into a large scrapbook.[8]

His first significant journey, in early 1871, took him to Auckland, Tauranga, Napier and the Hot Springs area, among other places. This last destination gave him the material for his first major talk to members of the Otago Institute: 'The hot springs of New Zealand', delivered on 28 August 1877 and printed a few days later in the *Saturday Advertiser*.[9] The 30 hand-written sheets for the lecture reveal his adventure, about which he was effusive: 'Surrounded as we are in this country of adoption by scenery of every kind & of most majestic description I yet know of none that so much excites our wonder & awe as that of the Lake District.' On tour he was thankful he met surveyor, soldier and interpreter Captain Gilbert Mair, who gave him a useful account of the district. He was less enthusiastic about others in the area: 'the remaining handful of Europeans are not of an intelligent stamp. Long residence amongst the Maories – indulgence in bad habits has utterly debased them.' After visiting Auckland, he went via steamer to Tauranga, and then inland through Horopi (Europe) and Maketu. Along the way, he noticed the 'modern' dress of Maori women: 'young girls bedecked with feathers and ribbons in their hair, and greenstone tiki around their neck, and heavy pendant earrings'.

His botanical interests were not left behind. He noticed 'a clump of half a dozen small trees called by the natives angiangi [beard lichen]. They are evidently of a great age & are twisted & grafted in a singular manner.' Then came a somewhat grisly discovery: 'the bleached fragments – but still recognisable – of human bones, many of them there of young children'. He also came across old carved lintels that were decaying. Conscious that 'much labour and art' had created these 'valuable memorials', he was keen to salvage them but local Maori would not allow this.[10]

Melding his 1871 experiences with others from a second trip to the area in 1875, he gave his listeners a good description of the surrounding mountain area of Ruapehu and Tongariro, the geysers, Ohinemutu, Rotomahana and the Pink and White Terraces, which, he prophesied, would face increased traffic and become a popular tourist enterprise like the German spas of the old world.

On that first trip of 1871 he called on the Rev. Seymour M. Spencer who lived close to Wairoa, near Lake Tarawera, and one night 'the natives favoured us with a peculiar dance of theirs called a haka & afterwards with a small war dance & certainly a more wonderful night of the kind I never saw'. The 40 or 50 men and women were led by 'the most ugly old woman I ever beheld – more dreadful than any of Macbeth's hags. It seemed as though the volcanic energies of the district had reigned them one & all … They sprang from the ground twisted right & left backwards & forwards in every direction, all keeping most accurate time …' His attitude to Maori was typical of the time:

> The Maories themselves are a most interesting people – full of fun
> & chatter – glad to see strangers & to do anything for them without
> expectation of reward – full of curiosity – free from impertinence because
> it is so child-like. And a great addition it is to have a dozen of them,
> men & women, accompanying oneself & guide to the various places of
> interest & camping out for two or three days together. They are invaluable
> paddling the canoes over the lakes carrying one through the smaller rivers
> & swamps & by night pitching the tent & seated around the camp fires
> incessantly talking in their most mellifluous of languages.

A less staccato and rather more human response is evident later, near the end of his first journey, when 10 Maori men and women, with names 'so musical' that Hocken copied them down, took him and his party down 'the lovely Tarawera' in a large canoe 'lined with fresh cut fern'. The 'fair Erenae' took Hocken 'under her special care & kindly carried me on her back whenever necessary throughout the journey & we became such excellent friends that I was promised an unlimited quantity of land if after settling affairs, I would go back & marry her'.[11]

Captain James Cook

Captain James Cook and his exploratory voyages had a powerful impact on many in the eighteenth and nineteenth centuries, and his travel accounts – full, abridged, pirated and translated – were avidly read.[12] There was also interest in other great explorers such as Vancouver, Bligh, La Pérouse, Duperrey and Dumont d'Urville; scientists such as Banks, Solander, Anderson and the Forsters; and artists such as Sydney Parkinson, William Hodges and John Webber. These men and their works also fascinated Hocken.

He delivered his first lecture, under the title 'The early history of New Zealand', on 31 August 1880, and with advance copy supplied it was printed in a supplement to the *Otago Daily Times* the following day. The so-called 'sketch' was wide-ranging in scope, and although there was more emphasis on Cook, it did allow Hocken to mention Marsden. The lecture was packed with information, as its successors would be – and it proved popular. Hocken later admitted proudly that the size of the audience necessitated a move to the basement cellar of the museum, where seats and benches were hurriedly arranged and illumination provided by kerosene lamps. He overturned an old wooden crate and stood on it so he could be seen.

He gave brief details of Cook's three voyages, noting – from the first – the reception of the visitors by the 'Indians' (Maori); the day Nicholas Young spied the southwest point of newly named 'Poverty Bay'; the teeming birdlife; the designated Maori names of the North and South Islands; Mercury Bay; 'Captain Cooker' pigs; examples of cannibalism; and the stay at Queen Charlotte's Sound, where possession of the South Island was claimed for King George III. To enhance his talk Hocken displayed a facsimile section of hydrographer Jean Rotz's map, which contained the east, west and northernmost part of Australia ('Terra Australis Incognita') sometime before 1542, and an 'excellent and faithful' copy of Captain Cook's first chart, which he had Edwin Hardy of the Survey Department draw up.[13] He also displayed a rare copper *Resolution* and *Adventure* medal borrowed from the widow of fellow Otago Institute member Peter Thomson.[14]

After talking specifically of having 'disentombed' his copy of Benjamin Franklin's proposed scheme for civilising New Zealand from his copy of Robert Dodsley's *Annual Register* of 1779, he made passing reference to Joel Samuel Polack's *New Zealand, being a Narrative of Travels* (1838) and Jean François Marie de Surville's account of Marion du Fresne's narrative in Julien Marie Crozet's *Nouveau voyage à la mer de sud* (1783), which was eventually translated by H. Ling Roth in 1891.[15] Hocken would eventually secure Roth's own copy of the translation, and it carries a cutting of the review he wrote for the *Otago Daily Times* plus a note on Abbé Alexis-Marie Rochon, the French astronomer and traveller who wrote about Madagascar.[16] The ferreting out of Franklin's work, which was originally published in 1771 as Alexander Dalrymple's *Scheme of a Voyage to Convey Conveniences of Life, Domestic Animals, Corn, Iron, etc to New*

Zealand, was something Hocken relished. And from what he quoted it is evident that by this time he already owned seminal works on Cook, including John Hawkesworth's three-volume *An Account of the Voyages Undertaken by the Order of His Present Majesty for Making Discoveries in the Southern Hemisphere* (1773), Cook's own *A Voyage Towards the South Pole and Round the World* (1777) and the third and final volume of Cook and James King's *A Voyage to the Pacific Ocean* (1784). (Hocken enthusiastically endorsed the second work: 'Well worth reading!')[17] He also owned a copy of Sydney Parkinson's *A Journal of a Voyage to the South Seas* (1773), two copies of the Parkinson reissue of 1784, Georg Forster's *A Voyage Round the World* (1777), Johann Reinhold Forster's *Observations Made During a Voyage Round the World* (1778) and the rare *A Journal of a Voyage Round the World in Her Majesty's Ship* Endeavour (1771).[18] Hocken could also point listeners to the copy of Nathaniel Dance-Holland's 1776 oil painting of Cook, which had been commissioned by James Rattray and presented to the province of Otago (and the Museum) in January 1876.[19]

Samuel Marsden

There were two main reasons why Hocken collected materials on and about the Rev. Samuel Marsden, who visited the country seven times between 1814 and 1837. He admired the man who 'introduced Christianity into New Zealand, and with it civilisation' and who planted 'the first germ of colonisation'.[20] As an important but later extension to his collecting, Hocken started writing a life of Marsden.[21]

In his August 1880 lecture Hocken praised the 'great Apostle of New Zealand', calling him 'a man of piety, strong judgment and common sense, great intrepidity, and firmness'. Yet it was Marsden's 'firmness' that tarnished his reputation, particularly in Australia, where he became known as the 'whipping parson'. Hocken acknowledged this characteristic by relating what he called 'an amusing instance' in which Marsden horsewhipped a newly married woman to cure her of supposed slackness in her wifely duties. Hocken's comment marks him out as a man of his age: 'It seems a pity that so simple and excellent a mode of dealing with refractory wives has passed out of fashion.'[22]

Hocken also collected works by and about Marsden's contemporaries and associates: men like John King, William Hall and Thomas Kendall of the Church Missionary Society (CMS). By natural extension he was also interested in the Rev. William Yate, John Gare Butler, George Clarke, William Wade, the Williams family, William Colenso and contemporary reporters such as Edward Markham.

In five later lectures on Marsden and the early New Zealand missionaries, given during 1905 and 1906, Hocken further promoted his hero whom he described fulsomely as 'this truly great and remarkable man', 'buoyant, cheerful, hopeful', 'sadly careless and inattentive to his personal appearance' and 'strongly built and of robust constitution'.[23] These talks were based on his ownership of manuscript journals of Marsden's visits to New Zealand, manuscripts by other missionaries and a much larger book collection.

> I have seized every opportunity through many years and from many sources of forming as intimate a knowledge of his [Marsden's] character as seems possible, with the result that it impresses me with profound reverence and admiration, with shame and sorrow that it should have been so aspersed, and with the desire to pay further tribute to that which was so tardily rendered, and then not until the latter years of his life, and after his death.[24]

Hocken delivered his second lecture on New Zealand's early history on 14 September 1880, and in anticipation of a larger crowd the venue was moved to the Oddfellows Hall in Albany Street.[25] This time the topics he touched on ranged from 'Missionary Work' and 'Maori Vocabulary' to 'Mr Busby appointed Resident' and the 'Ambition of Baron de Thierry'. (Charles Philippe Hippolyte de Thierry, who styled himself 'Baron', was an eccentric coloniser who attempted to establish a French colony in northern New Zealand.) In what would become a standard feature, Hocken exhibited items he owned for listeners to see and touch. They included a number of legal land documents displaying the moko and signature of local Maori – one was surely the declaration of ownership of Robucka (Ruapuke) Island, 28 March 1840, by 'John Touwaick' (Tuhawaiki, 'Bloody Jack')[26] – and a facsimile of the 1835 Declaration of the Independence of New Zealand (1877), the precursor to the 1840 Treaty of Waitangi.

Edward Gibbon Wakefield

There was a gap of four years before the third lecture was delivered. On 9 September 1884 Hocken began 'a short account of that great colonising movement', which had resulted in his listeners being the 'enviable possessors of one of the fairest countries upon earth – a Britain of the South'. This dovetailed with coloniser Edward Gibbon Wakefield's sentiments on New Zealand: 'the fittest country in the world for colonisation … the most beautiful country, with the finest climate and the most productive soil …'[27] Wakefield's name, which pervaded this New Zealand Company-oriented talk, was one that sparked contrasting reactions.[28] To some, like Justice H.S. Chapman, Wakefield was 'a man of great ability … endowed with many good qualities'; he could be unscrupulous and vindictive, but not mean.[29] To others he was an unscrupulous gold-digger, an Iago-cum-Machiavelli figure, dangerous and unpredictable.

Hocken considered Wakefield 'a man of undoubted genius, of indomitable perseverance, great foresight and resource, ready of pen and speech, and the author, amongst other works, of a new system of colonisation. No account of our early history would be complete without a reference to him.'[30] There was also the fact that the Wakefield clan and its associates stretched across those collecting fields that so interested Hocken. His net drew in the New Zealand Company; the *Colonial Gazette*, the *New Zealand Journal* and the *New Zealand Gazette*, which promoted it; the infant settlements of Wellington, Nelson, New Plymouth (Plymouth Company), Canterbury and Otago; the 'colonial reformers' such as Charles Buller, *Spectator* editor Robert Rintoul, and Charles Torlesse, Wakefield's nephew; premier and poet Alfred Domett; premier and artist William Fox; John Robert Godley, the 'founder of Canterbury'; and others such as Otago pioneer William Cargill.

Although Hocken did not formulate specific lectures on Wakefield himself, many of his articles and talks spoke of the spirit of

> this most clever and versatile man. Though his character has been aspersed, his honesty of purpose denied, and his great theory as to the 'sufficient price' for land derided, all who are acquainted with his writings recognise the charm of his language, the breadth and logic of his views on all matters connected with colonization, and can well believe the story of a fascination which, like a magnet or a spell laid all under his influence, and converted many into warm disciples of his doctrine.[31]

Hocken was not a snobbish collector. He was quite prepared to own copies or facsimiles of valuable originals. This content-based attitude is reflected in the items he brought along on the night of that third lecture. He displayed Edward Chaffers's chart of Port Nicholson, the first lithographic work undertaken in New Zealand, by Thomas Bluett in 1841, and the only known copy; the inaugural issue of the *New Zealand Gazette* (18 April 1840), the colony's first newspaper, edited by Samuel Revans; the first volume of the *New Zealand Journal*, edited by H.S. Chapman; various facsimiles, including the 1835 Declaration (again), and the Treaty of Waitangi; and early views of Kororareka (Russell).[32] He acknowledged Justice Chapman as a prime source of Wakefield material.

'A larger than usual' audience listened to Hocken's fourth lecture on 22 September 1885.[33] Its scope was the early history of Akaroa, New Plymouth and Nelson, and again he enlivened the talk with illustrative prints, including a lithograph by Thomas Allom of George Duppa's 'Part of the New Plymouth Settlement in the District of Taranaki' (February 1841) and Charles Heaphy's sketch of Port Nicholson (1841); a number of old New Zealand newspapers, including Henry Falwasser's *Auckland Times*; and his 'rare' Parisian copy of Raoul's *Choix de plantes de la Nouvelle-Zélande*.[34] And he sprinkled the talk with lighter moments: while visiting Nelson he had called it a 'sleepy hollow' and suggested to a friend living there that 'an infusion of some of our Otago energy' would be great for the town. His friend had replied: 'Ah, if you lived here for six months you would become as lazy as any of us.' Hocken commented dryly: 'and no doubt he was right'. Ending his talk with the settlement of 'Kororareka in flames', he offered an apology: 'I had intended to bring this lecture down to a much later date, but find the task of compression difficult. I do not wish to mutilate by excessive curtailment the narration of that war [the Northern], whose incidents are so various and interesting. With it I hope to commence my next lecture.'[35]

This, the fifth, was delivered a year later on 7 September 1886. The content outline of his posthumous *Early History* (1914) conveys the scope of this talk: 'Trouble between the Races – Heke's War – Troops from New South Wales – Enrolment of Militia – Capture of Pomare – Maori War-dance – The Okaihau Fight'. Again he used teaching aids, including George Thomas Clayton's 'Kororareka in the Bay of Islands', sketched on 10 March 1845 from the deck of a vessel before the town was destroyed; Joseph Jenner Merrett's 1846 pictures of Heke, his wife Harriett and Kawiti; maps of routes taken by soldiers to the scene of the war; and a manuscript 'Plan of Kawiti's Pa at Ruapekapeka' drawn by J.G. Nops and Midshipman Groves of the HMS *Racehorse* (1846).[36] Hocken had a strong sense of the dramatic, as was clear in his description of a haka he had seen during his trip north in 1871:

> Imagine a couple of hundred stalwart tattooed savages, six or eight abreast, clad in the *tatua* or war-girdle only, and holding some weapon aloft in their right hands. At a special signal given by a chief or perhaps by some ugly old woman more horrible in aspect than Fury, the whole party with one loud yell dashes forward for a few yards as one man, and with inconceivable speed …[37]

Hocken gave the concluding lecture in the series on 28 September 1886. The Northern War narrative ended with the appointment of Governor Sir George Grey and the fall of Ruapekapeka Pa. By now his listeners would have been accustomed to his format – lively historical matters illuminated by various objects. On this occasion he showed Lieutenant Wilmot's sketch of Ohaeawai Pa and two watercolour sketches by Sergeant John Williams depicting Ohaeawai and Pomare's pa in the north.[38]

All these lectures were written for a popular audience, designed to enthuse listeners and arouse interest. And from the very first Hocken was keen to explain why he embarked on them. He had often, he said, 'been surprised that so many intelligent and educated persons should be comparatively ignorant of the history of their adopted country – a country of surpassing interest to so many sections of cultivated men', whether they were geologists, zoologists, ethnologists, politicians or sociologists, 'and a large section of the British race, freed from the trammels and traditions of their former home, grappling under quite new conditions with social questions always and everywhere of the first importance to the success of the race'. To Hocken, 'these studies have ever had a great charm, and if I can but succeed in interesting you in them, and so in leading you to study them for yourselves, my object is gained, and

I am well repaid'.[39] His second lecture was full of sentiment (as collecting is) and a nostalgia for a recent past. It explained much about why Hocken was involved in collecting – to keep the records of human activity as a bulwark against erosion, disappearance, loss, the ravages of time. This was not a new thought. Back in 1871 while visiting Tauranga he had recorded an inscription carved on a decayed wooden slab at the head of the grave of a missionary's young wife who had died in 1834: 'I shall soon be with Him beyond that Star.' The fact that the slab had disappeared when Hocken visited in 1875 made the recollection more poignant. After describing the sad sights of abandoned mission stations – 'the bygone past of old New Zealand' – he explained that such scenes were 'the antiquities of New Zealand … Surely people unthinkingly say that New Zealand is too new a country, that it has as yet little or no historical interest and no antiquities. To my mind associations make antiquities, rather than great lapse of time.'

> When treading the steps that Captain Cook and Samuel Marsden and these old missionaries trod, I can readily see what they saw, hear what they said, and look upon the life that was around them. But the old abbey does not so readily recall to me the procession of cowl-clad monks whose solemn chants once filled their aisles. Perhaps I cannot see far enough through its stone walls: a prejudiced fondness for anything New Zealand may partly blind me; or perhaps, after all, my swans may be but little better than geese.[40]

The Southern Lectures

On 9 August 1887, less than a year after completing his first set of lectures, Hocken began another series on the history of Otago and Southland settlement. This was where his role of local antiquarian and annalist was truly defined. Portraits of early settlers such as George Rennie, Captain William Cargill and the Rev. Thomas Burns helped to contextualise the talk he gave at the Choral Hall.[41] He also displayed old 'favourites', such as the sketches by Sergeant Williams and by Nops and Groves and the map of New Zealand of 1841. Although some of the audience were more than likely early settlers who had experienced much of what he was describing, Hocken, typically confident and cocksure, maintained that 'much of the information to be presented to you this evening is quite new, and has been gathered from various sources …' He also suggested 'that whilst the facts of history should be written as they run, it may not be possible to accord them a just interpretation until long afterwards'. Even though he erred at times, he was a zealous promoter of New Zealand's early history, ever willing to put his adopted homeland 'in the broad sunshine'.[42] It is this role that has determined his importance as a collector in this country.

He gave the second 'Southern' lecture just over a month later on 15 September 1887. As usual, it was packed full of historical data. Part of the charm of Hocken's work was that he not only tied the various strands together to make one coherent narrative, but also grounded his story in accounts written by the early settlers and explorers. By then he possessed many such accounts, including Cook's voyages, Captain William Mein Smith's report to Colonel William Wakefield, John Wallis Barnicoat's journal (1843–44) and David Monro's *Selection of Site of Otago Settlement* (1844). He also asked his audience to follow the footsteps of Edward Shortland who, in September 1843, had journeyed south from Akaroa as interpreter at courts of inquiry into Maori land claims, traversing 'paths now well known to us but then surrounded by difficulty and adventure'.[43] Hocken then mentioned Frederick Tuckett, principal civil engineer and surveyor in Nelson for the New Zealand Company, who was mainly responsible for selecting the Otago block for the Scottish settlement of 'New Edinburgh' (Dunedin). Fortuitously, he was able to display one of his recently received 'treasures', an exact replica of a 'highly tattered, but none the less valuable explanatory map' drawn by Tuckett showing the site, which he had received from Samuel Hodgkinson in November 1886.[44] Another teaching aid held aloft was a portrait of missionary Johann Wohlers, who travelled with Tuckett on the *Deborah*; the painting was given to Hocken by Wohlers' widow. After dealing with Tuhawaiki's role in signing a deed of conveyance, and detailing the area of the Otago Block (400,000 acres or almost 162,000 ha) with the sum paid (£2400), Hocken finished his lecture, ending, as he always did, by saying: 'It but remains again to thank you for your patience and courteous attention.'[45]

He delivered his final six lectures to institute members over an eight-year period: on 14 August and 9 October 1888, 9 September 1891, 13 September 1892, 10 October 1893 and 3 September 1896. They covered everything from the formation of the Free Church Scheme in Glasgow and the arrival of the Otago immigrant ships *John Wickliffe* and *Philip Laing* to the French colonisation of Akaroa, the settlement of Canterbury, the troubled times for the New Zealand Company and much more. These talks would have been printed in the local newspapers as usual had they not been 'appropriated & printed in more than one North Island newspaper without any reference or acknowledgement'. Hocken took umbrage and wrote in his scrapbook at the end of the printed copy of his second Southern lecture: 'I therefore refused to allow the later ones to be printed & simply read them before the Otago Institute.'[46] Those not in the audience had to wait until the lectures were published in his *Contributions* (1898) and consolidated somewhat in the posthumous *Early History* (1914).

The Transactions

Hocken gave other talks, seven of which, to his satisfaction, were printed in the *Transactions* of the New Zealand Institute.[47] The first was 'Notes on the derelict ship in Facile Harbour, Dusky Sound', which he read before members of the Otago Institute on 14 June 1887, two months before beginning his 'Southern' series. It dealt with the notion that the hulk was Captain Cook's *Endeavour*, and was based on 'a few notes, the result of inquiries from many trustworthy people and further research'.[48] His informants included the reclusive William Docherty, who believed the wreck was the *Endeavour*; Ned Palmer, an old West Coast sealer who knew of the vessel; Captain Stevens of Riverton; Richard Henry of Resolution Island; Sir James Hector, who had seen the relic in 1863; Edward Ellis Morris, a Melbourne-based correspondent; and Captain John Fairchild, commander of the SS *Hinemoa*, who was keen to raise the hulk.[49] Hocken had visited the 'mysterious vessel' himself in 1877 and had attempted to verify its identity in London in 1882, without success. He finally made up his mind on the matter: 'I think there can now be no doubt that the enigma is satisfactorily solved, and that this derelict ship of Facile Harbour is none other than the *Endeavour* which was bound from Port Jackson to India — and that here has she lain for the last 93 years.'[50] In this he did not have the advantage of modern scholarship; one claim is that it was another *Endeavour*, commanded by William Bampton and abandoned there in 1795.[51]

Hocken had to wait seven years before his next address, 'Some account of the earliest literature and maps relating to New Zealand', appeared in the *Transactions*.[52] Read on 11 September 1894, this work was based on those voyage materials he owned including works by Alexander Dalrymple, James Burney and early Hakluyt publications. The Dutch documented the first authentic accounts relating to Australia and New Zealand, with seafarer and explorer Abel Tasman playing a prime role. Like many other collectors who pride themselves on owning works others do not have, Hocken crowed over his copy of Jacob Swart's edition of Tasman's journal, *Journaal van de Reis naar het Onbekende Zuidland, in den Jare 1642* (1860), which represented its first appearance in its entirety: 'The book is but little known apparently beyond Holland.'[53] Hocken impressed upon his listeners the collation work that he had undertaken with the *Journaal* and other narratives in Dalrymple and Burney. He then hinted at what was to come: 'Tasman's journal ... has not yet been put in English dress; but, with the assistance of a valued coadjutor, I can promise that the Institute shall soon have presented to it the first full English translation of Tasman's discoveries of Tasmania and New Zealand.'[54] This was a significant announcement and the project did see the light of day in 1895. After giving details on works by Hawkesworth, Cook and Parkinson, and showing off his Rotz map again, he mentioned the *Travels of Hildebrand Bowman* (1778), a book written in the manner and style of Swift's *Gulliver's Travels*, with satirical swipes at Cook, Banks and Solander. Often attributed to Dalrymple, *Travels* was, and is, a rare book and Hocken must have been pleased to secure it.

Six years later, on 11 September 1900, Hocken read 'Some account of the beginnings of literature in New Zealand: Part I, the Maori section', which was the result of his efforts that 'for some time he had been engaged in collecting and cataloguing'.[55] First mention went to the early CMS missionaries, many of whom were expert in the Maori language. Although not fluent in Maori himself, Hocken did have an understanding of phonetics and philological nuances, and maintained that he rehearsed the pronunciation of certain Maori words so as not to forget them. Tamati Parata, chief at Puketeraki, was one who aided his language acquisition; another was Robert Maunsell, from whom Hocken had the good fortune to learn 'the true sounding' of words when travelling in the Bay of Islands in 1880.[56] His rudimentary understanding of the language aided his documentation of the details of the development of Maori language publications. This paper was one of the first in the field.

In July 1901 Hocken delivered to institute members the second part of 'Some account of the beginnings of literature in New Zealand', which considered what he called 'the English newspapers'.[57] (A number of Maori language newspapers were published in New Zealand from the 1840s.) As usual, he laid out examples he had collected, which in some instances were old favourites such as Henry Falwasser's mangle-produced *Auckland Times*. Coverage was by locality, and he began with Revans' *New Zealand Gazette*. The last was the *Nelson Examiner and New Zealand Chronicle*, with Charles and James Elliott, George Rycroft Richardson and Alfred Domett involved in its production. Other printer-newspapermen on his list included Richard Davies Hanson, founder of the *New Zealand Colonist and Port Nicholson Advertiser*; the Rev. Barzillai Quaife, who started two newspapers in Northland; and Samuel McDonald Martin, editor of the *New Zealand Herald and Auckland Gazette* and later the *Southern Cross*. Always keen to demonstrate his efforts in salvaging, especially to complete a collection, Hocken told listeners of his attempt to secure the remains of the Columbia press that Revans had first used. He also revealed a number of print process tit-bits. For example, politician and naturalist Walter Mantell had carved woodcut blocks from a maire tree to create illustrations in the *Wellington Independent*, and the heavy ink required to print them gave the paper a 'smudgy appearance'. Some issues of the *New Zealand Spectator and Cook's Strait Guardian* were printed on red blotting paper (one was proudly displayed); the editor of the *Nelson Examiner* had once asked locals for treacle to assist the printing process.[58]

Hocken's last article to appear in the *Transactions*, in Volume 40, was given on 10 September 1907. 'Early visits of the French to New Zealand' acknowledged French contributions to the scientific knowledge of New Zealand: Hocken placed them ahead of Cook and Banks. In a rather pedestrian manner, he listed the major French visitors to New Zealand, beginning with Surville. He also covered the mystery surrounding the killing of Marion du Fresne and several of his men by Maori in 1772 and decided on the reason: 'in the present instant at least, no other explanation is required beyond that of the perfidy and rapacity which are such eminently marked traits of savage character.'[59] Hocken then focused on Dumont d'Urville, who visited New Zealand three times, in 1824, 1826–27 and 1840, when he ventured south in the *Astrolabe* and sailed inside the Otago Heads. As might be expected, Hocken owned *Voyage de la corvette l'*Astrolabe (1830), the multi-volume publication resulting from Dumont d'Urville's second journey. His copy of this 'magnificent work', as he termed it, contains the book label of Armand Joseph de Sibeud de Saint-Ferriol (1814–1877), whose travel books were sold in Grenoble in December 1881. Hocken probably acquired it while travelling in England or Europe between 1902 and 1903.[60]

Hocken then delivered brief details on Captain Jean-Baptiste Cécille's visit on *Héroïne* in April 1838, the arrival of Bishop Jean Baptiste Pompallier and the ensuing struggle for dominion over New Zealand. He finished with the French–British tug-of-war for Akaroa. Always keen to end on a positive note, he claimed there was now but one rivalry between the two great nations: 'that of best helping forward whatever advances the progress of humanity and knowledge'.

Hocken was not a connoisseur collector. He was more concerned with the content of a book, squeezing out the best and most interesting facts and figures for his talks and publications. He did, however, appreciate good quality. His copy of Cyrille Laplace's multi-volume *Voyage autour du monde par les mers de l'Inde et de Chine* (1833), which offers a description of the explorer's brief visit to the Bay of Islands in 1831, afforded him the chance not only to praise French publishing – these volumes were 'issued by the French Government in the same magnificent style of type and illustration' – but also to honour France herself, who stood 'in the foremost rank of cultivated nations' and demonstrated 'her splendid recognition and aid of scientific labour'.[61]

A Growing Authority

Through his lectures Hocken gradually became known as a good source of information on New Zealand history. Well-informed answers teased out of his increasing collection confirmed him as an authority. In August 1887, for example, printer and newspaperman William Craig of Invercargill wrote to the *Otago Daily Times* about Hocken's lecture on the early settlement of Otago: 'Those who have made New Zealand their adopted home should feel indebted to the doctor for the painstaking manner in which he is making us acquainted with its early history in an "intelligent, unbiased, and masterly manner".'[62] The next day the newspaper's editorial praised 'the exceedingly useful nature of Dr Hocken's investigations into the early history of New Zealand. Indeed, we question whether it would be possible to exaggerate the enthusiastic patriotism and untiring industry shown by the doctor in this matter, or to over-estimate the peculiar importance of his work.' He possessed 'the true historical instinct for research, combined with an agreeable manner of placing his materials before us'. Hocken would surely have agreed regarding the 'romantic element of early colonial life': 'At anyrate [sic] the appreciation of our country's oneness and continuity, and a lively interest in the details of its foundation and youth, are sentiments which should assuredly be cultivated ...'.[63] In November that year the gossip columnist of the *New Zealand Herald* bemoaned the lack of a 'good history of New Zealand' and suggested Hocken for the job, one 'who has devoted time, attention, and care to amassing knowledge on the subject, and he has all the necessary enthusiasm'.[64]

Hocken's industry in marshalling and disseminating the facts about historical New Zealand also won him kudos closer to home. William Martin, one of the first immigrants to Otago on the *Philip Laing*, attended Hocken's lecture on 9 October 1888. Pleased with what he heard, he moved a 'hearty vote of thanks', which was carried by acclamation.[65]

6
Cultivating Contacts

As a result of his keen interest in New Zealand history, Hocken made and cultivated contacts with key individuals throughout the country, many of whom had either lived through their own early settler experiences or were related to someone who had. With his social skills, his genuine regard for salvaging materials from a recent past and his outgoing personality, Hocken won over settlers, missionaries, surveyors and the like. Some were kindred spirits, ready and willing to help find ephemeral documents; many clarified historical details for him; others supplied him with books and manuscripts. They also formed additional lines of communication, leading to others who were also happy to assist. As one dedicated to 'treading the steps' that others had walked, Hocken also travelled widely, and his excursions are of immense importance in understanding him as a collector.[1] They satisfied his strong desire to 'touch recent history' and each connection afforded new information, albeit small or large, which he slowly amassed, recorded and kept. As we have seen, Hocken's first major New Zealand trip took place in 1871, but he was on the road again in 1875 and in 1879. (This last journey is covered in more detail below.) These domestic pilgrimages offer good evidence of his movements, the people he met and what, if anything, he obtained from them, be it manuscripts, books or historical gossip.

Bishop Henry Harper

On 15 May 1867, two months before his wedding day, Hocken received a letter written on 18 February that year by Henry John Chitty Harper, the first Anglican bishop of Christchurch, to Henry Selfe Selfe, legal adviser to the Canterbury Association chairman, Lord Lyttelton, and an active member himself. The letter recounted Harper's experiences as a traveller to the West Coast and the southern part of the South Island. More specifically it contained remarks on Hokitika, which he had visited in 1865, and the goldfields.[2] There is no evidence of when Harper first made contact with Hocken, but as the bishop's diocese then included Otago and Southland, it was certainly through the church. Harper obviously registered his fellow Anglican's keen interest in early New Zealand history and sent him the manuscript. Although small, it represented another first for Hocken's collection. In fact he placed it in the leading position in his compilation, '21 Important Letters, 1876–96'.[3] He also acquired a few of Harper's publications, including *Alms-giving: A sermon* (1858) and *Report of the Education Commissioners* [1864]. Hocken also obtained a copy of *Literary Foundlings* (1864), a small verse and prose publication compiled by the Rev. George Cotterill to raise funds for the Christchurch Orphan Asylum. Hocken identified many of the contributors, including Harper's own 'A Ketch' and Samuel Butler's 'A note on "The Tempest"'.⁴ Harper was a frequent and energetic traveller around New Zealand and may have served as a model for Hocken's own journeying.⁵

The Williams Family

In 1870 the Right Rev. William Williams, Bishop of Waiapu and author of *A Dictionary of the New Zealand Language* (1844), sent Hocken a copy of the Old Testament *Hexateuch* (1848). The following year he dispatched a copy of the fourth edition of the New Testament in Maori (1844) ⁶ Both were inscribed 'Dr Hockin'. An annotation by Hocken in a presentation copy of *The Murder of the Rev. C.S. Volkner* (1865) confirms an actual meeting with Williams and reveals that the church was but one link between the two men: '*W. Waiapu* was the first Bishop (of Napier afterwards). William Williams, *a dear old man* whom I learnt to know well during his prolonged stay with me .. '⁷ Williams had completed an apprenticeship as a surgeon in Nottinghamshire and they surely would have compared notes on their respective training. Philology may also have been discussed, especially the complexities surrounding the Maori language. In this, Williams was the right man. According to his brother, the Rev. Henry Williams, he was particularly fluent in Maori: 'He ... appears not to learn it; but it seems to flow naturally from him.'⁸

And items flowed gently to Hocken. In 1874 Williams sent a copy of the first complete Maori Bible (1868), which contains a note of origin: 'From Paihia Sunday School, Bay of Islands, April 1874'.⁹ This was one of two copies that Hocken would own. He also received a defective copy of *Three Letters* (1845), which contained Williams's defence of the missionaries from charges laid by the New Zealand Company. Hocken completed his copy by writing out the title page and imprint details. He also received a copy of *Remarks upon 'Ecce Homo'* (1867), which once belonged to the missionary John Hobbs, acquired a letter by Williams of 6 January 1835 to the Rev. William Jowett, clerical secretary of the CMS in London, and copied another letter Williams had received from the Rev. Richard Hill of Sydney dated 31 January 1835.¹⁰ Such copying was a sound strategy, especially if there was no likelihood of ever owning the original. It was also a sure-fire method of enhancing his collection; trust was implicit in each transaction.

Hocken was fortunate to forge a connection with the Williams family, who played such a major role in the establishment of the Anglican church in New Zealand. Although he had no direct contact with Henry Williams, he managed to secure and copy correspondence between him and New Zealand's first bishop, George Augustus Selwyn, and a letter from Henry's wife Marianne to their son Samuel.¹¹ His botanical interest was piqued by Henry Williams's 26 August 1836 letter to Dandeson Coates of the CMS in London, which contained manuscript excerpts on plants, especially the pittosporum.¹² Henry's third son – another Henry (1823–1904) – played his part by sending

Hocken copies of the Rev. Octavius Hadfield's pamphlet, *The Second Year of One of England's Little Wars* (1861), which appealed to the colonial secretary for justice concerning Maori land rights, and Auckland politician Walter Brodie's *New Zealand and the Constitution Act* (1861).[13]

Both William Williams's son Leonard and his grandson Herbert, who was also a fine Maori scholar, became bishops of Waiapu and frequently corresponded with Hocken. In June 1891 Hocken received a caustic letter from Leonard Williams, who severely criticised Edward Tregear's recently published *Maori-Polynesian Comparative Dictionary* (1891).[14] Hocken knew Tregear and worked with him on the Anthropology Section and the committee on 'Polynesian Bibliography, with special reference to Philology' under the auspices of the Australasian Association for the Advancement of Science (AAAS).[15] Hocken owned 24 works by Tregear, including three copies of his *Paumotuan Dictionary* (1893), one of which was a presentation copy dated June 1899. He was probably aware of the praise heaped on Tregear, especially by such eminent men as politicians Grey, John Ballance and Robert Stout, and ornithologist Walter Lawry Buller. In his copy of A.S. Atkinson's 'Notes on the Maori-Polynesian comparative dictionary of Mr E. Tregear' (1893), Hocken wrote: 'A biting criticism on Tregear's book & very valuable besides philologically', and repeated the sentiment in his *Bibliography* (1909): 'A severe, cynical, and accomplished criticism.'[16]

In 1893, Leonard Williams's letter reminding Hocken of lesser known missionary journeys throughout New Zealand reveals the interconnectedness made possible by increased and regular mail services. Williams wrote: 'Mr H.T. Kemp wrote to me a week or two ago to enquire about Mr Stewart who died at Poverty Bay. I gathered from what he said that you had perhaps applied to him for information on the subject. He was a friend of J.W. Harris, a prominent Poverty Bay landholder.[17] A year later, Williams sent Hocken two 'literary antiquities': Robert Maunsell's *Hints on Schools Amongst the Aborigines in Five Letters to the Lord Bishop of New Zealand* (1849) and a first edition of the Maori version of the service for the ordination of priests (c. 1860).[18] Williams also used the occasion to augment his own book collection. He recalled having seen copies of Sir William Martin's *A Series of Documents on the Proposed Church Constitution in the Colonies* (1854) in Hocken's own collection during a visit to Dunedin. In his May 1894 letter he asked, 'Do you happen to have a spare copy of No. 5?' and made an additional plea for a replacement copy of a pamphlet about the consecration of Bishop John Coleridge Patteson, which he had lost.[19] In return Williams supplied copies of synod reports when Hocken requested them in August 1894.[20]

Williams continued to filter books and pamphlets through to Hocken. In 1907 he sent two editions of the Church of England Hymns (c. 1860), a New Zealand Church *Almanac* (1845), his own *First Lessons in the Maori Language* (1862) and an item that Williams 'did not notice in your collection': *Te*

Tangata i Mate Ai Ona Hoa Noho Tata (1873), which contained translations by Colenso's wife, Elizabeth, of two moral stories called 'The man who killed his friends with kindness' and 'The lesson of the quilt'.[21] He later gave Hocken a copy of *He Kupu Whakamarama*, Nos 5, 6 and 9 (1898), a monthly Anglican newspaper translated as 'Words of Enlightenment', edited by the Rev. F.A. Bennett and published in Nelson.[22]

Hocken owned a copy of Hugh Carleton's two-volume *The Life of Henry Williams* (1874), a work he termed 'a valuable history of north New Zealand from 1822 ... until 1867'.[23] Numerous annotations and Hocken's ever-present cross-referencing reveal close reading and knowledge of events surrounding the Williams family. In the first volume, for example, Hocken added 11 February as Williams's birth date (page 12), and in reference to 'Takirau' in a footnote (page 23), he added: 'A mistake Tokerau is correct. This means smooth in contradistinction to the roughness of the west coast. So C.O. Davis tells me.' As was typical, Hocken added his initials 'T.M.H.' after many of the notes.

Charles Oliver Bond Davis

In late 1875 Hocken travelled north towards Tauranga and Taupo. While in Taupo, he met Charles Oliver Bond Davis, an important acquaintance especially in the field of Maori language and custom. Sydney-born Davis, who was a proficient Maori speaker, 'assisted in the meetings at Hokianga at which the Treaty of Waitangi was debated and signed'. He then became an interpreter and clerk to the office of the Protectorate of Aborigines and worked in the Native Secretary's Department. In 1855 he compiled *The Renowned Chief of Kawiti* and *Maori Mementos*, a translation of Maori songs and addresses to Grey. He was also instrumental in producing *Te Karere Maori* (*The Maori Messenger*), the official Maori newspaper. During the 1860s he fell 'out of official favour' and became a controversial figure. In 1873 he took a job as a land purchase agent, based in the Bay of Plenty and Taupo regions. By the time Hocken met him, Davis was living in Auckland and increasingly involved in the temperance movement.[24]

The first meeting between the two men clearly went well. When Hocken suggested a trip in 1876 Davis was not up to travelling, but was 'very glad to serve you and render all the help I can in your meditated tour'. Davis did offer to meet Hocken at Taupo, however, 'when you could determine as to further movements'. The older man was apologetic: 'Do not imagine that I feel indifferent as to your wishes. I very highly desire to aid you and add to your pleasure but when ill health breaks in upon us, we can hardly arrange matters with any degree of certainty.'[25] Instead, Hocken travelled locally in 1876 across to the west coast of the South Island, visiting Martins Bay, Lake McKerrow, Lake Alabaster, the Hollyford River, the Dart River and Lake Wakatipu. In his copy of R.P. Whitworth's *Martin's Bay Settlement West Coast of Otago* (1870), which was obviously a useful guidebook, he tipped in a hand-coloured map scaled to 2 inches to a mile. His note reads: 'Kindly drawn for me by the Survey Dept at Dunedin & showing my track when visiting the Lake in 1876.'[26]

On 28 October that year Davis sent his *Life and Times of Patuone* (1876) to Hocken for review in the Dunedin papers. He was despondent about its production – 'I think it would have been far better if I had arranged to have the work bound in boards' – and he did not want it to be at the total mercy of the Auckland reviewers, whom he called 'showy hurters'.[27] His cynicism was firmly entrenched. As Hocken noted in his copy of Davis's *The Renowned Chief of Kawiti*, 'Mr C.O. Davis tells me that though it was his intention to publish other parts relating to N.Z. warriors he abandoned it owing to various causes – one being the scanty sale of this part.'[28] Hocken also gave him medical advice. In this same letter, Davis wrote: 'I am glad to inform you that I am stronger ... Your medicines I still keep by me & take them when I feel the need & derive much benefit therefrom ...'[29] In December 1885 after Hocken had visited Davis in Auckland, he wrote: 'I cannot tell you how grateful I feel for your marked kindness since taking the medicines you were good enough to order for my health has much improved.' He continued: 'It is impossible for me to repay you, but I know that the blessed Lord we serve will abundantly shower upon you His benedictions.'[30] During that Auckland trip Hocken joined Davis on a historical jaunt which, Davis promised, 'will afford you much pleasure & some interesting matter for your lectures'.[31] While travelling north in 1879, Hocken acquired a copy of the 'Seal of the Maori King Potatau'. This fragile relic contains a note by Hocken that acknowledges input from Davis:

> One of the outcomes of the Maori King movement in the Waikato, about 1860, was the desire to have an official seal. The original Maori design was primitive and was drawn by a Maori hand for the engraver (Leach, I think of Shortland Street). The crest represents some bird (perhaps the Hokioi) and the sun. The central part the Maori flag, and below is a canoe &c. The finished seal however does not quite follow the native design, but is an artist's version of it (probably suggested by C.O. Davis). The bird is the kotuku, the tree probably a Puriri, the fish indicates whale industry.[32]

In 1886 Hocken saw Davis again. Although ill and nearly blind, Davis – described by a contemporary as 'a diminutive man of mummified appearance with a thin squeaky voice, destitute of one atom of personal charm' – made the journey south to Dunedin.[33] His reputation preceded him. A notice in the *Otago Witness* on 6 February announced the visit of 'the well-known Maori scholar' and that he would be a guest of Hocken. William Mason, the first mayor of Dunedin, wrote enthusiastically to Hocken from Queenstown: 'Mr Richards from Sydney who is the bearer of this note wishes an interview with C.B. Davis of Auckland who I learn is paying you a visit ... You have struck a *patch* as a gold digger would say.'[34]

Perhaps it was on this occasion that Hocken acquired more of Davis's publications, including *A Maori Phrase Book* [1863], *Temperance Songs in the Maori Language* (1873), a third edition of *Maori Lesson Book* (1874), *Te Honae* (1885) and works such as 'Maori names', 'Maori etiquette' (1882), 'Notes relating to the description of tikis, use and customs' and 'On the Maori word for the immortal principle in man' (1885).[35] Hocken had the first three bound together with an item by Leonard Williams under the pamphlet title 'Lessons in Maori'. In September 1886, in one of Davis's last letters south before his death in 1887, he painted an admirable interior scene of the Otago Museum: 'I am glad to hear that your Museum has been so nicely arranged – the Maori mats suspended from the ceiling & the other Maori carvings arranged around the walls, & those curious & valuable heirlooms of the Maoris, the heitikis & kurus, have been placed in a glass case.'[36]

Although their meetings were infrequent, Hocken regarded the older man as an authority, especially in matters Maori. At one stage they talked about tattooing, the catalyst perhaps being Arthur Thomson's 'On the peculiarities in figure, the disfigurations, and the customs of the New Zealanders', an article published in three issues of the *British-Foreign Medico-Chirurgical Review & Quarterly Journal*, No. 26 (April 1854, October 1854 and April 1855), which Hocken had acquired. As was typical, Hocken annotated his copy, adding various names for the moko on the face and referring to Davis's opinion, especially on Thomson's use and definition of 'Whakairo': 'C.O. Davis says this is a mistake. Whakairo referring to the carving on wood. Ta (to strike or tap) is the generic word for tattoo On other parts of the body than the face there are various names for the tattoo – puhoro.'[37] Hocken revisited this field of interest in later correspondence with General Horatio Robley.

Walter Baldock Durrant Mantell

Back in 1865 Hocken had organised a display of moa bones for the New Zealand Exhibition. One person who may have recognised his effort in this was politician and public servant Walter Baldock Durrant Mantell, known for his work in the late 1840s in purchasing Maori land and apportioning reserves to disenfranchised Maori. He was also a natural history collector. Mantell, who came to New Zealand in 1840, had strong scientific connections. Through his father Gideon, a London-based palaeontologist and geologist, he knew and corresponded with Darwin and Charles Lyell. While in Britain in 1856, young Mantell helped Richard Owen at the Natural History Museum to reconstruct a large moa skeleton. Mantell also knew Colenso, Hector and Haast, and was active in the New Zealand Institute.[38]

Sometime before 1876 Hocken left a reasonable sized moa skeleton of his own with the Colonial Museum in Wellington, of which Mantell was occasionally director when Hector was absent. As Hocken explained in a letter of 14 February 1876, he now wanted the skeleton back. 'I am wishful to take down with me to Dunedin the moa I deposited in your museum some years ago. I believe it is necessary to give a fortnight's notice of my wish. Our museum in Dunedin is now eventually advanced & there is at length excellent provision for safely keeping valuable specimens.'[39] Hocken was persistent. In this instance he was determined to see Mantell, using his acquaintance with Jane Hardwick, Mantell's recently married second wife, as a way to achieve this. Regarding this request, Mantell was action personified. His response, dated 19 February and scribbled on Hocken's letter, instructed his staff to carefully take the skeleton down, pack it up and send it to Hocken by the first available steamer.[40] This, however, was not the end of the matter. Frederick Hutton, curator of the Otago Museum and soon to be appointed professor of natural science at the University of Otago, noticed an omission while setting up the skeleton in March 1876. Hocken's moa lacked a pelvis, and one that belonged to the museum was used instead. In fact, Hocken's moa did have a pelvis, but because it was somehow defective it had been placed in a labelled case at the museum for safekeeping and had disappeared.[41]

This hiccup did not deter Hocken, who finally met Mantell. On 29 March 1888, while in Wellington, Hocken spent three or four hours with Mantell 'who was amusing as usual, though showing evident signs of decay'.[42] The next year, on 10 March, Hocken was in the capital again: 'Spent an hour or two with Mantell. Cynical and smart as ever and looks very well.'[43] Six years later, on 2 February 1895, only a few months before the 75-year-old Mantell's death, Hocken found him 'bright and intelligent as ever but nearly blind, full of fun and satire, takes too much whisky which unfortunately was medically ordered for him more than a year ago'.[44] It was Mantell who told Hocken that the first Wellington settlers objected to the name of Britannica, which was originally given to their town; they found it too metallic. Hocken dutifully recorded this delightful snippet in his 'New Zealand Notes', written between 1893 and 1897.[45] As well as enjoying gossip, the two men found common ground on aspects of anthropology and philology, as both were members of the anthropology section of the AAAS.[46] And of course they corresponded. In 1890 Mantell sent Hocken a mat he had obtained from England as an appreciation for his 'praiseworthy efforts' in the New Zealand Exhibition of 1889–90;[47] in April 1892 Mantell was unable to visit Hocken in Dunedin, but compensated by enthusing over his planned visit to the Catlins with George Fenwick;[48] and a month later Hocken was reminded of Mantell's 'steel', when he received a rather prompt letter criticising errors in the printed account of that trip, *A Holiday Trip to the Catlins District* (1892).[49]

Although Mantell did not publish much, he gave Hocken publications from his own personal collection, many of which were presentation copies. These included the *Rules of the New Zealand Society* (1851); Sir George Grey's *Address to Members of the New Zealand Society* (1851) with the inscription 'With Mantell's compliments';[50] William Rees's *The Effect of Native Lands Acts Upon*

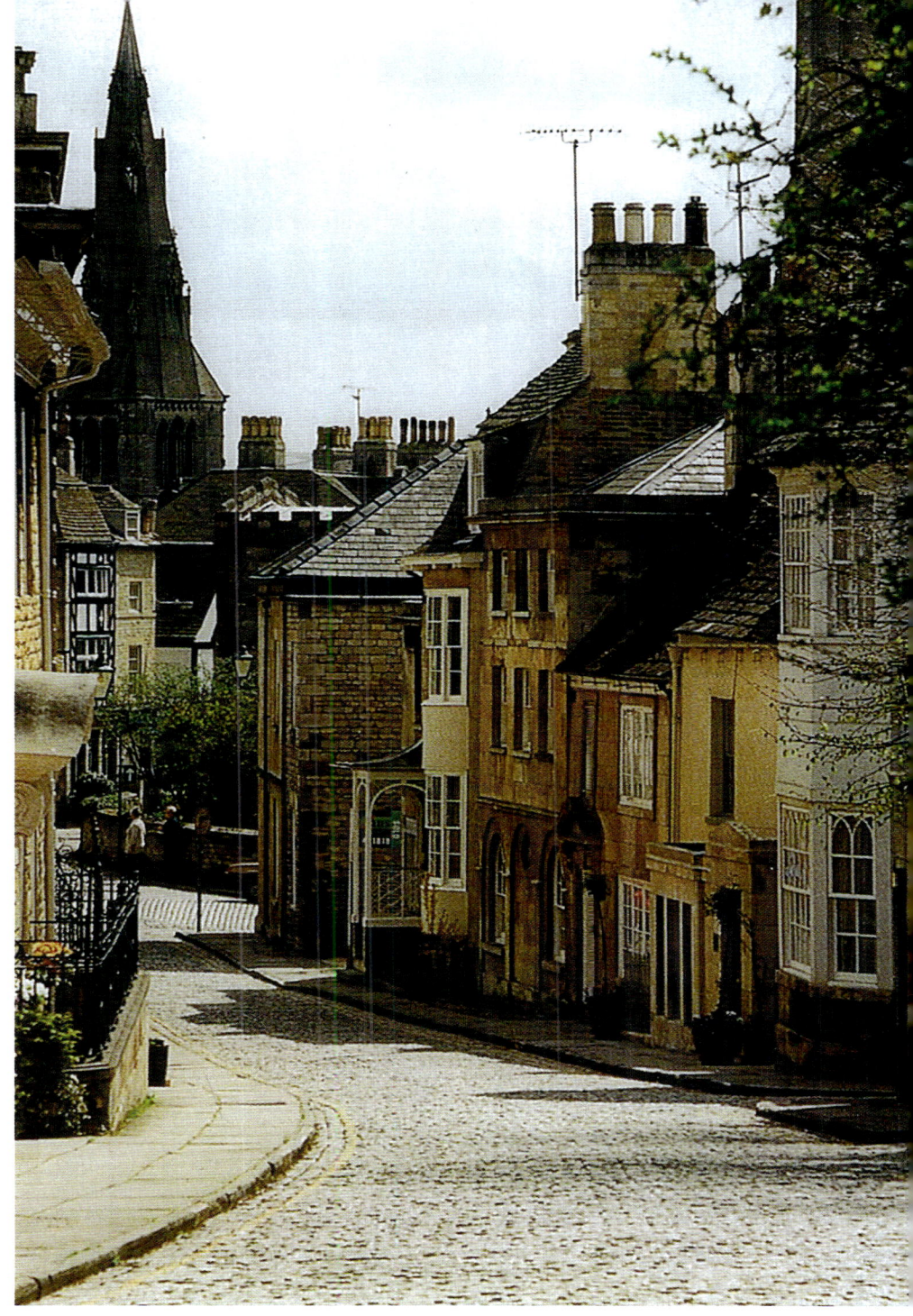

Stamford in Lincolnshire, a town of churches, was Hocken's birthplace, on 14 January 1836. *Private collection*

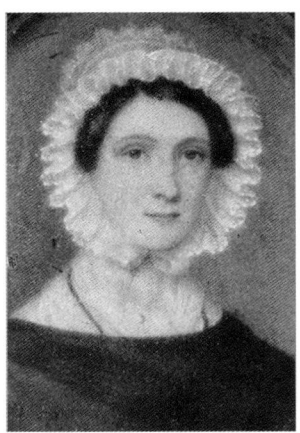

Yorkshire-born Anne Hocken Richardson married Joshua Hocken in Manchester in 1828. Both were aged 30. S14-298f, Hocken Collections, Uare Taoka o Hakena, University of Otago

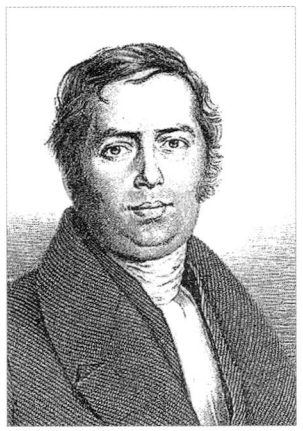

Joshua Hocken, itinerant Methodist preacher and author. Portrait engraving from *Methodist Magazine*, Vol. 70 (1847), p. 729. *Private collection*

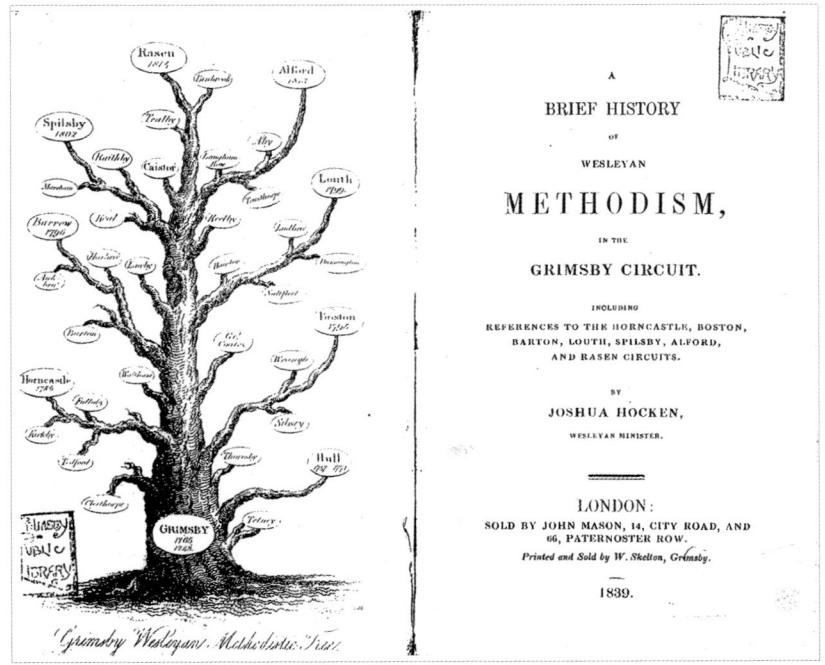

Joshua Hocken's first publication, *A Brief History of Wesleyan Methodism in the Grimsby Circuit* (1839), with its 'Grimsby Wesleyan Methodistic Tree'.
Private collection

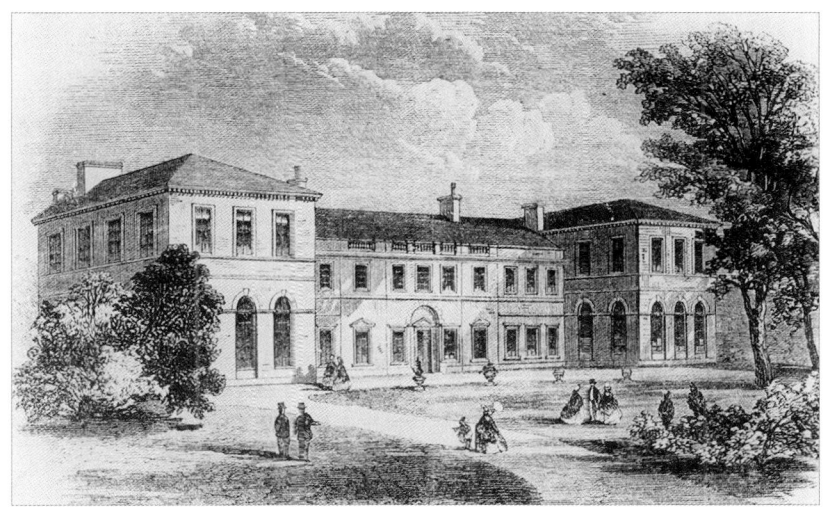

Woodhouse Grove School at Apperley Bridge, near Bradford and Leeds, in 1826. Hocken attended 'the Grove' from 1844 to 1850, as did his three brothers, James, Joshua and William. *S14-081e, Hocken Collections, Uare Taoka o Hakena, University of Otago*

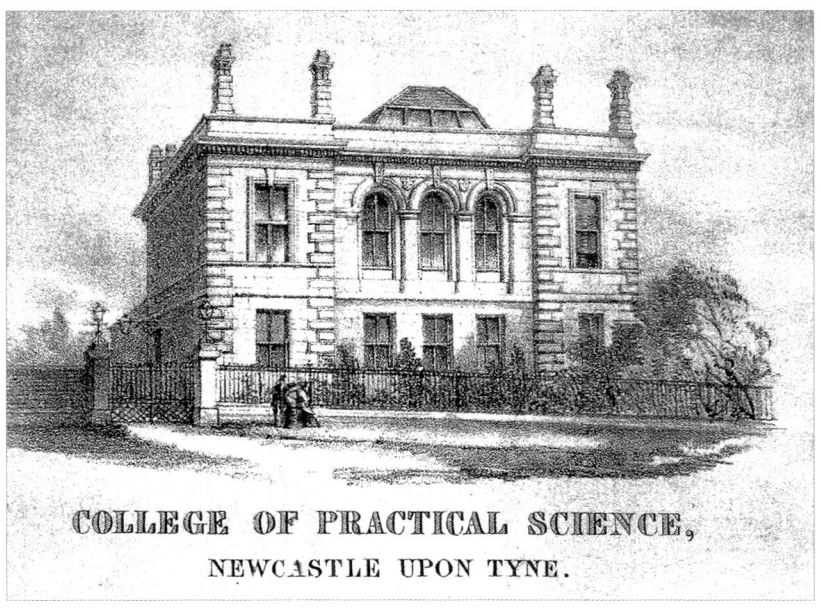

The Newcastle upon Tyne College of Practical Science, where Hocken attended lectures and practical tuition in medical and pre-medical sciences between 1854 and 1858. *Dennis Embleton Papers, University Arcaives, Robinson Library, University of Newcastle*

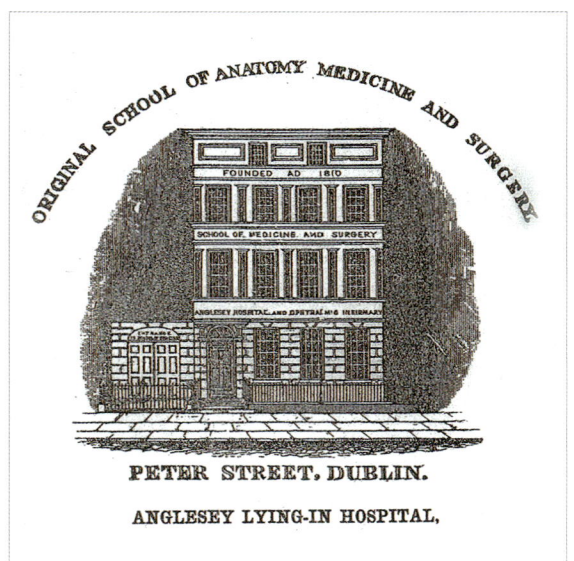

The Original School of Anatomy Medicine and Surgery, Peter Street, Dublin, where Hocken was a student from November 1858 to May 1859. This detail is reprinted from a medical course sheet at the Mercer Library, Royal College of Surgeons of Ireland, Dublin. *Private collection*

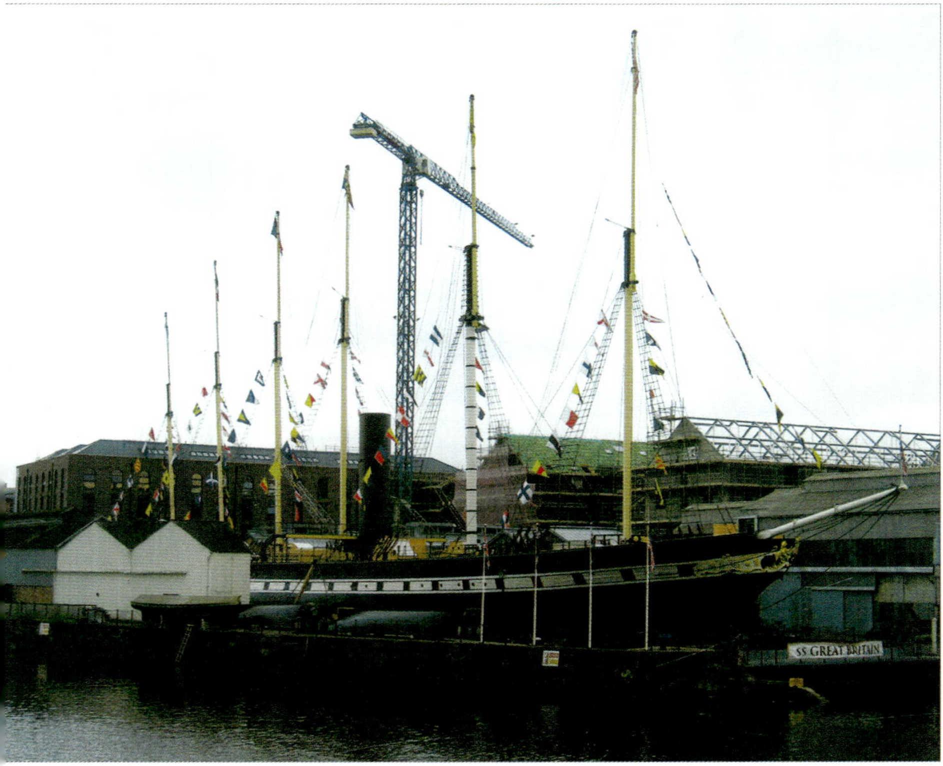

The great Isambard Kingdom Brunel–designed SS *Great Britain*. Hocken was surgeon-superintendent for three voyages between February 1861 and January 1862. The vessel is now dry docked at Bristol. *Private collection*

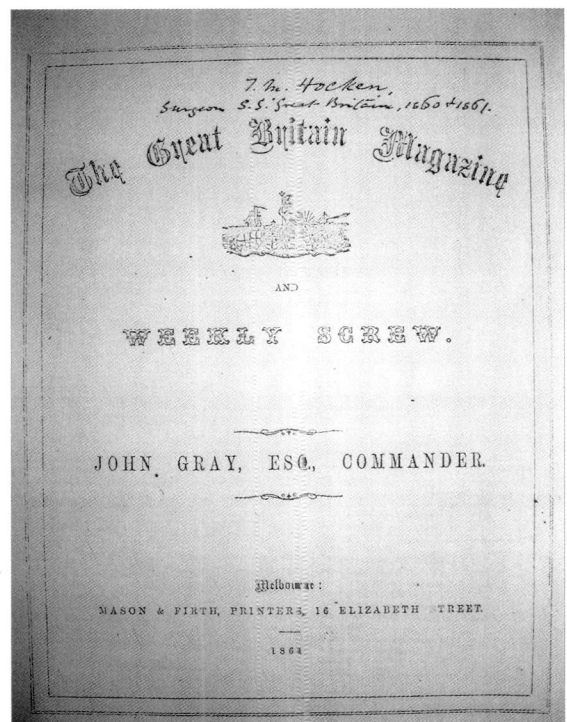

Hocken's own signed copy of the *Great Britain Magazine and Weekly Screw* (Melbourne, 1861), now in the SS Great Britain Archive at Bristol. He contributed much to this and other shipboard newspapers.
SS Great Britain Archive, Bristol

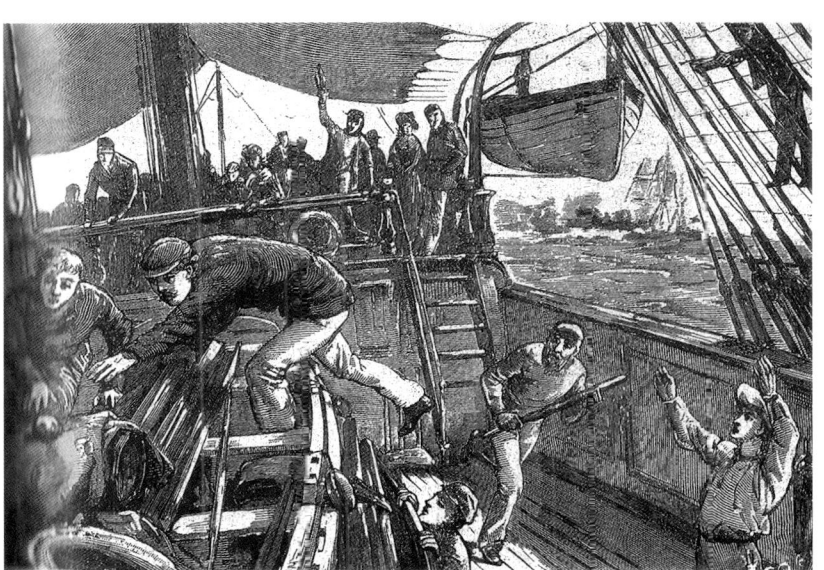

On Hocken's last voyage to Melbourne, in October 1861, the SS *Great Britain* carried the All England Eleven. He dealt with numerous injuries caused by playing shipboard cricket. *Private collection*

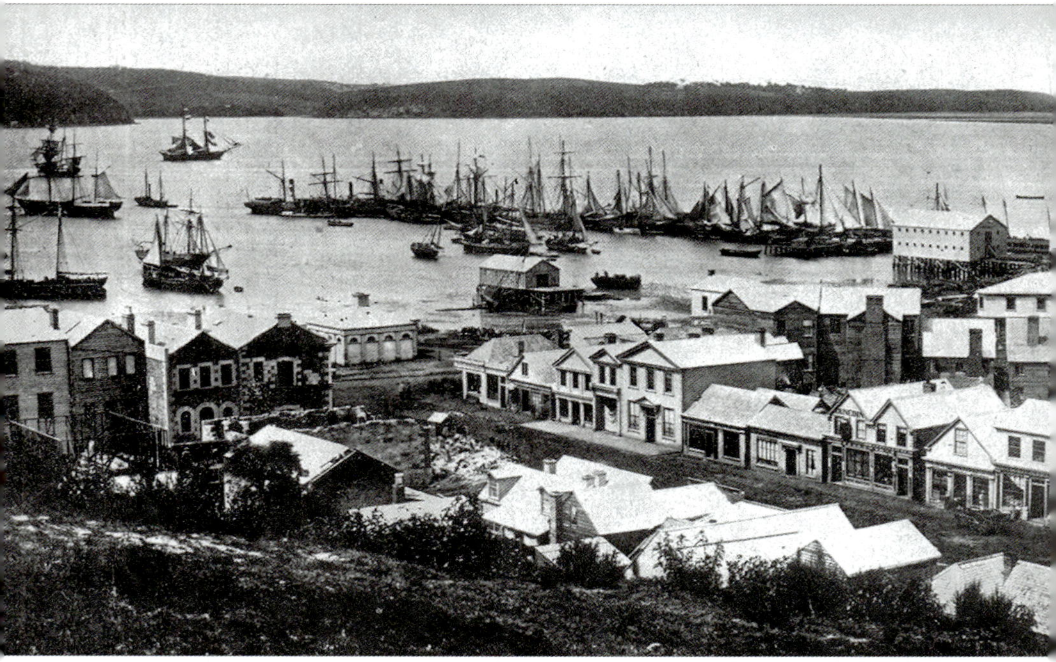

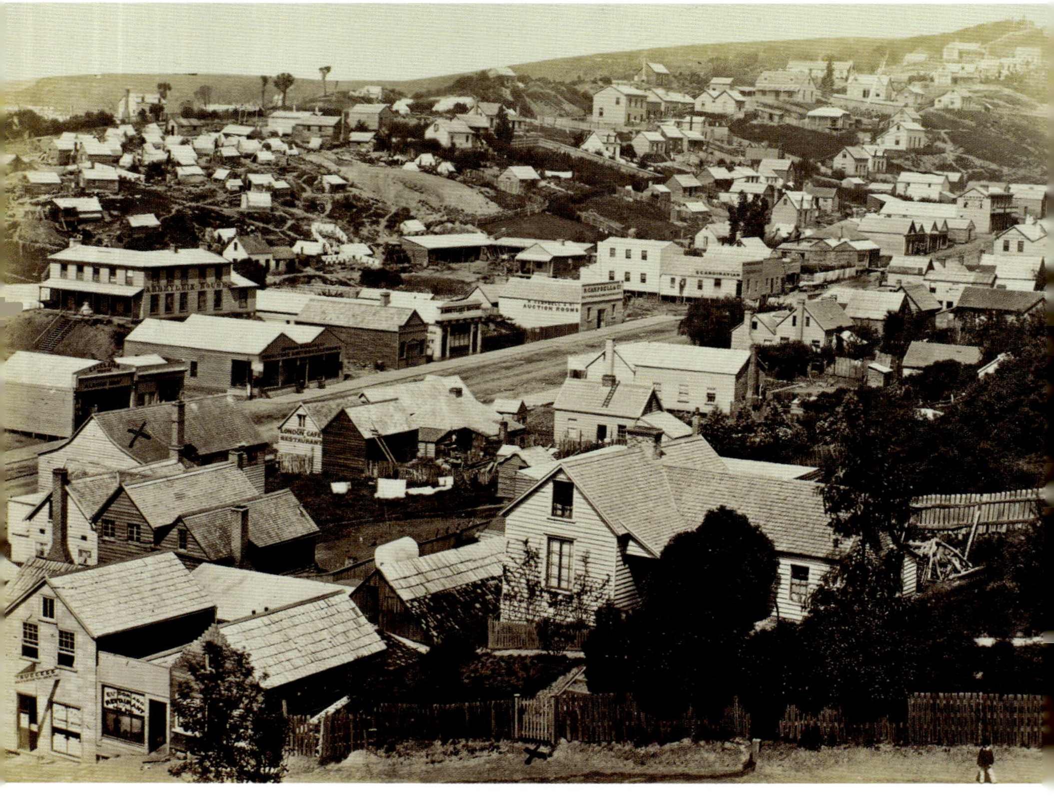

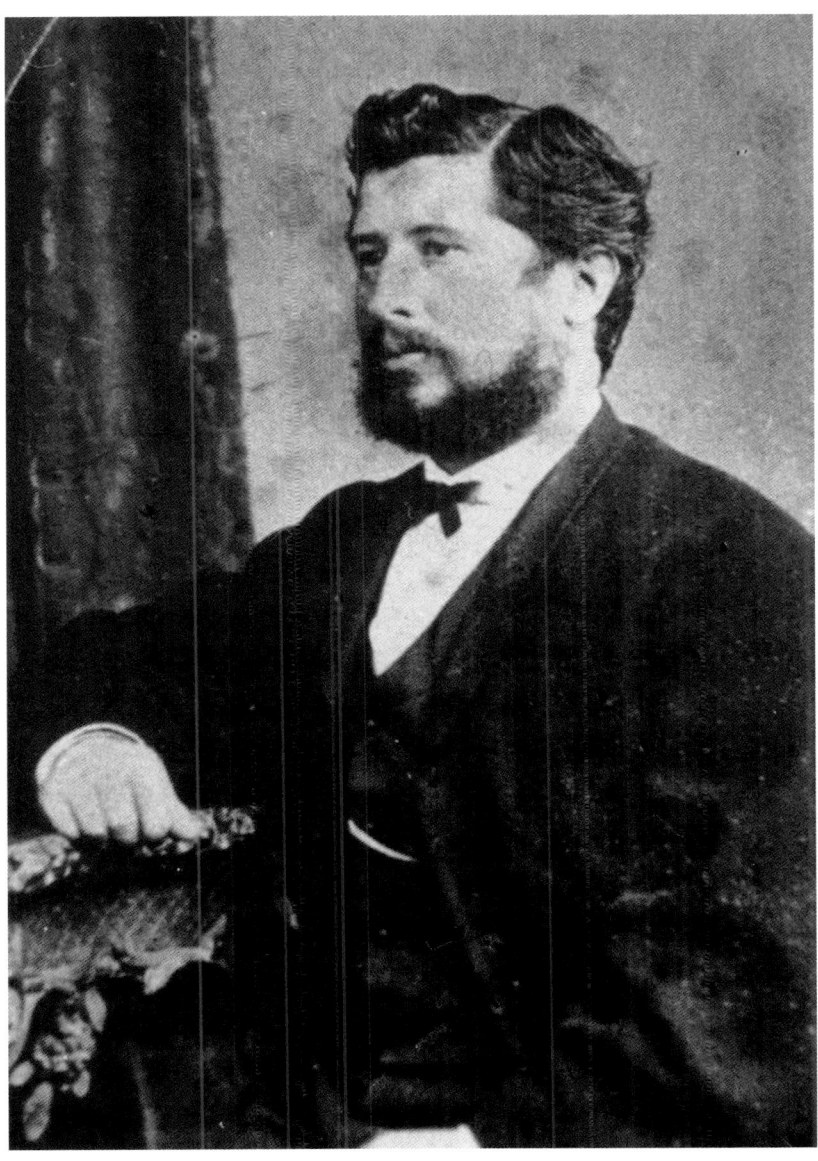

TOP LEFT: Princes Street, Dunedin, 1862. *A.H. McLintock,* History of Otago *(1949)*

ABOVE: A young Dr Morland Hocken. *S14-298b, Hocken Collections, Uare Taoka o Hakena, University of Otago*

LEFT: Hocken's first house in Rattray Street, Dunedin (at centre in front). *S14-081g, Hocken Collections, Uare Taoka o Hakena, University of Otago*

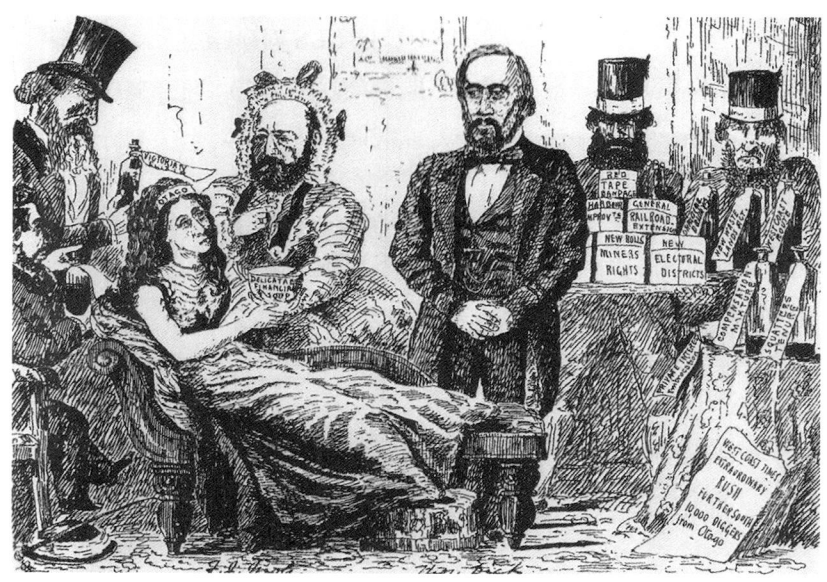

'Otago and her new doctors: A speedy cure anticipated', as depicted in *Dunedin Punch*. By 1865 the diminutive and bearded coroner, swinging his legs on his seat, was already an established 'identity'. *Private collection*

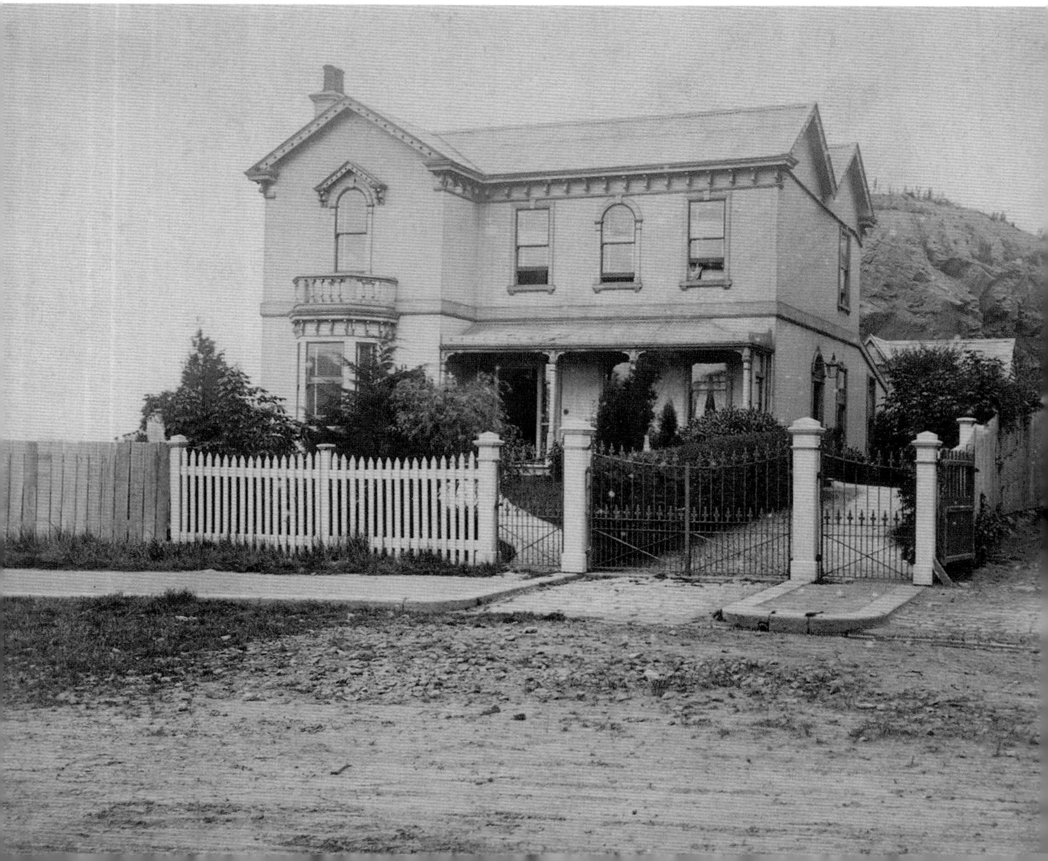

Hocken in his garden.
S14-298a, Hocken Collections, Uare Taoka o Hakena, University of Otago

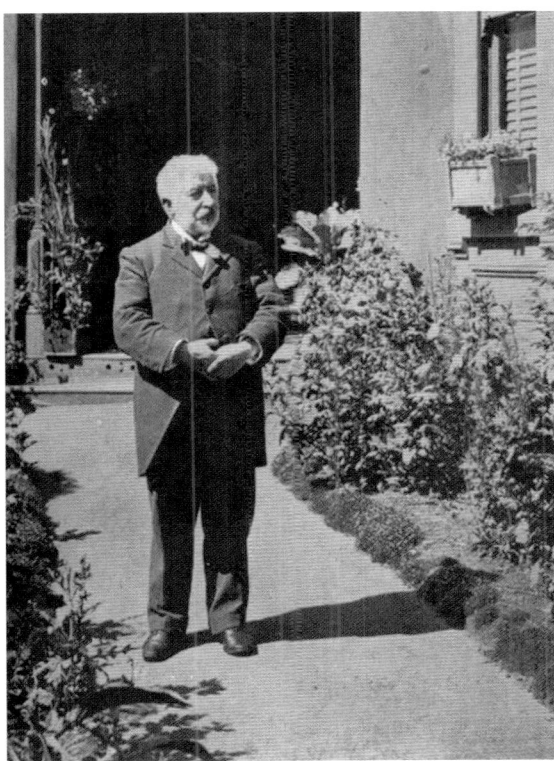

When in Auckland in 1879, Hocken made a conscious effort to collect books for his collection by placing this 'Wanted to Purchase' ad in Henry Brett's *Evening Star* on 29 March. *Private collection*

LEFT: Atahapara, on the corner of Moray Place and MacAndrew (now Burlington) Street, was Hocken's home from 1871. The house was designed by his friend Henry Frederick Hardy. *S14-081f, Hocken Collections, Uare Taoka o Hakena, University of Otago*

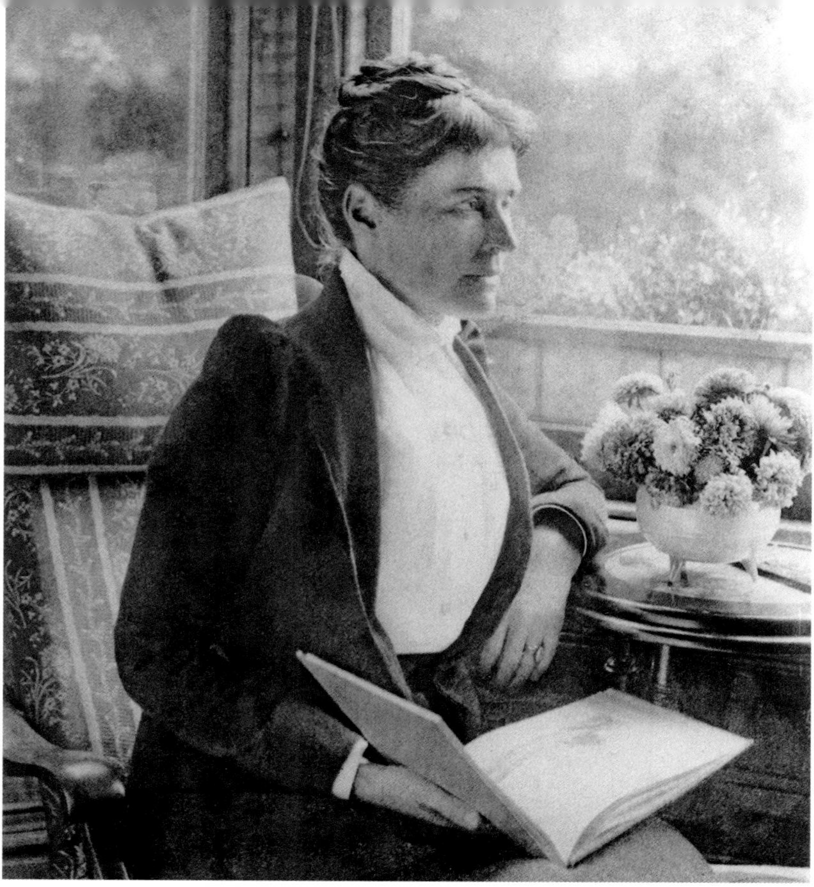

Elizabeth Mary (Bessie) Buckland (1848–1933) was 35 when she married Thomas Morland Hocken on 24 July 1883. She was well travelled, a linguist (Italian, German, French and Dutch) and, like her father William Thorne Buckland, knew Maori. She was musical, a more than competent photographer and sketched in oils and watercolour. Bessie was also a superb host who ran an excellent household. *S09-393d, Hocken Collections, Uare Taoka o Hakena, University of Otago*

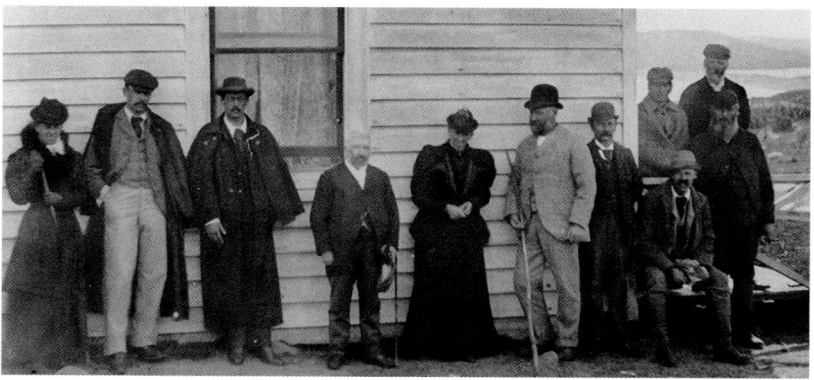

Hocken, centre stage, visiting Ruapuke in 1896.
S14-078a, Hocken Collections, Uare Taoka o Hakena, University of Otago

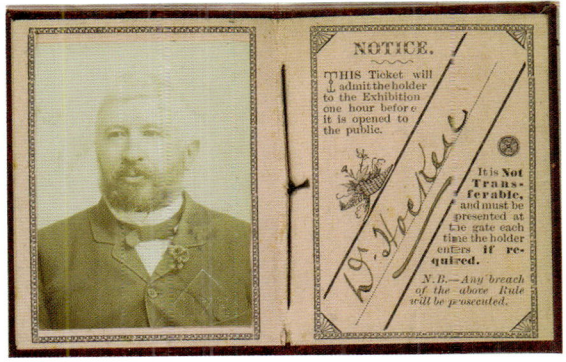
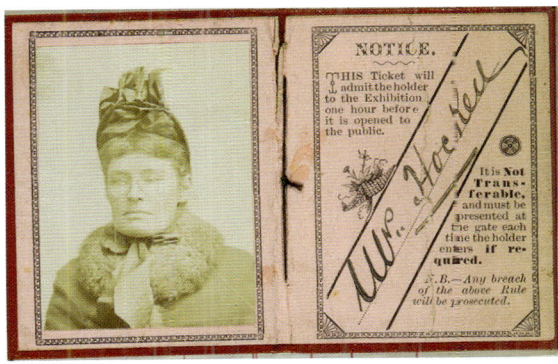
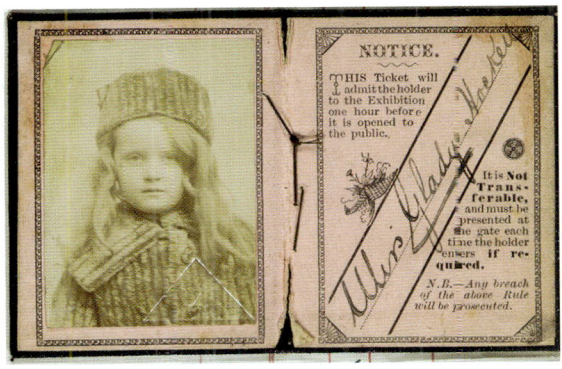

The Hocken family season tickets to the 1889–90
New Zealand and South Seas Exhibition, Dunedin.
*MS-0451/038: S14-298g, Hocken Collections, Uare Taoza o
Hakena, University of Otago*

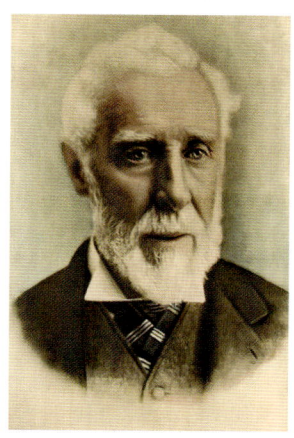

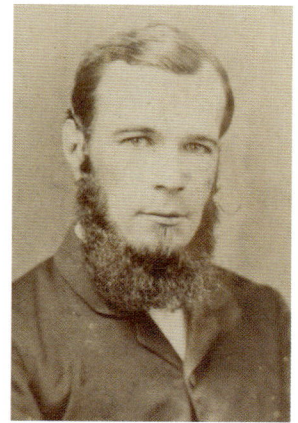

Sir George Grey (1812–1898), colonial governor and book collector, with whom Hocken corresponded and exchanged duplicate publications, and to whom he gave medical advice.
Private collection

Sydney book collector David Scott Mitchell (1836–1907), who not only corresponded about the details of gifting his collection, but also received a large number of duplicate publications from Hocken. *D.S. Mitchell, 19 December 1864. Safe 3/20: a928383, Mitchell Library, State Library of New South Wales*

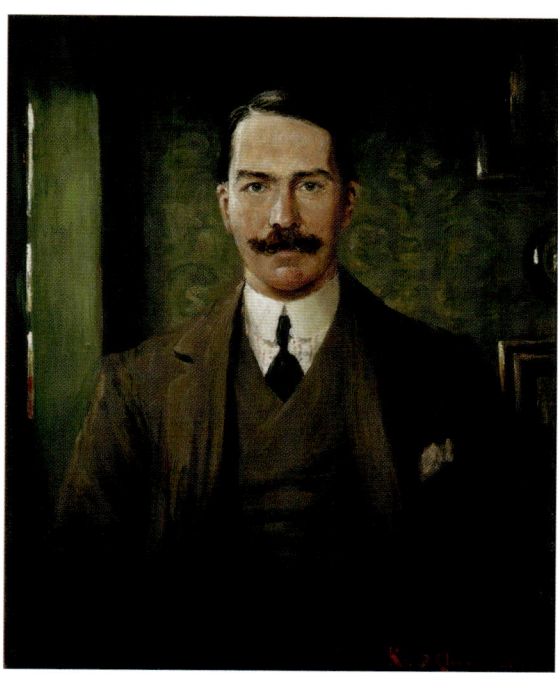

Alexander H. Turnbull (1868–1918), the Wellington-based book collector who, in April 1898, faced Hocken's 'crowing' over the acquisition of a number of items from Robert Louis Stevenson's library in Samoa.
Robert Stewart Clouston (1857–1911), Alexander Horsburgh Turnbull, 1909. Ref: G-600, Alexander Turnbull Library, Wellington

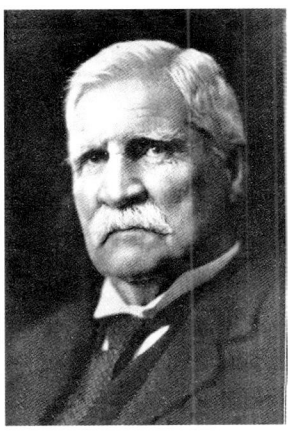

Judge Sir Frederick Chapman (1849–1936), a fellow Polynesian Society member, friend and collector of ethnographic materials, lived in Dunedin from 1872 to 1903. His large collection of pamphlets went to the Hocken Library. *S14-078b, Hocken Collections, Uare Taoka o Hakena, University of Otago*

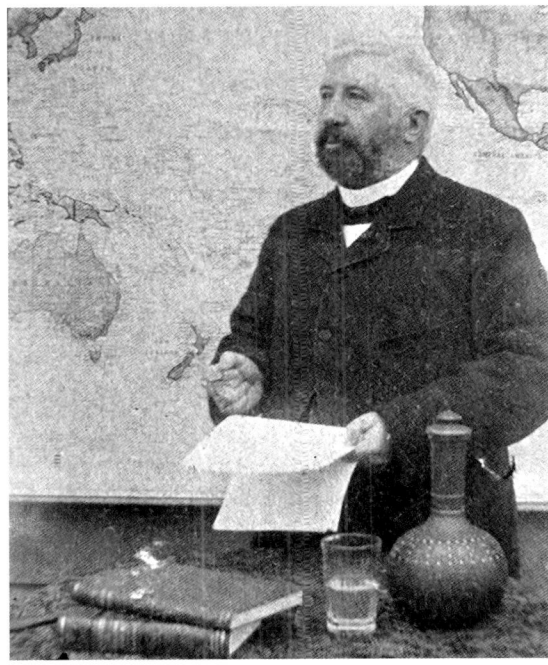

Poised to do what he did best – Hocken lecturing. *304-309d, Hocken Collections, Uare Taoka o Hakena, University of Otago*

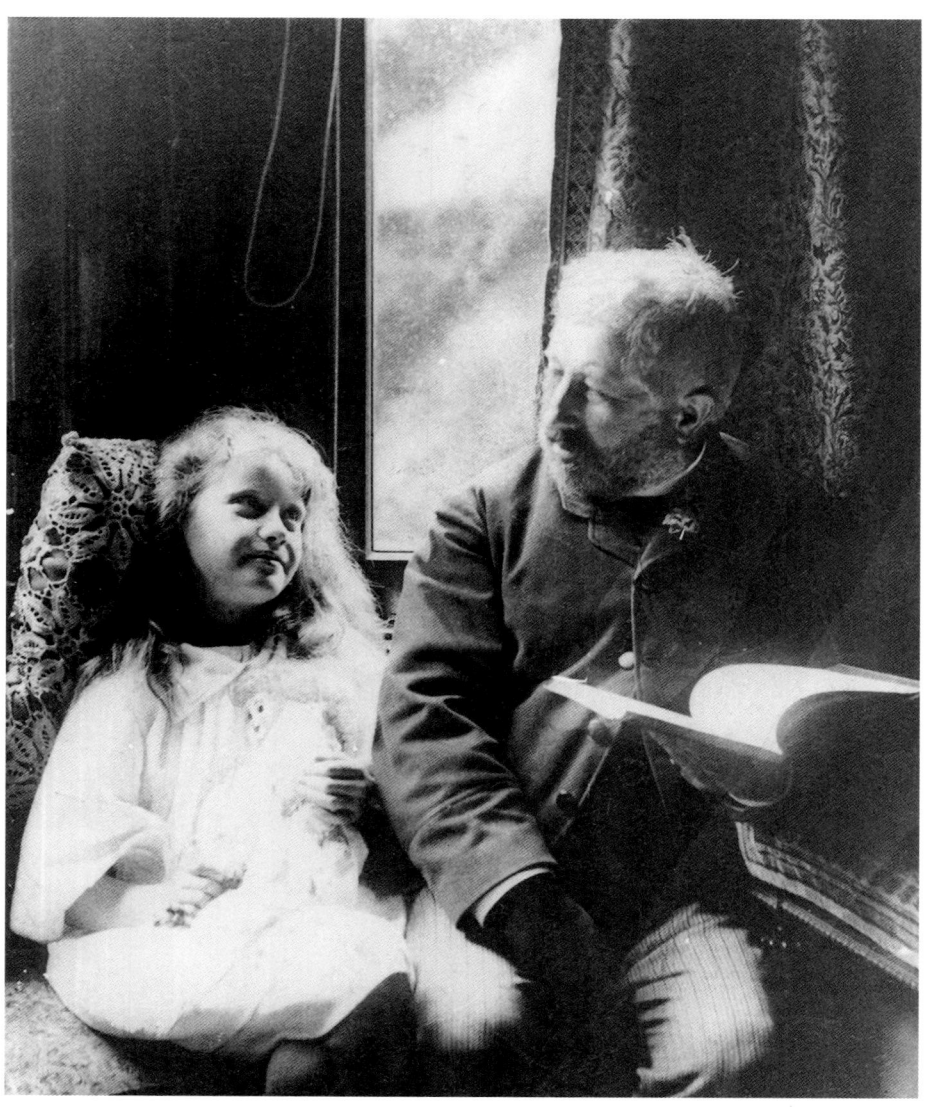

'Arrested Attention': Hocken and Gladys, his only child, in the reading room at Atahapara, photographed by Bessie. Born on 12 June 1884, Gladys was musical, painted and had an interest in photography. In March 1902, while travelling through the Mediterranean on the *Kawachi Maru*, she met Alan Le François, a merchant marine officer. They married in Yokohama in 1911.
S14-078c, Hocken Collections, Uare Taoka o Hakena, University of Otago

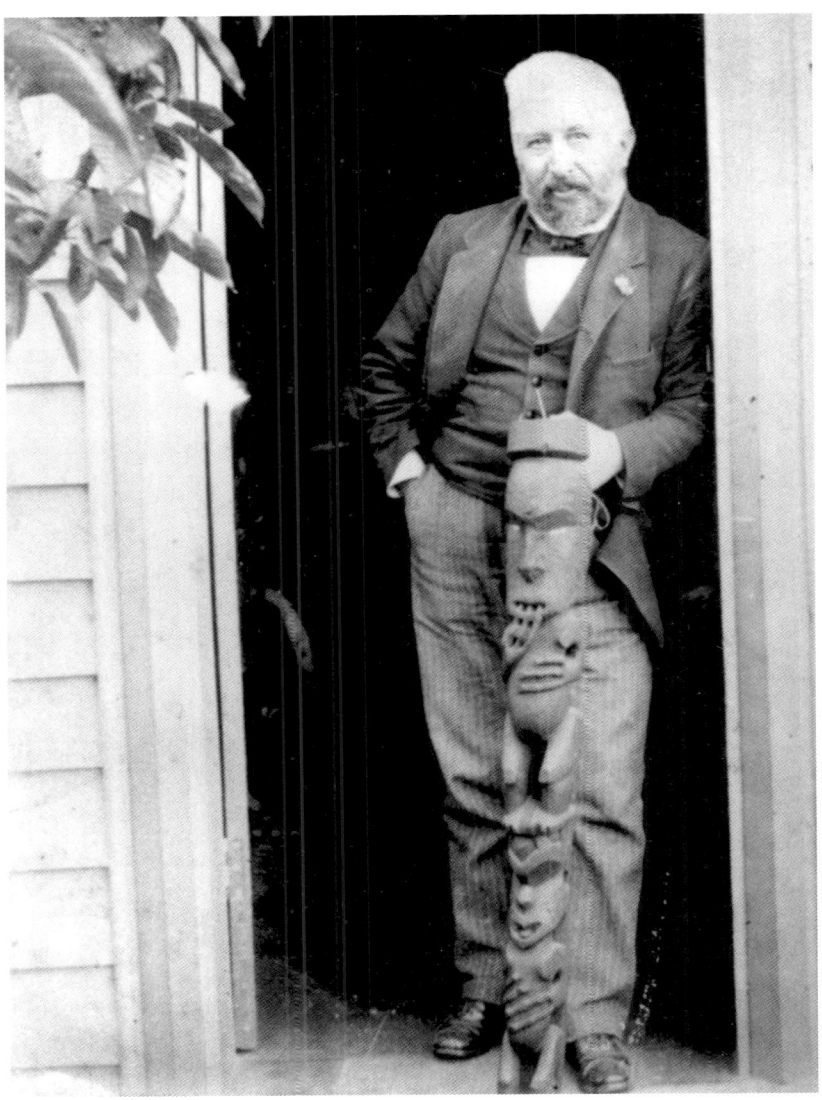

From his arrival in 1862 TMH collected Maori and Pacific carvings, statues and artefacts. The Hockens' gift of this material formed the basis of the ethnographic collection at the Otago Museum.
Hocken Collections, Uare Taoka o Hakena, University of Otago

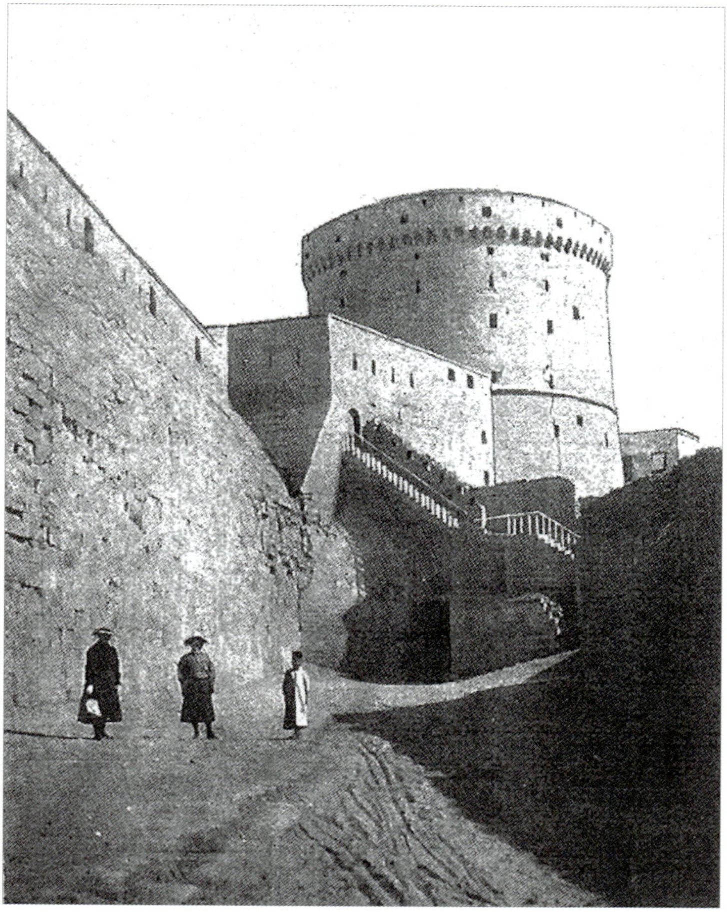

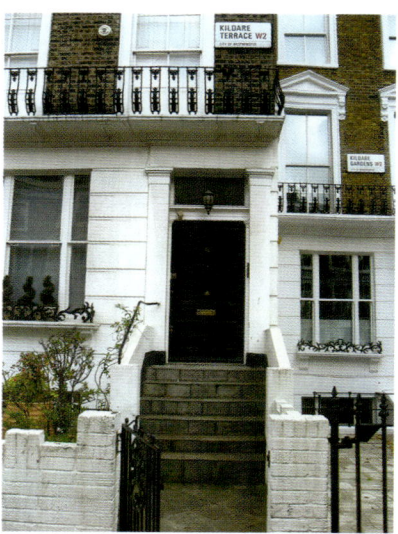

ABOVE: Bessie Hocken was a very competent photographer, winning a number of local photographic awards. She sent this image, named 'Citadel, Cairo', for publication in the *Otago Witness* on 4 March 1903.
Private collection

LEFT: 40 Kildare Terrace, Bayswater, London, where the Hocken family lived from June to December 1903.
Private collection

the *Colonization of the North Island of New Zealand* (1873);[51] Arthur Edward McDonogh's *To the Inhabitants of Wellington and its Vicinity* [1843];[52] Thomas Bowden's *A Memorial Upon Colonial Education* (1868);[53] Robert Donaldson's *Bush Lays and Rhymes* (1860);[54] George Henry Wilson's verse-work of Maori traditions and legends, *Ekino and Other Poems* (1869); John Plimmer's mythological *A Trip through Fairyland* (1884);[55] Walter Pearson's *In Memoriam: Sir John Richardson* (1879);[56] various religious publications, which Hocken bound up as 'Maori school books';[57] and an 1855 printed placard warning of outbreaks of tuberculosis and cholera in Nelson.[58] Items written by Mantell included *The Ostrich and Some Allied Birds Now Extinct* (1850) and a manuscript verse piece called 'Lay of the disappointed' (1851). Hocken also managed to obtain a copy of Mantell's father's *A Pictorial Atlas of Fossil Remains* (1850) and a separate manuscript note written by the geologist. For posterity, Hocken added a note to the latter: 'This is the handwriting of Dr Gideon Algernon Mantell, father of Mr W.D. [sic] Mantell one of the earliest & best known NZ settlers.'[59] Like many of his books, this work contains Hocken's efforts at immortality: it has his printed FLS bookplate, the hei tiki stamp, his signature on the preliminary pages, and the embossed coat-of-arms on page 35.

Johann Friedrich Heinrich Wohlers

Through his friendship with Riemenschneider, Hocken got to know Johann Wohlers, who had accompanied surveyor Frederick Tuckett on an expedition to find a site for the proposed New Edinburgh (Dunedin) settlement. Hocken read of Wohlers' experiences and activities on Ruapuke Island, with references to local Maori and the practical difficulties of running an isolated mission. Hocken, who liked to ground his historical work in fact, later visited the area and 'saw the dismantled remains of his old cottage & church, of which Mrs Hocken took sketches which are now in my collection. Tuckett was a pious Quaker & … a great supporter of his friend Wohlers.'[60] Hocken had 'a short correspondence on early day history' with the missionary. Conscious of the historical importance of this material, he wrote a small note on them: 'The letters I have carefully preserved. T.M. Hocken.' More Tuckett materials would come his way.

Hocken's 1879 Journey

Hocken's month-long trip of 1879 is the first he fully documented — and the diary covering his many travels north has survived.[61] Because this journey set a precedent for future excursions, it is worth examining in full. He covered a great deal of ground and did not linger long in one place.

Hocken left Dunedin on 13 February 1879, travelling by train to Oamaru and Christchurch. During his brief stop in Christchurch (Friday, 14 February), which he claimed was 'growing in extent and excellence of public and private building', he purchased for an unknown sum several old New Zealand books and pamphlets. He also called on William Reeves, owner and editor of the *Lyttelton Times*, and noted not only that the circulation of the newspaper was 3900, but that it was recovering from some dubious 'tactics' employed by owners of the *Press*.[62] It was just the sort of anecdote that Hocken enjoyed and happily recorded. He met, too, geologist and Canterbury Museum director Julius von Haast, who gave him what he described as 'Stanford's *Hints to Emigrants*', but was actually Charles Flinders Hursthouse's *New Zealandia or Zealandia: The Britain of the South* (Edward Stanford, 1857), a work that had induced Haast himself to visit New Zealand.[63] This meeting initiated a later exchange. On 7 February 1880 Hocken wrote to Haast offering an imperfect nine-volume set of Cook's *Voyages* along with 12 books on New Zealand, of which he had duplicates. They included Sir George Grey's *Ko Nga Moteatea* (1853), Edward Shortland's *The Southern Districts of New Zealand* (1851), a second edition of William Brown's *New Zealand and Its Aborigines* (1851), John Robert Godley's *Writings and Speeches* (1863) and J.S. Polack's *Manners and Customs of the New Zealanders* (1840). They were all offered for 'exchange', with Hocken's gentle reminder: 'I need hardly say how much obliged I should be to you for any documents, prints, pamphlets, books, &c relating to early N.Z.' It was a shrewd move, done in the hope that an exchange or purchase (perhaps cheaper than through normal channels) would result in the acquisition of an item he did not own. It also confirms his ownership of what was undoubtedly a growing book collection. As he proudly announced to Haast, 'If you pay a visit to Dunedin by all means let me have the pleasure of a visit from you, when I shall be quite happy to show you my possessions.'[64]

From Christchurch Hocken travelled on the *Hawea* to Wellington. On board he met Thomas Hooper, an old Nelson colonist, who had some strong and interesting opinions on the Wakefields which would have been grist to Hocken's mill. He found Wellington's main street and a few arterial roads passable but felt that the rest was of 'an extremely shabby unfinished appearance'. On the night of 16 February he heard Francis Redwood, the Roman Catholic Archbishop of Wellington, speak; an eloquent man, he was also a member of Wellington's Early Settlers' and Historical Society. The next day Hocken visited Robert Holt Carpenter, the eccentric bookbinder, bookseller and local politician who had started selling books in his Molesworth Street shop in the early 1850s. From Carpenter Hocken purchased, for an undisclosed sum, 'many old NZ documents', which may have been a number of Wellington almanacs that he had bound up in his pamphlet collection.[65]

The next morning he headed north through Featherston to Greytown, where he called on Samuel Revans, one of his first acquaintances in Dunedin and now retired. In 1865 during the exhibition celebrations, Revans had come down from Wellington with a 'special curiosity' to see what had transformed Dunedin from a plodding settlement to a bustling town. While there he became ill and was treated by Hocken, who described him thus: 'He was of rough exterior, careless in dress, and wore a conspicuously large Panama hat. His eyes were dark, penetrating, and deeply set, surmounted by thick, bushy eyebrows. His manner was restless, and his speech, though intelligent, often coarse. Some of those adjectives will apply as qualities of his leaders.'[66] Revans was primarily a newspaperman and had started the *New Zealand Gazette* in London in 1839, then printed the second issue in Wellington the following year: the country's first newspaper. It later became the *New Zealand Gazette and Britannia Spectator* and then the *New Zealand Gazette and Wellington Spectator*.[67] The two men had a 'long conversation' about the early days, especially about Revans' arch-foes, the Wakefields. Revans approved of Edward Gibbon's brother, Captain William Wakefield, but not of his 'intemperate and careless' son, Jerningham.[68] When Revans died on 14 July 1888 Hocken placed his obituary from the *Wairarapa Standard* in one of his F&J volumes.[69]

In Masterton, 'a thinning inland township dependent apparently on agriculture and sawmills', Hocken met Edward Riddiford, son of Daniel, the early pioneer runholder in the Wairarapa. By 20 February he was in Wanganui; the following day he sauntered about the town, his attention attracted by the hundreds of Maori in town 'engaged in selling land at the land Court ... squatting in tents on the right bank of the river'. (They were in fact investigating land claims.) Hocken carefully noted the inscription on the monument in the square – 'to the memory of the brave men who fell at Moutoa 14 May 1864 in defence of law and order against fanaticism and barbarism'. Hocken visited the 'old' Church of England cemetery, which contained the bodies of the Gilfillans who were 'murdered by Maoris in '47'. Four members of farmer and artist John Alexander Gilfillan's family were killed; he and his daughter were wounded. Perhaps this visit was the catalyst for Hocken's later interest in paintings by Gilfillan? He also visited the town's new cemetery to examine the graves of soldiers killed in the recent New Zealand Wars, and that of the Rev. Richard Taylor, missionary, naturalist and author of *Te Ika a Maui, or New Zealand and its Inhabitants* (1855), who had died in 1873. At Sandown Hocken met Taylor's widow, Caroline. In an effort to keep her husband's interests alive, she showed Hocken 'many curiosities of beautifully carved workmanship', which included 'godsticks', part of the many Maori artefacts that Taylor was known to have collected. Hocken, who may have met Taylor when the latter was in Dunedin for the 1865 exhibition, called them 'carved wooden curiosities' and recorded that they 'were thrust into the ground with a piece of string attached. Apparently the priest would sit close by, pulling on the string to arouse the attention of the Gods.' Hocken also visited Upongongaro, past Aramoho Pa, and settler homes such as that of Colonel Thomas Macdonnell.

On Saturday 22 February Hocken called at Putiki Pa on the south side of the river, where Taylor had been stationed as a missionary, and there met the Te Ati Haunui-a-Paparangi leader, politician and soldier Mete Kingi Te

Rangi Paetahi. He recorded his impressions: 'old house disappeared and school nearly so. Cave in cliff figured in Taylor's book with monument on top of hill. Garden gone to ruin – oranges, grapes and all fruit ripen in open air ... whares in terrible disrepair.'[70]

After Sunday in Wanganui, where he heard the Bishop of Wellington preach, he went on to Palmerston North and Fitzherbert, collecting an interesting piece of Wakefield gossip en route: 'Major Brown informed me on Wicksteed's authority that E.G. Wakefield had not intercourse with Miss Turner, whom he [kidnapped?] ... because of his having venereal disease.'[71] Te Kopua, near Dannevirke, was next on Hocken's itinerary before he passed through the 'magnificent Manawatu (beating heart) Gorge', though he noted, 'Not nearly equal to Otira.' He then travelled on to Napier where he visited 53-year-old John White, interpreter, linguist and author of *Te Rou: or the Maori at Home* (1874), who, just two months later, would be appointed to write what would become the multi-volume *The Ancient History of the Maori* (1887–91). White was another vital link, albeit an opinionated one. As Hocken wrote: 'he believes there were three distinct migrations to New Zealand of probably different people who found here a race distinct from the three. Mythologies are three too – one of the tribes north of Auckland ... second of those south inclusive of the Waikato district and third, those included in the above, that is, the pre-Maori peoples.'[72] As they talked, White showed Hocken a number of manuscripts that contained biographical details of individuals who lived in the north. White generously gave Hocken one that dealt with the Auckland area; although not an original, it was an excellent catch.

Two days later, on 28 February, Hocken travelled to Pakowhai Pa, near Napier, to attend the tangi of Ngati Kahungunu leader Karaitiana Takamoana (?–1879), who had been the MP for Eastern Maori.

> The body was in an ordinary coffin with glass plate let in to allow of features being seen and resting on his old flax mats some highly ornamented; at the head of the tent, under which the body lay were hung his two greenstone meres carved patu of hard wood and patu of whale bone. The coffin was ornamented with huia feathers. His four wives were seated on the floor of the tent keeping up an incessant wail or moan very similar to the moaning of the wind and accompanying this with wild gesticulations such as swaying sideways of the body clasping of the hands and weeping.

After describing the liberal provisions, including cooked meat, potatoes, bread, pipi and paua, Hocken wrote that the scene 'was rather one of festivity than of mourning'. He cast a critical eye over the structures: 'The pa is so modernized as to be uninteresting. Houses chiefly built European fashion and with very few carvings. Everything was dirty.'[73]

In the evening he visited the Tylees, who were related by marriage to

Richard Taylor, who gave him the already-mentioned copy of Potatau's seal and two wax impressions to which, according to Tylee, 'the rebel Maoris attach much importance'. Hocken was also introduced to the 'very pleasant' Samuel Locke and his wife, friends of Judge Frederick Maning, author of *Old New Zealand* (1863). And in proof that riches do abound in the most unlikely places, Hocken was shown a copy of Captain Cook's *A Voyage to the Pacific Ocean* (1784), which contained maps and engravings of the third voyage by John Webber. The following day Hocken left for Auckland travelling via Gisborne, which he called 'a miserable dusty town full of pumice sand'. Again determined to 'touch' history, he made a quick tour by boat to where Cook first landed in October 1769: 'Here the first Maori was shot in New Zealand.' Hocken also called on the Rev. Samuel Williams, who had founded Te Aute College for Maori boys and who had a local curiosity to display: 'hardened pumice stone where the foot prints of a moa were found'. In Tauranga he met a local identity, Oliver Quintal, who was a descendant of *Bounty* mutineer Matthew Quintal. Hocken's description has a medical flavour: 'Q is a pale lemon visaged man, thin, about 40 with scanty beard and moustache and washed out, almost colourless irises – was brought up by Sir W. Martin who for sometime allowed him £100 a year – now he practises as a solicitor in Tauranga.'

On 4 March Hocken arrived in a rainy Auckland. Even though it was a brief stay, he managed a visit to the Queen Street premises of the town's finest bookseller, George Chapman, where he purchased 'many old NZ books and pamphlets' with the tantalising 'promise of more'.[74] Chapman was chiefly known for his lending library of more than 4000 volumes and his influential *New Zealand Almanac*, first published in 1860.[75] He had spent his early years in the Otago region; here both men would have found common ground.

When Hocken arrived in Russell on 5 March he had with him a letter of introduction addressed to the widow of Dr Samuel Ford, New Zealand's first resident surgeon, who had witnessed the conflicts with Hone Heke. Hocken gleaned a few historical anecdotes from Martha Ford, who maintained: 'After their [the Maori] success they rushed in saying "we have mastered your Queen, we have mastered your Queen" and commenced according to Maori custom to run off with [my] goods thinking that friends, rather than foes should impound them.' She described Heke as 'a tall man, clever, splendid warrior and humane' and Kawiti as 'small repulsive looking, cunning and cruel'. Martha Ford had Wakefield connections: she used to spend some of her school holidays at Edward Gibbon Wakefield's mother's place in Ipswich.

Good fortune smiled on Hocken. Also staying at the Ford house was Archdeacon Robert Maunsell, who was making his first visit in 10 years to his old missionary stamping ground. On 6 March he and Hocken went to Paihia where they saw the ruins of the stone house built by the Williams family, and the spot where the first press was erected adjoining the church. They hired horses and rode to Pakaraka and through a 'dangerous mangrove swamp' to the Waitangi Falls Hotel. Then, because it was raining, they decided to return to Paihia and Kororareka. As they travelled Hocken collected opinions from his companion, including the latter's criticism of Colenso: 'an unprincipled man in consequence of his living with a Maori woman ... and quite unfit to compile the Maori dictionary as he was no philologist'. Hocken also learned that the newspaper editor, politician and writer Hugh Carleton, who had written a biography of Maunsell's father-in-law Henry Williams (which Hocken owned), 'was very reserved, a classic pedant' and had professed to the missionary 'an inviolate life'. Hocken also managed a walk over the area at Waitangi where the Treaty was signed, and while at Russell he examined the church, which still had bullet holes in it from the 1845 war. He visited the cemetery, unearthed an old 28-pounder lying near a small bay and visited the wife of Tamati Waka Nene, who was living in a one-roomed cottage: 'an old nearly blind ugly woman squatting on the floor near the fire with another Maori female'. Altogether, wrote Hocken, 'a deserted looking place'.[76] On 7 March Hocken ascended Flagstaff (Maiki) Hill and remarked on the 'magnificent prospect of Bay of Islands', with Rangihoua 'sitting on a small sandy beach with three or four houses about two miles inside to the right'. Hocken added Maunsell's claim for the correct spelling of Rangihoua to be Rangihona (signifying burrowing sky) and noted that Marsden had first preached the gospel there on Christmas Day, 1814.[77] Before Hocken left for Auckland he purchased from Joyce, a half-caste local with a handsome Maori wife, the three watercolours by John Williams, a soldier of the 58th Regiment, which he would later show to the audience at a September 1886 lecture. On 8 March Hocken was back in Auckland where once again he was busy. In the afternoon he went to Orakei to see hundreds of Maori perform a war dance that he called disappointing – 'a most inferior representation no time and not much spirit' – and in the evening went visiting. The next day he visited St Paul's Church, the oldest in Auckland, before dining with Maunsell that night at St Mary's in Parnell. Further conversation followed with this 'most intelligent and advanced man', who, Hocken recorded, did 'not believe that prior to the advent of the whites there [was] any spirit of or development towards a higher state of things than nature' and that the Maori 'were as much immersed in savagery as ever'. There was also time in Auckland to browse again Chapman's shelves and purchase 'many old works and pamphlets'; he also bought material from one Morton and from the bookseller and stationer Edward Wayte.

The journey was now telling on him. His entry for 11 March is the briefest: 'Visited with John Mills, Mr Burtt who has several Maori curiosities.' The next day he visited 'beautiful' Remuera: 'the fashionable locality, land about £100 an acre'. He met James Baker, who maintained that Augustus Earle, author of *A Narrative of a Nine Months' Residence in New Zealand* (1832), was a scamp, much addicted to Maori women. Hocken also paid for an advertisement in Henry Brett's *Auckland Star* – 'Wanted to Purchase, Books or Pamphlets relating to early New Zealand history' – and arranged for local accountant Thomas Leigh White to be the recipient of any forthcoming booty. Given that this plea appeared 16 days after Hocken's departure, and among 54 other 'Wanted' ads, any response was unlikely. Nevertheless, it revealed the lengths to which Hocken would go to collect, especially local books.

Although professional matters demanded his attention when he arrived home, Hocken did not let his data-gathering skills rust. On 12 July 1879 he had a conversation with Sydney-born brothers Edwin (George) and William (Bill) Palmer at Otokia, near Momona, south of Dunedin. Both men were sealers and whalers. Edwin had settled on Codfish Island in 1835 and had dealings with Johnny Jones, the successful whaler and merchant operating around Waikouaiti and Moeraki. William had worked at Preservation Inlet. Hocken managed to record brief details on the Palmers' lives and on the Otago area and the outlying islands. This early example of oral history was 'scribbled down by me under much difficulty, caused by the constant interruption of the two brothers and their cross memories'. It ended positively: 'remarkably fine stalwart open-faced men with splendid, visible teeth'.[78] With the claim that the information was 'quite new' and 'gathered from various sources', he wove it into his talks.[79] This was a process he would repeat in coming years.

7
Good Fortune, Dr Hocken, FLS

The year 1881 started on a positive note for Hocken. From the artist, retired surveyor, explorer and civil servant Charles Heaphy, he received not only a number of pamphlets but also permission to use them as best he could. Although Heaphy had no 'literary papers' relating to Frederick Tuckett's surveying or his own, he did refer Hocken to the files of the *Nelson Examiner* for information on the explorations of J.S. Cotterell, Thomas Brunner, William Fox, Frederick Weld and himself. The note ended cheerily: 'and if you need any specific information, I shall be very happy to afford it, so far as I can'.[1] It would not be long until Hocken saw Heaphy: he was planning another trip.

Hocken left Dunedin on 3 February, and as he travelled north through the Canterbury Plains, he 'saw abundant signs of progress in cultivation' and an increase in the size of small towns.[2] In Christchurch he visited Clark's sale room where he spied *Dr Evans and Mr Allwright Meeting the Maori Chiefs*, painted by his fellow Grovian James Smetham in 1863. Hocken was so taken with *The New Zealand Chiefs in Wesley's House*, as the painting came to be known, that despite the asking price of £700 he wrote to Mrs Burt, the owner, who lived in nearby Sumner. There is no record of a reply, but the painting would reappear later in Hocken's life.[3] A zig-zag walk over the Bridle Path from Heathcote to Lyttelton on 5 February offered 'a magnificent view of the plains in the front and the meandering Heathcote, Waimakariri and ranges of west coast in the distance'. Hocken proved his awareness of surveyor and draughtsman Edmund Norman's 1850s lithographs of the area – 'Norman's lithographs very accurate' – though now 'numerous plantations and cultivation would dot the whole of his picture'.

Art dominated Hocken's Christchurch visit. He attended the first Canterbury Society of Arts exhibition, which ran from 18 January to 12 February 1881 at Christchurch Boys' High School in Worcester Street. A hundred and five works were displayed: 18 oil paintings and 87 watercolours and drawings. Hocken noted James Peele's *Christchurch in 1852* and Captain E.F. Temple's *Early Settlers*; the latter, priced at £25, was 'well drawn' but, perhaps in reference to its condition, 'not well treated'. Other exhibitors included John Madden and his friends Gully and Hodgkins.[4]

In Wellington, on 7 February, Hocken called on George Sisson Cooper, one-time private secretary to Sir George Grey, whom he spurred into action: Cooper 'made a search of old things for me'. His next three visits – to Government Printer George Didsbury, long-time and distinguished civil servant Leonard Stowe and Charles Heaphy – proved disappointing as '[they] could get no useful information'.[5] But Hocken had more satisfaction in Nelson where, in a furniture shop in Trafalgar Street, he discovered a pen and ink sketch of the town by Heaphy. This was certainly *Nelson from the Gaol* (1859), which is now part of Hocken's original pictorial collection. He also obtained, from another source, copies of the *Wellington Spectator* for 1841 and 1842, and a copy of the *New Zealand Journal* for 1842. He visited John Gully, already an acquaintance from the very successful 1865 Dunedin Exhibition, and called on William Hough, an old Wesleyan lay missionary who once lived in a whare at Patea. Hough had definite views on the origin of the Maori, which he had put to readers of the *Nelson Examiner and New Zealand Chronicle*.[6] Hocken spent time copying down an old legend that had been passed to Hough by a Patea chief in 1844, which included mention of people living long ago at Patea who were 'black as Negros and with short curly hair, peaceful and harmless'. Hocken proclaimed Hough reliable, although he did pose the question: 'Is the legend viewed [through] his spectacles?'[7]

On 10 February Hocken travelled to Wanganui where he called on Richard Watson Woon, local resident magistrate and a member of the Wellington Philosophical Society. From Woon he obtained a copy of Sir George Grey's *Maori Proverbs* (Cape Town, 1857). In New Plymouth, which he described as 'apparently the poorest in NZ complain much of the native difficulty and want of access', he eventually made contact with the long-haired Thomas King, an original New Plymouth settler and former politician and bank manager.[8] Hocken had a letter of introduction to King from Isaac Newton Watt, a Dunedin sheriff and coroner, who described him as 'a good friend of mine, who is collecting material, for lectures on the early history of New Zealand, documentary & illustrative. If you can put him in the way of adding to his store or otherwise assist him I shall feel obliged.'[9] King, whom Hocken called 'most intelligent', eventually presented him with a copy of Hursthouse's *The Incorporation of Britain's Colonial with her Home Empire* [1866].

Hocken then travelled south skirting the coastline to Pungarehu, a small town between Okato and Opunake, near Parihaka. Led by the prophets Te Whiti o Rongomai and Tohu Kakahi, Parihaka – which was the biggest Maori community in New Zealand – was a pacifist settlement. Maori–Pakeha relations had become increasingly strained when, in 1878, the government started to survey the South Taranaki lands confiscated after the New Zealand Wars, in order to prepare them for European settlers. The men of Parihaka protested this development by ploughing up land and pulling out the surveyors' pegs.[10] The government responded with an increased military presence. Pungarehu was one of four main constabulary camps in the area; the others were at Rahotu, Egmont and Opunake.[11] Hocken's contacts at Pungarehu were mainly military – men like Lieutenant-Colonel John Mackintosh Roberts, Major Arthur Tuke and surveyor Wellington Carrington, who acted as interpreter for Te Whiti and Tohu. Roberts had been part of Gustavus von Tempsky's Forest Rangers and had fought in earlier campaigns at Patea; Carrington was a friend of Riemenschneider. For Hocken it was all too good to miss.

On the afternoon of 14 February he walked the 3 km to Parihaka 'through bush and papalli swamp'. His first impressions were not favourable: 'Village common, dirty, disorderly houses as though dropped over anywhere – built of raupo, flax, toi, and sticks – no carving or ornamentation whatever – mangy dogs and pigs abound.' He was fortunate to see Te Whiti:

> [He] was in a large whare with about 30 others who seemed to show him no respect ... Te W. quiet intelligent looking man, with cast in left eye – about 45 with black straight hair striated with grey – said not a word though frequently caught him looking at me when he thought I was engaged with the others – not exactly sullen but reserved and apparently thoughtful – perhaps playing a role. No one would interpret though several able to do so. Forehead just above nose very protuberant not unlike Sale altogether ... All consider [Te Whiti] to be a clever man but cannot understand him. Say that his policy of peace is fortunate for us and that Bryce's [Native Minister John Bryce] intention to seize him wrong in every way. Very argumentative but shifty in reaction. I do not think him the least insane, but fond of power – a sort of Mahomet – should not think it unlikely that his schemes are deeply laid ...

In November that year Bryce led an infamous invasion of Parihaka that resulted in the arrests of Te Whiti and Tohu and almost annihilated the settlement.

The next day Hocken rode out with Tuke to the 'beautifully situated' camp at Rahotu, built on the site of an old Maori fortification. While there, he spotted vertical stone structures that had curious figures like hei tiki and tattooed faces etched on them. Inspector Foster Goring, stationed at Rahotu, promised to take a rubbing of these relics for Hocken.

Just before leaving Dunedin, Hocken had written to Grey to say that he would be travelling north and would attempt to get across to Kawau Island and 'pay his respects'.[12] Hocken had also thanked Grey, now 69, for his feedback on the lectures he had sent and hinted at a proposal for another series that would deal with 'the rise & progress of scientific research in N.Z'. Of his collection he had written, 'The labour is with me one of love – the early history of this interesting country has ever had a singular charm & I entertain the purpose of publishing some contributions to it.' And there was the usual plea: 'I am sure you can render most valuable assistance & I should indeed be more than grateful for any old documents, pamphlets &c. which you may have & which you do not intend to use.'[13] Hocken actually stayed a week on Grey's island paradise, where he was shown the treasures that the former governor and premier liked to show off: his medieval Besançon Missal, the Richard Cromwell–John Thurloe letters and early printed books such as Caxton's printing of Jacobus de Voragine's *Golden Legend* and Richard Pynson's printing of Chaucer's *Canterbury Tales*. Hocken also successfully treated his host for piles and constipation. After Hocken returned home, Grey penned a note reporting that he was 'making extraordinary progress under your prescriptions'.[14]

There was excitement for Hocken back in Dunedin as he resumed his usual duties. On 1 October the previous year the Otago Institute Council, of which Hocken was now president, had sent Charles Darwin an illuminated address to celebrate the 21st anniversary of the publication of *On the Origin of Species*. Signed by Hocken and 10 prominent intellectuals, it read in part:

> However limited the field of our own labours may be, we cannot but be sensible of the influence which that work has had throughout the whole domain of Natural Science, and especially upon Biology, which, as one great comprehensive science may be said to owe its very existence to the fact that you made belief in Evolution possible by your theory of Natural Selection. We are glad to think that you have lived to see the almost universal acceptance of the great doctrine which it has been the work of your life to establish: it is hardly an exaggeration to say that every important Botanical or Zoological discovery of the last 21 years, particularly in the departments of Embryology and Palaeontology, has tended to fill up some gap in the evidence you had originally collected, and to make Evolution no longer a theory but an established doctrine of Science. We hope that you may long live to continue your labours and to see the further spread of their influence upon all scientific thought and upon all higher scientific work.[15]

A reply had come back from Darwin, written promptly on 21 February 1881, expressing his deep gratification for the 'great & unusual honour':

> This honour is particularly gratifying to me, as coming from New Zealand, the wonderful progress of which has interested me greatly. I have read every one of the volumes of the New Zealand Institute from the first … & always with admiration at the success & zeal with which Science is followed in a country, destined, as I believe, to be in the future the Greater Britain of the Southern Hemisphere. I beg leave to return to you personally my sincere thanks for your kind & courteous letter …[16]

Hocken would later read out this letter in one his lectures and he filed it in Volume 5 of his F&J.

Hocken did remove one obligation from his busy life: after 16 years' service he resigned from the position of honorary surgeon of the Dunedin Volunteer Naval Brigade. He continued with his duties as coroner and his involvement with the Benevolent Institute. The year ended sadly with Julia Hocken's death in early December.

Going 'Home'

Perhaps as a reaction to the loss of his wife, Hocken decided to go 'Home'. The first official notification of his wish to go was on 27 February 1882 when he wrote an application for leave to the Coroner's Office, announcing that he would leave for England via San Francisco on 25 March.[17] As was usual at the time, he was given a splendid send-off by friends the day before his departure, with over 40 people gathering for a dinner at the Imperial Hotel.[18] Speeches abounded and celebrations ended about 11 o'clock. The next day Hocken took passage on the *Wanaka*, which stopped at Wellington. While there he met Stephenson Percy Smith, a colleague of Edward Tregear at the Survey Department. It was the beginning of a long and fruitful friendship.

Hocken arrived in England in early May and stayed first in London. After an interval of 20 years he would have noted a great many changes in the city: the introduction of electricity (Dunedin would not have electric lighting until 1903), the increase in the number of newspapers and periodicals such as the *National Review* and the *Pall Mall Gazette*, and the increased variety of transport available. As a medical professional, Hocken visited hospitals and charitable organisations and felt that the Benevolent Institute in Dunedin compared favourably: 'Seeing as I did, whilst in England, something of the squalor and wretchedness amongst the poor, the conclusion was often forcibly impressed on with regard to the recipients of our own charity that their lives have indeed, comparatively speaking, fallen in pleasant places – well housed, fed and cared for.'[19]

But London was the centre of the book world, and its bibliophilic delights would have held far greater sway and attraction than hospitals. One item Hocken purchased on this trip was George French Angas's *New Zealanders Illustrated* – 'this magnificent work' – which contained superb hand-coloured engravings from the artist's original sketches and paintings and had been published by Thomas McLean in London in 1846.[20] In the course of several visits to McLean's son, another Thomas, at the firm's headquarters at No. 26 Haymarket, Hocken made his historical interests clear and drove home the fact that he had been searching for Angas's book for many years. McLean revealed that he did have a copy, but it was his father's and he was loath to part with it. On 8 August McLean wrote to Hocken confirming that the copy was available for £22 10s. Not only did this particular copy have an established provenance, but it was in the original 10 parts, never having been opened. For any collector, this is the perfect scenario; Hocken called it 'the best'. He secured it for £21. A January 1883 note in the front of the book says: 'We however became friendly & Mr McLean interested in my interest in, & account of New Zealand, at length consented to let me have his copy.'[21]

Hocken had been assiduous and persistent in his hunt for the Angas. Book agencies and sales in Dunedin, Wellington or Sydney may have satisfied some of his book needs, but they offered meagre pickings compared with what was available on the English book market.[22] About 1880 or even earlier, he was writing to British antiquarian booksellers Bernard Quaritch and Henry Sotheran, asking for their assistance in obtaining the Angas. The ledgers listing nineteenth-century buyers of books from Quaritch are in the British Library. On 4 June 1882 Quaritch, or one of his staff, wrote in one: 'Angas New Zealanders, folio Dr Hocken Dunedin, NZ'. In the margin is the note 'o.a.' (on approval), which further confirms Hocken's good standing with the firm.[23] Eight days later another entry lists 11 titles earmarked for him:

> Grammar and Vocab of NZ language (1820)
> Earle, Collection of lithographic drawings of NZ (1839)
> Beavan's Narrative of a voyage to NZ (1842)
> Fitzroy's Remarks on NZ (1846)
> Angas New Zealanders (1846)
> Oliver's Lithographic drawings from sketches of NZ (1852)
> NZ Company reports Nos 1–8 & 27 and after (1840)
> Tuckett's Report of an exploring expedition to Otago (1845)
> New Zealand Journal – any numbers of (1841 and after)
> Tancred, Notes in Natural History (1856)
> Bunyan's Pilgrim's Progress in Maori (1854).[24]

Presumably Hocken examined these titles in person and decided against the Quaritch Angas because he had already begun pursuing the superior McLean copy. He also decided against the Beavan, but paid for the other titles through his Colonial Bank of New Zealand account. He would have been pleased, especially on obtaining Kendall's early *Grammar*, the Earle (misdated) and Oliver's illustrative works.

Other Quaritch ledgers are arranged geographically. In the 'Asia, Africa Australia' ledger for 1899, Hocken is listed with 'Moray Place' scored out and 'The Octagon' replacing it. More importantly, there are indications of the collecting fields Hocken was interested in: 'F.A.' (Fine Arts), 'New Zealand' and 'Old Colonial Newspapers'.[25] He is not the only southern collector mentioned. Among the others are William Blaxland Benham, who was professor of biology at the University of Otago; prominent churchman the Rev. A.R. Fitchett; and Joseph Wood of the Supreme Court Library. Other New Zealand book collectors named included Sir George Grey, with 'in England' and then 'Dead' above his name, Invercargill's Robert McNab, Dr Young, the Southland Institute, Alexander Turnbull, Elsdon Best, and James Hector, representing the Colonial Museum in Wellington.

Hocken also called on Sotheran, Quaritch's leading opposition. There is no evidence of any purchases made, but he paid the firm's bookbinders £6 to bind the 10 parts of the Angas into one volume. He then took the bound copy back to McLean and asked if he could certify the details of the transaction on the firm's stationery. The tipped-in letter remains in the book today with the additional note by Hocken: 'This copy was the private property of the publisher. T. McLean Jr.'

On 23 June, about a month after he arrived, Hocken attended the ninth annual conversazione of the Royal Colonial Institute, held in the South Kensington Museum. On this grand occasion some 2000 people were present, including fellow 'Otagians' Mary and Elizabeth Hume, runholder and former politician Francis Rich and his wife, and Sir Francis and Lady Dillon Bell.[26] Hocken knew Bell, who was agent general for New Zealand in London and a fellow Mason. Some months before, when both men were in Dunedin, Bell had contacted Hocken about an appendix operation for a family member at Shag Valley Station, a run he owned near Dunedin.[27] This renewed acquaintance over tea proved a catalyst to Hocken's enquiries on the whereabouts of the New Zealand Company records. Bell was once a New Zealand Company clerk in the London office, and then an appointed agent in Nelson and New Plymouth. He was, however, unable to help. As he explained in a brief note to Hocken on 8 August 1882, the papers were not now in the Colonial Office: 'In all probability they were handed over, many years ago, to the [Public] Record office; but it is not certainly known whether this is the case.'[28] This is exactly what had happened, in June 1869 as Hocken would later discover.

Another unsuccessful sortie during this time was a search for the minute books of the Lay Association, an agency of the Free Church of Scotland established to promote the early settlement of Otago in conjunction with the New Zealand Company. The first meeting was held at the Eagle Tavern, Glasgow, on 16 May 1845 with individuals such as William and Allan Buchanan, the Rev. Thomas Burns, Andrew Aldcorn and William Cargill in attendance. Although Hocken later managed to obtain 'old papers' relating to the association, he failed to find the minutes, which 'must have contained much interesting historical detail'. He feared 'they had been destroyed many years before as useless rubbish!'[29]

Hocken also reconnected with family. His younger brother William lived in London at 48 Camberwell Road, Newington, Lambeth, and Joshua Jr was living in Liverpool where he was a successful chemist.[30] Hocken certainly went north, where he made one of his many pilgrimages to Farsley, near Leeds, which was the home village of Samuel Marsden. To find the actual birthplace of his hero Marsden relied on the Rev. James Maning – a relative of Judge Maning – who when the association was pointed out, replied, 'Yes, I believe I have some relative out in the colonies who has been there many years.' Aside from directing Hocken to 'Turner's fold', where Marsden was born, Maning, who was vicar from 1846 to 1891, gave him a copy of the *Proposed Memorial to the Late Rev. Samuel Marsden, at Farsley, near Leeds, 7 November 1866*, which details a printed list of donors to the memorial and a yellow leaflet headed

'Descriptions of windows at Farsley Church'.³¹ To keep these ephemeral items safe, Hocken filed them in his F&J Volume 6. Farsley, he discovered, was

> now of almost new growth – nearly all the old houses being replaced by very recent ones. A small block of four or five cottages alone remains with the date 1757 over them. It was behind these that Marsden was born in a small enclosure then called 'Turner's fold'. It was the practice then to keep a few sheep or cattle in such folds. This fold is now built over with a few dirty little cottages. It was situated on the right hand side of the street going up the incline but on the opposite side.

Hocken also visited nearby Calverley, some 3 km from Farsley, where Marsden was baptised at St Wilfred's Church. James Wright Hatton, the vicar, showed Hocken the baptismal registrar with Marsden's entry, and he stayed for the Sunday service.³² He then visited the nearby village of Stanningley where he had tea with woollen manufacturer Elijah Slater who, though interested in 'everything related to' Marsden, could not tell him anything new.

Hocken repeated all the above information, and more, in an October 1888 letter to Lizzie Betts, Marsden's granddaughter. He also conveyed to her his completist approach to collecting: 'no letter or document should be cast aside as too trivial for the purpose in view. It may contain but a grain of information, may supply a missing date, or may throw some light on something obscure.'³³ This approach applied equally to Hocken's pilgrimages, his need to touch history by walking the same paths, seeing the places and, as far as humanly possible, experiencing the worlds of those who interested him.

The Linnean Society, London

The Linnean Society, founded in 1788 and named after the Swedish botanist Carl Linnaeus (1707–1778), is situated in the west wing of Burlington House on Piccadilly in London. The society acquired the botanical, zoological and library collections of Linnaeus, that extraordinary systematist, in 1829 via the first president, founder and collector Sir James Edward Smith (1759–1828). One day in 1882 Hocken walked up the steps of this august building. His name had been put forward to become a member, a Fellow of the Linnean Society of London. Candidacy involved three nominators and he was at Burlington House to secure the signatures of eminent entomologist Robert McLachlan, Benjamin Daydon Jackson, a respected botanical bibliographer who was also secretary of the society, and Edward Augustus Petherick, an English collector raised in Australia, who was back in London as the British buyer for Australian bookseller George Robertson.

Hocken may have known the other two men by reputation, but Petherick was his key acquaintance. The bookseller, publisher and collector of Australiana was riding high.³⁴ As well as the Linnean Society, Petherick belonged to the Royal Geographical Society, the Hakluyt Society, the Library Association and the Royal Colonial Institute. His intention was to create a bibliography of printed works about Australia. As he wrote in 1878, 'the business of the London department being well organised, I took up the work again; but finding I could do little without the books, I began to collect them – as they came within my grasp, and the savings of a limited salary.'[35] Further employment came as bibliographer for Stephen William Silver's York Gate Library, which was housed at Silver's fashionable John Nash-designed townhouse at 3 York Gate, Regent's Park. Silver had taken over his father's exporting and banking business and produced a very successful *Emigrants' Guide to Australia, New Zealand, The Cape of Good Hope* (1859). He was chairman of the India-Rubber and Telegraph Company, Deputy-Lieutenant of the City of London, Governor of St Thomas's, St Bartholomew's and Bridewell hospitals and a Fellow of the Linnean, Botanic, Zoological, Colonial, Bible and Geographical societies. He also had land holdings near Marton in New Zealand.[36] Silver's 5000-volume library, which was accessible to visitors and researchers, included many treasures, such as rare collections of Hakluyt and Purchas, many original editions of accounts by early travellers, a perfect copy of the Latin de Bry, manuscript diaries of Joseph Banks's voyages to Newfoundland and Labrador in 1766, relics of Captain Cook's expeditions, a coloured copy of the 1598 edition of *Theatrum Orbis Terrarum* by Abraham Ortelius and the very rare Arnold Colom's *Zee-atlas*, showing the earth's sea coasts (Amsterdam, 1658). It is not clear whether Hocken saw Silver's library in 1882, but he certainly did so in December 1903 during an extended visit to England.[37]

In September 1882 Petherick was celebrating the fruit of his labours: the privately printed octavo *Catalogue of the York Gate Geographical and Colonial Library*. Its appearance boosted his standing in literary and antiquarian circles and prompted Silver to commission a supplement, a second edition called *An Index to the Literature of Geography, Maritime and Inland Discovery, Commerce and Civilization*, which was later published by John Murray in 1886. Hocken was on hand to share Petherick's joy. He was with the bibliographer on 25 September when the initial copies of the 1882 *Catalogue* arrived, and he secured one, as the note in the front confirms: 'This copy (one of the two first printed) was given to me by Mr Petherick on its receipt from the printer this day. Mr Petherick had much [all] to do in the cataloguing, & he revised, if he did not write, the preface. The prolegomena at least are his selection.' This was not the only book Hocken received from Petherick. When Benjamin Franklin's *Scheme of a Voyage to Convey the Conveniences of Life, Domestic Animals, Corn, Iron, etc. to New Zealand* (1771) was reprinted in a limited edition of 50 copies in 1882, Hocken secured two copies from him, Nos 23 and 49.[38]

Confirmation of membership of august societies can often be glacially slow. Hocken was back in Dunedin before he learned that his Linnean Society candidacy was successful. On 1 March 1883 he officially became a Fellow on the grounds of his 'Attachment to the study of natural history, especially that of New Zealand and Polynesia'. Coincidentally, that same month Petherick became a member of the Otago Institute, and in later years he sent Hocken copies of his own compilations, *The Colonial Book Circular and Bibliographical Record* (September 1887) and *The Torch and Colonial Book Circular* (December 1887; 31 March 1890), which are filed as part of Hocken's pamphlet collection.[39]

As a Fellow of the Linnean Society, Hocken joined a long line of distinguished individuals such as Darwin, Charles Lyell, Alfred Russel Wallace and Robert Brown. There was also the New Zealand contingent: William Swainson, George French Angas, Walter Buller, Thomas Kirk and Alexander Turnbull, the latter elected on 19 February 1891.[40] Membership was updated regularly, as were subscriptions for the *Transactions*. A recently discovered letter at the archives of the Linnean Society documents Hocken forwarding his £6 for both 1885 and 1886, and giving his address to ensure receipt of the volumes and those he had not got the previous year.[41] Hocken took immense pride in being an 'FLS'. As already mentioned, he created a specific bookplate and added the initials in ink to the bookplates already in hundreds of his books. Hocken was never shy about self-promotion, and recognised that such actions aid immortality.

Before his return to New Zealand Hocken pottered about in London, persisting with 'pertinent enquiries' about the derelict ship lying in Dusky Bay.[42] He visited the offices of Shaw Savill line but to no avail. He also made 'minute but unavailing inquiry' about John Gilfillan's *Interior of a Native Village or Pa in New Zealand*, and even walked 'end to end' of Arundel Street in the Strand asking for information on Captain F. Moore, who had organised lithographic copies of the original to be made.[43] Part of this inquiry led him back to Shaw Savill, but again he found nothing.

It was time to go home. After travelling via Melbourne he arrived back in Dunedin on 23 December 1882. It is easy to imagine the pleasure he took in re-examining the books he had obtained overseas and in anticipating those that had yet to arrive.

8
In Her Own Right

Within seven months of returning from England, on 24 July 1883, Hocken married Elizabeth (Bessie) Mary Buckland at St John's Church, Invercargill.[1] He was 47, she 34. The newspaper notice of the marriage included Hocken's newly acquired status of 'FLS'.

The couple may have met when Bessie Buckland was visiting her brothers in the south: her older brother, John Channing Buckland, was a farmer, and MP for Waikouaiti from 1884 to 1887; her third brother, Henry, had a run in that district. A.G. Hocken suggests that Hocken and Bessie crossed paths while she was travelling in Europe during 1879 to 1881, but this is an unlikely scenario as Hocken himself did not go to England until early 1882.[2] However they met, it was, as Hocken wrote in an 1890 birthday message to his 'dearest wife', 'a propitious fate' that linked them together.[3] There was obviously a strong attraction between the diminutive doctor and the taller Bessie, a fact that is borne out in their surviving correspondence, which is amorous, playful and full of gossip.

Bessie Buckland was born in Auckland on 25 October 1848. She had nine siblings — five brothers and four sisters — and was a wealthy woman in her own right: in 1882 she owned land in Auckland to the value of £2500.[4] The first Buckland to arrive in New Zealand was her father, William Thorne Buckland (1820–1876), who came to New Zealand from Adelaide in 1841. He became involved in house building, purchased land in 1850 and supplied beef stock to the troops during the war of the 1860s. He was president of the Auckland and New Ulster Agricultural and Horticultural Society (later the Agricultural and Pastoral Association), and represented Raglan and Franklin on the Auckland Provincial Council and the House of Representatives.[5] Buckland was also a skilled linguist, and his facility in Maori helped him to negotiate the lease and subsequent purchase of land near Cambridge in the Waikato. He went on to become a major landowner in the area.[6] Buckland was described as 'of a bright intellect, keen perceptions, strong physique and undaunted courage', and local Maori nicknamed him 'Te Pukeran' (The Buckland) because of his pioneering and 'Toa' (warrior) spirit.[7] He was also said to be fair and just. His brother Alfred, who arrived in New Zealand and as an auctioneer had extensive connections in the wool trade, built Highwic, now a notable historical home in Auckland.

In recognition of Bessie's personal wealth, the couple drew up what we would now call a pre-nuptial agreement the day before their wedding:

> To Miss Elizabeth Buckland
> In consideration of the marriage shortly to be solemnized between you and myself I hereby convey transfer assign and give to you all my real and

personal property of every kind and description and wheresoever the same may be for your own sole and separate use and benefit and to be dispersed of by deed will or other writing as you or your absolute discretion shall think fit. And I declare that all real and personal property now and hereafter possessed by you shall remain your separate estate. And I agree when required by you to execute all necessary documents to complete this agreement and to vest all such property in yourself.
Thomas Morland Hocken; Elizabeth Mary Buckland.[8]

Very little is known of Bessie's formative years, but her life changed drastically on 4 September 1871 when her mother Susan, aged 50, committed suicide by stabbing herself in the neck with her own nail scissors. Twenty-three-year-old Bessie and her older sister Marianne had been looking after Susan, who was 'subject to great mental despondency'.[9] It was Bessie who first went into her mother's bedroom and discovered the bloodied body. Then, despite becoming 'slightly insensible', she instructed her sister to get the family physician. The next day she and Marianne relived the experience by giving depositions at the inquest held at the family home at Pine Terrace House, Grafton. There had been warning signs: Susan Buckland had been depressed, hardly eating. She had also attempted suicide six years before, when the family was living in the Waikato. They had then all promised to look after her, never leaving her alone.

It is impossible to gauge the impact of such a tragedy on a young woman, but this event may help to explain Bessie's overprotective attitude towards her husband and their only child Gladys, who was born on 12 June 1884. As photographs show, Bessie had strong angular features and, although not beautiful, was distinguished — more than the 'plain comely wife' she claimed to be.[10] Dunedin writer C.R. Allen called her 'plain', but he also called Hocken 'dwarfish' and 'almost grotesque' so his opinion must be regarded with some caution.[11] From all accounts Bessie always presented herself well. For example, at an evening party at Heriot Row in April 1894, her dress was described as 'black silk stylishly trimmed with yellow veiled in black lace, black floral bonnet', while at the 'Daffodil Ball' in September 1897, where on behalf of the St Paul's Cathedral Guild she provided and arranged the entertainment, she was dressed in 'black with lace and jet'.[12] But Bessie was much more than just a fine hostess, fulfilling all the social duties expected of the wife of a notable Dunedin identity: she was highly cultured, well educated, a linguist, a competent musician and a talented artist.

Bessie belonged to a number of associations and organisations. There was the Kahanga Club, a Dunedin ladies' group of about 120, which held regular meetings in members' homes. Cards (whist, euchre), music and informal lectures provided the usual entertainments. At a meeting held at Atahapara in August 1896 it was reported that 'Mrs Hocken's large rooms were strained to their utmost to find accommodation for all. A most enjoyable evening was spent.' On this occasion Miss Towsey gave a pianoforte solo, Mrs Sale gave an 'instructive' reading, Miss Lily Shand delivered a vocal solo, Mrs Shand imitated an old Scotch woman, Miss Ethel Neill and Mrs Monkman sang some songs and Miss S. Bartleman and Miss Greenwood closed with a 'clever little dialogue'. There were 'delicious refreshments' during the interval.[13] At another meeting Bessie read Banjo Patterson's poem, 'Clancy of the Overflow', which was 'new to most of the audience, and most pathetic'.[14]

Bessie also belonged to the Free Kindergarten Association along with Sir Robert and Lady Stout, among others.[15] In January 1893 she was present at a meeting of the Jubilee Convalescent Fund, which was dedicated to sending five girls to the country for rest and change. She gave £1 towards the enterprise.[16] In 1905 Bessie was an active member of the Dunedin branch of the Victoria League, inaugurated as a memorial to the late monarch, which supported and assisted any scheme leading to a more intimate understanding between subjects in Britain and the empire. Practical work was encouraged by sponsoring visits and scholarships, holding lectures, preparing small popular histories and offering prizes in colonial schools. In May 1905 she was voted in as secretary. She looked after the 'Newton' lantern slides, which were sent as promotional materials from London, and she actively promoted Canadian Tercentenary celebration picture cards to local schools.[17] In May 1909 she and Hocken became subscribers to the newly formed Society for the Promotion of the Health of Women and Children.[18]

As early as March 1887 Bessie was registered as a Ladies Committee member of the Otago Society for the Prevention of Cruelty to Animals; by 1896 her daughter Gladys was a subscriber, giving 10s 6d.[19] She was a proud pet owner, having at one time cats, dogs, parrots and ponies. In September 1894 when Bessie was holidaying with Gladys at Kinloch, at the head of Lake Wakatipu, Hocken wrote assuring them that all the animals were well.[20] Bessie also seemed to have her own collecting penchant: teaspoons. She received examples from James Hector and local friend John Halliday Scott, who reported to his daughters in 1909: 'on Sunday I dined with the Hockens and gave Mrs Hocken her spoon with which she seemed pleased'.[21] Like most women of her time and class, Bessie did needlework and embroidery. Her tablecloth in the Hocken Collection is embroidered with the signatures of significant donors and acquaintances. It is but one outstanding example of her work.

As would have been expected, especially given her husband's standing in the community, Bessie attended 'at homes' and accompanied him to events such as a farewell function for the Governor and Countess of Onslow in February 1892. In the same month she attended an afternoon tea at Mrs Joachim's, which welcomed back Professor and Mrs Sale. On 26 April 1893 she was present at the marriage ceremony of William H. Field and Isabel Jane Hodgkins (sister of the more famous Frances). Bessie was also a capable organiser of entertainment. In May 1893, for example, she helped to oversee a ball for visiting Cantabrians at the Pirates Football Club and received an honourable mention: [she] 'gave very valuable assistance, left nothing to be desired'.[22]

Bessie suffered bouts of ill-health which may have been nervous breakdowns or – as A.G. Hocken suggests – she became something of a cardiac neurotic.[23] Many of her visits to Kinloch were taken for recovery and rejuvenation, even though she still had to care for Gladys. On one occasion, Hocken wrote: 'So often through the day do I think of you & *yearn* after you – but with my desire for your return, for I picture to myself how much rest & health you must be gaining in that delightful mountain air & with our troublesome little girl by your side. Drink plenty of milk & don't forget your medicine.'[24]

Bessie ran an excellent household and gave frequent dinner and luncheon parties for the wealthy circle to which the Hockens belonged. According to Ruby Neill, one of Gladys's childhood friends, the food was good and the company stimulating. And because the Hockens were considered 'rather exclusive', there was a certain *cachet* in being invited.[25] Bessie not only mingled with the cultural and intellectual elite, including such notables as visiting satirist Mark Twain and the English 'Prince of Journalists' and gastronomic buff, Augustus Sala, but also held her own, especially in male company. She knew and corresponded with Sir George Arney (New Zealand's second chief justice, who died in 1883); interpreter and writer C.O.B. Davis; Thomas Pratt (Tame Parata of Pukiteraki); Samuel Tarratt Nevill, the first Anglican bishop of Dunedin; Professor William Benham; Stephenson Percy Smith in Wellington; the Australian-based ex-Dunedin civil engineer L.O. Beal; G.W. Pogson, an ex-Strath Taieri runholder based in Tasmania; and woolbroker John Sutcliffe Horsfall of Narrandera, New South Wales, who was a pastoral adviser to the New Zealand Loan and Mercantile Agency.[26] Obviously proud of her husband's achievements, she also bore the brunt of his enthusiasms and knew the right time to leave him to his passions. James Backhouse Walker, an Australian solicitor and historian and one of Hocken's correspondents, has left a personal glimpse of a night at the Hockens' on 6 March 1898:

> Back to Hotel, changed & to Dr Hocken's for dinner. Very little round man with grey hair. Mrs Hocken very charming. Daughter nice girl but shy. Sat over wine talking about Hot Lakes & what to see, the Dr having been there several times. Also abt Hone Heke war & comp'd a/cs of Toby Philpots death & Okiwai pah, Despard &c Ruapekapeka with Geo. Clarke – found they agreed remarkably. To select him partics from G.C.'s lecture. Then to his study & joined Mrs H. He showed me 4 drawings by Sergt Williams of Hone Heke – the attack on Owikauai & Ruapekapeka. Talk abt books & comp. notes. Mrs H's signs not to speak of books he hadn't got. He shewed me Hob[art]. Spectator as bribe for NZ Festival litho. Talk abt Frank Pogson. Mrs H. retired. The Dr finally showed us his splendid coll'n of Maori relics &c.[27]

Bessie was sometimes a reluctant companion. In June 1892 Hocken booked tickets for them both to hear the visiting explorer Henry M. Stanley's last lecture on African pygmies. Fearing her reluctance to attend, he enticed her: 'I shall have everything comfortable & cosy for you & a nice warm bath. Won't it be delightful to get back?'[28] There was also some playful disparagement about his collecting, hinted at by Hocken in a letter from Wellington in February 1894: 'I have been as usual principally with Mantell & have got quite a boxful of "rubbish" as you will call it.'[29]

Bessie had land investments and, like her husband, owned stocks and shares.[30] It is possible that both perused the pamphlets and prospectuses that now form a pamphlet volume headed 'Manufacturers' in Hocken's collection. This includes an ex-General Assembly Library copy of *Outline History of the Gold, Coal, and Other Known Mineral Resources of New Zealand* (1886), Walter Pearson's *The Financial Position of the Colony of NZ* (1887), and L.O. Beal's *Guide for Gold Mining Investors* (1889).[31] Bessie was also financially involved with her husband in the New Era dredge operation at the Port of Otago.

Gladys was the Hockens' only child, and very close to her mother. 'Father and I never seem to be able to get on well ... and mother acts as a kind of go between. She has been a mother, companion and sister all in one.'[32] Bessie delighted in photographing her daughter, who was considered lovely.[33] Observers, however, recognised the overindulgence lavished on an only child. As John Halliday Scott wrote in 1910, 'I have seen Mrs Hocken on several occasions. Her plans I find are very vague, and she does not know how long she will be away. She is quite under Gladys' thumb in such things and while that young lady talks at one time of being away for three years, next day she will say that she could not think of leaving for more than eighteen months at the very outside.'[34] Hocken, as the lone male, was often the butt of humour by his womenfolk. This is evident in his response to a suitor's intentions towards Gladys, captured amusingly by Bessie in a letter to her daughter in January 1907. She had been out and came home to find Hocken 'sitting white & fierce with the letter before him'. According to Bessie, he said at once, 'Read this!' He then 'considered it right to ring up [John] White & tell him what he thought of him, & then the fun began'. Bessie described the phone call:

> 'Is that Mr White? I wish to say that we are much pained – my daughter & I – at your extraordinary behaviour – much pained – I beg your pardon – what did you say? I can't hear you – speak louder! Misapprehension? There's no misapprehension & I have to beg that you'll desist – what did you say? Christchurch? Are you saying that you are going to Chch? I hope so – can't hear what you say – that you will write me? I don't want your letters!' (here I thought that Williams between his anxiety not to miss any of the conversation & his wild efforts to stop laughing, would choke & die). 'No. I don't want that. What do you say? Christchurch? Very well, you are going on to Chch. Then Good Night!' (This last like a fierce

threat). And off he rang! ... This morning Dad said to me 'What I dislike about the whole thing is that he should put such ideas into our little girl's head.'[35]

When Bessie married she gave 'London' as her place of residence. It is not known when or how long she stayed there, but it was perhaps in England or at a European finishing school like one that Gladys eventually attended that Bessie acquired her abilities in Italian, German, French and Dutch. They stood her in good stead, especially as she was the key translator-cum-communicator when visiting the Mediterranean, the Middle East and Europe with her husband between 1901 and 1904. Bessie continued to read Italian, getting the occasional Italian paper delivered to Moray Place, and in later years owned a copy of Giuseppe Capra's *L'Australia nei suoi rapporti con l'Italia* (1910).[36] She read French, as did Gladys, and even supplied French novels to her friends.[37]

In December 1893 Percy Smith, one of Hocken's most prolific correspondents, wrote asking if he could enlist the services of 'your niece Miss Hocken' to translate some Dutch passages that his friend Elsdon Best was finding hard to decipher in his work on the alphabet of Malaysia.[38] The 'niece' was actually Bessie. The work was done, and represented a precursor to a much larger and more important undertaking. Smith's thanks appear in a letter tipped into Hocken's copy of George Windsor Earl's *The Eastern Seas* (1837) – one of the few occasions that Bessie is given credit for her work:

> My dear Dr Hocken,
> How am I to thank you and Mrs Hocken sufficiently for your kindness in translating that long Dutch passage? I have not had time to see Mr Best yet but I am quite sure he will feel deeply indebted to you. He has been making a study of the Malaysian alphabet for some years and has a great deal of information about them which he will not I think allow to rust in a cupboard. Really it was exceedingly kind of Mrs Hocken to take so much trouble. By glancing into it I see the paper is very interesting ...[39]

Bessie's Dutch translation skills came to the fore with her work on 'Abel Tasman and his journal', the project that Hocken had announced to his listeners during his 11 September 1894 lecture to the Otago Institute. Bessie was that 'valued coadjutor' who gave the collated voyage component an 'English dress'. That month she was entrusted with the manuscript while on holiday at Moeraki. On 2 September Hocken was imploring her to finish 'the full & proper translation'. The bad weather was surely a help: 'I fancy you would have been glad to have taken the material out with you in this weather.'[40] The following day another letter arrived: 'You will see the black mark in Tasman indicating the N.Z. portion. If you have time after completing it you might do the Tasmanian (Van Diemen's Land) portion which just precedes. This would make the translation very interesting & perfect.' His postscript read 'Take *great care* of Tasman.'[41] 'Abel Tasman and his journal' was eventually read to Otago Institute members on 10 September 1895 and published in Volume 28 of the *Transactions* that year.[42] It was an important publication, gaining international recognition by scholars in Holland and experts on Tasman in Australia.

Bessie's work was not acknowledged, and in fact Hocken claimed credit for the translation on at least one occasion. While interviewing Hocken in 1908 Annie Trimble asked him: 'But this is English … Who translated it?' Her article went on: '"I did," replied the Doctor, modestly. "There was no English translation, so I learnt Dutch, in order to find out for myself all about it." He laughed. "And as soon as I had finished I promptly forgot all my Dutch."'[43] Full credit for Bessie's efforts would come later.

Hocken corresponded with – and eventually met, in Europe and in Dunedin in 1906 – C.A. de Fleurieu, a descendant of the French explorer and hydrographer Charles Pierre Claret de Fleurieu. All of Fleurieu's long letters dealing with French expeditions to the Pacific, historical errors on maps and other matters, were written in French and Bessie again came to the fore, providing useful extracts and translations.[44]

It also seems that Bessie, like her father, had knowledge of Maori. She once owned a copy of the *New Testament* in Maori (W233) in Hocken's collection, which previously belonged to politician, pastoralist and writer Josiah C. Firth and was then given to one Manihera on 23 March 1867. It was then gifted by Manihera to 'Elisabeth Meri Pulkanal' [Buckland] at Taupo in 1868. Her initials 'E.M.B.' are on a preliminary page.[45] Although the possession of one book does not constitute hard evidence of any language skills, there is a hint that she had some competency. On 16 June 1892 she attended a Kahanga Club meeting where, in front of 50 others including Gladys, she gave 'an interesting reading from a Maori translation'.[46]

Bessie was also musical. She played the piano part for Mendelssohn's 'Romance' at a conversazione of the Early History Society of Otago on 17 April 1885, and played at the Dresden Pianoforte Company City Hall's Grand Tableaux Concert in aid of funds for St Paul's pro-cathedral (and later gave £5).[47] Her skill as a pianist did not, however, seem to extend to care of her instrument: in 1907 she wrote to Gladys: 'Piano tuner came yesterday & said the piano was *very* dusty inside. Showed me how to dust keyboard.' She enjoyed going to theatre and musical performances. In the same letter she told her daughter: 'I forgot to say that we got good seats at the Band, but it was packed. I liked the encores best.'[48]

Morland and Bessie were very close. Their letters speak of their deep affection and how much they missed each other when apart. Writing to Bessie from Dunedin on 24 January 1888, Hocken addresses her as 'Dearest Sweetheart' and blames 'something peculiar about the mails' for not having heard from her for a week: 'This is my third letter.' After telling her all his news he ends: 'And now darling good bye & many kisses. I know you often think of me & wish I were by your side. I am sure I do. Won't it be delightful when we can take our trips together. Ever yours Morland.'⁴⁹

The following January Bessie is away again, at Wanaka, and Hocken sits down at 10 o'clock on a Sunday night 'to enjoy a chat with my dear sweetheart'. He relates all that has been going on and assures her that 'Everything is going well here so thoroughly enjoy yourself.' Her 'most welcome & long looked for letter came yesterday after our separation of 8 days … It was so pleasant … to know that you were so thoroughly enjoying your surroundings. Do go to the Diamond Lake & other places of interest.' Ever the collector, he asks: 'Try to bring a few native plants back with you. The rata is metrosideros – your species is probably lucida but of course I could not be certain without examining a specimen. Now, dearest, good night & for more pleasant dreams of you (& I have had some already). Your loving husband Morland.'⁵⁰

In March of that same year Hocken is in Auckland, writing to his 'Dearest Geliebte [beloved]' from the Northern Club. 'What will my darling sweetheart say to all this long silence! The fact is it was simply unavoidable since the last scrap of a postcard from Oneroa & until this morning I have been in places the most inaccessible & out of the way & where there has been no post office, nor mail, nor telegraph, nor any sign of civilization.' But, despite the longest silence that has ever elapsed between us' she must not 'fancy for a moment that pleasant thoughts & longings for your dear self have ever been absent. Constantly have I wondered what you are doing, how you were, & how delightful above all things it would be to be by your side & kiss you. It would be useless as impossible to tell you what I have been doing; all this must be reserved for our pleasant chats.' He tells her all the places he has visited: 'By far the pleasantest trip I have ever had because so complete.' He has walked many kilometres each day and is 'as brown as a berry & as high spirited as possible. It will require all your wifely efforts to reduce me to a proper & modest condition again. I should like to say a good deal on this point but perhaps had better not. It is sufficient to say that length of absence does but make me grow warmer, truer if possible, & more desirous of being with you.'⁵¹

When writing to Bessie from Moray Place late on the evening of 25 May 1890 he can report that he has 'been working at the congenial task of the catalogue & now for a rest before going to bed I chat with you. Everything has gone on perfectly well. When I came back from the station Gladys was dressing her doll & I am glad to say was not distressed by your departure – nor indeed has she been since.' Bessie is in Kinloch caring for a sick friend, Janine. Gladys has company, a school chum called Lyndon. The latter is 'of course as good as gold. Gladys is as usual quarrelsome & unruly, however I am looking after her.' Dinner was 'famous … The children stuffing to repletion.' They have been doing 'a great deal of painting & upsetting of water. They send you the enclosed – how to be distributed I forget.' He discusses the best place to address his next letter – 'you will leave Kinloch on Friday noon reaching Queenstown at 3 so I will address it to Eichardt's' [hotel] – and reports that the children 'have given me about a thousand kisses to be distributed amongst you. The weather is fine & lovely & a bright starlight night. And now my own Geliebte adieu. I constantly think of what you are doing & am so pleased that our separation is of so short duration. Kisses to you all over & much love. I send the Star & £1. Thine ever Morland.'[52]

Bessie's reply, from Queenstown, assures Hocken that Janine is 'much better' and 'I certainly shall come back myself to my treasures': 'For where your treasure is there will your heart be also.' She gives news of friends then writes: 'You cannot think how I long all day to have that magic glass of our Arabian nights friend, & keep on you all, and yet you were cruel enough not to send a telegram today. But you never will understand what it is to be anxious.' After sending a 'hundred kisses to be divided between Gladys & Lyndon' she ends: 'Do you love me? Ever your Gebliechte [sic].'[53]

✳   ✳   ✳

Bessie Hocken's greatest talent lay in her abilities as an artist in oils and watercolour, and as a photographer. And in these activities her achievements were recognised. She regularly exhibited with the Otago Art Society from 1887 to 1914 and was a council member in 1899 and again in 1908.[54]

Natural landscapes and botanical subjects seemed to dominate her oeuvre. She exhibited a flower painting in November 1888, for example, followed by *Broad Leaf, Purakanui* in February 1890 and works such as *Yellow Kowhai and Native Orchids* and *Ribbonwood Blossom and Native Orchids* in November 1891. Her *Study of Black Pine*, shown in December 1892, was described as 'a very meritorious example'. (Eight-year-old Gladys also had a painting on display in this show.) Further exhibitions included pictures such as *Evening, the Nuggets* and *All Day Bay* in November 1896; *Vavau Harbour* and *Waimanu, Rewa River, Fiji* in November 1898; and *Forest Glade, Kaka Point* and *Beach Avenue, Paradise* in December 1907. The last two works were described, respectively, as 'a careful and detailed study of old wind-clipped trees dwarfed by the strong sea breezes' and 'a difficult theme carefully and conscientiously rendered, unaided by trickery of exaggerated lights or colour'.[55] She won an award for flower painting at the 1889–90 New Zealand and South Seas Exhibition in Dunedin.[56] Bessie was also generous with the works of others. On her return from visiting Japan in 1904, she exhibited a number of paintings by the Japanese artists Nakamura and Shusen, which the *Otago Witness* classed as 'interesting'.[57]

A small number of Bessie's works are in her husband's collection, including the oil painting of the takahe (*Notornis mantelli*) and three 'J.F. Wohlers' works: *Ruins of the Rev. J.F. Wohlers' House*, *Mr Wohlers' Church and School House* and *Mr Wohlers' Grave, Ringaringa Point, Stewart Island*. The first was painted in

March 1895 when Hocken and Bessie travelled together to Stewart Island. The others were done a year later on another visit. Another watercolour, *The Old Mission Station at Waikouaiti*, is particularly important because it represents one of Bessie's earliest works, sketched in September 1887. In recognition of the house's historical importance as the first European house built in Otago, Hocken supplied an extensive note including dimensions and plans.[58]

Bessie Hocken was also a good amateur photographer, a skill she shared with the family of her older brother John, and especially his daughter Jessie, who became an extremely accomplished photographer. Bessie joined the Dunedin Photographic Society in 1892, two years after it was established. A few of her prints survive including a portrait photograph of Riria Potiki, daughter of Ngai Tahu chief Karetai, taken about 1889, possibly for the New Zealand and South Seas Exhibition.[59] Others include *Arrested Attention*, the well-known image of Hocken and Gladys sitting together at Atahapara, and the *Old Mission Station, Waikouaiti*.[60]

Annual exhibitions often held in conjunction with camera clubs from Nelson, Christchurch and Wellington offered Bessie and her fellow society members opportunities to exhibit their work. In April 1894, for example, she displayed *In the Forest Green* which had a 'nice atmospheric effect', and in May 1897 the 'pick' of the several photographs she showed was the 'very pleasing and soft' *New Zealand Flowers*; other prints were deemed 'somewhat over-exposed'.[61] She also showed a series of photographs at the Otago Agricultural and Pastoral Society show in December 1900, and some of her overseas photographs appeared in the *Otago Witness*.[62]

Bessie even received correspondence about potential subjects, in one case from early conservationist and explorer Richard Henry of Resolution Island: 'You cannot get a shot looking into Cook Creek in Pickersgill Harbour except out of the boat & the movement of the boat spoils them; & looking out of the creek gives a poor picture.'[63] In 1895 she won First Prize Figure Subject in a competition run by the *Australasian* magazine with *Mother's Treasure Box*, a photograph of 11-year-old Gladys sitting on a small chair in front of a dressing-table, holding a hand-mirror and bedecked in finery. Hocken encouraged Bessie's talents – 'I hope you will be able to do a little photography though I fear no sketching owing to the cold' – and recognised subjects that might appeal to her: 'I only regretted that you could not have taken the scene in the garden with the camera. It was perfectly lovely for the snow fell with much gentleness & absence of wind that the snow was deposited quite thickly on every individual leaf, with most exquisite result.'[64]

Bessie's artistic and photographic skills greatly enhanced her husband's collection. Although Hocken always stressed the need for information over aesthetics – 'The value of a picture in itself is but little if there is no full description of that to which it refers. With this description, its educational value is vastly increased' – he found Bessie's copies of the material he collected invaluable.⁶⁵ Her illustrations also appeared in his historical publications, particularly his *Contributions* (1898). The copies she made not only provided him with working copies but also valuable second copies in case of loss. They were often the next best thing to the original, particularly when he knew that the original was held elsewhere and that he would never own it. In 1879 he secured three sketches by John Williams and missed out on the fourth sketch of Okaihau, which was bought by Judge Maning and promptly passed through to the Auckland Institute and Museum. Hocken wrote to museum director Thomas Cheeseman:

> I am naturally serious that this series should remain unbroken & that its severed member should be restored. With this in view I beg to offer this proposal to the Council of your Institute:– that if they will give me their picture I will undertake to have a copy made of each of the four pictures & have them framed similarly to the quaint framing of the originals … [and] … that four copies shall be transmitted to the Institute as an exchange.⁶⁶

By March 1889 he was asking just to take a copy of the Okaihau sketch: 'As you know I have the other three pictures painted by him representing the destruction of Pomare's pa, Ohaeawai, & Ruapekepeke & it seems a pity that the series should not be completed. It is needless to say that I shall take every care of so valuable a picture & shall speedily return it.'⁶⁷ Progress was slow: it was not until April 1905 that Hocken could thank Cheeseman for 'the ragged roll you so kindly lent me which I hereby return by this mail. You would not know it in the new dress as done by Mrs Hocken.'⁶⁸

In 1892 when Hocken obtained George Baird Shaw's *View of Dunedin from Church Hill, 1851* for £3, he had Bessie provide a 'key plan' showing the houses of prominent citizens and the location of various services (No. 14: Henry Mayo, grocer; No. 58: John Proudfoot, boot-maker), streets and places. This featured 'for the first time' in his *Contributions*.⁶⁹

A year later, in 1893, he obtained from the estate of Sir William Fox a sketchbook containing some of his 118 sketches and watercolours. Bessie copied a few of these, including views of Lyttelton, the Canterbury Plains and Dunedin. About this time, she also copied H.T. Cridland's early depiction of Riccarton. Surveyor Charles Henry Kettle (1820–1862) played an integral part in the early development of southern New Zealand. In March 1898 Bessie not only made a pen and ink key plan of his *Lower Harbour and Port Chalmers* but also later copied his 1849 *View of Dunedin* and provided a key sketch to it for her husband's *Contributions*. She also provided keys to James Smetham's 1889 *The New Zealand Chiefs in Wesley's House (1863)* and Stoddart's *New Plymouth, Taranaki (1859)*. Other copying included a watercolour copy of John Alexander Gilfillan's *Sketch of the Chief Hone Heke Pokai* (c. 1845) from an unknown officer's sketch book; a 1903 copy of William Holmes's *The Canterbury Plains from the Heathcote River* (1851); a pen and ink and wash portrait copy of George Rennie, the chief originator of the New Edinburgh or Otago scheme; a copy of Joseph Jenner Merrett's *Ohinemutu Pa on Lake Rotorua*; and a number of watercolours by John Johnson. As was typical, Hocken added historical information that contextualised the item. On Johnson's sepia wash of Government House in Auckland he wrote: 'Government House was brought out in framework from Manning's establishment in Holborn & was erected on the present site of Government House about the end of 1840. It was accidentally burnt down in 1848. The front view faces the North Shore, Mount Eden is behind. TMH.' He noted, too, that Bessie had copied these 'most interesting sketches' from Eliza Hobson's album.

Images from printed publications did not escape Bessie's attention. She copied Sydney Parkinson's painting of Mt Taranaki from his *A Journal of a Voyage to the South Seas* (1773) and selected plate 16, *A War Canoe of New Zealand with a View of Gable End Foreland*, from Volume III of John Hawkesworth's compilation voyages book, also published in 1773. She signed the latter.

Her contribution did not stop there. She transcribed many pages of manuscript text, a tedious task that required patient deciphering and a high degree of accuracy. Manuscripts such as Hocken's fourth southern lecture (9 October 1888) and the journals of the Rev. William Richard Wade, John Wallis Barnicoat and Colonel Charles Stapp contain samples of her hand. The last named was copied from the original in May 1897.[70]

After Hocken's death in 1910, Bessie, as one of his trustees, along with John Halliday Scott, was committed to advancing her husband's legacy. She remained in touch with library and Otago Museum developments, and in 1913 and 1920 she donated further items, including Fox's *Dunedin*, the Parkinson mentioned above, a lithographic copy of George Duppa's *Part of the New Plymouth Settlement, in the District of Taranaki, New Zealand* (n.d.) and a watercolour copy of Merrett's *Three Maoris Seated in Front of a Whare* (1850).

Hocken was a man of his times, reluctant to fully acknowledge his wife's contributions to his work. He did, however, dedicate his *Contributions* to her in 1898. After initial attempts, including 'my wife by whom invaluable counsel & assistance I have always been aided I owe so much', he settled on: 'To My Wife To Whose Counsel and Help I owe So Much.'[71]

9
A Reputation Established

In 1889 schoolmaster John Blair presented Hocken with a copy of his newly published *Lays of the Old Identities*. It was more than just another book destined for a growing collection. The dedication read:

> This volume is respectfully dedicated to Dr Hocken, M.R.C.S., F.L.S., who has laid the community under a deep debt of gratitude for his Lectures on the Early History of New Zealand, and the Otago Settlement in particular. The Doctor has not spared himself in unearthing many valuable documents bearing upon the History of the Good Old Times, which would otherwise have been lost; and I believe, as a friend of mine expressed it the other day, that his name will descend to posterity as the Herodotus of New Zealand.

By the late 1880s Hocken's reputation as a local historian of New Zealand was secure. He had become an authority, primarily through the delivery and printing of his lectures. He was also planning a history of New Zealand. There were public acknowledgements: William Craig's fulsome praise in a letter to the editor of the *Otago Daily Times* – 'Dr Hocken gives us the result of his researches on the early settlement of New Zealand in a more intelligent, unbiased, and masterly manner than those who have previously written on this subject, and it is only fair he should receive public acknowledgement for it' – and an editorial in the *Otago Witness* paying tribute to his 'true historical instinct for research, combined with an agreeable manner of placing his material before us'.[1]

Hocken was also known as a collector of books, maps and manuscripts relating to the early history, development and settlement of New Zealand. Indeed, by September 1885 his collection was sufficiently large to attract George Augustus Sala, who made arrangements to see it.[2] From Auckland, recently retired hospital superintendent Dr Thomas M. Philson presumed Hocken was in 'possession of "The Story of New Zealand" by the late A.S. Thomson', while closer to home, Dean Henry Jacobs of Christchurch wrote to Hocken on 30 April 1887, asking if among his 'treasures' he had a copy of the Rev. William Yate's *An Account of New Zealand* (1835) and, if so, could he supply details on the missionary's arrival in the Bay of Islands.[3] Despite his busy professional schedule Hocken soon replied to Jacobs, who responded within three weeks thanking him for the information, which would be useful for his forthcoming book on church history.[4] Of course there was criticism. After reading an account of one of Hocken's lectures, Agnes J. Burns, daughter of the Rev. Thomas Burns, wrote to put Hocken straight on the naming of Dunedin and John McGlashan's involvement in it 'as I heard it from my late Father'. Hocken, with a mounting armoury of reference and manuscript materials at hand, made a private annotation on the letter: 'Most of this is quite wrong. The name was given by W. Chambers in a letter to the N.Z. Journal dated Oct 30/43 (appeared Nov. 11). Mr McGlashan had nothing whatever to do with N.Z. until 1847 when he was appointed Sec?'[5] But not everyone was aware of Hocken's collection. When Englishman C.W. Holgate toured the chief libraries throughout New Zealand in 1885, accumulating notes that were published the following year as *An Account of the Chief Libraries of New Zealand*, a description of Hocken's collection was noticeably absent.[6] This was perhaps to be expected, given that Holgate was rather derisive of provincial, especially southern, library collections. Hocken owned a copy of Holgate's slim work, which he filed in Volume 48 of his Pamphlet Collection.

Early Accumulations

There is very little hard evidence on when and from whom Hocken obtained his books. His collection lacks a cache of book dealer invoices, and he seemed reluctant to write such details in his books. A physical examination of his entire collection has revealed a few clues to actual acquisition, but his habit of going back to a book or manuscript, annotating it and dating that annotation muddies the acquisitional waters. Most evidence for when he acquired an item is revealed in his correspondence, his travel notes and his printed articles.

One of Hocken's earliest contacts, and a man who played an important role in advancing his collecting and his reputation, was John Webster (1818–1912), the Hokianga-based trader, merchant and settler who was a friend of Judge Frederick Maning, the 'Pakeha-Maori'.[7] After Hocken met Webster early in 1874 the trader, obviously impressed, sent documents on 21 February:

> I found amongst my old papers a chart without date but I have reason to believe it was taken between 1820/28. My father-in-law Mr Russell [timber trader George Frederick Russell] had it in his possession. I send it to you with the old almanack you refer to … If I ever go south I will certainly avail myself of your hospitable offer to visit you. I would I am sure be delighted & equally so if you could again visit me.[8]

Their correspondence continued until Hocken's death in 1910.

The 'Plan of Kawiti's Pa at Ruapekapeka' (1846) was another northern acquisition, obtained early in 1875. It, too, was a gift, given to Hocken by the widow of Major Henry Matson of Parnell. Not only did Hocken get Bessie to create a copy suitable for framing, but he revealed in one of his 'New Zealand' notebooks a family connection: 'Matson's 1st wife was de Thierry's only daughter [Isabel] who died with the infant soon after her first confinement; the present Mrs. M was Miss [Amelia] Buckland, my wife's aunt, & sister of William Thorne Buckland M.H.R.'[9]

An ephemeral item he received as he passed through Wellington about 1880 was a hand-written newspaper that featured original works by Judge C.D.R. Ward, runholder and politician Robert Pharazyn, William Fox and Bethia Featherston who, as Isaac Featherston's wife, is identified by Hocken as 'a Miss Scott [actually Campbell Scott] of Edinburgh'. In the 1850s, these 'scribblers' formed a budding literary group that met regularly in Wellington. The manuscript was given to Hocken by a former governess to the Featherston children.[10]

A local acquisition was the 'convict' bell used at the Wesleyan mission station at Waikouaiti until 1848. In 1880, Hocken paid £1 for this 'sweet-toned' relic with its strong local provenance. Once on a Botany Bay convict vessel, it was obtained by the trader-entrepreneur Johnny Jones, who used it on his whaling brig *Magnet*. He then placed it at the mission, before it was positioned on the church reserve called Bell Hill. It then passed to John Cargill and to John Hyde Harris, from whom Hocken bought it.[11] Another local item was the Letterbook of Charles Henry Kettle, Chief Surveyor of the Settlement of Otago, which was given to Hocken in 1882 by W. John Cargill, son of Captain William Cargill.[12] The manuscript, which spans the years 1846 to 1850, contains letters to Colonel William Wakefield and William Cargill as agents of the New Zealand Company and documents the personal differences between the two. In 1884 Hocken received from Henry Wynyard, son of Colonel Robert Henry Wynyard, a manuscript that detailed the latter's career as an officer and colonial administrator in New Zealand.[13]

By September 1886 Hocken also owned George Thomas Clayton's 'Kororareka in the Bay of Islands, New Zealand' (1845), the inaugural issue of the *New Zealand Gazette* (18 April 1840), the first New Zealand newspaper, a rare issue of Edward Chaffers's survey chart of Port Nicholson (1841), the *New Zealand Journal* (1840), a facsimile copy of the Treaty of Waitangi, Raoul's *Choix des plantes* (1846), Heaphy's 'View of Nelson Haven, in Tasman's Gulf, New Zealand' (1841), a copy of Henry Falwasser's *Auckland Times* produced in 1842 on a clothes mangle, John Williams's three sketches (purchased in 1879), and Lieutenant Wilmot's *Sketch of Heke's Pah at Owhaiawai*.[14] He also secured, in Wellington in 1885, manuscript notes on the manufacture of ammunition and the operation of artillery. These came from C.T. Batkin, whom Hocken described privately as 'a curious looking man, constantly half closing or winking his eyes and sniffing through his nose'. Batkin had been chief clerk and cashier for the central government in Auckland and then assistant controller and auditor general in Wellington. The manuscript 'had been sitting about on shelves of [Batkin's] office as long as he could remember & had probably been brought down from Auckland when the seat of Government was changed'.[15] Hocken's earlier notation that 'It probably belonged to some officer who had been engaged in Hone Heke's war' was later amended to verify attribution to Lieutenant Wilmot.[16] This small gift represented another occasion of generosity that he experienced throughout his collecting career.

Presentation Copies

As we have seen, Hocken gladly accepted presentation copies. By the 1880s his wide-ranging collection included the Rev. Gideon Smales's *Whitby Authors and their Publications* (1867), received 'with the author's best wishes' on 28 February 1881; a copy of *Hinemoa: A love song* (1881) from Maning; a copy of James Stewart's *On the Establishment of a Grand Hotel and Sanatorium in the Rotorua District* (1884), given to him in Auckland on 26 October 1885; a copy of H.A. de Latour's *Education in Relation to Public Health* (Oamaru, 1887); and, given in 1883, T.S. Ralph's *On the Occurrence of Bacteria (Bacilli) in Living Plants* [1883], bound with *Observations and Experiments with the Microscope on the Effects of Various Chemical Agents on the Blood* (1866). Hocken left a matter-of-fact note on his fellow medico who, as detailed earlier, sold him a number of botanical books in December 1885: 'Dr Ralph was an old Wellington settler of considerable attainments. He, conjointly with Mr W.B.D. Mantell, was secretary of the Wellington Society & one of its chief founders, instituted in July 1851. He also drew the illustrations for the Maori translations of 'Pilgrim's Progress' & Robinson Crusoe issued by the Government in 1852 & 1854. He finally practised in Victoria & died at Kew a suburb.'[17] Hocken was generous enough to subscribe to three copies of William Colenso's *An Account of Visits to, and Crossings Over, the Ruahine Mountain Range, Hawke's Bay, New Zealand: and of the Natural History of that Region; Performed in 1845–1847*, published in 1884. He eventually received his three copies, which either he or Trimble filed in three different pamphlet volumes.

Early Pictorial Illustrations

There was a grain of truth in J.M. Philson's claim of Hocken's insatiable itch to write: *cacoethes scribendi*.[18] Publications did bolster his reputation and helped to satisfy the educative role he so strongly believed in. The writing process also had benefits. It required the sifting and sorting of sketches, maps and illustrations, thereby clarifying what he actually owned. In early 1884 Hocken penned 'Early pictorial illustrations of New Zealand' for the *New Zealand Educational and Literary Monthly*, which duly appeared in the 14 June issue.[19] This periodical was edited by James Horsburgh, a Dunedin bookseller and stationer who specialised in educational works. He supplied books to schools, published titles such as James Copland's *The Origin and Spiritual Nature of Man* (1885) and Professor Black's *Chemistry for the Goldfields* (1885), and used the London-based firm of Sampson Low, Marston & Co. as book suppliers. This firm was to publish Hocken's *Contributions* in 1898.

Hocken's two-page account of early illustrations of New Zealand described the visual records he owned up to 1884, thereby confirming the fine arts interest noted by Quaritch. Because of his collecting interests, the focus of the article was mainly on the New Zealand Company which, he maintained, 'spared no pains or expense in its efforts to colonise New Zealand'.[20]

Hocken would have agreed with later comments by Eric McCormick, himself a Hocken Library devotee, who wrote that 'in spite of its errors and sins, for more than a decade and particularly in its early prosperous years, the Company acted as a generous patron of the arts, organising expeditions into the interior, encouraging its servants to record what they saw, publishing the results in handsome books and lavish folios'.[21] Hocken owned many of these handsome books.

Charles Heaphy was first. In addition to the 'entirely agreeable' sketch of *Nelson Haven* (1841), and *Nelson from the Gaol* (1859), Hocken owned the artist's two views of Wellington, published by Smith Elder in 1841.[22] These had 'an air of calm beauty' and 'a general romantic, out-of-the way effect' calculated to stir a potential settler into action. He not only pointed out the rarity of these 'faithful delineations of our magnificent New Zealand scenery' but also used to good effect Heaphy's own words on their scarcity. He would eventually own 13 pieces by the decorated soldier-settler.

The next pair of images was entitled *Part of the New Plymouth Settlement in the District of Taranake, New Zealand. Mount Egmont 30 Miles Distant*. Both were executed by the artist George Duppa and lithographed by Thomas Allom. The larger one is hand coloured and dated 1841; the smaller is undated. To the former, Hocken added his typical factual note:

> This view was taken from the deck of the *Brougham* represented in the picture by Mr George Duppa in February 1841 immediately after the selection of the site for the settlement of New Plymouth. Mr Duppa came out in the *Oriental* in 1840 from Hollingbourne House, Kent. He finally settled in Nelson & early imported valuable stock. He was one of the first to take up sheep country in the Wairau & Amuri where he held 100,000 acres which afterwards sold for £150,000. He founded a scholarship at Nelson College & returned to England in 1863.

The undated lithograph was not part of Hocken's original gift in 1910; it was returned to the collection by Bessie Hocken in 1913.[23]

On a more local note, Hocken then described his own copy of Charles Kettle's *View of Dunedin Taken from the Upper Part of Stafford Street*. He called it 'artistically chosen' and added that the 'customary cows' lying contentedly in mid-street gave the picture a bucolic feel. He contrasted the image with Kettle's woodcut of the *Lower Harbour at Port Chalmers*, published in the August 1852 issue of the *Otago Journal*. On one occasion, however, he was not uncritical of Duppa and Kettle. On top of his own copy of 'Early pictorial illustrations' he wrote in reference to their drawings the words 'very crude'.[24] He was, however, more enamoured of the skills of the lithographer Thomas Allom, who readied the images for publication. Because of Hocken's interest in the New Zealand Company, Allom's son Albert would later become a frequent correspondent.

Hocken then moved on to Canterbury, briefly describing his copies of Edmund Norman's 'cleverly depicted' drawing of the panoramic *Port Hills*, and two smaller lithographs entitled *Town of Lyttelton* (1852), and *Lyttelton, Port of Victoria* (1852).[25] Auckland did not get a mention apart from a disparaging comment on P.J. Hogan's four views of the city, which Hocken admitted were of 'historical interest' but 'inferior in conception and execution'. He then passed judgement on British lithographers William Day and Louis Haghe's illustrations for Edward Jerningham Wakefield's *Adventures in New Zealand* (1845), calling them a 'style of high art'.

To tantalise his readers Hocken finished by mentioning the 'quaint views' in Tasman's journal, the 'interesting engravings' in Cook's *Voyages* and the 'truly magnificent coloured lithographs' in Angas's *The New Zealanders Illustrated*. A 'to be continued' note was printed at the end of the article, but as he recorded: 'There was no continuation. Either the paper expired, or there was no further application for my contribution to it.'[26] The last issue of Horsburgh's periodical appeared on 1 May 1885.

Tuckett Papers

William Gladstone claimed there were six qualifications for a collector: 'appetite, leisure, wealth, knowledge, discrimination, and perseverance'.[27] Of these, Gladstone claimed for himself the first and last. One particular collection Hocken secured in the 1880s reveals his perseverance and desire, plus a mixture of plain good fortune and timeliness.

Hocken had already secured letters by surveyor Frederick Tuckett but he coveted more, especially Tuckett's diaries and journals. Initial enquiries made to Wohlers resulted in Hocken receiving in May 1884 Alexander Mackay's *Memorandum ... on Origin of New Zealand Company's 'Tenths' Native Reserves* (1873) and his *Land Purchases, Middle Island: Report* (1875), sent to aid the compilation of a history that Hocken was planning.[28] In September that year Hocken had more luck. Wohlers sent through letters written by Tuckett but reported he did not know anything of any report or diary.[29] Correspondence continued, with Wohlers' letter of 17 November 1884 eventually providing an interesting morsel.

> In our correspondence about the history of the Otago Settlement, I had forgotten (old people are forgetful you know) that in 1857 Mr Tuckett had sent me a book from London part of a work named *The British Colonies* by [Robert] Montgomery Martin which book contains a great deal of information about the commencement of the settlement of New Zealand. I would have sent it you the book (it is a little heavy) only I thought you might have the work, but if you have not you will kindly let me know and I will send it. I will transcribe here what it says about Mr Tucketts transactions in Otago ...[30]

Hocken did not then own the multi-volume Martin work. Through a prompt by Southland settler W.B. Scandrett, Dr Samuel Hodgkinson, a former fellow surgeon-superintendent and local MP, contacted Hocken in late November 1886 about 'any notes and information that might be useful to you in compiling your history of New Zealand'.[31] Hodgkinson not only gave personal details on his career and friendships with Frederick Tuckett, Sir George Grey and prominent Taranaki settler and writer Charles Hursthouse, but also included a few printed pamphlets. These included his own *Provincialism versus Centralism* (1868), and three by Hursthouse: *Letters on Colonisation* (1866), *New Zealand, or, Zealandia, the Britain of the South* (1857) and the second edition of *New Zealand, The Britain of the South* (1861), to which Hodgkinson added a small bibliographical note:

> You will notice the name 'Zealandia' on the title page of my little pamphlets on Canterbury Province. I suggested the name to Mr Charles Hursthouse when he was preparing his book *New Zealand the Britain of the South* – and at the end of 1st volume of the 1st edition of 1857 he appended a note repeating the name – a copy of which I enclose. I do not like the old name which to me is always associated with Cannibalism & perhaps from scurvy when a child [sic] read Captain Cook's voyages.[32]

Hodgkinson also included a manuscript letter and a plan, which 'I think be interesting as it relates to the first settlement of Otago & is written by a man formerly well-known in New Zealand'. This was Tuckett's letter to Hodgkinson, written on 16 August 1844 immediately after selecting the site for settlement. The plan was a sketch of the rural district of 'New Edinburgh', dated 1844, which Hocken had copied.[33] Their correspondence was timely. Hodgkinson admitted to Hocken that he had considered depositing both items in a 'Home Museum or Library'. Hocken thought the letter important and did it proud. It eventually appeared as Appendix B in his *Contributions*.[34]

'Despite unceasing enquiries', Hocken could not locate Tuckett's diary and journal. He feared the worst, that they were long gone – destroyed.[35] But then he had another stroke of luck. Some months before he delivered his 15 September 1887 lecture to the Otago Institute, he was contacted by a Miss McGlashan, who had a copy of Tuckett's journals. As he proclaimed to his audience that night: 'Imagine then my delight when ... through the kindness of Miss McGlashan, a copy came into my hands.' However, his delight was tempered somewhat: 'As is often the case with much-coveted articles, where possession does not equal anticipation, the much-prized journal proved on perusal by no means to fulfil the great expectations formed of its contents.'[36] This did not stop him from making it available to a wider audience: it was copied and reproduced as Appendix A to his *Contributions*.[37]

While preparing the lecture, however, 'in the most unexpected manner ... I procured information which led me to hear of and at once communicate with a gentleman who is a relation and executor of Mr Tuckett, and who possesses papers'.[38] This was the Bristol-based Frederick F. Tuckett, nephew of the surveyor. As usual, Hocken, in a 12 August 1887 letter, inundated him with enclosures that not only described his uncle's activities in New Zealand, but also promoted his own bibliophilic work. Tuckett's reply, written on 25 October, spoke of the serendipity that often surrounds collecting:

> Luckily, only yesterday morning, while looking for something else, I discovered a bundle of old New Zealand letters addressed to my father through a range of several years including the period when my uncle was surveyor at Otago. There are about 2 doz. in all & I think 3 (marked in pencil with a X) referring to Otago. With one of these is a tracing of the original survey, which I think may possess an interest in your eyes. The entire series, together with a map of Nelson & plans of the City &c, and sundry other documents shall be forwarded to you tomorrow thro' Messrs Sutton & Co. and I hope will reach you safely.

He asked Hocken to use his 'judgment and discretion concerning any 'references to personal or family matters, or to third parties, which should be strictly private', but otherwise gave him carte blanche to 'keep any of the contents of the parcel (including all the maps) which you think of sufficient value or interest either for your own collection of documents or for any one public destination'. He would, though, ask for the return of the photograph, 'which is the only portrait of my uncle in existence so far as I am aware'. Tuckett also promised to send Hocken anything else that might turn up, though he had 'ransacked every likely hole and corner'. He also possessed 'a very considerable number of letters to my uncle, written by various friends of his, mostly, I think, in Nelson and dating after 1850, or perhaps up to 1865 or so', but had not sent these as he felt unsure that he should 'let them go out of my hands, as some of the writers as well as of those referred to, may be still living or have left relatives in the colony'. If Hocken was interested in these, Tuckett would check them.

> In conclusion, let me thank you very heartily for sending me the 2 papers with reports of your two most lucid and valuable lectures. I have read every word of them with the greatest attention and interest and hope that they will some day appear in a more permanent form. I fear I shall have bored you with this long yarn, but it may serve to get you into training for the deciphering of my uncle's with more lengthy enumerations which I will not imitate by crossing this as he frequently did ...[39]

Hocken was prompt in copying the documents and sending them back. After a four-month holiday in the Mediterranean, Tuckett finally responded: 'I was rejoiced to learn that you were pleased to have [the documents], & that you had been so persevering as to decipher the mass of crabbed MS which I ventured to inflict on you.' He was also delighted to learn that Hocken had 'succeeded in discovering a copy of my uncle's journal of exploration in the southern island'. He was particularly interested to hear 'that his friends Dr Hodgkinson & Mr Barnicoat are still living. I believe that I have several letters from the latter, as well as from some of his other friends, written to my uncle *after* his return to this country, and, if you thought it likely that they might contain matter of interest either to yourself or the writers, I would willingly forward them to the latter, if living, & ask them to communicate them to you if they felt willing to do so.'[40]

In the main, Hocken was scrupulous about returning items to their rightful owner. He was also generous, as in this instance when he posted back an additional copy of the original photograph Tuckett had supplied. 'The copy is really admirably done,' Tuckett replied, '& in fact superior to the original because more distinct & effective. I shall value it much.'[41]

Hocken would not abandon his Tuckett searches. Back in 1885 he had made contact with John Wallis Barnicoat, another member of the original survey team, and sent him a copy of his lecture on the 'Early history of New Zealand', along, certainly, with a request for historical documents.[42] In August 1887 Hocken wrote again, including copies of his lectures and asking about Tuckett's diary. In his reply Barnicoat was 'glad to hear of the probability of your successful search', and included a brief overview and the status of some of the personnel in the original survey team, including David Monro and William Davison.[43] Barnicoat also later sent his own private journal for copying, though there were problems as Hocken's long note on the copied text, dated February 1888, explains:

> The following is a copy of Mr Barnicoat's journal. The journal was given to me by Mr Barnicoat, but he afterwards regretted his gift & desired to have it returned. To this I of course assented & returned the two volumes to him on the occasion of his visiting Dunedin in 1888 as a member of the General Synod. I however copied this valuable contribution to early N.Z. history first, the only portion omitted (for want of time) being the nine months of 1842. The interspaces contained in the original little plans & sketches some of which are here reproduced. My wife & I & a hired penman completed the copy in two days.

He went on to explain that Barnicoat, a Cornishman, had lived in Nelson during his 'almost lifelong' residence in New Zealand. 'I have frequently corresponded with him on historical matters & once spent a day at his house at Richmond. He was a quiet, reserved, almost uncommunicative man, but of good memory, very intelligent, & polite.' Hocken ended with details of Barnicoat's wife's family.[44] The effort and time involved in the copying was well worth it. As Hocken wrote of the manuscript, 'Its value and interest are considerable, containing as it does, a great deal of reference to matters directly connected with the exploration, and which are not elsewhere referred to.'[45]

Hocken later collected the obituary on Tuckett and contemplated completing the circle by obtaining the journal of David (later Sir David) Monro.[46] Here at least the quarry was easier to find. Monro's journal had been published in the *Nelson Examiner* of 1844 and copied into the *New Zealand Journal* of 1845. These were resources Hocken could readily lay his hands on.

The Early History Society of Otago

On Saturday 19 April 1884 an advertisement appeared in the *Otago Daily Times* calling for a meeting the following Wednesday at the Education Office in the Colonial Bank Buildings for those interested in the formation of an Early History Society of Otago. It was signed 'T.M. Hocken'. On the next page, the newspaper was encouraging about the idea:

> The subject is undoubtedly one of great interest, and it behoves those who are desirous of gathering together and placing on record all matters relating to our early history to do so without delay. The number of our early pioneers is year by year being reduced, and now its members form but a comparatively small band. We are glad to observe as convenor of the meeting the name of a gentleman who, it is well known, has long taken an interest in everything connected with early New Zealand history.[47]

Some 50 postcards were also sent out to individuals considered to be interested in forming such an organisation.[48]

Hocken, the driving force, eventually became vice-president, with colourful former provincial superintendent James Macandrew as president; colonist and writer James Barr became the first secretary. On 23 April 40 men assembled at the Education Office for a meeting chaired by Hocken, who delivered a short address. After some discussion, those present agreed on the Early History Society of Otago as a name and sorted out the constitution and bylaws. On 16 May, with Hocken again in the chair, the rules and regulations of the society were adopted The main objective of the society was determined and fixed in print: 'to collect, classify, and preserve all information, documents, or relics connected with the early history of the Otago Settlement'.[49] There was an entrance fee of 5s for all members plus a yearly subscription of the same amount, paid 'in advance'.

The June meeting fine-tuned the research process. Eight committees were formed to concentrate on specific areas of research, with some personnel overlap. Presbyterian minister and educationalist Donald Stuart, treasurer of the Dunedin Presbytery Edmund Smith and accountant and prohibitionist A.C. Begg were to procure documents and information from the Free Kirk of Scotland and elsewhere respecting the Otago Settlements. Teacher and former Milton lawyer James Elder Brown and lawyer J.A.D. Adams, along with Smith,

James Barr and C.C. Kettle (son of the surveyor) were asked to obtain information, memoirs and diaries relevant to the first ships and their passengers. Local businessman James Rattray, Presbyterian church leader the Rev. William Bannerman and Donald Stuart were to acquire materials on the early churches and their congregations. Schools and the educational development of the region were allocated to Mainwaring Brown (a Professor of English at Otago University), school principal Alexander Wilson, Begg and Edward Bowes Cargill (William Cargill's son). Civil institutions, including the asylum, the gaol and the hospital, fell to Alexander Rennie, an active member of the Benevolent Institute, Professor Brown and printer John McIndoe. Kettle, Hocken and the lawyer, judge and ethnologist Frederick Revans Chapman were given the early or 'pre-historic' period before the foundation of the Otago settlement, while Rattray, Cargill, James Brown and Professor Brown were to examine the early Otago industries. Finally, lawyer and MP William Downie Stewart, former Otago superintendent John Hyde Harris, Kettle and Chapman were to find materials on the early administration of justice in the region.

With a prospectus drawn up and 'Conversazione' evenings planned for 7 October 1884 and 17 April 1885, it was a solid start. On these occasions lectures were delivered by Macandrew (the Otago Association), Stuart (kindred societies), Begg (progress of the province since 1851) and Hocken, who talked about the exhibits he had on display, including Maori and Moriori carvings, early newspapers, the seal of Potatau and pencil caricatures by James Brown. (Hocken eventually owned 48 individual drawings by Brown, New Zealand's first cartoonist, and wrote notes on each explaining who the public figures were and the occasions lampooned.) At the beginning of each lecture Hocken's 'convict' bell was rung. Bessie and four other women provided musical interludes.

The initial research results of the society were mixed. Edward Petherick, Hocken's friend in England, wrote to James Caffin on 2 July 1884 about early passenger lists, which were passed to Hocken, who noted on 23 October 1884: 'I forward this correspondence to the Sub-Committee of the E. H. Soc? I think however I have documents in my possession which will give the desired information.' He tried to make headway himself, sending letters to Alfred Chetham Strode, one-time resident magistrate and sub-treasurer for Otago, then living in England. The reply was not encouraging:

> I have now made enquiries at, I think, every likely place in London, and have been unable to hear of one of the old 'New Zealand Journals'. I remember the paper well, as it commenced its career just at the time I first went to N.Z. and my father used to send me copies of it as long as it was published. Indeed all the old records of the N.Z. Company seem to have been utterly extinguished, as after making numerous enquiries from the most likely people in London, I am told that there is no such thing to be had.[50]

The death of James Barr, a poor turnout at the meeting on 19 May 1885, the failure of members to gather materials and the deferring of a November 1885 conversazione sounded the death-knell of the society. As Hocken noted, it 'came to an abrupt end'.

> The work devolved on two or three persons but it was found impossible to galvanize the old identities into any mood to give information or personal reminiscences in writing. Many lived at a considerable distance from town & it was difficult to visit them. If visited the interview consisted of little more than twaddling personal details. Altogether the movement ended in a fiasco. Mr F.R. Chapman & myself have worked informally & have thus gradually gathered together that which the Society set itself to do.[51]

Although the enterprise was short-lived, its existence provided Hocken with more contacts and gave him further impetus to continue his collecting. And the experience showed him that if the hunting down of historical materials were to continue, the responsibility to secure them was his alone. It would not be the last time that Hocken confronted inertia in others.

Draft Catalogue 1887

In this period, too, Hocken created a catalogue of all his books, pamphlets, newspapers and manuscripts. His starting date is unknown, but the painstaking task was certainly completed by 1887. He transcribed author, title and publication details into a 300-page catalogue arranged chronologically, with bibliographical details extending to pagination and publication formats (folio, quarto, octavo) only. He provided no provenance information. The sum total was some 1100 books, pamphlets, maps and manuscripts.

Although it is only a bare-bones list, the draft catalogue stands as a significant document. It not only confirms what Hocken owned at this point but reflects his own pride in his collection. It was also an excellent way in which to revisit each item and recall the events associated with its acquisition and, of course, an admirable excuse to play. He called the draft: 'Catalogue of books, pamphlets, maps, newspapers, prints &c relating to New Zealand. In the Library of Dr. T.M. Hocken of Dunedin, N.Z.'.[52]

It is instructive to briefly examine some of the pre-1830 publications relating to New Zealand that he then owned, in comparison with his more complete *Bibliography* published in 1909. The latter lists 93 books or article entries up to 1830, many including extensive bibliographical descriptions. The draft catalogue of 1887 contains 56 entries, of which the first is the very brief *Terra Australis Cognita* (1766) and the last is *Narrative and Successful Result of a Voyage in the South Seas* (1829), with the attached note: 'To ascertain the fate of La Pérouse's Expedition &c. By the Chevalier Cap. P. Dillon. Vols II.

London Hunt, Chance & Co.'[53] In between are many standard Pacific voyage titles: the already-mentioned Hawkesworth, Cook's *Voyages*, Parkinson, works by Johann and George Forster, Alexander Dalrymple's *Historical Collection*, Andrew Kippis's first biography on Cook, French and English editions of George Vancouver's *Voyages*, David Collins's *Account of the English Colony in New South Wales*, Burney's work, botanist Jacques Labillardière's *Voyage*, John Webber's *Views in the South Seas*, J.L. Nicholas's *Narrative of a Voyage to New Zealand*, Amasa Delano's *Narrative of Voyages*, and specific New Zealand titles such as Kendall's *Grammar and Vocabulary* (1820). A notable title listed in the draft catalogue was Alexander Shaw's *Catalogue of the Different Specimens of Cloth* (1787), which contained 39 tapa cloth samples gathered by Cook and his men on the three Pacific voyages. It is most likely that Hocken obtained this exceedingly rare and valuable item in 1882 when visiting England. Unfortunately Hocken's copy is now missing from his collection.

The predominance of English language publications in the catalogue is understandable. Hocken no doubt found such editions easier to read and work with, especially bibliographically. And despite their wider antiquarian coverage and wares, the book dealers he bought from were predominantly Anglophiles. He later broadened his sources, as is possibly suggested by the presence of Parisian book labels pasted in the endpapers of his dumpy green volumes of de Brosses's *Histoire des navigations aux Terres Australes* (1756) and Rochon's *Voyages aux Indes Orientales et en Afrique* (1807). Sometime after 1887, and perhaps during his trip to Europe between 1901 and 1904, he also secured his copy of Thévenot's *Relations de divers voyages curieux* (1696) and the atlas volume *Histoire du voyage* by Duperrey.[54]

Travels in the 1880s

Hocken travelled north on two foraging expeditions during this period, in 1885 and 1888. As already mentioned in Chapter 4, an added incentive for the first trip, which began in Timaru on 19 October, was the cheap return fare of 80s offered to those attending the New Zealand Industrial Exhibition in Wellington. In Christchurch he visited Haast at the Canterbury Museum and called at the local library where he met met Dean Jacobs, who regaled Hocken with gossip about the fiasco of the bishop designate, the Rev. Thomas Jackson. At Clark's sale rooms he saw again James Smetham's painting, which had remained unsold since his last visit in 1881. He was cheeky enough to offer 25 guineas for it, which was not accepted.

On 21 October Hocken arrived in Wellington, where he packed a great deal into his two-day visit. He called on John Howard Wallace, an early settler who was preparing his *Manual of New Zealand* for publication. His description was somewhat disparaging: 'hale old man, bow legged, talkative, uneducated, & preparing a publication of his reminiscences which will have little interest beyond that afforded by the subject itself.' Nevertheless, Hocken acquired the book shortly after its publication in 1886, as it is listed in his 1887 draft catalogue. He also visited 64-year-old William Seed, the Secretary of Customs, who had once been a clerk in the New Zealand Company office and was 'full of life and fire while describing old days'.[55] On Friday 23 October Hocken went to the exhibition, which he claimed was 'highly creditable'. He also met the new government librarian and bibliographer James Collier, John Plimmer, an early settler who at 74 was 'fresh and intelligent', and Johnny Martin, 'a wealthy, healthy vulgar purse prune old man, but energetic'. Among all this socialising, book chasing was not forgotten, though the results were poor. Driven by a tantalising hint from George Sisson Cooper that a box in the old Provincial Buildings contained some New Zealand Company documents, Hocken 'raked' through it all. This effort bore 'little success', however, and the old land orders and a number of company reports that he rescued were of 'very little value'. Cooper made amends the following year when he visited Dunedin: he gave Hocken a copy of his *Journal of an Overland Expedition from Auckland to Taranaki* (1851), which detailed the trip that Cooper made with Sir George Grey, Te Heu Heu Iwikau (paramount chief of the Tuwharetoa tribe), the artist Cuthbert Clarke, interpreter Pirikawau and 'a train of wives and followers' during the Christmas period of 1849–50.[56] The *Journal* has Hocken's signature on the title page and his embossed coat of arms on page 35.

Hocken left Wellington for Picton on the Friday. Judge Richmond and his wife were fellow passengers on board, and the Treaty of Waitangi was one topic of conversation during their five and a half-hour journey, as were the Wakefields. Hocken also noticed Richmond's features, remarking on his 'lantern jaws and parchment visaged but expressive and intellectual face'. After finding nothing of note in Picton or Nelson, Hocken left for Taranaki and Auckland on 25 October. This date was also Bessie's birthday, and while passing the time chatting to 'various intelligent people' he noted, 'I wish she was here.' In Auckland he visited her brothers Alfred and Frank Buckland, and with the latter drove through to Kohimarama 'where dear Bessie was born'.

Although his diary for the 1885 journey ends at this juncture, he did remain in Auckland for a few more days. He met Grey and C.O.B. Davis, who gave Hocken a copy of his own compilation *Te Honae* (1885), the enlarged second edition of temperance and sacred melodies. Hocken met Maunsell again, and G.B. Owen, who knew J.S. Polack, author of *New Zealand Being a Narrative of Travels and Adventures During a Residence in that Country Between the Years 1831 and 1837* (1838) and *Manners and Customs of the New Zealanders* (1840).[57]

At the end of March 1888 Hocken was on the road again, heading up to Wanganui via Wellington. At Clark's auction house in Christchurch he purchased copies of the *Lyttelton Times* spanning 1851 to 1859 'for the most moderate sum of £7'. He was particularly pleased with their provenance, since they came from the library of naturalist and pioneering conservationist

T.H. Potts. He did, however, find it 'inexplicable' that 'this valuable and almost unique copy of the "Times" should have been allowed to remain on sale for a fortnight without a purchaser'. After a disappointing visit to Government Buildings, where there was 'nothing of historical interest or importance', Hocken made an astute comment: 'Each successive yearly travel shows me how diminishing is the interest taken in early history matters and the older settlers here past away or are indifferent, whilst the younger ones devote themselves almost entirely to outdoor sports.'

On 30 March he was in Wellington where he saw Mantell again and left him his draft catalogue (or a copy) for perusal. It was a significant occasion. Hocken also met W.H. Kirk, a 'rising young scientist' at the museum, whom he recognised would 'worthily tread in his father's [Thomas Kirk's] footsteps'. Kirk gave him a few pamphlets, which, sadly, are unidentifiable. Hocken spent that evening with 'the oldest printer in the colony', one Thomas McKenzie, who had assisted Samuel Revans in his printing of the *New Zealand Gazette*. From McKenzie, Hocken gathered more historical trivia, including the sources of paper for printing and the fact that the first printing office had been a tent. Hocken also called on Bishop Octavius Hadfield, who had lived in the Wellington area for well over 50 years. In an effort to obtain first-hand information from someone who had seen so much, Hocken 'begged him' to write down his reminiscences. Hadfield, however, knew his own abilities, claiming he had contributed 'trifles' to New Zealand literature, and declined the opportunity. In September 1900 Hocken wrote to Hadfield, then living in England, asking for any spare copies of *Te Karere* and other pamphlets, and again for any reminiscences. Hadfield reiterated his stance that he had limited output outside expected ecclesiastical exertions.[58] Hocken again called on John Howard Wallace, and visited the painter Charles D. Barraud, who had exhibited at the 1865 New Zealand Exhibition in Dunedin. Although he made no comment on the artist's work, he was dismissive of his family: 'all his relatives have the artistic afflatus'. Hocken could be extremely judgmental, especially if he did not recognise someone as a kindred spirit. This unprofessional yet private comment is but one of many on record.

After Wellington Hocken travelled on to Wanganui, where he met Samuel Drew, a jeweller and watchmaker who had amassed a collection of natural history objects and Maori curiosities, and who, over a number of years, had exchanged specimens with collectors like Haast.[59] Hocken admitted many of those on display were 'quite new to me', including two cylindrical wooden flutes that had the skin of a chief's penis stretched over them. This was, as Hocken wrote, 'the greatest indignity that could be passed on the body of a conquered chief'. Despite finding Drew 'intelligent though uneducated and quite an enthusiast', Hocken had misgivings about his knowledge of Maori customs, feeling it was 'not quite reliable'. This did not, however, prevent him from accepting an old iron tool that was dated to Cook's arrival, and walking over to the site of Putiki Pa. Perhaps grudgingly, Hocken admitted, '[Drew] was able to point out much more to me than I had previously seen.' The Austrian collector Andreas Reischek was also there 'arranging and stuffing etc his birds'. Although 'most garrulous in conversation' and 'deficient in scientific knowledge', he was judged 'a good observer of the habits of animals' and 'a nice simple fellow'.

Hocken also called on local solicitor Francis Matthews Betts, a grandson of Samuel Marsden, but was not impressed: 'Betts seems lost an unmarried man, of 35 – Cambridge man, has attempted to drown himself in Wanganui, is intemperate, cynical, cannot understand my interest in his grandfather, or pretends so, of whom he speaks in the most disparaging, disaffected way.'[60] Hocken was shown an album of Marsden family photographs, to which he responded privately: 'Betts's mother alone seemed to me to have any resemblance to the celebrated father and that was through the bottle nose on the old gentleman's engraving.'[61] Although he 'could gather *nothing* from the grandson of his grandfather', he did secure the address of Elizabeth (Lizzie), Betts's unmarried sister and Marsden's granddaughter.[62] After a lengthy and assiduous correspondence with her, Hocken eventually obtained 'a valuable box' of material containing some of Marsden's journals, a collection of letters and further family contacts to approach.[63] Throughout these exchanges he was prompt in reply.

Robert Maunsell and Stephenson Percy Smith

During the 1880s two correspondents, each in their own way, confirmed Hocken's growing authority in the field of early New Zealand history: the Rev. Robert Maunsell, who played an important part in the history of early European New Zealand, and Percy Smith, as he was known, the amateur scholar who played a large part in rejuvenating interest in New Zealand history. Maunsell was nearing the end of a long career: he died in 1894. Smith was a new breed of researcher, who would correspond with Hocken until the latter's death in 1910.

As mentioned earlier, Hocken first met Maunsell in 1879 and although they met infrequently, they obviously liked each other. The old missionary farewelled Hocken on his trip to England in 1882; his 'travel-well' letter is safely tipped in Hocken's second edition of Maunsell's *Grammar of the New Zealand Language* (1862).[64] They met again in Auckland in 1885, when one topic of discussion was the pronunciation of Maori, something in which the former missionary was well versed. In 1905 as Hocken worked through his copy of Edward Markham's manuscript, 'New Zealand or recollections of it', he noted that the 'letters R, D, & L were so lightly pronounced in some words it was difficult to say which was used. Take for instance the word 'kauri'; in some old publications it is spelt kaudi & kauli showing the difficulty of apportioning a well marked consonantal sound. An apostrophe might almost take the place of the letter as kau'i.' He added: 'Archdeacon Maunsell explained this to me 20 years ago.'[65]

Maunsell also gave Hocken a number of items. In 1887 he sent a document hand-written by Bishop Selwyn and witnessed by John Kinder, announcing Maunsell's elevation to archdeacon on 25 January 1860.[66] Other manuscripts included a copy of Benjamin Thornton Dudley's September 1858 'Journal of 4th Melanesian Voyage in the "Southern Cross"', and Maunsell's own 'Journal of a Winter Spent on Amota Bank's Island, 24 May 1860'.[67] He also may have sent Hocken a copy of the Rev. A.W. Murray's *The Bible in the Pacific* (1888). A letter tipped in this work highlights the amount of trouble others went to on Hocken's behalf. That the search for this book was carried out by Maunsell, who by 1881 had started experiencing fainting attacks, by 1882 was termed 'eccentric' and by 1888, when the letter was written, was 78 and 'too old to travel', makes it more significant. On 3 October, the day after a September 1888 letter from Hocken, Maunsell called on two fellow clergymen seeking information and was able to report that Archdeacon Williams of Gisborne was 'forming a collection of old C.M.S publications'.[68] The process, of course, was reciprocal. Maunsell was another recipient of Hocken's printed lectures, about which he was most complimentary: 'I don't think that I ever read anything on New Zealand so well written. I, of course, was well aware of the event there recorded; & yet so graphic was the style, & so well told was the story, that I seemed to be reading a narrative of recent events.'[69]

Hocken met Smith in 1882, on his way to England. The surveyor, ethnologist, writer and collector had been nine when he arrived in Wellington in December 1849. After schooling in Taranaki, where his family settled, Smith had joined the provincial surveying department in 1855 and helped to survey the land around New Plymouth.[70] He had served in the militia in 1857 and was further employed in surveying in Waitara (where he made sketches of the stockades), the Kaipara, Northern Wairoa and Coromandel, and was involved in the surveys of Waiuku (1864), Taranaki (1865–66) and Pitt Island (1868). Through active service, he rose to the position of surveyor-general and secretary for lands and mines. Fluent in Maori, he was an interpreter and a keen collector. With Edward Tregear, he was the co-founder and co-editor of the *Journal of Polynesian Society* (*JPS*), which was established in 1892. Like Hocken, he was a 'gentleman-scholar' who published his findings, many of them in the pages of the *JPS*. Some of his monographs included *Hawaiki: The Whence of the Maori* (1898), *History and Traditions of the Maoris of the West Coast, North Island of New Zealand Prior to 1840* (1910) and *The Lore of the Whare-wananga* (1913–15). Apart from his stint in Wellington, Taranaki was home for Smith, where he died on 19 April 1922.

Bound in volume 47 of Hocken's Pamphlet Collection is Smith's *The Kermadec Islands* (1887), which contains a tipped-in letter dated 9 October 1887, the first of some 30 or so the two men exchanged. It not only indicates

Hocken's willingness to assist a fellow researcher but also documents the earliest mention of his intention to write a 'History'. From Judges Bay in Auckland, Smith thanked Hocken 'very much indeed for your great kindness in sending me (through Mr Adams) the information about the Kermadec Islands. I am especially obliged for the extracts from d'Entrecasteaux voyage – the reference to d'Urville's visit & reference to Pollack.' After reminding Hocken that they had met, Smith wrote: 'If I can at any time be of any assistance to you in getting information as to points connected with this northern part of NZ, pray let me know and I will do the best I can. I have always taken an interest in such subjects and during my 37 years residence here have of course met with many interesting facts connected with its history – but unfortunately have kept few notes.' He added: 'I also passed 13 months at the Chatham Islands in 1868–69 and learned some few things of interest from the Moriori, such as they are they are at your service, though I fear they would be too few & too brief to be of much value.'[71] In later years Smith's work on the Kermadecs came under scrutiny: allegations were made about the use of fraudulent pictures and misinformation about the land and its capabilities. With typical thoroughness, Hocken secured this information and filed it in one of his Variae files.[72]

As a surveyor Smith had much practical experience and had rubbed shoulders with many people, especially in the more remote areas of New Zealand. He proved to be not only a valuable connection in the burgeoning New Zealand ethnology network but also an important sounding board for Hocken's own personal researches.

10
'A Very Big Affair Indeed'

During the second half of the nineteenth century, exhibitions appeared in rapid succession throughout the western world, most patterned on Prince Albert's Great Exhibition of 1851, an extravaganza that effectively showed off Britain's achievements in the fields of manufacturing, science and the arts. A reflection of Victoria's empire, it also encompassed the industrial and cultural works of other nations. From Ireland to Sydney, from Philadelphia to Paris, the exhibitions were many and varied, and New Zealand, too, caught the fever. There was the Dunedin Exhibition of 1865, the Dunedin Industrial Exhibition of 1881, the Christchurch Exhibition of 1882 and the New Zealand Industrial Exhibition in Wellington in 1885. Hocken contributed to the first occasion and managed to salvage various scarce ephemeral items relating to it, many of them filed carefully away in Volume 11 of his F&J collection.[1] He did not participate in the Dunedin Industrial Exhibition, held at Garrison Hall in 1881, but did visit the 1885 New Zealand Industrial Exhibition held in Wellington and commented briefly on its achievements. He also amassed a number of catalogues from overseas exhibitions.[2]

The year 1890 marked 50 years of British sovereignty over New Zealand. The first proposal to hold an exhibition in Dunedin to celebrate the jubilee, and to illustrate the progress of the colony, came during the Adelaide Jubilee Exhibition of November 1887. With the date of late 1889 in mind, discussion followed on whether it would be an international or inter-colonial exhibition. There was also a suggestion that it be a New Zealand exhibition, which would increase the likelihood of government funding. Local support was poor initially but by October 1888 there was a new momentum for the concept, and financial contributions followed. By 26 October it was decided to form a guarantee company (not for profit) with a capital of £10,000 in £1 shares.[3] Executive officers were appointed, shares were allotted in November and permanent office-bearers were appointed. Almost simultaneously, political lobbying began. After convincing Wellington that the exhibition should be recognised as the colony's jubilee celebration – stressing features such as the loan of an art collection from Melbourne, support from other countries, a willingness to undertake the expenses connected with early history, Maori and South Seas exhibits and the procuring of a building that would contain government exhibits and a picture gallery – the government finally agreed to give £10,000, reminding the organising committee to spend it wisely. In fact, the government did much more by offering the free use of post and telegraph offices for exhibition business, granting free passes on the railways and giving grants to cover both the use of electric lights in the gardens and fernery, and the cost of sending through the English pictures.[4]

A 12-acre (5 ha) site on Crawford Street was approved, clinched by the generous 'free of cost' gift of land from the harbour board. The proposed building would cover 10 of those acres (4 ha); the rest of the area would be filled by sideshows, gardens and open spaces. R.E.N. Twopeny, editor of the *Otago Daily Times* and executive commissioner of the exhibition, undertook a promotional tour to Sydney and Melbourne, which led to the three principal colonies of New South Wales, Victoria and South Australia committing their involvement.

For the citizens of Dunedin the New Zealand and South Seas Exhibition, as it became known, became real when the foundation stone was laid on 20 March 1889 by chief patron Governor Sir William F. Drummond Jervois, who announced that the exhibition doors would open on 26 November 1889. The other patron was His Excellency the Earl of Onslow, with vice-presidential dignitaries including Sir F. Dillon Bell, Sir George Grey, Sir James Hector, Sir Robert Stout, Sir Julius Vogel and Dunedin mayor Hugh Gourley. There were to be some 10,500 exhibits, subdivided into 36 sections and 203 classes, for which 107 jurors had to be appointed. The exhibits would come from countries such as Mauritius, Fiji, Samoa, Tonga, Costa Rica, Britain, the United States, France, Germany, Austria, Italy, Belgium, Japan, the Australian states mentioned above, and of course New Zealand.[5] There was much work to be done.

How Hocken became involved in the preparations for this enterprise is unknown, but it was the sort of project he relished. He was already searching for materials by late March 1888, and on 24 April 1889, at the fourth meeting of the Early History, Maori and South Seas (EHMSS) Court Committee, he reported that he had 'been very successful in procuring promises of support & of loans in every place visited except in Auckland where a very bitter & hostile spirit had been evinced by the Mayor'.[6] As the *Otago Daily Times* noted on 26 April – Hocken kept the clipping pinned next to the meeting minutes – he had been, in his own words, keeping 'matters relating to the forthcoming exhibition constantly in view'. He explained how, 'in the least likely and most out-of-the-way places', he had found 'many objects of value and interest, and many small industries struggling for existence, but quite susceptible of considerable development' In the Hokianga, for example, he had seen hats made of lacebark 'which for lightness and beauty of texture rivalled, if they did not surpass, any of those made by fancy straw, and which, if exhibited in any fashionable shop window, would speedily have found customers'. He had also convinced the Northern Steam Ship Company 'to convey exhibits free to and from those ports visited by the fleet'.[7]

The Early History Society of Otago had given a real boost to Hocken's collecting, but the South Seas Exhibition was far more important. It not only provided a greater catalyst, but gave Hocken licence to contact people for exhibits (and other materials) with a circular 'New Zealand Exhibition

1889–90 Dunedin' stamp on every letter. And he was able to exhibit portions of his own collection. He was unanimously elected as chairman at the first EHMSS Court Committee meeting on 8 January 1889 and later became the secretary. He saved the minutes of each meeting and three associated letterbooks.[8]

Aside from the committees representing Auckland, Wellington, Nelson, Greymouth, Canterbury, Invercargill and smaller districts such as Waihemo, Taieri and Vincent, there were 13 special committees, all dedicated to specific tasks or themes, and each committed to have everything ready for the 1 October 1889 deadline. The first meeting was one of general discussion, the eight members focusing on how best to achieve their objectives. It was suggested that they all make enquiries to those known to possess articles suitable for exhibition. For an avid correspondent with an already large number of contacts, Hocken was in his element. At the second meeting, on 6 March 1889, two sub-sections were formed: one to take charge of the Early History and Maori and the other the South Seas Islands. Hocken was on both. The third (27 March) and fourth (24 April) meetings saw further feverish activity. A programme was approved, printed and directed to individuals and institutions, with an overriding pledge by the committee to look after all exhibits received.

Although it was not recorded in the minutes, Hocken was making inroads locally. In response to a letter of 31 January 1889 Octavius Harwood, manager of the Weller Brothers' whaling station at the Otago Heads, sent him a canoe head, some stones from Portobello and a simple chart showing fishing areas nearby. The canoe head was particularly significant in that it came from a double-headed fishing canoe which had been given to the old whaler by 'Bogany', a local Maori chief.[9] Although it was a gift, Hocken sent Harwood £2. The canoe head was eventually listed as item No. 45, under 'Bone Implements, Ornaments, etc' in the exhibition catalogue.[10]

Hocken also travelled to Auckland in March, and to Wanganui in early April 1889, seeing key people and promoting the exhibition. Indeed, his efforts on smoothing Northern waters were later recognised: 'Auckland came to the party, through Hocken's work.'[11] While in Auckland, he saw Cheeseman at the Auckland Institute and Museum, from whom he secured the original picture of 'Okaihow [Okaihau] by Sergeant Williams' for copying. He saw this work – and the others he owned – as eminently displayable, and they subsequently became items 39 to 42 in the exhibition catalogue.[12] While he was in Wanganui, Hocken received from the exhibition organisers a telegram congratulating him on his 'energetic work'.[13]

By early June, the EHMSS members had developed further strategies to gain more exhibits and increase participant involvement. More letters were sent to institutions and museums, and all the living ex-governors were contacted and asked for portraits to display. To combat Auckland's initial reluctance about the exhibition, the committee would write directly to Sir George

Grey to secure something of his Maori collection for display. It was also suggested that the exhibition president, John Roberts, should visit Auckland. Thomas Cook, the tourist operator, wrote expressing a desire to help. Some offers, however, seemed more trouble than they were worth: a Mr Coxhead had 20 enlarged views of Dunedin which he would allow to be shown if the committee framed them. But one matter did require attention: Augustus Hamilton, ethnologist and future Otago Museum director, had written from Hawke's Bay explaining his 'great fear' about not getting a Maori house that Hocken regarded as an exhibit of paramount importance. As chairman, Hocken promptly responded, telegraphing Hamilton 'to use increased efforts to procure' it.[14]

Hocken was extremely busy. On 4 June 1889 he wrote apologetically to John Webster: 'It has weighed long on my mind that I should have written you much earlier. But I must plead a constant series of engagements, not merely professional but also those connected with our forthcoming Exhibition. This promises to be a very big affair indeed & I do hope that you will make arrangements to visit it with your children.' Even though it was over a year since his last visit to Northland, he took credit for galvanising a local 'exhibitions' group in Russell and, he told Webster, 'I have asked them to communicate with you. This they doubtless have done. At any rate I am about to write them & shall speak of this.' He hoped that

> you will send us from amongst yourselves a goodly number of objects of interest. Perhaps your sons would take some special trouble in procuring the old armour which formerly belonged to Hongi & Waikato. I think you said it was in some wahi tapu. Every care will be taken of whatever is entrusted to us. In my court we have engaged careful packers & have numbers of well locked strong glass cases. The Northern S.S. Co will take your packages free of all charges. I enclose a programme relating to the court in which I am specially interested. Can you entrust to us those pictures of yours taken on the 'Wanderer'? They would be a great feature.[15]

The armour was never found. Hocken also mentioned the lacebark hats, asking that samples, plus jars of preserved fruit, be sent to Dunedin.[16] Displayed under the 'Unclassified Exhibits', No. 4, the hats and fruit had mixed fortunes in the exhibition.[17] As he explained later, 'the bottled fruits looked splendid but from some unexplained cause they soon became covered with mould & one bottle burst' The hats were a success, and their makers, Miss Webster and Miss Bryers, won an award for their 'universally admired' exhibits.[18]

Nothing, it seemed, escaped Hocken's attention, especially if it was old, needed salvaging and was displayable. Almost as an afterthought, he asked Webster 'whether the pilot would let me have the old chart of 'Jokeheshanger', which Hocken had obviously seen while in the Far North.[19] The pilot was John Martin and the 'Jokeheshanger' was an English corruption of the Hokianga, first surveyed by Captain Herd in 1827. Hocken's persistence paid off: the chart was displayed as part of the 'Maps, Charts and Plans' section of the Early History Court.[20]

Persistence also paid off with James Smetham's *The New Zealand Chiefs in Wesley's House*, which was painted in 1863 to celebrate the fortieth anniversary of the Wesleyan mission in New Zealand.[21] Set in the home of John Wesley, the painting depicted William Jenkins, a defrocked lay preacher; the Rev. F.J. Jobson, treasurer of the Wesleyan Methodist Foreign Missionary Society and his wife; Wiremu Te Wana, one of Hongi's generals; Takarei Ngawaka, grandson of Te Heu Heu; Hare Pomare and his wife Hariata Tutapuiti; and 10 others.[22] Hocken had seen the painting twice in Christchurch and by November 1887, 'after a curious history', it was in his possession, secured for an unknown sum, although this may have been about 'two hundred guineas'.[23] And of course, as was typical of him, he diligently formulated biographical data on the individuals in the painting, recorded the minutiae of the occasion and dispelled misconceptions surrounding the English tour undertaken by Jenkins and the iwi representatives. Underscoring the latter, he was emphatic:

> The expedition was undertaken with the sanction of the New Zealand Government. It received the most hospitable reception from the Queen and the highest persons in the kingdom. The Queen was god-mother to a Maori boy born during the visit – Nov. 1863. The picture indicates the meeting of the civilized Maori with the missionary to whose labours his advancement is due. It was intended that it should hang in the Mission Hall and Mr Swales, a publisher in Darlington, undertook to publish a Jubilee print from it, but the scheme fell through. *The chiefs travelled through the country giving exhibitions and soon became demoralized by their mode of living. Then they were discredited and finally became stranded. Ultimately they were sent back to New Zealand by charitable people.* In another hand there is a marginal note: 'These three clauses are incorrect.'[24]

By the time he wrote this the exhibition was well over and Hocken had managed to communicate with Smetham's widow, Sarah, who not only told him that the portraits were all careful likenesses, but also gave him more information which he recorded: 'Jenkins & the natives left London in the *Surat* June 20th 1864, arrived at Auckland Oct. 4th. Two of the natives died at sea of consumption. A short account is in the *Nelson Examiner* of Dec 8 in which Jenkins does not shine.'[25] He filed away her letter of 12 April 1899 in which she wrote: 'I am glad to hear that it [the painting] is at present in such good hands and has the prospect of an honourable future.'[26]

Even during his final illness Hocken was pursuing information about the painting. In September 1909 he dictated a letter to W.N. Jenkins asking for the journal that his father had written while in England. 'I propose to give it to the Dominion in December next together with my large collection of books, manuscripts, documents and pictures.' He continued: 'Of course it should be interesting from an historical point of view, and moreover it has much relation to the subject of Smetham's picture which it assists in interpreting. Can you see your way to letting me have this. In such case I should have it well bound and refer to it as having been given me by the son of Mr Jenkins.' He added a comment immediately recognisable to modern scholars, archivists and librarians: 'I dare say you know the too often final fate of such journals if left in private hands. They become fingered useless & finally lost & destroyed.'[27] Luck was not with him on this occasion; the original journal was presented to the Alexander Turnbull Library by Mrs A. Jenkins of Eltham in 1934.

Exhibition business meant casting his net wide. From Hobart, James Backhouse Walker feared there was 'not much to be done for your exhibition' but promised to spread the news and even gave hints on other contacts: 'I mentioned the matter to the Rev. George Clarke, a friend of mine, who was in the Hone Heke war, and with Sir Geo. Grey in the old days. It might be worth your while to write him on the subject. He is a brother of Archdeacon Clarke of Waimate.'[28] Walker also presented Hocken with a copy of his *List of Books relating to Tasmania* (1884), provided bibliographical information on the *Tasmanian Journal* and offered biographical details on the painter Joseph Lycett.

By the committee's eighth meeting, on 19 June, Hamilton was 'more hopeful' of the Maori house and offered his services at 15s per day to erect it in Dunedin. This was accepted, as was a suggestion to bring down a troupe of Islanders, including a musical band of 15 from Tonga. A telegram from Mr Ford, secretary of the Russell Society, stating that the local committee had no funds to pay for space, packing and postage. eliciting the succinct response 'Indolent' from Hocken, who sent a letter urging Ford to 'diligence & again drawing his attention to procuring exhibits of special interest such as the armour of Hongi & Waikato'.[29]

The July and August meetings involved further decision-making and the firming up of arrangements, made even harder by limited finances. To force the issue, the EHMSS compiled a list of costs that included bringing people from Tonga, Samoa and Fiji, plus the Tongan band, plus 'Maories', the house and other expenses. The total came to £900, which was sent to the executive commissioners of the exhibition who, unsurprisingly, did not agree to the sum asked for.[30] They disallowed £150 for 10 Samoans ('five of each sex') and offered only £60. The Tongan band was seen as an attraction, but it was given £100, not the suggested £170. There was some good news, however: 'After infinite difficulty & lengthy correspondence the Maori whare had been secured for Exhibition.'[31]

On 7 September 1889 Hocken wrote to Sir George Grey asking for 'some valuable assistance' towards the exhibition. 'I would more especially seek your aid, & doubtless this is the one which would most engage your interest. Will you entrust to us any exhibits of the sort now indicated? Anything connected with the early history of the colony? Any old maps, plans, pictures, papers, documents, etc?' Given that Grey's collection was now in the public domain, Hocken did not press the trustees of the Auckland Free Library until he had Grey's permission. He also asked for 'any of the Maori carvings presented by you to the institution. Every care will be taken of such loans, which will be exhibited (unless too large) in secure slope cases, insured, & have freight paid both ways at our expense.' Hocken also requested a recent portrait, and even though he claimed 'considerable success' with those he had already contacted, he appealed to Grey for help: 'Will you be so good as to favour me with the names of anyone possessed of articles similar for our purpose & relating to early New Zealand? A request and a word from yourself to such persons would be very valuable.' Hocken added enthusiastically: 'Of course you will visit us.'[32]

Little came from this personal appeal. Grey submitted a portrait and a cast of a whakapakoko haukakenga, or god of the harvest, but nothing else.[33] Hocken had to rely on others, including Archdeacon Williams in Gisborne, the Colonial and Native Offices, the Otago Church Settlement Group, F.R. Chapman, John Webster, Auckland's John Logan Campbell, Gilbert Mair, Augustus Hamilton and Sir Walter Buller.

After the two October meetings further sub-committees were formed to deal with specific themes: the Decorative, Early History, Maori and South Seas exhibits, the pressing problem of showcases, and taking charge of the visiting 'Natives'. Once again, Hocken was on them all. October was significant, too, because the first lots arrived – framed portraits of Maori. Augustus Hamilton finally reached Dunedin and was asked to document all the exhibits and take charge of their arrangement in the court. More cabinets were needed, so another appeal went to the executive. On 6 November 1889 Hocken wrote to Cheeseman thanking him for the exhibits that arrived and pressing him for more old views and photographs of Auckland. He did not forget his personal agenda: 'When you come down please bring the loose newspapers with you & we will then arrange an exchange for the pamphlets. Bring all except the Sn X [*Southern Cross*] which I have. The nos. of the N.Zers wanted which I know you have are 1, 3 & 34, & of the Govt Gazette nos. 12 & 19.' As he pointed out, 'It is far better to make one complete set such as mine rather than have a few scattered numbers which will sure be destroyed.'[34]

With time running out November saw more disappointments, concessions and hurried approvals. There were problems with bringing the Tongans and Fijians to Dunedin, and with the Fijian exhibits. Hocken almost certainly had a hand in writing the entries and descriptions in the EHMSS section of the exhibition catalogue, and one can imagine his disappointment on penning these words:

> Most of the Fiji exhibits did not arrive until many weeks had elapsed after the opening of the Exhibition. The lists accompanying them

were somewhat imperfect – perhaps unavoidably so Hence it has not been possible to collate and catalogue them with much approach to completeness. It is further a matter of regret that so few articles came forward illustrative of native arts and customs.³⁵

The Maori house continued to cause difficulties. When there was concern that it would look ridiculous, especially with a pine roof, it was suggested that it be displayed unerected, in panel form. An additional problem was further labour costs, even though some costs might be recovered by selling the framework at the close of the exhibition. Over the next two days Hocken and a colleague called on the executive, asking for a much-needed £250; they were given £200. Eventually it was decided that the slats would be displayed and the sides of the house built using a combination of felt, manuka wattle, plain wood and Chinese matting. Hocken asked an Invercargill lumber house to supply slats with bark on, the edges cut straight and not too heavy: 'Count on your efforts to help us. Reply prompt. State price & how you can deliver.'³⁶ Pressure was obviously telling. The slats were ordered; the government refused to send down the original Treaty of Waitangi because it was too fragile.

The opening date of 26 November finally arrived. It was a fine day, and the exhibition was launched with pomp and ceremony and processions – friendly societies, Hussars, songs and psalms, and the statutory three cheers. The occasion was crowned by the reading of a congratulatory message from Queen Victoria. The principal feature of the new building was an impressive dome with four square turrets and two octagonal towers. There were four large annexes. The eastern one, for example, measured 1090 by 45 ft (30.4 by 13.7 m) and housed, among others, a British court, a foreign court, Victorian, New South Wales and South Australian courts, a concert hall, Hodgkins' art gallery, a New Zealand government court, a court devoted to education and home industries, and local courts for Otago and Southland, Auckland, Napier, the West Coast and Nelson. Flags and bunting gave 'an air of festivity to the building'.³⁷

William Hodgkins, an artist himself and father to talented daughters Frances and Isabel, was the driving force of the Fine Arts Committee for the exhibition. In 1884, he had founded an art gallery in Dunedin to house a public collection of art. Using his contacts and enthusiasm, he managed to get some 1571 works, many by Scottish artists, transported to New Zealand for display. It was a significant 'Art' event, and New Zealand's first exhibition of British and European art. Of the 236 works that were finally sold, four were purchased by a committee of citizens and then presented to the city's art gallery.³⁸ One of the local exhibitors was Bessie Hocken, who showed her *Kowhai and Ribbonwood*.³⁹

Richard Combe Miller, an overseas traveller passing through Dunedin, made three visits to the exhibition in December:

As you enter the building an excellent statue of Her Majesty faces you, and then, proceeding along the corridors, some admirable specimens of carved furniture in native woods attracted my attention. I also observed some most beautiful specimens of native pottery; two vases of cream-coloured basket-work china … some splendidly finished canoes; the original charter granted by Her Majesty, under her sign manual, establishing New Zealand as a colony, and other later documents granting extended powers and boundaries; a beautiful fernery, most tastefully arranged … samples of every kind of coal, and various specimens of gold, found in New Zealand; a few English carriages; exhibits from Her Majesty's prisons, consisting of writing cabinet, military chest of drawers, camp-desk, made of Rimu and Kauri woods, &c; and finally, models of a Samoan canoe, Samoan house, Samoan coral, and Samoan baskets.[40]

Miller's mention of the exhibits in the EHMSS court would have delighted Hocken. Of the more than 1565 items in this court listed in the exhibition catalogue, some 368 – almost 25 per cent of what was on display – belonged to Hocken. He owned 29 of the 35 maps, 32 of the 34 early newspapers, 12 of the 14 documents relating to the history and development of settlement and 86 of the 90 illustrative materials such as prints and sketches. Thirteen of the 40 documents pertinent to Otago's early settlement were his; he was 'beaten' by his friend Chapman, who scored 14.

The EHMSS catalogue also gave the first listing of Hocken's artefacts, many of which were described separately, such as 'Flint-lock musket, from the armoury of the French corvette *L'Aube*', 'relics of the Wairau massacre in 1843' (found 34 years later, rusted and decayed), 'Seven greenstone Hei tikis', 'three carved wooden tobacco pipes' (one belonged to Hone Heke), 'two carved walking sticks' and 'Portion of Copper Sheathing from the *Bounty*, with description in the hand-writing of Baron de Thierry'. Some appeared in multiples, for example, 'long slender chisels, of several distinct types' and 'a collection of splinters taken from a Maori workshop, Riverton, Western Otago'. Overall Hocken had fewer Maori implements on display – only 148 out of some 800 listed. From a total of some 450 South Seas items, Hocken exhibited 26, including clubs, a wooden pillow, bows and arrows, two looms from the Santa Cruz and New Hebrides group, and a spear, a kadjo (tomahawk) and three boomerangs from Western Australia.

Preceding the EHMSS court item descriptions is an unsigned nine-page introduction. In another printed version of the official catalogue the introduction is spaced more leisurely, as are the entries, and carries Hocken's name at the end. To further validate his authorship, he has added in his own copy the words 'Written by' beside 'T.M. Hocken, Chairman'. The text is an historical overview from Magellan's naming of the Pacific in 1520, Tasman's skirting of 'Staten Land' in 1642 and James Cook's celebrated navigation and mapping of

New Zealand to the arrival of the British and American whalers. It includes brief descriptions of key figures such as Marsden, Wakefield and Hobson, and the legacy of the Treaty of Waitangi up to Parihaka in 1881. It was all familiar material to Hocken, and he no doubt cobbled it together from lectures and talks already given, and his not inconsiderable printed and manuscript resources. He made sure to convey the positive spirit behind the exhibition: 'With the healthiest climate in the world and the lowest death-rate, richly abounding in minerals, and with the most fertile soil, it is certain that ere long New Zealand will earn the oft-applied title – Britain of the South. Nature has poured upon her the horn of plenty, and her only enemies have been those within her own border.'[41]

Writing about the smallest component of the exhibition, the materials from the South Seas, he alluded to the 'discovery' of the Pacific Islands and not only gave a simplistic breakdown of the Melanesian, Micronesian and Polynesian regions, but also of their racial and ethnic attributes and the mystery of their origins. Research had already begun and he hoped that the materials in the EHMSS court would contribute something to the field. And while acknowledging the artistry of the South Seas Islanders, he praised the Maori – 'foremost of the savage race' – for the perfect workmanship of materials on display. He made one final point: 'The stone age through which Europe long ago passed yet survives in Polynesia.'[42]

Hocken played a major role in the success of the court and the exhibition. He prompted many of the individuals and institutions to be exhibitors, and he was the prime initiator and conduit for their involvement – as he felt he needed to be. 'Very early it became plain that the members of this committee took but little interest in the business. Under the circumstances I found it quite necessary to discharge the duties of Secretary as well as Chairman. This I did, transacting almost the entire business. The Court was perhaps the most interesting & successful of the whole Exhibition.'[43] This disappointment also found its way into the conclusion of his catalogue introduction: 'regret must be expressed that many others have lacked the willingness to assist an interesting department of a truly Colonial undertaking, and one which may not recur until New Zealand shall celebrate her centenary.'[44]

In 1889–90 the population of Dunedin was 45,898. During the 125 days the exhibition was open, 625,248 people went through the turnstiles. On 19 February 1890 alone a total of 7908 people went through, 5880 of them paying cash for admission; others had season tickets and passes.[45] On 1 April, the Tuesday before Easter, a 'Monster Cavalcade' brought some 5000 passengers in eight trains from Christchurch. For everyone spilling out of the carriages and into the exhibition, there were the official daily programmes announcing attractions and events and giving information on the various courts. For instance, those attending on 20 December 1889 would have read about the Jubilee Bell, the Eiffel Tower Otis Elevator (adults were charged

6d and children 3d to go up and down), the parachutist Professor Jackson who would descend 1000 ft (300 m) in the air, the Alexander Brothers who were tightrope walkers and a number of visiting Samoans, including two girls who made mats, tapa and kava on site. There was also a 'Lost and Found' column, concert announcements and the necessary map of the exhibition layout. Hocken collected an almost full run of these ephemeral programmes, plus numerous pamphlets advertising the exhibition such as the *New Zealand Jubilee and Exhibition Chronicle* of 29 January 1890, which has his annotations explaining the Dunedin photographs.[46] He also owned two copies of the official exhibition catalogue that he had specially bound with interleaved blank pages to which he added additional factual information on the sub-committees, various trades and professions. In his collection, too, were Jules Joubert's *Proposed New Zealand Exhibition in London* (1890) and his *Shavings & Scrapes* (1890). The former was a presentation copy in which Hocken wrote: 'Jules Joubert who with R.E. Twopeny supervised the erection of the NZ Exhibition at Dunedin of 1889–90.'[47]

As Hocken told John Webster, 'The Exhibition … was an immense success – more than the number of N.Z. inhabitants having passed through the turnstiles. We had visitors from all parts of the world & all were astonished & pleased. There can be no doubt but that it will prove of benefit to the colony generally.' He then went on to describe the 'special & interesting features which marked it & which prevented it from being merely a huge bazaar', noting

> the splendid exhibit of Early History, Maori & South Seas things to which as you know I devoted all my energy, & the reward & success were all that could be desired. Such a collection of Maori carvings & implements &c was never seen before – case after case of all sizes being filled with them – the Early History things alone occupying a space of 250 x 8 feet [76.2 x 2.4 m] of wall space besides flat cases all being glassed in. My own collection formed a great portion of this & for it I received special mention & a special award. In this Department were hung your old almanacks & Martin's Chart also specimens of poor Maning's letters.[48]

Hocken's collection of early history manuscripts, charts, sketches and maps was outside the scope of a jury award but it was noted as 'extremely valuable and interesting'. However, the Judging and Awards Committee, headed by Hocken's friend George Fenwick, decided to award him a special certificate.[49] He was also formally thanked at the last meeting of the EHMSS committee on 2 October 1890, even though only three other members were present. His reply was discreet and tactful: he expressed his 'sincere regret … to know that this was the last of those interesting meetings at which each member had vied with his neighbour to make the Early History, Maori & South Seas court a distinguishing feature of the New Zealand & South Seas Exhibition'.[50]

At this meeting, too, Hocken reported that everything had been returned satisfactorily with the exception of 'two trifling articles'. The adjective was perhaps a little flippant, given that one of the objects belonged to the Auckland Institute and Museum. After offering 'grateful thanks' for the loan of the exhibits, Hocken wrote in May: 'I need hardly say that they formed a most conspicuous & admired feature of the Maori court. Every care has been taken of them & I shall be glad to know that they reach you safely.'[51] Unfortunately, however, Cheeseman replied by return mail that one exhibit was damaged. Six weeks later, after reiterating his personal requirements – 'Do not forget the specimens of the preserved kumara hou nor any other papers you may come across' – Hocken wrote: 'I spared no pains whatever in sending things back safe & from several people have received warm letters of thanks. But of course all this is no consolation to you. I am deeply sorry. How did the "head" get back? I saw it packed myself.'[52]

In a more formal letter written on the same day, Hocken explained that the packer was an experienced person and there had been no other complaints. He included a report from George Davie, the person in charge of unpacking and packing, who pointed out that the 'large figure was very much cracked & had been patched before coming to the Exhibition'. Its legs, bolted on, had been 'unfastened because it stood too high in the court'. The framework it came in was 'very much broken' and Davie had to build a new one, which was 'well nailed & braced & the two pieces securely fastened in side'. It was 'sound' when it left Dunedin '& nothing but very rough or careless handling could have broken any part of it'. Portions of the carved figureheads sent from Auckland were found to be broken when they were unpacked, 'but they were glued & mended'. Davie blamed 'the very rough handling of goods by the sailors on board the steamers'.[53]

Hocken also questioned the captain of the ship that transported the goods, contacted Augustus Hamilton for a report and was determined to hold his unassailable position: 'Of course you will not forget that sentence in my last which informed you that when the exhibits arrived from Auckland there were portions broken off from them.' Eventually, armed with Hamilton's report, Hocken wrote to Cheeseman in July 1890, reiterating that the exhibits had been 'carefully packed under [Hamilton's] superintendence & were further fitted with hay so as to diminish the chance of injury'. Although 'deploring as much as ever that the articles you so kindly lent us have received damage', Hocken hoped that the museum would 'now entirely absolve [the exhibition] from any charge of blame & carelessness'.[54] Happily the saga ended here.

Another whom he had to placate was Thomas Ritchie who, writing on behalf of a number of Chatham Islanders, was 'quite surprised' that Hocken had lost 'the God', a carved 4 ft (1.2 m) statue-like figure of akeake wood. As late as 30 June 1891 Ritchie informed Hocken that visiting Chatham Islanders had seen the figure at the exhibition, and that 'he met with an accident by having his penis knocked off. I mention this so that it might lead to his discovery.'⁵⁵ There is no further correspondence on this mystery.

On 21 May 1890 a letter written by Hocken appeared in the *Otago Daily Times* under the title 'A Maori House for Dunedin'. This was his plea to the citizens of Dunedin to buy, through subscription, for 'the most moderate price of £200', the carved slabs 'which recently formed the interior of the Maori house in the exhibition grounds'.⁵⁶ But there was 'no response to this suggestion'. As he wrote privately, 'There never was much public spirit in Dunedin & people had spent largely during Exhibition time.' The slabs 'were carved near Napier for the celebrated Hawkes Bay chief, Karaitiana, who proposed erecting with them in Whare-Runanga. But he died in 188–? & the slabs were left lying.⁵⁷ I heard of them & received their loan for the N.Z. Exhibition of 1889–90 where they were erected in a house.' When 'an effort was made to purchase the carvings & send them to Paris', Hocken 'stept into the breach as no time was to be lost'.⁵⁸ He purchased the slabs, presented a couple to the Otago Museum, gave two to the Adelaide Museum and two or three to Augustus Hamilton and wrote to D.H. Hastings, to whom the idea of the Exhibition was first mooted back in 1887, that he had 'reserved four or five for myself'.⁵⁹

Hocken's interest in exhibitions did not abate. Ever the energetic enthusiast, he continued to collect and amass more materials, which today form valuable resources in the study of exhibitions, museology and developing nationhood. He was also involved in another such event, serving on the general committee of the 1898 Jubilee Industrial Exhibition; because of his acknowledged interest in the field, he sat on the 'Historical and Maori' sub-committee.

11
Bibliographic Connections

Sir George Grey and Alexander Horsburgh Turnbull, along with Hocken, form the Holy Trinity of book collectors in New Zealand. Their counterparts across the Tasman were David Scott Mitchell and Sir William Dixson. The connections and exchanges between Hocken and both Grey and Turnbull are known; those between Hocken, Mitchell and Dixson are less so.

The Antipodean interrelationships could be fascinating. Robert Louis Stevenson visited Sydney four times between February 1890 and March 1893. During one trip, probably the first, from 13 February to 11 April 1890, he is said to have called on Mitchell at his terraced house at 17 (now 65) Darlinghurst Road. According to legend, Mitchell refused to see 'Stevenson of Samoa'. Asked years later if he regretted this decision, Mitchell replied, 'Yes, because I might have got a copy of "Father Damien" from him for nothing, instead of having to pay £5 for it.'[1] George Robertson, of Angus & Robertson, heard a slightly different version: 'Stevenson wishes to call upon me, but I have heard that he wears long hair, doesn't wash, and smokes cigarettes all day at the Metropole. I won't see him.'[2]

Three years later on 25 February 1893 Stevenson, accompanied by his wife and his stepdaughter, Isobel Strong, called on Grey in Auckland to ask his advice on Samoan affairs.[3] Stevenson found the 81-year-old politician 'a wonderful old historic figure to be walking on your arm and recalling ancient events and instances! It makes a man small, and yet the extent to which he approved what I had done – or rather have tried to do – encouraged me. Sir George is an expert at least, he knows these races.'[4] Isobel Strong was also amused that Grey had treated the novelist as a politician and not a word had been said about his books, while her stepfather had complimented the politician on his literary success. Grey later ordered the entire Edinburgh Edition of Stevenson's works from Chatto & Windus, a firm outside his normal book contacts.[5]

Stevenson died on 3 December 1894. Four years later in April 1898 Hocken and Bessie visited Fiji and Samoa with their friend Dr Daniel Colquhoun, lecturer in medicine at the University of Otago. While at Apia they visited Stevenson's library at Villa Vailima (now a museum), climbing the steep Mt Vaea to the Scot's last resting place. While there, Hocken was able to secure a number of unidentified volumes from Stevenson's library and a single hand-written sheet in the author's hand, an item he held in high regard. He noted the details about how and when he acquired it, then filed it in his F&J Volume 5 along with the other 'famed and named' documents.[6] On their return to New Zealand the Hockens passed through Wellington and spent an evening with Turnbull, to whom Hocken showed off his Stevenson acquisitions. Spurred into action, Turnbull wrote to Hocken's Samoan contact on 10 May 1898, stating that he too was 'anxious to secure a few souvenirs of Stevenson, and ask you to send me a few volumes. Will you do so? If you let me know what the cost will be I can remit you the money.'[7]

Sir George Grey

Sandhurst-educated George Grey (1812–1898) had a strong interest in languages, an area of collecting that is evident in the collections he left to Cape Town and Auckland. His contact with the indigenous people of Western Australia led to his first publication, *Vocabulary of the Dialects Spoken by the Aboriginal Races of S.W. Australia* (1839). The results of his two expeditions along the coast of Western Australia were written up in his *Journal of Two Expeditions of Discovery in North-west and Western Australia* and published in 1841. After serving as resident magistrate at King George Sound and then governor of South Australia, Grey became governor of New Zealand in 1845.[8] He continued his philological and linguistic work in Auckland, extending his knowledge to the Maori language. A major setback to his collecting was the severe loss of materials in the Government House fire of 23 June 1848. His determination to carry on collecting was evident in a letter to the naturalist Richard Owen, dated 3 November 1848: 'I lost all my plate, china, linen, wine, and the most valuable of my books, various collections of curiosities, native songs of different countries, objects of natural history, which I have been many years collecting ... but I will in course of this summer endeavour to collect again as much as I can.'[9] And Grey's persistence bought results. He collected, compiled and had translated writings that were eventually published as *Ko nga Moteatea, me nga Hakirara o nga Maori* (1853) and *Ko nga Mahinga a nga Tupuna Maori* (1854). Both remain classics in their field. He also had contact with individuals in New Zealand such as Bishop Selwyn, Chief Justice William Martin, Maunsell and, later, Hocken. Such men, keen collectors themselves, not only aided him in collecting such indigenous language materials but also extended the scope to include Pacific region languages such as Hawaiian, Tongan and Samoan.

By December 1854 Grey was in Cape Town, beginning his post as governor of the Cape Colony and high commissioner for South Africa. There he continued his book-collecting activities and his interest in philology. He actively collected African language materials, and in 1856, with the arrival of Wilhelm Bleek, the first trained philologist in Africa, the collecting increased dramatically. Bleek catalogued Grey's books and compiled the various language catalogues covering areas such as South Africa, North Africa, Madagascar, Australia and Polynesia (1858–59), and two others: *Manuscripts and Incunables* (1862) and *Early Printed Books* (1867).[10] On 21 October 1861, 18 days after he was again sworn in as governor of New Zealand, Grey sent a letter to South Africa's Judge E.B. Watermeyer, informing the latter of his intention to gift his library of some 5200 books to Cape Town. The collection consisted of medieval manuscripts, incunabula and other rarities such as a Shakespeare First Folio (1623) and Isaac Newton's *Principia Mathematica* (1687).[11]

Back in New Zealand Grey purchased Kawau, an island in the Hauraki Gulf north of Auckland where, between 1862 and 1888, he not only rebuilt what is now Mansion House but also created an island paradise by importing rare animals and plants. He also built up his second collection, which has been described by Christopher de Hamel as 'the world's most remote library'.[12] In 1882 Grey announced his intention of gifting his library to the citizens of Auckland, and on 26 March 1887 he was present to address and open the new Auckland Free Public Library. Grey returned to England in 1894 and died there in 1898. The remainder of his collection, barring some personal papers that were burnt, was sent to Auckland. The final collection totalled 15,000 books and manuscripts.

Apart from four brief returns in 1840, 1854, 1860 and 1869, Grey was absent from England for some 50 years. However, he knew many of the London booksellers and bought from their catalogues, his main method of purchasing books and manuscripts. The firms he dealt with read like a roll-call of the English antiquarian book scene: Joseph Lilly, H.G. Bohn, T. & W. Boone, Willis & Sotheran, George Bumstead, Ellis & Elvey, Bernard Quaritch, Nicholas Trübner, Lionel Booth, John Murray, Adolf Asher, J. Tregaskis, Francis Edwards, Elliot Stock and Chatto & Windus.[13] And, like most Antipodean collectors, he had the two necessary attributes: persistence and an ability to wait.

Alexander Horsburgh Turnbull

Alexander Horsburgh Turnbull was born in Wellington on 14 September 1868.[14] After attending London's Dulwich College from 1881 to 1884, Alick, as he was known, started work in the family wholesale drapery firm. In 1885 and 1886 he made long return visits to New Zealand and on the second trip bought J.H. Kerry-Nicholl's *The King Country; or Explorations in New Zealand* (1884). This volume, dedicated to Sir George Grey, was an important purchase, 'the first book of my collection'.[15] His first manuscript purchase would be 'The Old Dramatists from Lillis to Dryden', bought in London in 1890.[16]

Back in London, Turnbull developed further his passion for collecting, especially 'New Zealandiana'. In late 1887, for example, he purchased an eight-volume *Cook's Voyages*, Parkinson's *South Seas*, and a two-volume *Dampier's Voyages* for £9 12s 6d.[17] With the sale of the family business providing the necessary finances, Turnbull's collection grew. During the winters of 1889 and 1890 he travelled to Smyrna, Constantinople and Algiers. He received catalogues from the London antiquarian book dealers Quaritch, Sotheran and Dulau & Co., directed business to a number of provincial booksellers such as Georges of Bristol, Meehans of Bath and William Brown in Edinburgh, and took advice from fellow collector Charles Rooking Carter. Continental,

American and Australian sellers also received requests. Like Hocken, Turnbull wrote to and commissioned individuals to help chase down a specific item: for example, he enlisted the aid of H.R. Russell, the Hawke's Bay politician and landowner, to hunt down Rusden's *Tragedies in New Zealand*.[18]

In February 1891 Turnbull was elected a Fellow of the Linnean Society, and in July arms were attached to his family.[19] To cap off these niceties, Turnbull commissioned the British artist Walter Crane to design an ex-libris bookplate with his name and the motto: 'Fortuna favet audaci' (Fortune favours the brave).[20] All of these activities were in preparation for his return to New Zealand in 1892 to join the firm of merchants founded by his father. Before leaving he asked Quaritch, the 'Napoleon of booksellers', to value his collection, which was estimated to be worth the substantial amount of £1500. In preparation for the move Turnbull wrote to his brother Robert in Wellington: 'I do not wish the books unpacked until my arrival, but I wish them insured against damage whilst waiting.'[21]

Back in New Zealand he continued to collect books and mingle with a select group of bibliophiles: Augustus Hamilton; insurance company director C.A. Ewen; ethnologists Elsdon Best and Stephenson Percy Smith; Charles Wilson, librarian of the General Assembly Library; and Robert McNab and George Fowlds, both MPs. On 23 May 1893 Turnbull wrote to Dulau & Co.: 'Anything whatever relating to this Colony, on its history, flora, fauna, geology, & inhabitants, will be fish for my net, from as early a date as possible until now.'[22] This was his defining collection development policy in relation to New Zealand, extending to the Pacific Islands and voyaging to the Pacific. Other areas of interest included Australiana (many purchased from Angus & Robertson), John Ruskin, British nineteenth-century fiction, works on Scotland, English drama, a standing order for William Morris's Kelmscott Press editions, and works by the poet John Milton. Turnbull's demand for clean, perfect copies reflected his attitude towards his collection generally. He was particular.

Although he worked competently and conscientiously, his heart was not in the family business and it went gently into decline. By 1916 it had to be sold and liquidated. During this time, however, there was a positive. In June 1914 he was in the throes of house building, planning accommodation for himself and his books at the now familiar Bowen Street building. Fellow collector Robert McNab urged that he 'make it big enough for the large number of Accessions you have'.[23] Turnbull's collection at this time was about 40,000 volumes, and he responded to the empty shelves in the new house by filling them. As his long-time housekeeper, Emily Brouard, remembered, Turnbull 'lived only for his books. He was very reserved, almost a man of silence. Sometimes I've seen him go for days without saying a thing … Cases of books came every other mail. He had his agents everywhere buying for him. Books filled his mind.'[24]

Turnbull was not a scholar collector like Grey or Hocken. He attempted some rudimentary bibliographical listings, but these attempts petered out. He did, however, help others by making his collection accessible, and he was concerned about the future of his collection, which by the early years of the twentieth century numbered 55,000 books and manuscripts. About 1910 he noted Hocken's and David Scott Mitchell's arrangements for their libraries and discussed the problem with Percy Smith and Robert McNab (the latter, in 1914, would give his book collection to the city of Dunedin).[25] In 1916, aged 48, Turnbull made a decision: the collection would go to the state rather than to Victoria University College, Wellington, as originally set out in his will. He added a codicil to that effect on 1 March 1918; on 28 June that year New Zealand's prime book collector died.

David Scott Mitchell

David Scott Mitchell was Hocken's near exact contemporary, born on 19 March 1836. Unlike Hocken and Grey he was a true Antipodean, born in Sydney, the only son of a Scots-born army surgeon who had settled there in 1821. Mitchell's wealthy father was, among other things, a founding member and at times vice-president and president of the Australian Subscription Library, which would eventually become the State Library of New South Wales. Mitchell and his two older sisters grew up in a leisured environment, and an atmosphere of culture and learning. In 1856 the future bibliophile graduated from the newly established University of Sydney with a BA with honours in classics, and an MA in 1859. In December 1858 he was admitted to the Bar, but never practised law. By this time he had other obsessions, and because he had independent means, he could indulge them.

School book prizes and an edition of *Robinson Crusoe* (1837) given to him by his father on his seventh birthday formed the small nucleus of a book collection. Legend has it that he acquired a number of old surplus volumes from his father's library, took them to his room and provided shelves for them – and thus began the Mitchell Library.[26] He eventually inherited the family's Hunter Valley land and after a short while moved to his Darlinghurst Road property where he remained for the rest of his life. Except for Mondays, when at 9.30 am he hired a hansom cab and made a round of the bookshops until 1.30 pm, his daily routine was the same. At 10.30 each morning he would come down the stairs from his bedroom and sit in his armchair, poring over books and manuscripts until bedtime. He ate two meals, both consisting of grilled chops, at 11 am and 8 pm.

Mitchell's collecting interests were wide: medieval manuscripts; early printed books; Elizabethan drama and voyage material; standard eighteenth-century authors; nineteenth-century poetry; drama and fiction; and contemporary French literature such as works by Baudelaire and Stendhal. By 1900 Mitchell owned 10,000 volumes of English literature.[27]

And then there was the Australiana, which he recognised as important to collect: 'I generally get all the Australiana literature I come across not so much for intrinsic merit which I am unpatriotic enough not to find in them as that I think some day anything like a complete collection of Australian books will be curious.'[28] Mitchell cast his net wide, contacting George Robertson and other Australian booksellers such as James Tyrrell and William Dymock and overseas dealers such as Quaritch, Sotheran, Maggs Bros Ltd and Francis Edwards. Tyrrell left an account of Mitchell, who never married:

> In manner and appearance, Mitchell was a typical book collector ... Even his beard, short and turning black to grey, was somehow in character for the part. His usual dress included a black bowler hat, black-cloth paget coat, matching black trousers and black elastic-side boots. His loose change he carried distributed in his vest pockets – sovereigns in one; half sovereigns in another and silver change in his coat pockets![29]

Like Hocken across the Tasman, Mitchell understood the importance of salvaging documents and books relating to the early history and development of his country: 'The main thing is to get the records. We're too near our own past to view it properly, but in a few generations the convict past will take its proper place in the perspective, and our historians will pay better attention to the pioneers.'[30] He became obsessive – 'I must have the damn thing if only to show how bad it is' – and uttered a common refrain: 'the night cometh when no man can collect'.[31]

And material kept pouring in, growing to a collection of well over 40,000 books and an enormous range of manuscripts, maps, pictures and prints. Alan Ventress, one-time Mitchell librarian, was correct: as a collector Mitchell was the right man in the right place at the right time. He was wealthy, he was single, he had time on his hands, he had space in his house (although this rapidly diminished) and he had identified a market in which few were interested. He appears to have settled on his mission in life and from that point did not waver. He had a prodigious memory for the contents of his books and their location within his house.

Mitchell was also conscious of what would happen to his collection after his death. Aware of Sir George Grey's benefaction, he got in touch with Hocken about his deed of gift. Mitchell had verbally agreed on the 17 October 1898 to bequeath his collection to the trustees of the public library, but only if a new building were provided to house the collection separately as the Mitchell Library. Mitchell also offered an endowment of £30,000, later increased to £70,000, for the purchase of additional books, manuscripts and binding.[32]

A site was chosen – next to parliament, facing the botanic gardens and the domain – but there was the inevitable procrastination. A frustrated and ill Mitchell announced that if something did not happen the collection would be given to the University of Sydney or sold. Galvanised into action, the premier commissioned an architect, and the foundation stone was eventually laid on 11 September 1906. Mitchell was too ill to attend the ceremony and never saw the building complete. He died at the age of 71 on 24 July 1907. The Mitchell Library, the grand repository for the history of Australia, was opened on 8 March 1910. Like the Grey Collection in Auckland, Mitchell's gift enthused others, providing a source of inspiration that formed a strong bibliophilic legacy.

Sir William Dixson

William Dixson was born in Sydney on 18 April 1870, the eldest son of a prominent horticulturalist, businessman and philanthropist. After being educated in Australia from 1889 to 1895, he lived in Scotland where he qualified as an engineer. In 1896 he returned to Sydney and worked for Norman Selfe, the engineer and educationalist who became known for his work on steamships. Dixson finally entered the family business and eventually became director of a number of companies. He played golf, was a competent photographer (as evidenced by various albums in his collection), enjoyed gardening and liked travel.[33] Unlike Mitchell, he was a genial host.

His collecting started mildly – a mere hobby – but then grew and absorbed him. He was an inveterate list-maker, detailing the names of sailors on Cook's voyage and those of early Australian artists and Sydney's upper echelon, including their nicknames. Fortunately, his interests remained wide: he gathered maps, coins, stamps, curios, relics, manuscripts and books. Like Grey, but not like Hocken, and much less than Turnbull, Dixson acquired traditional European collector items such as a book of hours, a medieval missal and incunables. Over the years he amassed some 20,000 printed books, which included the *Works* of Chaucer (1532), for which he had a fondness, Holinshed's *Chronicles* (1587), a Geneva Bible (1598), Jonathan Swift's *Gulliver's Travels* (1726), a Benares edition of *The Arabian Nights* (1885–88), a rare *Pickwick* in parts and a first edition of Tennyson's *In Memoriam*. Works by Carroll, Trollope and Kipling were also included. He was particularly interested in books in original bindings, including fore-edge paintings, significant rebindings, association copies or works that contained annotations or letters.

Dixson also had a strong interest in the exploration of the Pacific and works by the maritime explorers, as well as Australiana. Literary manuscripts by Henry Lawson and Henry Kendall, a vast collection surrounding the Tichborne case (a Victorian legal cause célèbre), official papers, warrants and dispatches relating to New South Wales and Van Diemen's Land (Tasmania), original letters by Marsden, choice manuscripts from the First Fleet and French accounts of Pacific exploration were also in the collection. Many of the latter, including works by Freycinet, Bougainville and Dumont d'Urville, were translated by Dixson himself.

A.H. Spencer, the Melbourne antiquarian book dealer, recalled Dixson's excitement on first seeing original charts drawn by Captain Cook:

Quickly, as I had done when I first saw the charts, he spread them on his office floor, and, as I had done, he got down on hands and knees and almost ate the charts! To see the 'points' he excitedly made, my wife, too, was obliged to kneel, and it was a very laughing office that afternoon. There is the picture – the King of Collectors, and my wife kneeling with Captain Cook.[34]

When Dixson learned that Mitchell's bequest to the then public library could not be spent on pictures and prints, he realised that here was an opportunity to shine. He acquired valuable paintings and prints of historical interest, including works by Webber, Hodges and Parkinson, artists who had accompanied Cook on his voyages, and endowed the collection so that more could be bought.

In 1919 Dixson offered some of his pictures to the state, repeating the offer in 1924 and adding that he would also bequeath the rest under similar conditions to those required by Mitchell. The Dixson Gallery opened on 21 October 1929 with some 360 historical pictures and prints relating to Australia, New Zealand and the Pacific on show. Like Grey, Hocken and Mitchell, Dixson was conscious of what would happen to his collection. His books, after all, were 'personal friends'.[35] He left the entire collection to the trustees of the public library and enabled the establishment of a permanent fund, the William Dixson Foundation, which allowed the reproduction of manuscripts relating to Australasia and the Pacific, and for those that needed translations into English. Dixson, who never married, was knighted in 1939 and died on 17 August 1952. The Dixson Library was opened seven years after his death. Although there was some duplication of materials, the Dixson, very much a closed collection, supplemented that of the larger and ongoing Mitchell Library.

✳   ✳   ✳

Hocken and Grey were corresponding during the 1880s. When Grey left New Zealand in 1894, a flurry of correspondence began between Hocken and Turnbull. In fact, that was the year they met. About 1896 and 1897, when Hocken was considering his own deed of gift, Mitchell contacted him about similar matters. Few letters between Hocken and Mitchell have survived, even though Hocken sent his Australian counterpart a large number of books and pamphlets. Dixson was also a recipient of Hocken's generosity, but no correspondence remains.

Hocken and Grey

The first recorded contact between Hocken and Grey is documented in a letter of 28 October 1880, tipped into 'Historical narrative of an attempt to form a settlement in New Zealand', a manuscript written by Charles,

Baron de Thierry and now in the Alexander Turnbull Library, Wellington. Grey began by explaining that he was writing in pencil as he was lying down, having been 'very unwell'. He had just read Hocken's second lecture, 'which I presume you sent me', 'with the best interest and delight − I regard it as most excellent. I hope you will continue your lectures, and make them into a continuous link which would be very valuable.' He did feel, however, that Hocken had 'a little misunderstood Baron de Thierry' and explained that he had paid the eccentric coloniser to write his autobiography:

> He began with the New Zealand part of his life, which he finished a few weeks before his death. His illness was very short. This part of the narrative was supported by the original document [s] which I have. From these I clearly understand that all he claimed here was a small tract of land, in fact a small estate, and he contended that within those limits, until a regular Government was set up, he could exercise the rights of a chief and that he was one of the Sovereign Chiefs of New Zealand, not the Sovereign Chief. I am sorry he did not live to complete the early part of his life, for it was very curious.[36]

As we have seen, Hocken called on Grey in his island home in 1881 and returned to Kawau in November 1885. The book talk that eventuated from this last visit was a catalyst for action by Grey. On 10 November he wrote: 'Dear Hocken, I shall always say you have treated me badly. The first day I have had to myself at home, I have had to search through musty books and papers, for some things you wanted ... but as yet I have only found one − *The New Zealand Journal* for 1841. I send you that by book-post.'[37] Hocken had asked specifically about duplicate New Zealand Company reports, but Grey found only '18th Report 9th May 1845 with supplement of 62 pages − and the 12th Report 1844, without supplement'. And, just in case, Grey listed his own desiderata: 'The numbers I am deficient are 2, 4, 6, 9, 13, 15, 16, 19, 20. If my duplicates are of any use I will send them on.' He reiterated his desire to assist in filling gaps by asking for a list of New Zealand pamphlets that Hocken did not have. The search would continue but, sounding somewhat harassed, the old bibliophile wrote: 'I leave it to the servants now. You will soon be odious in their eyes − so do not come for a month or two, until this uproar is forgotten.'[38] Grey also sent a copy of Lord Lyttelton's 1854 *Memorandum*, which contained his reply to the many charges made against him while in office.[39]

Less than a month later, on 7 December 1885, Hocken replied apologising for his tardy response, saying he had been waiting to receive further reports, possibly duplicates, from Wellington. He did, however, dispatch three New Zealand Company reports (Nos 13, 19 and 20) to fill gaps in Grey's collection and also thanked him for the *New Zealand Journal* and Lyttelton's *Memorandum*, which was being bound up into one pamphlet volume with a number of his other speeches.[40] (Clearly, by December 1885 Hocken had made some headway in personally arranging his pamphlet collections for binding; it was a task he would not complete.) Ever persistent, he repeated his liking for duplicates and stressed his willingness to reciprocate. He was also confident enough about his collection to invite Grey to examine it when next in Dunedin. When Grey gifted his library to the citizens of Auckland in March 1887 Hocken asked again for a list of the pamphlets that Grey had given to the library; he had made many requests for this: 'You will confer a great favour in producing one for me.' At the time, Hocken had 50 bound volumes of pamphlets, totalling some 672 individually published items: 'it is very probable that I do not possess many that are noted in your list & which I should be delighted to receive.' He also squeezed in a postscript: 'Have you a spare copy of Cap. Fitzroy's "Remarks on N.Z."?'[41] Grey's response to this letter is lost, but Hocken seemed to have forgotten that he already owned a copy of FitzRoy's scarce pamphlet bound up in Volume 41 of his pamphlet collection. According to the signature within, it was acquired from the Williams family.[42]

Three months later, on 19 September 1888, Hocken sent Grey another instalment of his lectures on the early history of New Zealand and promised to forward another portion. Although conscious of Grey's political obligations, Hocken reminded him of his promise: 'You were kind enough to say that you would make further search for any spare copies of the N.Z. Journal you might have & you may remember that I wrote to you shortly before the Session on the point.' And then he added his requests: 'I have not got any numbers of the years 43/44/45 & my numbers in the succeeding years have many deficiencies.' And, of course, 'I shall be very grateful to you for anything you could let me have in the old history way.'[43] Again, there is no known response from Grey, a silence that continued until the New Zealand and South Seas Exhibition of 1889–90 prompted Hocken to write to him asking for loans and help in gathering materials for it. As noted earlier, little came from this personal appeal.[44] No further letters between the two collectors have survived, but given their bookish connection, it is unlikely that correspondence ended here.

Hocken and Turnbull

In early February 1894 Turnbull wrote to Grey asking for help over the New Zealand-related manuscripts in the Grey Collection at Cape Town. Grey encouraged him to contact the Cape Town librarian to ask for estimates of the cost of transcribing some of the most important works. Although this initiative fell through, Turnbull's letter to the librarian is of interest regarding his philosophy of collecting New Zealand material: the copying 'would contain information of great value to students of folklore and mythology but now practically inaccessible to them. A faithful transcript in New Zealand would place the material in reach of those [to] whom it would be a real benefit.'[45] Turnbull's desire to get his hands on the manuscripts remained strong: 'I am Sinless with regard to coveting Sir George Grey's splendid series of Maori

MSS for my own library but I do break the tenth commandment on behalf of the people of New Zealand.'[46]

Later that month Turnbull wrote to his Uncle Robert:

> A Dr Hocken of Dunedin has been visiting me lately, he is a great collector of New Zealand books & we have had many a long talk already over our respective libraries. Dr Hocken is supposed to have the finest series of works on this country there is. He is a most entertaining little man & during his stay in Wellington has been most instructive to me.[47]

The correspondence between Turnbull and Hocken, both proud of what they secured and ever eager to obtain that one last item, remained fairly constant until the latter's death in 1910. Their letters are full of the inevitable crowing and the inevitable desiderata.

Although they first met in 1894, Turnbull made an earlier reference to Hocken in a letter to bookman William Brown of Edinburgh on 2 November 1893. Somehow the southern collector had secured a copy of the *Album of New Zealand Views* (c. 1880), which he was instructed by Brown to send on to Turnbull in Wellington. Turnbull confirmed its arrival and stressed that he 'should be very glad if you would keep a look out for anything original or unique or very scarce relating to the Colony of New Zealand'.[48] With Hocken now in the loop Turnbull was quick to make further contact, writing to him in May 1894 to say that he had 'discovered a small parcel of duplicate pamphlets in one of my cupboards; it must have escaped my notice when I was disposing of my duplicates before leaving Home.' He goes on to list them:

1. Catechism of the Constitution of N.Z. by a member of a Provincial Council. Lyttelton, 1855. 12mo. Pamphlet. pp. 8.
2. Report of the Settlement of Nelson, N.Z. by Wm Fox. London, 1849.
3. Handbook of N.Z. & the Australian Continent by John Bright. London, 1841. 8vo. pp. 210 (wants 2 pp. of addenda).
4. Hints to intending sheep farmers in N.Z. by F.A. Weld. Fourth edition, London, 1864. cr. 8vo. Pamphlet. pp. 40.
5. N.Z & the N.Z. Coy. In answer to a pamphlet entitled How to Colonize by T. Heale. London, 1842. 8vo. Pamphlet. pp. 63.
6. N.Z. as a field for emigration by Rev. J. Berry. London, 1879. cr. 8vo. Pamphlet. pp. 40 with map.
7. Information relative to N.Z. for the use of Colonists. London, 1839. 8vo. Pamphlet. pp. 80 with map.
8. Memorial to his Grace the Secretary of State for the Colonies together with a vindication of the character of the missionaries & native Christians. London, 1861. 8vo. Pamphlet. pp. xi & 35.
9. Further Remarks on N.Z. Affairs. London, 1861. 8vo. Pamphlet. pp. 30
10. The case of the war in N.Z. by E.H. Browne. Cambridge, 1860. 8vo. Pamphlet. pp. 51.

Turnbull was 'very happy to effect exchanges [for a] number of pamphlets not in my collection' and his letter also included the inevitable queries: 'Do you have a duplicate of the first number of the *Otago Journal*, as you thought you did when we met in Wellington? And could you spare a copy of the New Zealand Company's "Fat Book"?' Hocken did: one of Turnbull's two copies of the *Supplement to the 12th Report of the New Zealand Company* (April 1844), a work of some 1000 pages, has Hocken's signature on the title page. When he wrote, Turnbull had just returned from Auckland and detailed some of his booty for Hocken: 'some good carvings, a very old hei tiki, early Maori printing from the Catholic Mission press, and a number of pamphlets'.[49]

The following year between 17 and 20 May Turnbull was in Dunedin, and although there are no details of this visit, he surely called on Hocken and viewed his collection. And given their future contact, it seems rather strange that in November 1897 Turnbull asked one of his London booksellers to 'keep an eye open for a work by Dr. T.M. Hocken on the early history of Otago, New Zealand, to be published by Low I think'.[50] The next exchange was in 1899. Hocken had just completed some housekeeping, specifically the sorting of his holdings of newspapers, and discovered that he had duplicates of the *New Zealand Spectator*, the *Wellington Independent*, the *Nelson Examiner* and the *Otago Witness*, which he offered to Turnbull for 'exchanges or purchases'. Hocken wrote that he was after 'old Kororareka ones (/40 to /43) & some of the early Southern Crosses. But you might let me know what you have, what you want, & what you think would be the value of these old records.' As usual, Hocken's postscript was full of more requests.[51] A flurry of correspondence over duplicate newspapers followed. Although his financial situation was at times precarious, Turnbull was certainly wealthier than Grey or Hocken. Like many collectors, he liked bargains and often pushed for a lesser price for a desired item. With Hocken, however, he met his match. On 30 May 1899 Turnbull responded to Hocken's list of duplicates and his asking price of £200: 'I am obliged to you for the trouble you have taken in compiling it but I was not prepared for so high a figure being put upon the papers and my idea of the value would be nearer £100 seeing that some of the sets are incomplete.'[52] Turnbull then suggested seeing the items, for which he was prepared to pay postage costs to Wellington. Four days later he acknowledged the scarcity of such newspapers and expressed concern for their safe arrival.[53] When the first consignment reached his home, Elibank, Turnbull 'became all bustle – excitement' and after documenting various discrepancies and missing issues, he agreed that £200 was fair. A cheque would follow but was preceded by the usual list of wants, including proceedings of provincial councils, of which he had 'very few'. 'Of course these latter I look upon as distinct from the newspapers and will be very glad to pay for them. I wish I had some duplicates to exchange with you, so as to avoid the "money" difficulty but you have everything in your library that I have in duplicate so there is no chance for me.'[54]

A week later on 26 June 1899 Turnbull again documented gaps in his own collection that he hoped Hocken could fill: 'I am much obliged to you for your promise of the Otago Gazette & proceedings: of Nelson I possess nothing. I have never seen "Otago Punch" nor have I any numbers of "Dunedin Punch".'[55] There was reciprocation: Turnbull offered to Hocken duplicate copies of 'Auckland Punch', a number of the Wellington Provincial Council reports and a copy of 'a work called "Jewlius Rex", a pamphlet published at Gisborne, lampooning Sir Julius Vogel & others'.[56] Hocken's copy of this anonymous work is in Volume 86 of his pamphlet collection; there is no indication that it came from Turnbull.

On 4 July 1899 the second 'newspaper' consignment arrived, for which Turnbull offered his sincere thanks. As he had other sources of supply, he also kept Hocken informed of what he had acquired. After assuring Hocken that he was not the other 'A.H. Turnbull', 'an ardent book collector' in Auckland who owned a 'tall folio Shakespeare', Turnbull mentioned that he owned Thévenot's rare *Rucueli de voyages* (1681) and *Relations de divers voyages curieux* (1696), the first important travel collection in French.[57] Hocken owned a copy of the latter. Turnbull then offered Hocken more duplicates. The two men had a contrasting approach to such items, as revealed in a letter by Turnbull to William Downie Stewart in 1908: 'Dr Hocken is a bit of a miser with regard to his duplicates. He pursues a different policy in this matter to what I do. I am not sure he is not right because I never seem to have duplicates to give away when they are much wanted whereas the Dr always has some up his sleeve to distribute or exchange when necessary.'[58]

On 21 August 1899 newspapers continued to be a topic of discussion, and Turnbull's announcement that he had secured J. Pratt's 1827 Manchester printing of *Abduction: The King v. Wakefields & Thevenot: A report of the proceedings on the trial of Edward Gibbon Wakefield, William Wakefield, Edward Thevenot, Edward Wakefield, and Frances Wakefield, for a conspiracy, for the abduction of Miss. E. Turner, before Mr. Baron Hullock, on Friday, the 23rd. of March, 1827, at Lancaster Assizes* must have forced Hocken, a collector of Wakefield material, to recognise a gap.[59]

Items continued to go back and forth between Dunedin and Wellington. In April 1900 Hocken gave Sissy Turnbull, who lived in Dunedin, some 'valuable papers', a view of Auckland and a plan of Dunedin to pass to her brother. A contrite Turnbull wrote apologising for his tardy response: 'I am ashamed to look you in the face – even by means of a letter as it were.'[60] Apart from informing Hocken that he had acquired a few Milton items to fill gaps, the hot topic was the sale of William Larnach's library, which occurred in Dunedin on 30 April.[61] Hocken attended and bought what were considered bargains, including the two-volume edition of Flinders' *Voyage to Australia* (1814), for which he paid £9.[62] Not being on the spot, Turnbull was less fortunate, complaining that the Park, Reynolds & Co. catalogue of the sale was 'an utterly useless document to anyone at a distance because no proper description is given of the books, the dates of publication in the greater number of instances are omitted as well as the edition and no indication is given as to "condition"'. There were, though, one or two lots he might bid for 'on spec'.[63] Although Hocken gave Turnbull a number of pamphlets he had purchased from the sale, this act of generosity did not stop the Wellington collector from continuing his complaint in a May letter: 'The sale must have been horribly mismanaged and the catalogue was without exception the worst one I have seen of a library containing so many books of colonial interest.'[64]

The process of sorting out holdings in a large collection can be a taxing business especially if they are newspapers, with their complex issue sequences, pagination (or not) and the invariable title or format changes. As dedicated collectors, both Hocken and Turnbull understood the necessity of this activity; they also recognised the importance of newspapers as historical documents and actively collated their holdings. And informing a kindred spirit of the gaps revealed was but a common and intelligent strategy. In sorting out his large collection of J.G.S. Grant material and his recent acquisition of copies of the *Hawke's Bay Herald*, the *Hawke's Bay Times* and the *New Zealand Spectator* from William Colenso's collection, Turnbull pressed his southern friend with questions: 'Were there any more issues of [Grant's *Saturday Review*] after that date?', 'Do you happen to possess duplicates [of the *Hawke's Bay Times*]?' and the enticer: 'If there are any missing parts in your set of *Spectator* please let me know, because I might be able to find them.'[65]

Hocken's absence from New Zealand between 1901 and 1904 explains a gap in their correspondence, and it was not until early June 1905 that Turnbull wrote, including a copy of a letter by Edward von Dadelszen, printer of *Te Pihoihoi Mokemoke* (1863), and the offer to supply any deficiencies in his holdings. As Hocken was able to secure one of the two rare proofs of this paper, he had Turnbull's letter and the Dadelszen letter bound with issues of *Te Pihoihoi* and *Te Hokioi*, the first Maori-language newspaper produced entirely by Maori.[66]

Four years later Turnbull wrote again, having read about Hocken's intention to gift his library to the University of Otago: 'I am sending you a copy of the *Evening Post* dated 3rd inst. containing an article by Mr Stephens on your collection ... So far as I can recollect this is the first proper description of your collection, as a whole, I have seen & I am glad it has appeared because it will give the public some idea of what you are presenting to the Dominion &, I hope, will make them realize what sacrifices in time & money you have endured to make your library so perfect.'[67]

And the hunting continued, each man keeping an eye out for materials that would satisfy the other. Hocken spurred Turnbull's interest in Samuel Butler, especially in reference to his writings in the Christchurch publication *Literary Foundlings* (1864). For Turnbull this event resulted in correspondence with Henry Festing Jones, Butler's biographer.[68] When Hocken's *Bibliography* appeared in 1909 it caused a flurry in Wellington book circles, and Turnbull actively spread the news about it to other collectors.[69] Turnbull's last letters to Hocken have disappeared but we have a reply from Hocken written in February 1910 when he was dying: 'My dear Turnbull, I must not allow a second of your kind letters to pass unanswered though I am in a sadly crippled condition & do not know what the end may be.' He was pleased that Turnbull had found the bibliography useful; he himself believed it was of 'great value'.[70] He was too ill to supervise the distribution of his books and pictures into the newly built Hocken Wing: 'Few can understand this but you will most thoroughly.' He also apologised for not calling on Turnbull during his last Wellington visit: 'I was too ill to leave the ship. You know how much I should enjoy a long talk & browse with you. Let us hope the day may come again.'[71] When Turnbull, sometimes called 'reserved' and 'almost a man of silence', heard how critically ill Hocken was he wrote: 'All this makes me very sad and think of Thomson's lines: "Whether man's life or heart it be/Which yields thee harvest, must thy harvest fields/Be dunged with rotten death."'[72]

A few weeks after Hocken's death, Turnbull received a cache of duplicates from Bessie Hocken. Pressing his fortune a little further, he asked if she knew of any other newspapers, pamphlets, Maori works and engravings that could be spared. A list of such items, he added, would be helpful.[73] Bessie's reply is not known.

Hocken and Mitchell

On 8 April 1899 in his only letter to Hocken, David Scott Mitchell wrote: 'Should you visit Sydney I shall be glad to show you anything I have.'[74] Hocken did visit Sydney a number of times, but it is not known whether he called on Mitchell. Although the latter never went to New Zealand, he approved of Hocken's collection and his approach: 'It seems to me that you are entirely right in taking all possible precautions for the further care & preservation of your library, which I have always understood to be the finest & completest in existence in all matters relating to New Zealand.' This was high praise indeed. In fact, Mitchell added, 'Such a collection, could probably never be got together again, & should be scrupulously cared for.'[75] And in response to Hocken's letter, now lost, Mitchell succinctly detailed the conditions he had laid down for the gifting of his own collection to the Public (later the State) Library of New South Wales. (Hocken actually knew this, as two weeks earlier he had received a letter from Henry Anderson, principal librarian, detailing formally the conditions laid out by Mitchell; the go-between for this information had been George Robertson.)[76] Mitchell did sound a warning: 'It is a matter of interest to all book-lovers that such a library as yours should not be left to the tender mercies of those who might not know its value.'

There was a little-known exchange of materials between Hocken and Mitchell sometime about 1899: housed in the Mitchell Library are 145 books and pamphlets that were once owned by Hocken. Excluding seven pamphlet volumes that contain publications without any provenance details, there are 87 titles that are duplicates, once housed in Hocken's library. In the world of rare books there is no such thing as a duplicate, each volume containing its own unique provenance and features. Yet Hocken chose to give these items away, including Lieutenant-Colonel Porter's *Major Ropata Wahawaha, NZC, MLC: The story of his life and times* (1897), which he had been given by William Waller relatively soon after publication, and Philip Philips's own *Memories of the Past* (1888), a presentation copy 'With P.A. Philips compts' received on 5 April 1897. Some of the titles contained Hocken's own handiwork, as if they were to be retained. The relatively scarce bilingual printing of George Sisson Cooper's *Journal of an Expedition Overland from Auckland to Taranaki, by Way of Rotorua, Taupo, and the West Coast* (1851) was but one, with the title page bearing Hocken's name and on page 35 his embossed arms. W.T. Cunningham's edited *New Zealand as a Tourist & Health Resort: A handbook to the hot lakes* [1893] not only contains annotations by Hocken but also his green Hakena stamp, which shows that by 1899, at least, he had had the stamp created and had started using the Maori form of his name.

Given Hocken's acquisitional tendencies, it is surprising that he also released publications of which he did not have doubles. Some of these 46 non-duplicate titles now in the Mitchell include Robert Maunsell's *Hints on Schools amongst the Aborigines* (1849), Henry Jordan's *Emigration to the New Colony of Australia* (1860), G.W. Rusden's *Lecture on the Character of Falstaff* (1870), Octavius Hadfield's *A Reply to the Question: Is a miracle opposed to reason?* (1875), Theo H. Davies' *Letter to His Grace the Archbishop of Canterbury* (1886) and Charles Hursthouse's *The New Zealand Handbook* (1866). The Falstaff item was certainly more in keeping with Mitchell's scope, while the others were within the throw of Hocken's collecting net. And again there were provenance details. One possible justification for dispatching duplicates and non-duplicates was that Hocken was deferring to Mitchell: here was a chance to impress the great Australian collector. Another possible reason was money.

Hocken also sent Mitchell various issues of the *New Zealand Spectator and Cook's Strait Guardian* (1844–65). His letter of early October 1899 to Angus & Robertson hints that some of the titles mentioned above were not outright gifts.

> By this mail I am sending you the case of newspapers together with a collection of other papers & books which I have gathered together & which I make no doubt you will appreciate. Their value & price I leave to your judgement. I have many holes & corners yet to search & shall doubtless find something further to send you.

The newspapers herewith sent are of great rarity & value & are sent in lieu of those which Mr Robertson saw when in Dunedin. Those papers were unbound & there were many missing & imperfect numbers, nor were they of such old date as those now sent. I could hardly make up my mind to part with them but on the whole have decided to let you have them. The price I will leave to be fixed by yourself & Mr Mitchell.[77]

Gifts or no, Mitchell did respond. Embedded in Hocken's pamphlet collection are two small publications that the Australian collector presented to him. Intriguingly, they are both closely associated with Mitchell. The first was Patrick Scott's *The Farewell and Other Poems* (London, 1827), which Hocken duly annotated: 'Patrick Scott, natural uncle of Mr David Mitchell of Sydney. He was an Indian Civil Servant & visited NSW two or three times where his relative, Dr Scott (his father) lived.'[78] The second concerned Mitchell's father: the *Statement of the Case of Jas. Mitchell, Esq, Late Surgeon on the Civil Establishment of New South Wales* (Sydney, [1838]), which Hocken bound into Pamphlet Volume 175, along with 22 other items.

Hocken and Dixson

There is no known correspondence between William Dixson and Hocken, yet the former's library contains five publications that were once in Hocken's. The two duplicates and three non-duplicates show varying degrees of ownership determined by Hocken before being dispatched, either as gifts or purchases. The first duplicate is G.W. Rusden's *Curiosities of Colonization* (1874), a work dealing with Holt and Margaret, political convicts of New South Wales, and containing some reference to Samuel Marsden and Wakefield's theory of colonisation. It has Hocken's signature on the title page. The other duplicate is John Ward's *Supplementary Information Relative to New-Zealand: Comprising despatches and journals of the Company's officers of the first expedition* (1840). This work by the first secretary of the New Zealand Company contains Colonel Wakefield's first dispatch from New Zealand on 1 September 1839, and has information dealing with the settlement of Port Nicholson and Cloudy Bay. It contains Hocken's signature on the title page, his embossed arms on page 35 and evidence of earlier ownership: 'N.Z. Book Room, Wellington'.

The first non-duplicate publication is James Larnach's *A Bibliographical History of Australia: Read before the Historical Society of Australasia on Friday, 27th November, 1885* (1885), which has Hocken's signature on the title page and evidence of earlier ownership: 'James M. Larnach 1886' or 'W.J.M. Larnach, 1886'. Perhaps this was one of the items Hocken purchased at the Larnach sale of April 1900. If so, he owned this item for a very short time. The second is a Philadelphia printing of the Rev. Donald MacDougall's *The Conversion of the Maoris* (1899), which contains Hocken's signature and his small note on the author. The last non-duplicate item was *Journal of a Cruise among the Islands of the Western Pacific* (1853) by John Elphinstone Erskine. It is surprising that Hocken released this classic nineteenth-century account of Pacific exploration, which was with him long enough to bear his signature and bookplate.

※ ※ ※

The lives of these five collectors span some 140 years, from the Peninsular War to the death of King George VI and the accession to the throne by Princess Elizabeth. Their combined generosity has given Australia and New Zealand lasting book and manuscript treasures. In all this, Hocken was a key figure: gregarious, generous and aptly placed chronologically between Grey and Dixson.

12
The Fieldwork Continues

Hocken continued to be busy throughout the 1890s. In 1894 he travelled to Oamaru and Christchurch, and in 1895 he travelled twice, once to the north and south to the Stewart Island region. In 1897 he ventured north again, and while in Auckland went on a harbour excursion with Auckland members of the New Zealand Journalists' Institute.[1] On the local front he was active in church affairs. He was a member of the synod for Otepopo and Hampden in 1891, a parishioners' churchwarden and secretary for St Paul's in 1894, and a member of the church's governance committee in 1896. In early February 1896 he was involved in the Inter-Colonial Medical Congress and, as already mentioned, in 1898 was a commissioner and sub-committee member for the 'Historical and Maori' section of the Otago Jubilee Industrial Exhibition.

In 1893 Hocken started his 'Historical notes' and 'New Zealand notes', two manuscripts of 12 and 85 leaves respectively that form an important link with many of his published writings and the books and manuscripts acquired up to and including 1899.[2] 'Historical notes' contains brief chronologies of the lives of Thomas Kendall and the Rev. John Butler, the names of their children, a rather detailed account of Maori names used by Marsden and a fairly graphic account of Captain Jarvey's death in 1865, which Hocken attended as coroner. The larger manuscript contains the small beginnings of a bibliographical listing of pamphlets owned and factual information on the early New Zealand newspapers, as well as anecdotes about Sir George Grey, the Wakefields, surveyors Theophilus Heale and J.T. Thomson, Mantell and the Akaroa Resident Magistrate Charles Barrington Robinson, who 'cheated at cards at Wakefield Club. Wellington'. Also included were the derivation of names surrounding Dunedin (Goat-Hill, Vauxhall, Forbury). Interspersed throughout are Hocken's notes identifying those from whom he obtained the gossipy historical information. William Mason, Sir William Fox and W.H. Pearson, an early Southland settler, were but three.

Compilations such as these involve both time and effort. The process of sifting and sorting the mound of historical information and marshalling it into a coherent form was a necessary activity, especially if, as was clearly evident, publication was intended. Hocken also wrote down anecdotes and facts to help solidify in his mind the events, dates and people involved. He liked documenting; indeed, he scrupulously recorded, in a British Medical Association booklet designed for the purpose, Gladys's growth from birth to the age of 19.[3]

Percy Smith and the Polynesian Society

In 1858, when he was only 18, Stephenson Percy Smith and four companions – his cousin Charles Wilson Hursthouse (a fellow cadet in the Survey Office), F. Murray, J. McKellar and H. Standish – made a 965-km journey from Taranaki to Mokau. It was an arduous venture, accomplished before seasoned geologist–explorers such as Hochstetter and Haast. Smith's journey was written up and published by the *Taranaki News* office. Many years later in 1890 he sent a copy to Hocken, unaware that there was already one on the shelves at Atahapara.[4] Despite being a duplicate, this small item signalled the beginning of a trickle south that included, among other things, a manuscript letter by F.A. Carrington headed 'New Plymouth Harbour', dated 1 March 1880; Carrington's *A Synoptical Account of the Making of the Harbour at New Plymouth* (1888); Elsdon Best's *In Ancient Maoriland* (1896); and Smith's own *The Eruption of Tarawera* (1887), *Hawaiki* (1898), *The Peopling of the North* (1898) and *Wars of the Northern against the Southern Tribes of New Zealand in the Nineteenth Century* (1904), plus his notes on the 'Pedigree of Hursthouse'.[5] Coincidentally, these items signal some of Hocken's unique collection arrangements. The first two titles are in Pamphlet Volume 46, Smith's three titles – all presentation copies – are in Pamphlet Volume 114 and the manuscript notes on Hursthouse are in Variae Volume 3.

More significantly, from the early 1890s onward Smith became a valuable contact in Wellington, especially with the access provided by his jobs as surveyor-general and secretary for lands and mines. In September 1890 Smith sent Hocken

> two postal maps which might be adapted to your purpose after alteration. All the colors & tables can be stopped out and many of the names if you think the maps will suit. If they will, you might run your pen through any thing you think unnecessary, and I can send you a print from it. The [lithographic] stone can then be kept and have any information you may wish to add placed on it when the time comes for printing.

He also announced his intention of visiting Dunedin in October and hoped to 'do myself the pleasure of calling on you for it would be a very great treat [for] me to see your collection'.[6] No evidence of such an occasion exists, but one – perhaps the first – did occur in July 1892 when, after visiting Hocken and meeting Bessie and Gladys, Smith exclaimed: 'It was indeed a treat to me to go thru' your library.'[7] One 'prize' that Hocken certainly showed off was his copy of John Rochfort's *The Adventures of a Surveyor in New Zealand* (1853), a work that Smith had heard about but not seen.

Although feeling poorly, Hocken attended the AAAS conference in Christchurch in January 1891. Participants at this important third meeting of the association included Mantell (vice-president), Edward Tregear (secretary), Augustus Hamilton, the Rev. J.W. Stack (curate of the Diocesan Maori

Mission) and many others. Hocken had hoped that John White, compiler of *The Ancient History of the Maori*, would be there, but he had died while travelling to a court sitting at Whakatane.[8] Also present at the conference was Chatham Island-based Alexander Shand, who was involved in his own research into the Moriori spurred on, as Hugh Stringer has suggested, by Percy Smith.[9] A correspondence between Shand and Hocken resulted. In between asking Hocken for medical and dietary advice for an unknown Moriori friend and trying to induce him to move to the Chathams because of the shortage of doctors, Shand mentioned Smith's idea of forming a Polynesian Society.[10]

Hocken, a great supporter of efforts to get the society off the ground, played his part by exchanging information with Smith. On 2 February 1891 just after the AAAS conference, Smith wrote asking if Hocken could copy specific extracts on the 'Philomele' (nightingale), as described by Lesson on Gambier Island near Tahiti and found in Dumont d'Urville's multi-volume *Voyage de la corvette l'Astrolabe* (1830–35). According to Smith, the only copy of this work in New Zealand was at either the university or the museum library in Dunedin. Smith added a postscript: if there was anything on the bird, he preferred the original French.[11] Smith was probably unprepared for the prompt and complex reply, and a raft of copied extracts.

> Of d'Urville's magnificent work I am the fortunate possessor & it has given me the greatest pleasure to search it for you though I am conscious it is to little avail. However I thought it best to make the entire extracts from it & from Duperrey as well. Neither Duperrey nor d'Urville visited the Low Archipelago on these voyages so that I am at a loss to know when Lesson wrote his 'Iles Mangarewa' [Mangareva]. Give me a little more information on this point & I will make further search in other directions. What is his date? The nearest approach to your Philomele (where do you get this name?) is the *Philedon bouroensis* [*bouruensis*] from one of the Moluccas. The figure of this bird as given in d'Urville is very similar to that in Buller – but of course it is not coloured. On d'Urville's 2nd voyage in the *Astrolabe* 'Au Pole Sud' in /37 to /40, Hombron & Jaquinot were the naturalists, Lesson was not one. On this occasion the Poumoton archipelago [Tuamotu] was visited & Manga Rewa explored, but there is not a word of the Anthornis under any of its names (Philedon &c) …[12]

Hocken ended by offering to 'translate this chapter for you – easier than transcribing the original French', which of course meant that Bessie would do it. Smith's response of 16 February was equally prompt and included a reference to his idea: 'How badly we want a "Polynesian Society" to take these matters up, based on the lines of the Asiatic Society – with correspondents at the various islands.'[13]

One result from the AAAS conference was the formation of a committee on 'Polynesian Bibliography, with special reference to Philology'. Hocken was already a member of the anthropology section along with Mantell and Tregear, among others, and duly received the association's reports, which he filed in his collection.[14] In reality, philology was outside his expertise; the benefits from networking were far more important. Smith, however, continued to press home Hocken's involvement: 'You do not say if you will take charge of my contribution to Polynesian Bibliography. I have got 45 works not mentioned in that of the Association. I have no doubt you could add many others.'[15] Perhaps because of the fear of overcommitment and thoughts towards his own projects, Hocken was noticeably quiet on this.

Smith did, however, have a 'captive' audience and he bombarded Hocken with his thoughts on the Polynesian Society, especially on the proposed quarterly publication: 'I will however put my ideas into shape and then send the notes to you for criticism.' The 'Bibliography' project also came tumbling in, with Smith sending his list of works to Hocken and stressing again the need for publication. There was also gossip: 'I see that Dr Fraser is again Secretary. Now unless either you or Tregear, or Mr Stack move in the matter, I expect nothing will be done.'[16] In Smith's eyes, at least, Hocken was considered a man who started and completed tasks. Smith and Tregear co-founded the society in 1892, and it was to become very important to Hocken. He was a paid-up member, as evidenced in a letter to Smith in June 1906: 'I enclose my Polynesian subscription which as you see I have made payable for *two* years instead of the current one alone.'[17]

As already indicated, Hocken was generous to kindred collectors and extremely acquisitive. In July 1892 Hocken sent Smith a work on the 'Maori King Movement', and asked about some volumes on 'Old Maori deeds', no doubt emanating from their discussion in his library. The latter was most certainly H. Hanson Turton's *Maori Deeds of Land Purchases in the North Island* (1877–78), of which Smith complained: 'someone has walked off with the spare copy I had in the office, but it will come back I have no doubt and then you shall have it.'[18] By November 1892 Hocken was not only the owner of Malcolm Ross's *Aorangi, Or, The Heart of the Southern Alps, New Zealand* (1892), but also the proud possessor of the first volume of Turton '& one Vol. plans of old Maori purchases', with promises from Smith 'to not forget you' when it came to finding the other volumes.[19] In that November letter Smith also thanked Hocken for 'the loan of C.O. Davis MSS', and ended on a pleasing high with news about the recently formed Polynesian Society: 'We shall have a very interesting No. of the Journal for Jany. – the best yet out – and papers come in faster than we can make use of them. There are 8 new members & the election next meeting of the Journal – so the Society will be a success.'[20]

No matter how interesting the world of textual analysis and philological specifics was, Hocken's inclination was towards collecting. Unlike Smith, he had neither the time nor the language skills to concentrate on aspects such as the evidential reliability of recorded waiata and poems. Indeed, on occasions,

Hocken relied on Smith's linguistic judgement. An annotation in his copy of the Maori language edition of John Bunyan's *Pilgrim's Progress* (1854), suitably signed on the preliminary pages and with his 'F.L.S.' signed bookplate, reads: 'Part of Governor Grey's native policy was to publish interesting books in the Maori language ... These books are rare' and 'Mr S. Percy Smith tells me that these translations (Crusoe and Bunyan) are in most excellent Maori.'

Yet Hocken did dabble in linguistic matters. In June 1893 he sent his own language compilation to Smith along with a précis on the *Alligator*'s mission culled from William B. Marshall's *A Personal Narrative of Two Visits to New Zealand in His Majesty's Ship* Alligator (1836), and Marshall's own *N.Z. the Vocabulary of South Island Words*.[21] Hocken's effort was a rudimentary one, as Smith commented: 'I have your vocabulary quite safe. I have been hoping to find time to copy it out and arrange it alphabetically, but have not done so yet.' He then stated the obvious: 'It requires a good deal of work put into it for I am convinced many words are wrong.' More significantly, Smith's December letter mentions another of Hocken's projects, one that actually came to fruition: 'I am glad to hear you are progressing with the Bibliography. It will be most valuable, and who so well able to do it as yourself?'[22]

The Network Spreads

Smith's letters were not the only ones that made demands on Hocken, and, as usual, he spread himself over a wide variety of activities including, it must not be forgotten, his professional and family obligations. In late January 1891 he was fielding correspondence from Edward Charles Stirling at the South Australian Museum in Adelaide and dealing with the receipt and payment for the carved slabs left over from the exhibition.[23] About 11 May that year Hocken received a rather belated catalogue of books dealing with Australia and New Zealand from James Miller, Market Street, Melbourne, in the hope 'that it will afford you some interest', and later, a copy of Thomas Cass's memoirs, *Canterbury Times*.[24] Hocken considered Cass an old friend, and in early February 1894 while travelling through Christchurch he met the 76-year-old surveyor, who had worked with Torlesse for the Canterbury Association.[25] On 18 May 1891 Hocken wrote to Cheeseman at the Auckland Institute and Museum asking for a possible exchange of 'oldest numbers of the *Nelson Examiner* – 1842 to 1845 or of the *Port Nicholson Gazette* – 1840, for your earliest Auckland papers the *Standard*, *Chronicle*, *Times*, etc.' To courier the booty south, Hocken offered the services of his brother-in-law Frank Buckland, who was then visiting Auckland.[26] Hocken wrote to Cheeseman again on 8 July and included news of his collection:

> I shall be much obliged if you will not forget but will at any time send me anything in the old history way ... I should much like you to see my N.Z. library & you would indeed then assist in making any additions to it in

your power. The pamphlets alone number 60 thick volumes & they do not consist (as so many of Grey's do) of collections of Chamber of Commerce, & other similar yearly Reports, but are really historical ones.

He also revealed to Cheeseman that he was 'just now engaged in writing the history of the Canterbury Province' and asked: 'Do you come across any of the Canterbury Pamphlets?'[27] In September 1891 Hocken wrote again, informing Cheeseman of his recent purchase of pamphlets from Whitaker's sale and offered to sell some for 'the price paid'.[28]

Hocken was also corresponding with John Fraser, his fellow 'Polynesian Bibliography' member, on Samoan customs. On 11 May 1891 the Sydney-based Fraser pressed Hocken and fellow members Tregear and Stack to compile a parallel paper 'from one who knows the Maori race'.[29] Fraser added: 'I do not know which of you may have leisure or inclination for that labour!'[30] In September that year Hocken finished the draft of his first lecture on Canterbury (28 foolscap pages). In March 1892 he received a copy of *A Letter Addressed to the Most Rev. The Primate of New Zealand on the Establishment of Cathedrals in Colonial Dioceses* (1886) from Bishop Samuel Tarratt Nevill, but not without having to read Nevill's outpourings on the fact that had he known he would be bishop for 21 years without a cathedral, he would not have accepted the appointment.[31] Four months later Hocken was receiving answers from the Rev. Thomas Godfrey Hammond, who had consulted Phillip Tapsell from the East Coast, on his own query about the bone 'papa toe ake' (or 'papa tikonga or 'papa pu hope') and the differentiation between and meanings of 'kuri' (dog) and 'pero' (also dog).[32] And in December 1892 Hocken met the Rev. William George Lawes, the first resident European missionary to Niue, who was passing through Dunedin as part of his 'world' lecture tour. Their meeting resulted in Lawes sending his 1888 edition *Grammar and Vocabulary of Language spoken by Motu Tribe, New Guinea*.[33]

Good Fortune

Hocken had his share of luck. In August 1891, in response to one of his 'searching' letters, he received a letter from G. Gerard Shaw, the nephew of artist G.B. Shaw.[34] Shaw gave the details of 'colonial pamphlets' asked for, mentioned various duplicates of early South Australian and Victorian books that he was prepared to exchange, and offered a brief list of books 'relating to your colony' that Hocken could have if he did not have them already. The titles (some imperfect) included Charles Terry's *New Zealand, Its Advantages and Prospects* (1842), C.W. Adams's *A Spring in the Canterbury Settlement* (1853), Julius Vogel's *Official Handbook of New Zealand* (1875) and Anthony Trollope's *Australia and New Zealand* (1873). Shaw's prime message, however, was to thank Hocken for the list of tokens he had sent. These metal discs – with devices, inscriptions, or more commonly both, impressed upon them by specially cut stamps or dies – were ordered and circulated in considerable quantities by mercantile firms, banks, public companies and others as currency. Tasmania had led the way with some minted as early as 1823; Christchurch was last in 1883.[35] Hocken collected these scarce relics and eventually gave some 80 to the Otago Museum.[36] Most notably, the postscript to Shaw's long letter read: 'N.B.: I have a very interesting memento of Dunedin in the shape of a watercolor painting of that town in 1851. The view is taken from Church Hill looking towards Ocean Beach, the size is 19 x 15.'[37]

Hocken responded promptly, asking more about the painting. By October 1892 the 'long hunt of many years' was over and Hocken had acquired the watercolour for £3.[38] The 'long hunt' may have been an exaggeration, but Hocken was certainly aware quite early on of the painting's existence. He had found notice of it in the *Otago Witness* of 29 November 1851 and discovered that it had been on display at a Princes Street office. There was also high praise for the painting from H.F. Hardy and John Hyde Harris, both of whom supplied details of names and descriptions for the eventual key plan. Because the painting was an excellent depiction of Dunedin in 1851, Hocken included a copy of it in his *Contributions*. It also warranted display at the Otago Jubilee Industrial Exhibition of 1898 along with some 116 portraits and views, 40 of which belonged to Hocken.

Again, the catalogue for this exhibition is important because it documents what he then owned.[39] His contributions included the *Map of the Settlement of Otakou* (1847); Kettle's *Map of Suburban Lands in Settlement of Otago* (1849) and *View of part of Dunedin from Stafford Street* (1849); Edward Immyns Abbott's *Dunedin from Little Paisley* (1849); Thomas Redmayne's pencil drawing of Dunedin (1864); George O'Brien's *The Taieri Plains* (1867); and of course Shaw's view of Dunedin from Church Hill, with the key plan executed by Bessie. Among other items were portraits of Frederick Tuckett and the Rev. Thomas Burns; photographic views of Oamaru (1865) and Waikouaiti (1865); £1 promissory notes of James Macandrew (1853) and John Jones (1855); specimens of deeds with tattoo signatures; and the usual run of early newspapers such as the *Otago Daily Times* (November 1861) and the *Evening Star* (May 1863).[40] For Hocken, the exhibition provided another opportunity to shine.

Further Additions

In 1893 Hocken exchanged letters with Henry Tacy Kemp, who was the son of missionaries James and Charlotte Kemp of Kerikeri and a Maori interpreter and writer. Kemp had witnessed the signing of the Treaty of Waitangi and was purchaser, for the Crown, of most of the South Island from Ngai Tahu in 1848. On 29 July 1893, in reply to Hocken's queries about Captain Stewart of Stewart Island, Captain James Herd's visit in the *Rosanna* to the Hokianga in 1826 and the availability of any early newspapers, Kemp wrote: 'I have already written to some old friends to furnish particulars as they can & have every reason to believe they can & will do it cheerfully.'[41] Two 'old friends' responded. One was William Leonard Williams; his letter brought information on Stewart as well as book gifts.[42] The other was William Webster of Kohu Kohu, Hokianga, who provided details on the New Zealand Company and Captain Herd. This document was transferred to Hocken and is filed in his '21 Important Letters' volume.[43]

Penning his letters from his library at Atahapara, Hocken extended his network to anyone remotely linked to the subject or topic he was concentrating on. Replies reaching him often carried further leads. Occasionally there was a jolt. In May 1894 Alithea Symonds cast aspersions on his collecting activities. There had certainly been a misunderstanding, as she wrote: 'I have safely received the Parcel which you sent me and I was delighted to get those Books in my possession again. I am sorry you made a mistake and that you were under the impression that I gave them to you. I could not do so.'[44] Two years later, James Heberley, the first harbour pilot for Port Nicholson and the first European to stand on the summit of Mount Taranaki (Egmont), on Christmas Day 1839, told Hocken that he could not have a particular manuscript as requested because it was going to his wife, who was going to publish it.[45]

There were other disappointments and reality checks. In August 1894 Bishop John Richardson Selwyn, son of George Augustus, Bishop of New Zealand, wrote to say that the sermons Hocken was asking about were out of print.[46] In November 1896 Albert Allom wrote clarifying the historical accuracy of a particular painted view of Port Chalmers and verifying his voyage south on the schooner *Carbon* when he and Richard (later Sir) Nicholson had travelled to meet Tuckett and Davison to survey the Otago Block. The ex-surveyor was also adamant about the accuracy of his recollections: 'When I tell you anything it will be fact – not matter of belief only.'[47] And because Allom was travelling, he enlisted help from Hocken and his 'treasures', accessing copies of the *Spectator* to further verify the date of Edward Gibbon Wakefield's involvement in the settlement of South Australia.[48] Allom was an important Wakefield connection who assisted Hocken in later years.

Hocken also continued to lend out material, including copies of George Vancouver's *Voyages* to Richard Henry, who later responded with his interpretation of the harsh and arduous conditions faced by Maori and early whalers at Dusky Sound. Of the Maori he commented: 'Fancy them coming over here with their bare shins braving the sandflies & the storm & wet of this place for the feast & the finery to take home to their wives & sweethearts.'[49] And Percy Smith was not forgotten: in May 1895, after enquiring about the *Missionary Register* and its relative scarcity in New Zealand, Hocken bundled up 11 volumes covering 1815 to 1825 and sent them to him.[50] Smith later acknowledged Hocken in his *Wars of the Northern against the Southern Tribes of New Zealand in the Nineteenth Century* (1904): 'I am sincerely grateful to Dr

T.M. Hocken F.L.S. of Dunedin, for a loan of the latter work. So far as I know there are very few copies in the Colony – hence the value of Dr Hocken's copy and his great kindness in lending it.'[51]

In May 1896 Hocken received from Paddy Gilroy, a Bluff resident, a reply containing personal anecdotes about the trader Captain William Anglem, to which, as evidence of close reading of a book owned, Hocken appended a note: 'This old whaler – Gilroy – died at the Bluff in April 1903. He is referred to in the closing chapters of Bullen's *Cruise of the Cachalot*. T.M. Hocken.'[52] Hocken often repeated similar or additional information in other files, as instanced in his 'New Zealand notes':

> In March 1895 I visited Stewart Island with a view to learn something of Cap. Anglem. At the Bluff I found old Gilroy – at 84 – who came in 1835 as a whaler. He married Anglem's half-caste daughter with whom I conversed. Her father died at the Neck, Stewart Island in 1846 when she was 17 years old. She does not know what became of his papers &c – perhaps they were buried with him ... Old Joyce – a half-caste – showed me where he was buried on the neck.[53]

From Dunedin resident Arabella Valpy, Hocken received manuscript materials containing purchases and expenses incurred by the Valpy family before their departure for Otago on the *Ajax*.[54] On 27 May 1896 he received notification from William B. Taylor, who had just accepted on behalf of the city the portrait of George Rennie, originator of the movement that eventuated in the settlement of Otago.[55] This particular gift was the direct response from Hocken's own correspondence with Rennie's son, Sir Richard.

Hocken also found time to attend an auction of 'Maori Relics' on 20 May 1896 at Park, Reynolds & Co.'s premises in Dunedin. On this occasion for £7 5s 6d he bought 14 items, including a flax hat, a bird snare, a greenstone adze, two ear pendants and a 'tattooing instrument'. Most of these artefacts, along with some 430 others, were gifted to the Otago Museum by Hocken or his wife, Bessie.[56]

North Again

At the end of January 1895 Hocken travelled north again, reflecting on 'the difference in travelling accommodation within the last 25 years when I commenced my trips'.[57] In Wellington he reconnected with the 'bright and intelligent ... but nearly blind' Mantell. While at Napier, he called on Henry T. Hill: school inspector, educationalist, Fellow of the Geological Society (1887) and member of the Hawke's Bay Philosophical Institute (later a branch of the Royal Society of New Zealand). He viewed Hill's 'very fine' collection of greenstone, mats and old carvings. One represented John Rutherford, the tattooed 'White New Zealander', with an immense penis. Hill maintained that the penises of Maori were small compared with those of Europeans, 'a fact well known and appreciated by the Maori women'. Hocken scribbled in his diary: 'I failed to recognise this and do not believe it.' At Gisborne, he called to see the Rev. Herbert Williams and, more importantly, teamed up with Augustus Hamilton, his 'saviour' during the 1889–90 exhibition, who was in his fifth year as registrar at the University of Otago.

It was a fruitful excursion. Hocken asked Hamilton, a keen photographer, to record carvings, and at Turanga he photographed eminent Ngati Porou leader Hirini Te Kani in a white dog-skin cloak.[58] At Tokomaru Hamilton took a photograph of the 76-year-old Hori White, said to be the son of Barnet Burns (c. 1805–1860), the English sailor–trader who lived for some years as a Pakeha–Maori on the East Coast of the North Island.[59] At Pakirikiri in Poverty Bay Hocken was given a carved tokotoko stick, a sinker and a rare form of oval fern-root beater. On this journey he perceived a change in the local Maori: 'The natives however, have almost lost their habits of industry and their good qualities, they are thriftless, lazy, and happy and have no care for the future.'

The results of the meeting with Hori White highlight Hocken's collecting impulse and reveal the quirky nature of where such incidental occurrences can lead a collector. He owned a copy of *A Brief Narrative of a New Zealand Chief* (1844) written by Barnet Burns, who returned to England and Europe about the 1830s and spent his time delivering lectures on his experiences in New Zealand and the customs of the Maori. He was heavily tattooed, which no doubt enhanced his performance. Although Hocken would eventually decide that, 'like Rutherford's, much of this story is probably fictitious', he did try to find out more about Burns' activities.[60] The catalysts were his receiving a copy of the *Kidderminster Shuttle & Worcestershire Mercury* that mentioned the tattooed performer and his recent contact with Burns' supposed son. Acting promptly, as was typical, on 20 March 1895 Hocken penned a letter to the editor of the newspaper.

> An extract from the Athenaeum records would be of interest, and perhaps of value. It is probable that a few of your townsfolk – young men in 1842 – might remember the incident, and may have conversed with Burns himself. I should like to know what age he was, where he resided and died, whether he had any family, and what became of his implements, etc, and indeed, any incidents that are trustworthy.

He explained that he had 'just returned from a holiday ramble along the east Coast of New Zealand' and that he 'made search for Burns and his antecedents, and with interesting results'. Burns's son was 'now an old man of 76, [living] with his family in a Maori village or kainga, called Tokomaru. He is entirely native in habits and customs, and is accounted a great chief.' In addition, on collating the dates and incidents in Burns' *Brief Narrative* 'with those given by my Maori friend serious discrepancies arise, and I must conclude that he is not one of the wise men who knows his own father'. Hocken was keen for 'any biographical information beyond that contained in his pamphlet, of the putative father, Barnet Burns'.[61]

Hocken actually owned a printed broadside that advertised lectures by Burns at the Lecture Hall, Derby, in April 1842, and a printed poster featuring him at London's Royal Adelaide Gallery in May 1849.[62] Although there is no known response from the editor at Kidderminster, Hocken may have turned to a more local resource. Alexander Turnbull owned a broadside that advertised lectures by Burns in the town's Athenæum, Assembly Room, Lion Hotel, on 4 and 8 March 1842.

Publications

Hocken had to balance constant letter writing and tracking the flow of books and manuscripts into Atahapara with his own efforts to write. On 14 January 1891 he completed 'Some account of the earliest explorations in New Zealand', which was constructed as a talk for the AAAS conference and later published in their *Australasian Association for the Advancement of Science, Report of the Third Meeting: Transactions of Section E*, 3 (1891). The 24-page draft ended up in the hands of Robert M. Laing, the honorary secretary of the Philosophical Institute of Canterbury (and subsequently in the archives of the Museum of New Zealand Te Papa Tongarewa).[63] With such a wealth of information to be squeezed into the talk, Hocken was faced with a dilemma: 'To compress these written required limits is indeed to give but a mere catalogue of names & dates or to present with rapid succession a list of explorations divested of all those little incidents which give to travel its very soul & spirit. However in an evil moment I accepted the task & rather than lack faith have now to bespeak your consideration for shortcomings which to me seemed unavoidable.'[64] The result, most of which was culled from his other writings, was a rather pedestrian overview of exploration from Abel Tasman onward.

The second publication in this period came from more arduous activities. In 1892 Hocken and his two good friends, George Fenwick and H.F. Hardy, made a short excursion to the Catlins area via Willsher Bay. This 'boys-only romp' was written up in the *Otago Daily Times* and reprinted as *A Holiday Trip to the Catlins District (via Willsher Bay)* that year. By train, buggy, horse, boat and foot, the three men, each carrying 'a small Gladstone bag containing the barest travelling necessaries', trekked to the Nuggets, Port Molyneux and Catlins Lake and then by skirting the coast to Chaslands Mistake went on to the Waikawa track, and then via Tahakopa Bay, Ratanui and Catlins Bridge to Owaka. A push through to Balclutha meant they caught an early train back to Dunedin. The round-trip 'adventure' took the best part of 10 days. Billy tea, rustic hospitality including home-made biscuits and scones, river trips on 'flatties' (flat-bottom boats), early morning rises, roaring fires and dawn choruses of the pihoihoi and kaka combined with historical information on whaling captain Edward Catlin; chiefs Tuhawaiki (Bloody Jack) and Karetai (Jacky White); sealer, whaler and pilot Tommy Chasland; and whaler Edwin Palmer. There were views of the 'Blowhole', unparalleled bush vegetation and the finding of wild-bee honey. While on the Catlins River, Hocken and his friends came across the remains of Guthrie and Larnach's 'big mill', once a household word in the area but now a 'picture of ruin and desolation'.[65]

The most important work Hocken produced during this period was *Abel Tasman and His Journal*, which he read to Otago Institute members on 10 September 1895, and which was published in Volume 28 of the *Transactions* in 1895.[66] His promise to put Tasman's journal 'in English dress' was now fulfilled, following Bessie's translation efforts while staying at Moeraki.[67] Publication had its usual benefits: it alerted those in the field of Tasman studies to an English translation, albeit restricted to New Zealand; it initiated correspondence from those interested in such matters; and it allowed Hocken another opportunity for self-promotion. As was usual, copies of the text accompanied letters to correspondents old and new. Among those recipients was Hobart-based James Backhouse Walker, who wrote in January 1896 to thank Hocken for 'your kindness in sending me your papers on Tasman and Early NZ literature'.[68] Indeed, it seemed that Hocken's translation had arrived just in time. Walker was undertaking his own work on Tasman, which included his own English version of the New Zealand portion. Although it was at the press for printing, Walker expressed interest in wanting to use an extract from Hocken's translation and eventually sent a presentation copy of *Abel Janszoon Tasman: His life and voyages* (1896), which Hocken read closely, marking passages used from his own (and Bessie's) work.

Walker also alerted Hocken to a proposal by Blackwoods to publish Basil Thomson's translation of the whole journal and Frederik Müller's facsimile edition, edited by J.E. Heeres. Walker ended his letter with a useful collegial suggestion: 'If you cared to send a copy of your Tasman paper to Mr E. Heeres, Het Rijkes-Archief, 's Gravenhage, Holland, I am sure he would be very grateful for it, and he might – possibly make use of it for the forthcoming Journal.' Hocken needed no prompting. He was already in touch with Müller, asking about the proposed facsimile and other in-house titles. In March 1896 Hocken heard from Heeres, who thanked him for 'your papers about Tasman and about the earliest literature relating to New Zealand, which was unknown to me … It is very interesting, that in New Zealand or Tasmania both the voyage of my famous countryman excite in the same time so much interest.'[69] Further correspondence resulted, all of which is tipped into Hocken's facsimile copy of *Abel Janszoon Tasman's Journal*, published in Amsterdam by Frederik Müller in 1898. On receiving this large work, Hocken proudly added a note: 'I was fortunate enough to have some of my work regarding Tasman inserted into this magnificent volume & was, so far as I can learn, the first to translate into

English that portion of his journal relating to New Zealand. This appeared in Vol. XXVIII of the Transactions of the N.Z. Institute. T.M.H.'[70] Of course, some things had lives of their own. In Walker's papers in Tasmania there is a letter from Edward E. Morris, another of Hocken's Australian correspondents, which suggested another project: 'Dear Mr Walker, Let me thank you very warmly for your kindness in sending me your most interesting paper on Tasman. You and Dr Hocken ought to combine your forces and bring out a book on the subject, you taking the Tasmanian part and he the New Zealand ... '[71] Perhaps if Hocken had known about this, and lived long enough, such a work might have eventuated.

13
A Gift, a 'Literary Venture' and the South Seas

Over 1895 and 1896 Hocken honed his general knowledge of New Zealand history by completing two small 'Christmas' articles for the *Otago Witness*. One was his 'Early statesmen and public men of New Zealand', which covered 15 luminaries such as Grey, Selwyn, Featherston, Bell, Domett and Justice Henry Samuel Chapman. Photographs were included in what was a rather balanced assessment.[1] The other was 'The governors of New Zealand', which contained 18 biographies, from Hobson, FitzRoy, Grey (again) and Gore Browne through to Sir William Jervois and the Earl of Glasgow.[2] Hocken also dealt with lesser 'governors', such as Busby, Willoughby Shortland and Edward Eyre. The act of completing these articles helped him to get the historical data right for his own *History*.

Hocken travelled north again in January and February 1897. While in Wellington he called on Sir Francis Dillon Bell, who regaled him with stories. In Otaki James McMillan, the CMS missionary, gave Hocken Tamihana Te Rauparaha's Bible, *Ko te tahi wahi o te Kawenata Tawhito*, one of 10,000 seen through the British Foreign Bible Society press in 1848 by John Telford and then Edwin Norris, the English philologist. It was given to Tamihana when he visited London in 1851 and contains his signature and a tipped-in brightly coloured map of the Holy Land between pages 96 and 97.[3] Sometime after 1909 Hocken revisited this item and added provenance details and a perfunctory note, including reference to his own work: 'This is the first volume of the Holy Scriptures printed by the British and Foreign Bible Society in 1848. Vide my Bibliography of literature of New Zealand – Maori section.' By 15 February Hocken was in Auckland, where he was shown letters and rare sketches of war canoes, weapons and moko. Such was his standing as an authority on historical matters that C.W. Greenwood, the owner, allowed him to take the sketches back to Dunedin for further investigation. Not only did he write out a full historical report, but he had Bessie make facsimiles of the originals, which were returned and then eventually housed in the Grey Collection in Auckland.[4]

Just after his return from the north, Hocken announced his intention to gift his collection to the nation so that it would be a public resource in Dunedin. The announcement was first made at a meeting on 18 March 1897 where other Dunedin notables were gathered at the City Chambers to discuss how best to celebrate the anniversary day of the settlement of Otago. His intention to do this was apparently a deep secret. Indeed, it has often been said that Bessie found out about the gifting of the collection by reading the public announcement in the *Otago Daily Times* the next day, though given their very close relationship, this scenario is unlikely.[5]

Importantly, at least to Hocken, the proposal provided an ideal opportunity to make the forthcoming celebrations significant. If Dunedin undertook to construct a building to house historical documents and Maori carvings, 'he would be proud to present the library and other possessions he had accumulated during many years to such an institution'. It was crucial that it be of the right quality: he would 'certainly not allow his library to go to any inferior object at all'.[6]

A major catalyst had been his visit to the new Free Public Library and Art Gallery in Auckland, where he was visibly impressed by the building that housed Sir George Grey's collection. In fact, he was so taken with what he saw that he packed up 47 pamphlets and various New Zealand Company reports, dated from 1838 to 1892, and presented them to the Auckland library. These items – all deemed 'of great rarity, and difficult to obtain' – are listed in an uncatalogued letterbook headed 'Books bought in America by John D. Enys' as part of the Auckland Library Archives.[7]

Another catalyst was the obvious educational role fulfilled by such a collection. When visiting Auckland Hocken had asked 'two intelligent youths' where Hobson was buried. The fact that they could not answer this question and did not know that Hobson was the first governor of the colony shocked him. He was acutely aware that 'very little or nothing was known amongst the young of the romantic history that attached to this and to other settlements' and hoped that access to his collection and all it contained would cause 'the young people to take pride in the deeds of their forefathers'.[8] On 20 March he wrote a long letter to the editor of the *Otago Witness*, which appeared five days later, to 'state ... explicitly ... my views and desires with regard to this gift'.[9] He referred proudly to the 'many thousands of books and pamphlets relating to the history of New Zealand from its earliest days', 'pretty well complete sets of nearly all the newspapers of this colony' and old letters, documents, journals, maps and other manuscripts. There was a judicious use of 'rare' and 'unique'. His major point, however, was that he wanted to keep the collection intact; it was not to be dispersed. Although he placed its monetary value at 'many thousand pounds', it was its historical and instructive value that really mattered. He also emphasised that he had spent 'many happy years, and, indeed, the best part of my life' in Dunedin. This was his payment for that debt.

He made two other points. First, Dunedin deserved such a library: 'It would mark our culture and forward our advancement', especially with the forthcoming Jubilee celebrations. Second, he could not hand over his library yet. It was a working library, 'an absolute necessity' for his ongoing projects, especially his 'history of the colony'. In a note familiar to most modern-day researchers, he wrote: 'The work of writing my book necessitates constant reference to the old records and books in my possession, and it is work that cannot be hurried, for amidst the taxing duties of a busy professional life spare time for historical writing is, unfortunately, all too short.' The book was his *Contributions to the Early History of New Zealand* which, as detailed below, would appear as promised in 1898, just in time for the Otago celebrations.

The Publishing of Contributions

Embedded in the middle of one of Hocken's letterbooks of the 1889–90 exhibition are 15 letters concerning the publication of *Contributions*, his 'history of the colony'.[10] This little-known cache is significant because it constitutes a snapshot of late nineteenth-century book production processes, made more complex because of the distance between the client (Hocken) and the publisher, the London-based firm of Sampson Low, Marston & Co., whose archive was destroyed in the Blitz on the night of 29–30 December 1940.[11] Although the correspondence is one-sided, it remains a valuable glimpse of an author's personal concern for his first literary publication.

The book's gestation, from initial contact to publication, lasted 32 months, and considering the problems of distance and the slight changes that occurred, it was a relatively smooth process. Even though Hocken pleaded ignorance on book publishing matters, he had firm ideas on what he wanted and of the potential for sales – and he was a quick learner. All this was certainly understandable as he was paying the bills for its entire production.

The search for a publisher began in June 1895. Hocken heard that local book dealer James Horsburgh was travelling back to England and asked him a 'great favour': when approaching publishers in England, could he mention the project? Even though Hocken claimed that the publication had 'not taken any special shape, chiefly from ignorance of the best mode of procedure', he had an exemplar in mind and a working title. The model was Arthur S. Thomson's *Story of New Zealand*, published by John Murray in 1859. Hocken liked 'the get up' of Thomson's book, and settled on the volume being a 'demy 8vo & the type long Primer, & the binding cloth bound'. The title was to be 'Contributions to the early history of New Zealand, together with a history of the Otago Settlement'; the illustrations would come from his own collection. And again, although 'quite at sea' about the process, he was adamant about the images: 'These [old views, sketches of Hone Heke's war] I think should be in folded plates as the page size is of same as quarto would be small plates. I could have these photographed for reproduction at home. Of course the illustrations should not be trashy; a few samples would be of use.'[12] Naturally, his 'at home' photographer was Bessie.

He had two publishers in mind: Macmillan, who had been good to his friend T. Jeffrey Parker with his *Textbook of Zoology* (1897), and Sampson Low, Marston and Co., who were supply agents for Horsburgh. Aware that publishers were often reluctant to fund relatively unknown ventures, Hocken stressed that he would meet the entire costs. In summary, and for Horsburgh's benefit, he asked for an estimated cost of a book of 400 or 500 pages with a dozen or so illustrations. After talking to Fenwick, he added issue numbers and extras:

'the price for 1000 & 2000 copies & for each subsequent 500. Also price with 8to [octavo] pica leads & without leads. To be gilt lettered on back; edges uncut. Price of paper at 48 & at 44 lb, double demy.'[13]

The next letter was written 18 months later in January 1897 to Sampson Low in response to the firm's estimate of production costs, which were obviously higher than those Hocken calculated. He had initially considered a larger book with content covering both New Zealand history and the more specific Otago-related material, but was forced to pare the project down – 'modify' was the word he used. He was now thinking of 'two or three parts or volumes, which will be quite independent of each other, & which can therefore be published at intervals of say a year or more'.[14] He reiterated the format of this new version: 'demy 8vo. 1000 copies; Paper, 48 lbs dble demy; Type, small pica solid & no leads between paragraphs; Binding, cloth, gilt lettering on back.' He was still lost about the illustrations and indeed had misplaced the reproductions the firm had sent him. To help facilitate action, he sent them negatives for reproduction, which he presumed would be half-toned images. Awaiting their instructions, he pleaded ignorance:

> I know nothing of these matters & therefore shall be obliged by you sending me fuller information on what would be better a specimen of a reproduction from one or two of the photographs sent – say a portrait & a view. For this of course I should pay & if suitable would go for the book. There could be seven or eight portraits & perhaps the same number of views, with one or two plans which last would perhaps do better lithographed.

The traffic of letters accelerated. On 17 March 1897 he informed the firm that a box of negatives and black and white prints of the proposed illustrations had been dispatched; colour was ruled out because it was too expensive.[15] He had also labelled them clearly. 'Can you inform me approximately how long it would require to have the book ready for sale? I should like it to appear *here* about Xmas next. If I sent you manuscript in say two months hence would you have time to send me proof & then to have the consulted copy returned to you for final printing.'[15]

On 14 April Hocken replied to the publisher's letter of 7 March. He acknowledged the sensible decision to separate the work into two, agreed to the dropping of the words 'Volume' or 'Part' in the title and included a £70 draft. This was partly a goodwill payment towards production, but also to cover the increased number of illustrations he wanted to include.[17] Twelve days later he sent through information on the key plans, expertly drawn by Bessie, for Kettle's and Fox's views of Dunedin.[18]

By the end of May Hocken had completed 54 pages of manuscript, which 'I have the pleasure herewith of forwarding for my book'.[19] He also posted off copies of 'Mr Tuckett's diary', 'A letter from Mr Tuckett to Dr

Hodgkinson, Otakou, 16 August 1844', David Monro's 'Notes of a journey through a part of the middle island of New Zealand' and a letter by 'Colonel Wakefield to the Secretary of the [New Zealand] Company, New Edinburgh [Dunedin]', which would form four appendices totalling 73 tightly packed pages of text. Monro's 'Notes' had been extracted from various copies of the *Nelson Examiner*, and in order to guarantee exact reproduction, Hocken sent them to the firm, asking for their safe return as they 'form part of a valuable set'. This letter is significant because it reflects his growing awareness of the complexities involved in shaping the book for publication, especially from so far away. To this end he informed the firm that he had engaged a friend in London to superintend the proofs. This was his brother-in-law, James Buckland, who was given full credit for his work in the preface. One other Buckland also received full, proper and permanent credit: he had posted off the dedication to Bessie.

Hocken's work on the manuscript proceeded quickly. Within the next 10 days he completed another 37 pages of the text proper and compiled another appendix of eight pages: 'Arrangements for the establishment of a settlement and for disposal of the lands of the New Zealand Company at Otago.' He was conscious of the need to get things right and valued the publisher's experience: 'I have done my best to make everything plain & intelligible & trust that you will have no difficulty in following the arrangement ... I do not know whether you consider the chapters too short; if so perhaps your intelligent reader could re-divide them without much trouble. But doubtless your letter that I am anxiously expecting, will give me some hints of directions.'[20]

In early July, despite a severe bout of flu, he posted Chapter XVIII. He also sent photograph and lantern-slide images of the 'Mission House' and 'Ferntree Cottage at Half Way Bush', both taken by William Livingstone. On 26 May Hocken had written to Sampson Low but did not receive their reply until just over six weeks later, on 12 July. It was this letter and the accompanying sample pulls of illustrations that caused him consternation. He wrote his stern volley-like response the very next day:

> I was much distressed with them with the exception of the portraits & the old church (No. 16). I am sure that they must be re-done. Perhaps I was not explicit enough in my first directions. Whilst they are pretty, they are far too small & convey little to a curious reader. I am desirous that they should be definite & diagrammatic & with this view it must be evident that at present they are of little or no service. This is especially the case with Nos. 12 (Shaw's Dunedin) & its key (No. 14) which if you remember I asked should be of double plate size (folded) so that the houses could be identified from the numbers of the key, but these are pretty well obliterated in the process of reproduction. No. 17 (Plan of Settlement) is simply unintelligible & as it appears would be a blot in my work.

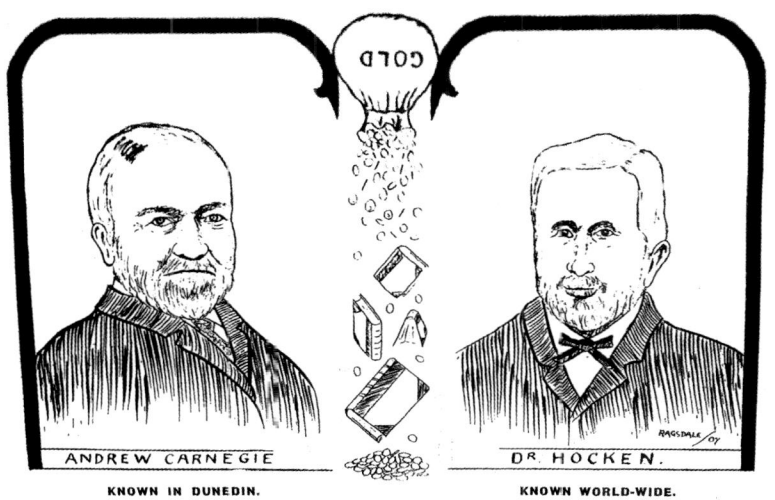

Ragsdale's cartoon of Andrew Carnegie and Hocken in the 1907 *Otago University Capping Magazine*, about the time of the 'Hocken Collection' dilemma. *Private collection*

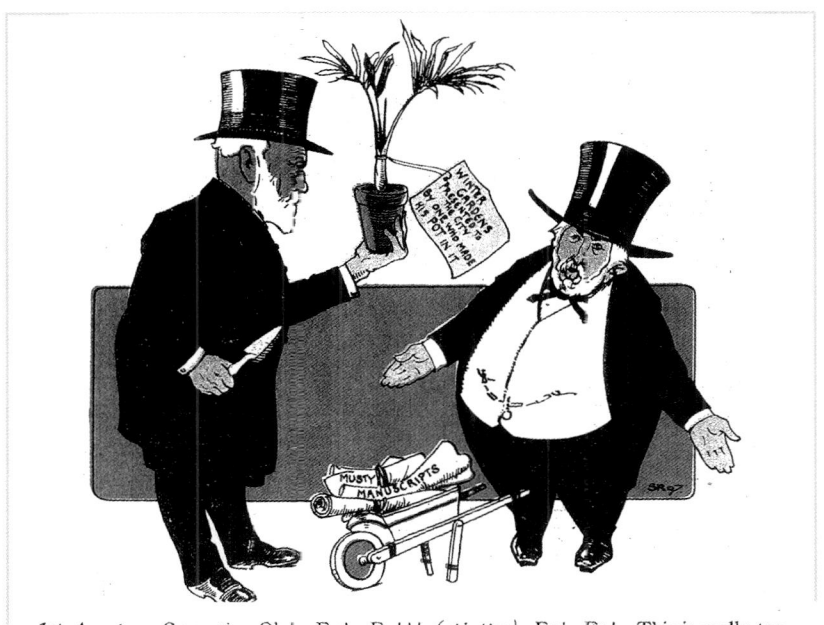

SR's cartoon of Andrew Carnegie and Hocken in the *Tickler for Otago and Southland* (c. 1907). *Private collection*

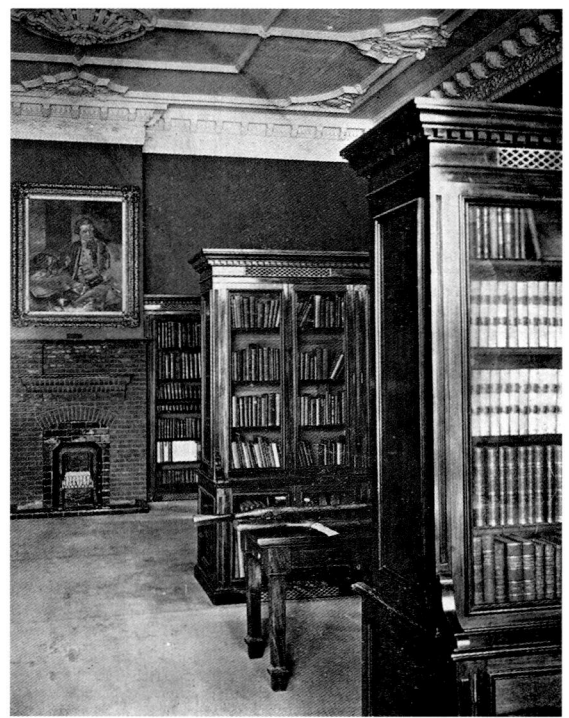

LEFT: Hocken's books on the red pine shelves in the Hocken Wing, Otago Museum. Note the James Cook portrait, a gift from James Rattray to the city in 1876. *Otago Witness* (6 April 1910).
S10-074a, Hocken Collections, Uare Taoka o Hakena, University of Otago

BELOW: The arrangement of Hocken's framed prints and sketches on the southern wall of the Otago Museum. *Otago Witness* (6 April 1910).
S10-074c, Hocken Collections, Uare Taoka o Hakena, University of Otago

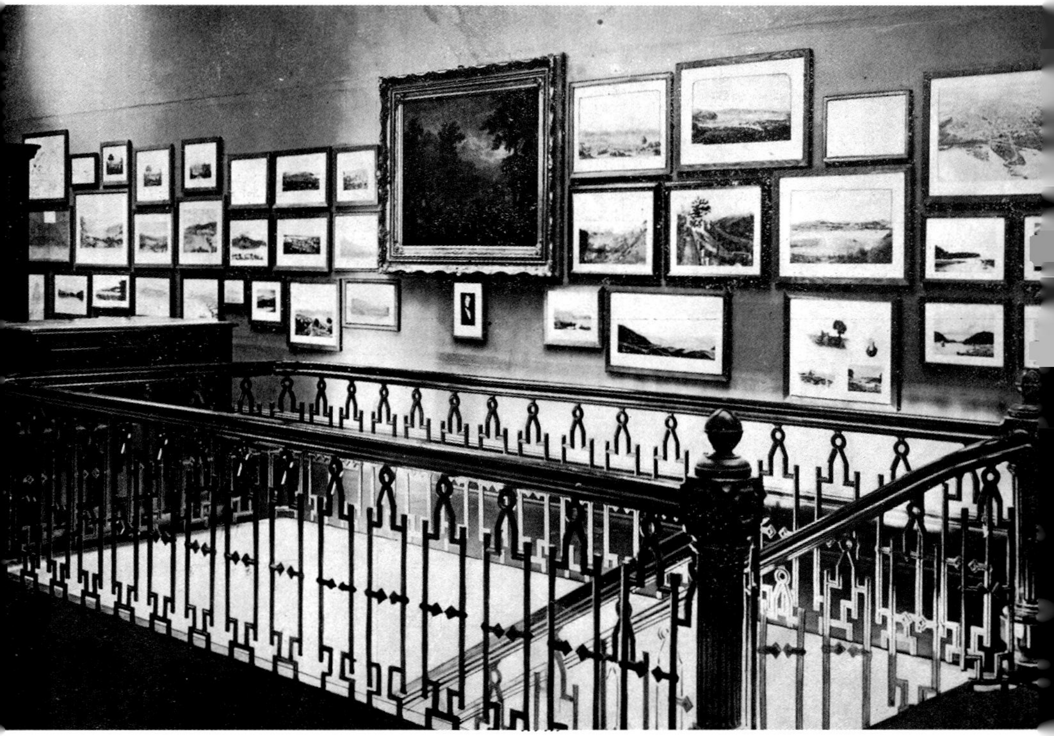

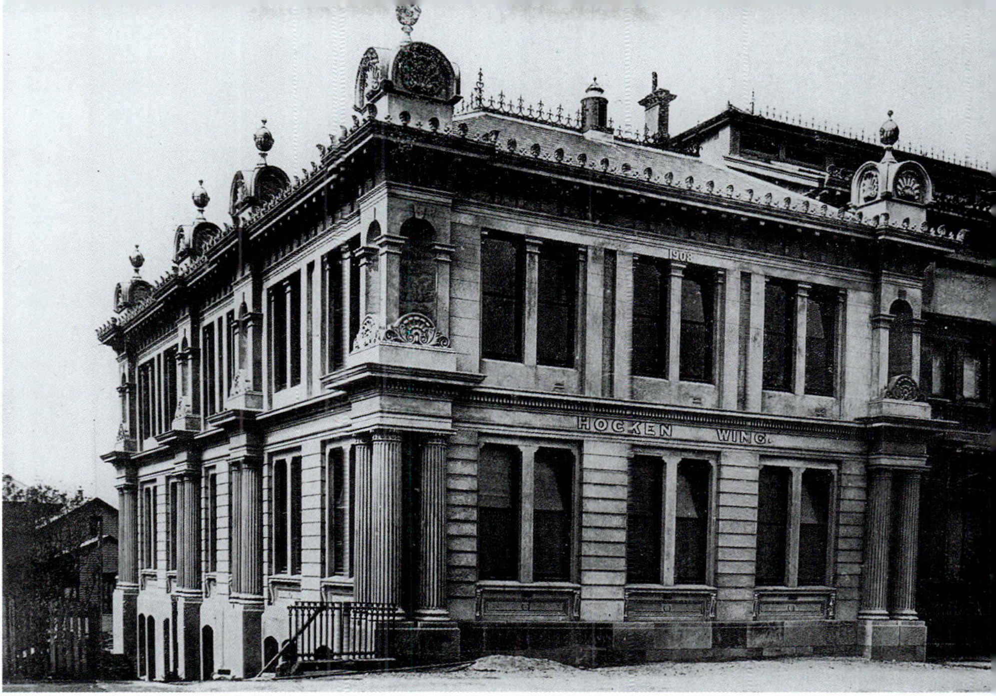

On 9 January 1908 Dunedin architect John Burnside was appointed to design the extension to the Otago Museum that would house Hocken's collection of books, manuscripts and pictures. The Hocken Wing, the first substantial addition to the museum, was opened by Lord Plunket on 31 March 1910. The books and manuscripts were held on the upper floor, and a Maori Hall on the lower level held artefacts Hocken had collected. *Otago Witness* (6 April 1910).

S14-078d, Hocken Collections, Uare Taoka o Hakena, University of Otago

CONTRIBUTIONS

TO

THE EARLY HISTORY

OF

NEW ZEALAND

[*SETTLEMENT OF OTAGO*]

BY

THOMAS MORLAND HOCKEN, M.R.C.S. ENG., F.L.S.,

MEMBER OF THE OTAGO UNIVERSITY COUNCIL

"—*forsan et haec olim meminisse juvabit.*"—*Virg.*

"Much with hoary men
He walked conversing, and sedately glad
Heard stories which escaped historic pen."
Allan Cunningham

WITH PORTRAITS AND OTHER ILLUSTRATIONS

LONDON

SAMPSON LOW, MARSTON AND COMPANY

LIMITED

St. Dunstan's House

FETTER LANE, FLEET STREET, E.C.

1898

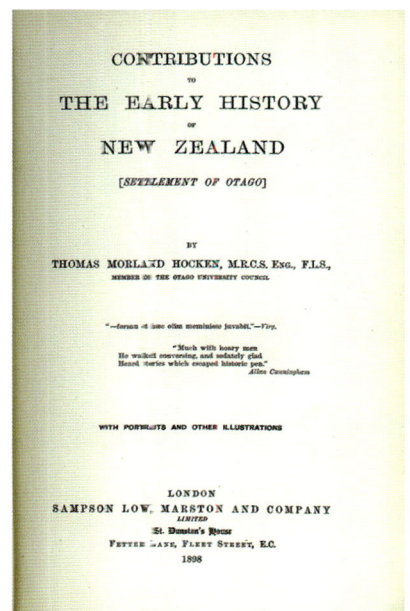

Hocken's first 'literary' endeavour, *Contributions to the Early History of New Zealand [Settlement of Otago]* (1898).

Private collection

36.

1786 | Dissertatio Inauguralis (Botanico-Medica) de Plantis Esculentis Insularum Oceani Australis &c. Auctore Georgius Forster &c. Halæ ad Salam Typis Grunertianis, MDCCLXXXVI. Sm 8vo Pp. 8vo

1786 | Another issue with different title page & other variations

1786 | Florulæ Insularum Australium Prodromus Auctore Georgio Forster M.D. serenissimo Regi Poloniæ &c. Gottingæ Typis Joann. Christian. Dieterich MDCCLXXXVI - 8vo Pp 8 - 103

1787 | A Catalogue of the Different Specimens of Cloth collected in the three Voyages of Captain Cook to the Southern Hemisphere; with a Particular Account of the Manner of the Manufacturing the same in the various Islands of the South Seas; partly extracted from Mr Anderson and Reinhold Forster's Observations, and the verbal Accounts of some of the most knowing of the Navigators: with some Anecdotes that happened to them among the Natives. Now first arranged & printed for Alexander Shaw, no 379, Strand, London sm. 4to. Pp 8 & 20 n.p. leaves containing tapa specimens

The | Life | Of | Captain James Cook . | — |
Totique maris vastique exhausta Pericula Terrae.
Virg. | — | By | Andrew Kippis, D.D. F.R.S. and S.A.
— | London: | Printed for G. Nicol, Bookseller
To His Majesty, | In Pall Mall ;| and G.C.J.
and J. Robinson, Pater-noster Row . |
M.DCC.LXXXVIII.

4to pp. xlj & 527

Entries for Alexander Shaw's tapa specimen book (1787) and Dr Kippis's *Life of Captain James Cook* (1788) in Hocken's draft 'Bibliography' of 1887, which he began compiling as early as 1885. The tapa cloth book is now missing from the collection. MS-0044: S14-298c, Hocken Collections, Uare Taoka o Hakena, University of Otago

A

BIBLIOGRAPHY

OF THE LITERATURE RELATING TO

NEW ZEALAND.

BY

T. M. HOCKEN,

M.R.C.S. ENG., F.L.S., F.R.G.S., FELL. ROY. ANTHROP. INST., F.J.S., MEMBER OF THE COUNCIL OF THE UNIVERSITY OF OTAGO;
AUTHOR OF "CONTRIBUTIONS TO THE EARLY HISTORY OF NEW ZEALAND," ETC.

"HE MAHI NUI RAWA ATU."
—Maori saying.

Wellington, N.Z.:
PRINTED BY JOHN MACKAY, GOVERNMENT PRINTER.
1909.

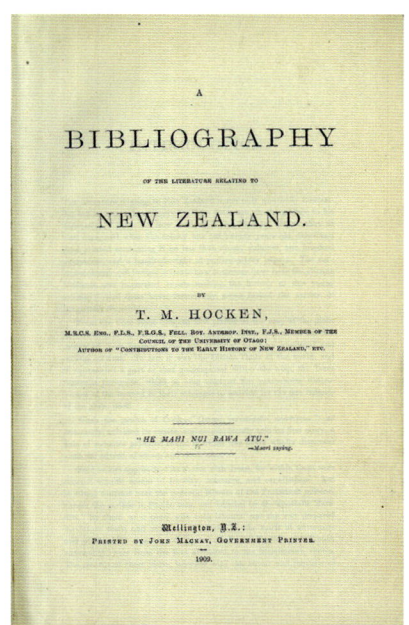

Hocken's *A Bibliography of the Literature Relating to New Zealand* appeared in late July 1909 in a functional brown buckram case, with gold-tooled title on the spine and three rectangular blind impressed rules on the back and front. At 632 pages, this solid, plain book retailed for 10s. On the title page Hocken's fulsome credentials sat above a Maori motto: 'He mahi nui rawa atu', translated as 'Truly, this is a very laborious deed', which no doubt it was. *Private collection*

DR. T. M. HOCKEN.

THE

EARLY HISTORY

OF

NEW ZEALAND.

BEING A SERIES OF LECTURES DELIVERED BEFORE THE OTAGO INSTITUTE;

ALSO A

LECTURETTE ON THE MAORIS OF THE SOUTH ISLAND.

BY

THE LATE DR. T. M. HOCKEN.

WELLINGTON, N.Z.
JOHN MACKAY, GOVERNMENT PRINTER.
1914.

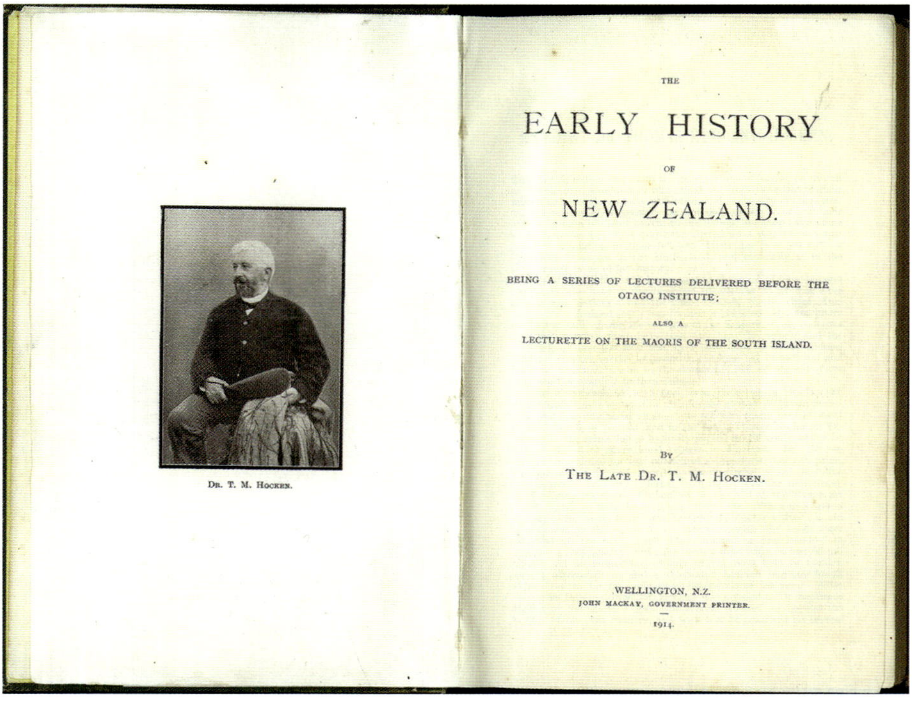

Hocken's *The Early History of New Zealand* (1914), a posthumous publication that appeared in print through the efforts of his wife Bessie. *Private collection*

W.H. Trimble, *Catalogue of the Hocken Library* (1912), the first accessible record of Hocken's book and manuscript collection.
Private collection

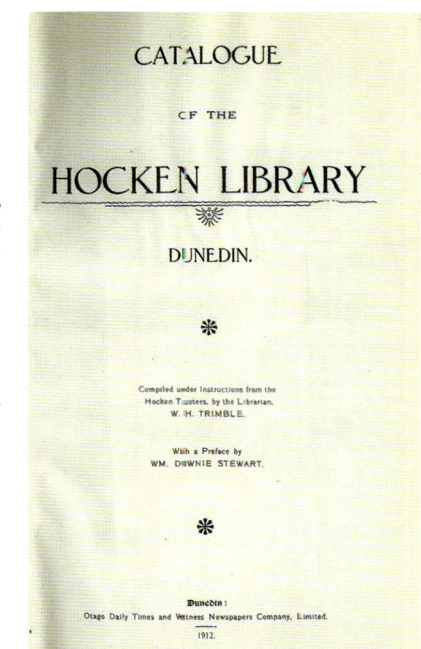

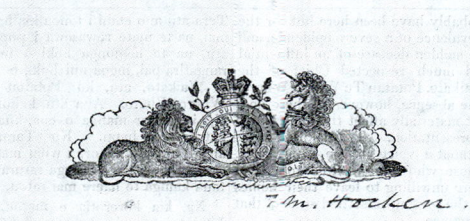

Hocken wrote to Thomas Cheeseman, John Kinder, Bishop Hadfield, John Webster and others in order to secure a full set of the *Maori Messenger: Te Karere Maori*. This is his copy of 'The Kohimarama Conference' in the issue of 14 July 1860.

S14-298e, Hocken Collections, Uare Taoka o Hakena, University of Otago

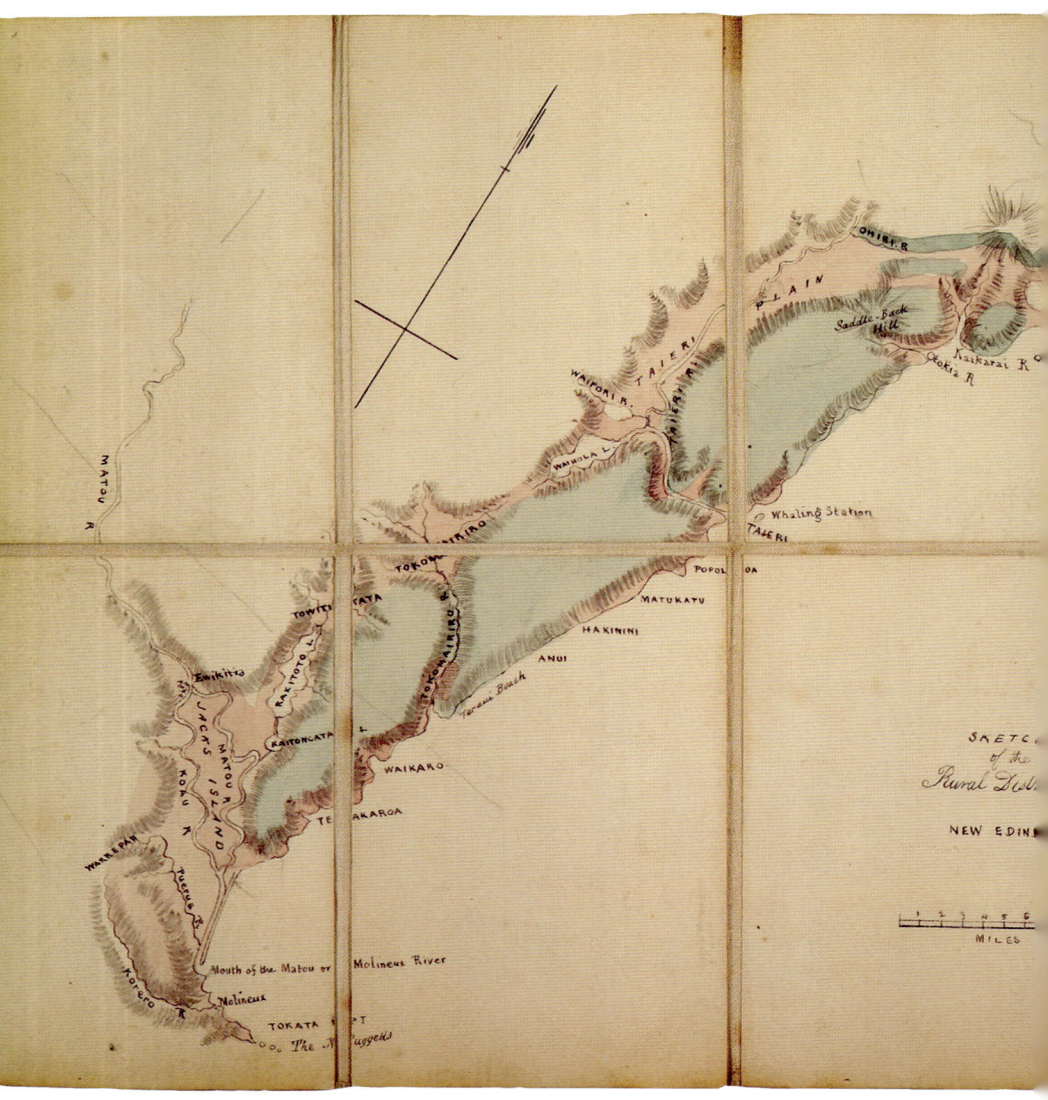

Frederick Tuckett, *Sketch of the Rural District of New Edinburgh* (1844). Tuckett was the New Zealand Company's principal surveyor, charged with finding a site for the projected 'New Edinburgh' in the South Island. Hocken acquired this map from Samuel Hodgkinson in November 1886.

S14-077b, Hocken Collections, Uare Taoka o Hakena, University of Otago

Samuel Marsden, *An Answer to Certain Calumnies in the Late Governor Macquarie's Pamphlet and the Third Edition of Mr Wentworth's Account of Australasia* (1826). Hocken collected books and manuscripts on Marsden, and intended to write his biography, though this did not eventuate. One work collected to support this project was Marsden's *An Answer to Certain Calumnies*, published in 1826 as a defence of his conduct in Australia. Pamphlet Vol. 80, No. 2: S14-524i, Hocken Collections, Uare Taoka o Hakena, University of Otago

KO TE

RONGO PAI

I

TUHITUHIA

E

RUKA.

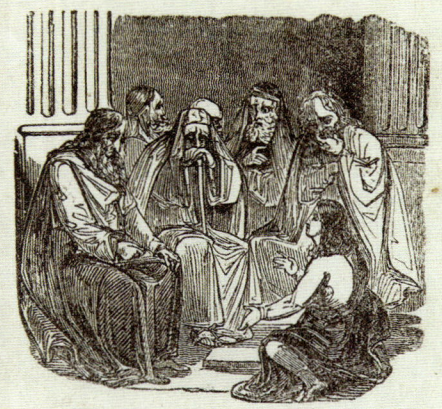

Upoko 2, 46.

PAIHIA:

HE MEA TA I TE PEREHI O NGA MIHANERE O TE
HAHI O INGARANI.

1835.

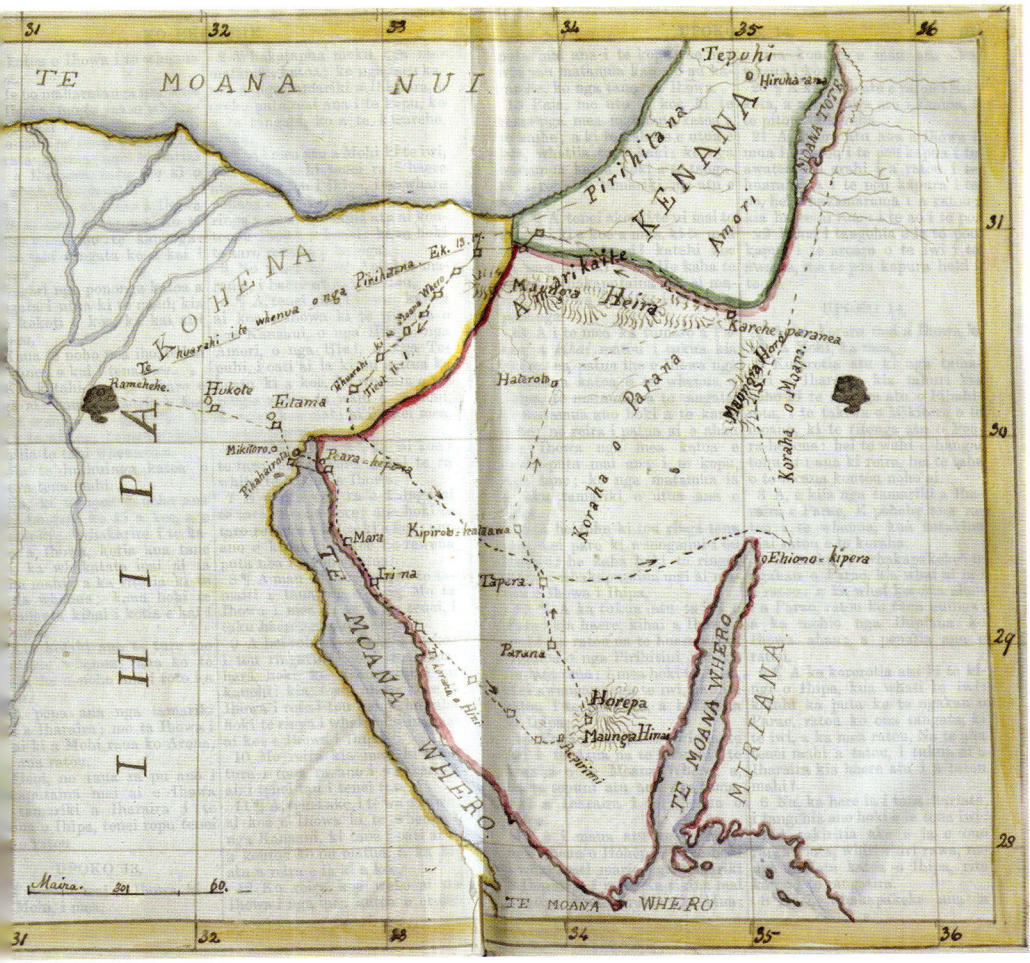

LEFT: *Ko te Rongo Pai i Tuhituhia e Ruka [Luke]*, (Paihia, 1835). Despite poor equipment and a lack of good paper, William Colenso's early print productions were a considerable achievement. His first work was a 16-page translation into Maori of the *Epistles of Paul to the Philippians and to the Ephesians*, which appeared on 17 February 1835. *The Gospel of Luke*, translated by the Rev. William Williams, was his second publication. Typically, Hocken has affixed his signature to the title page.
W17: S14-077c, Hocken Collections, Uare Taoka o Hakena, University of Otago

ABOVE: This coloured map of the Red Sea is tipped into *Ko te Tahi Wahi o te Kawenata Tawhito*, the Maori language edition of the Old Testament, printed in London in 1848. Hocken obtained this copy, given to Tamihana Te Rauparaha when he visited London in 1851, while in Otaki in January 1897.
W167, copy 2: S14-524h, Hocken Collections, Uare Taoka o Hakena, University of Otago

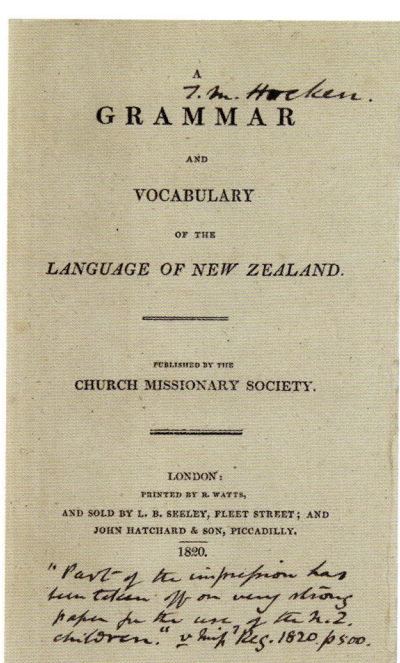

Hocken obtained his 'strong paper' copy of Thomas Kendall and Samuel Lee, *A Grammar and Vocabulary of the Language of New Zealand* (1820) from book dealer Bernard Quaritch in London in 1882. Kendall compiled this grammar and vocabulary under the direction of Professor Samuel Lee, oriental linguist, at Cambridge, England, with the assistance of Hongi Hika and Waikato.
W3ii: S14-524a, Hocken Collections, Uare Taoka o Hakena, University of Otago

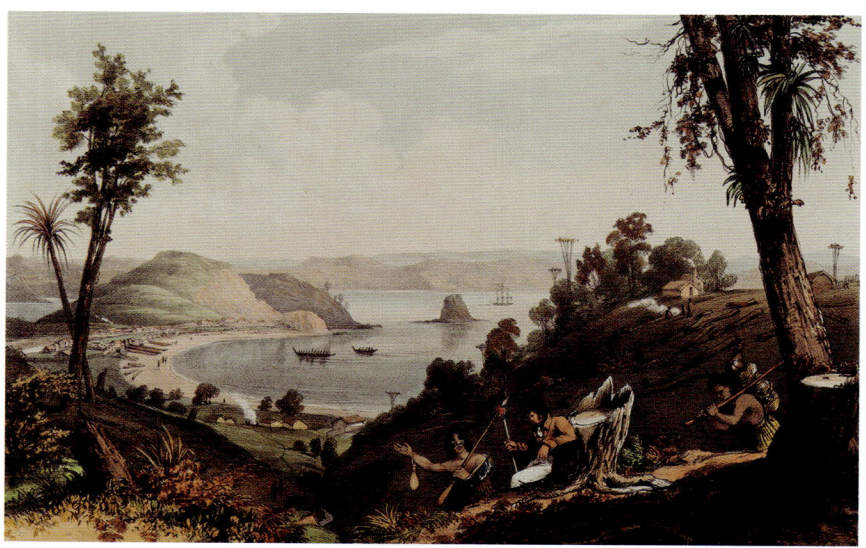

Augustus Earle's *Kororahika Beach* from his *Sketches Illustrative of the Native Inhabitants and Islands of New Zealand*, London, 1838. Earle was the first trained artist to visit New Zealand and live for any length of time among Northland Maori. Those of his paintings that survived a fire in Australia in May 1828 form a remarkable commentary on early New Zealand. Hocken bought this copy from Quaritch for an undisclosed sum in June 1882.
S14-298d, Hocken Collections, Uare Taoka o Hakena, University of Otago

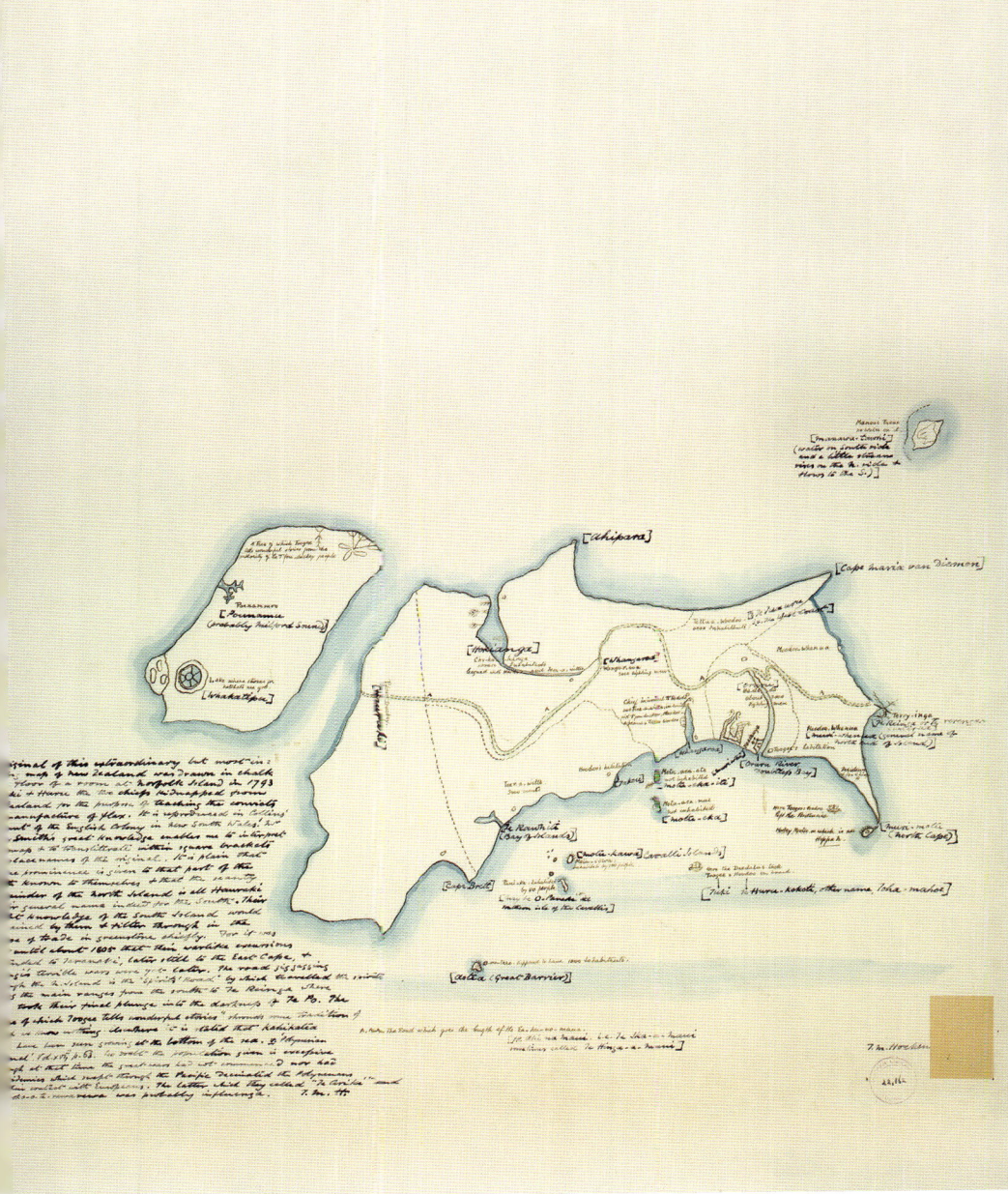

Hocken's extensive annotations on his copy of the 'Mind-Map' of New Zealand, originally drawn in chalk on the floor in Government House, Norfolk Island, by Tuki Tahua and Ngahuruhuru in 1793. 'Poenammoo' (Te Wai Pounamu, the South Island) is identified with two natural features, a tree and a lake. The original paper version is held in the Public Record Office in London. S14-077t. *Hocken Collections, Uare Taoka o Hakena, University of Otago*

The Revd W Slick (an able Maori scholar) tells me that the 'f' vice the 'wh' sound, which frequently appears in this vocabulary, was introduced by the Whalers & is depraved Maori. Also that the feature of the South Island speech was its roughness as compared with the smoothness of the north, in the wcab.

Most of the words are the same as those in the N.

May 1895. T. M. Hocken.

1

Tangata.	A man
Wahine	Woman
Tamaiti	Children
— tane	Male Child
— Wahine	Female Do
Tāgata Bōla.	White man
Waka Bōla.	Ship
Waka.	Canoe
Mikara.	Knife
Fara.	Fork
Rauhamon."	Book Paper
Kakahu.	Dress
Uakai iroiro.	Writing, Carving
Uare.	House
Uai.	Water Uai moti fresh Do
Tai.	The Sea. Moana
Ra.	The Sun
Marama.	The moon
Wetu.	The Stars.
Brero.	The Tongue.

Hocken acquired James Watkin's 'Vocabulary of Maori words compiled at Waikouaiti, 1840–1844' from his son, the Rev. Edwin Watkin of Melbourne, in March 1893.

MS-0031: S14-077e, Hocken Collections, Uare Taoka o Hakena, University of Otago

xxx

George Albert Hansard, 'Voyage of the *Acheron*, Part 3rd' (1849–51). Hocken was given this manuscript – one third of the original dealing with New Zealand – by Mrs Samson, the daughter of John Lort Stokes, captain of the *Acheron*.

MS-0157: S14-081a, Hocken Collections, Uare Taoka o Hakena, University of Otago

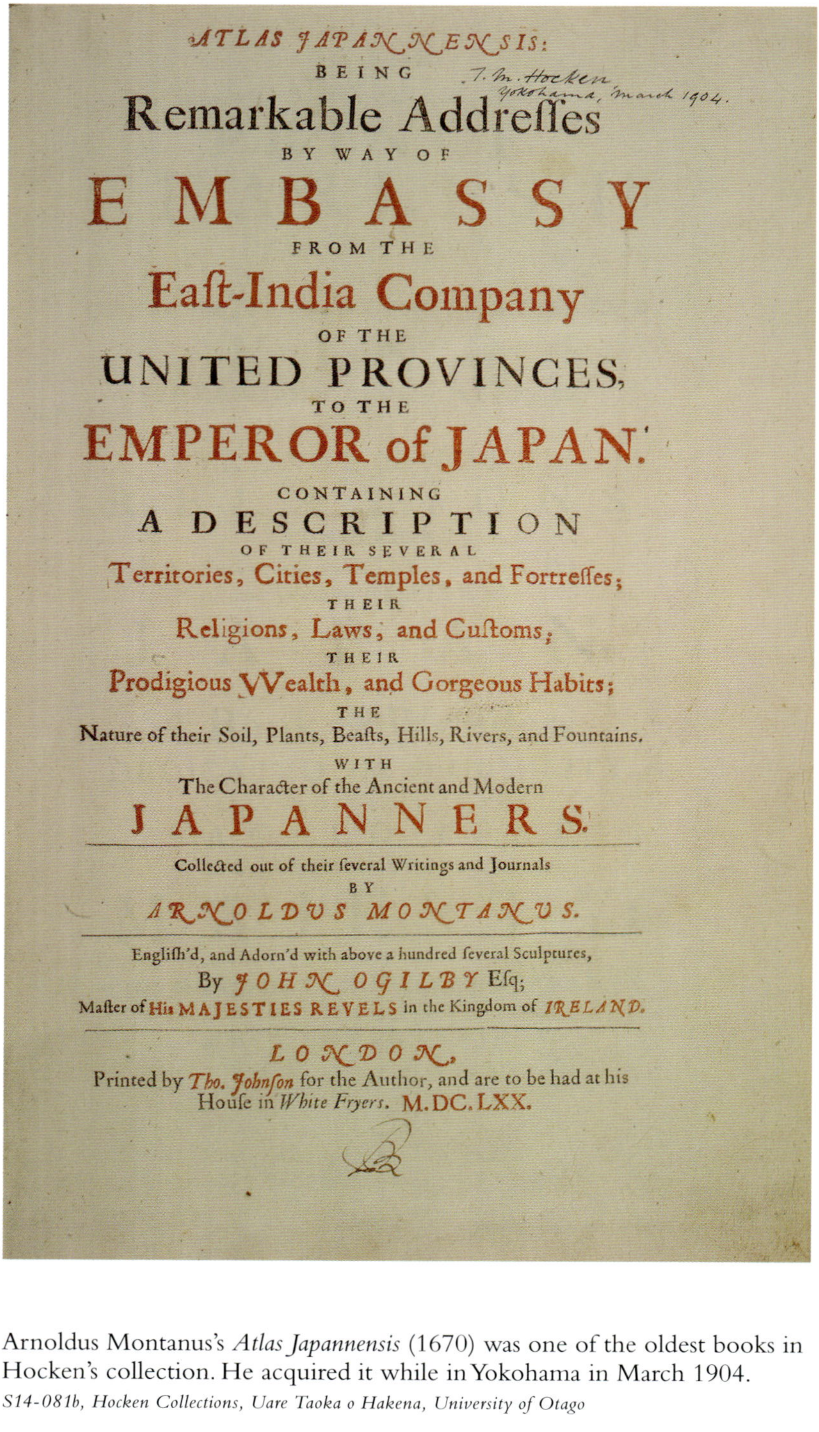

ATLAS JAPANNENSIS:
BEING
Remarkable Addresses
BY WAY OF
EMBASSY
FROM THE
East-India Company
OF THE
UNITED PROVINCES,
TO THE
EMPEROR of JAPAN.
CONTAINING
A DESCRIPTION
OF THEIR SEVERAL
Territories, Cities, Temples, and Fortresses;
THEIR
Religions, Laws, and Customs;
THEIR
Prodigious Wealth, and Gorgeous Habits;
THE
Nature of their Soil, Plants, Beasts, Hills, Rivers, and Fountains.
WITH
The Character of the Ancient and Modern
JAPANNERS.

Collected out of their several Writings and Journals
BY
ARNOLDUS MONTANUS.

Englissh'd, and Adorn'd with above a hundred several Sculptures,
By JOHN OGILBY Esq;
Master of His MAJESTIES REVELS in the Kingdom of IRELAND.

LONDON,
Printed by Tho. Johnson for the Author, and are to be had at his
House in White Fryers. M.DC.LXX.

T. M. Hocken
Yokohama, March 1904.

Arnoldus Montanus's *Atlas Japannensis* (1670) was one of the oldest books in Hocken's collection. He acquired it while in Yokohama in March 1904.
S14-081b, Hocken Collections, Uare Taoka o Hakena, University of Otago

Although he had known the illustrations could not be 'full plate', he had hoped they could be reduced 'as little as possible'. In order to have the illustrations as large as possible, he asked if the book could be uncut and untrimmed. 'Of course I must undertake the extra expense that all this involves.' Time constraints also meant that he would not see any new proofs: 'I must now trust to those further details & to the intelligent carrying them out of your artist.'[21]

Three weeks later a perfunctory letter was sent to London with three more chapters, totalling some 40 printed pages. After briefly mentioning his disappointment over the illustrations, he asked: 'Is it proposed to gilt letter the back of the book? If so, would this be too much to put on ... "Contributions/ Early History/ New Zealand./ [Otago]/ Dr Hocken./ Sampson Low/".'[22] The publishers happily complied with this request.

By mid-September 1897 Hocken had received proofs of all chapters up to XIX and appendices A to E. The turnaround was prompt. He sent the proofs back a few days later with additional and final appendices F and G, a total of 58 pages in the final printing. His statement that the preparation of these particular appendices was 'difficult work' was correct.[23] Appendix F, 'Vessels dispatched from Great Britain for the settlement of Otago from 1847 to 1850 inclusive; together with a list of emigrants', lists 19 vessels. Collating the names of passengers (including children and servants), their ages, occupations and, in some instances, place of residence in Otago, represented a large amount of dogged and tedious labour. Compiling Appendix G, 'Principal events which have occurred in Otago from 1840', involved the same sifting and sorting processes. The tabulation of events, dates, personalities and seemingly unimportant data such as the cost of potatoes in December 1848 or criminal assaults in November 1851 was a huge undertaking. Hocken used extracts from the *Otago Daily Times*, dutifully credited. He also used his own resources, including runs of early newspapers, early Dunedin publications, information culled from interviews with 'Old Identities' and manuscript materials. Despite errors, the results are a godsend to modern-day genealogists and local historians who are grateful for this information, 'much of which seems now trivial [but] will prove interesting and perhaps valuable hereafter'.[24]

Hocken knew the work had grown. Almost as a postscript to his September 1897 letter he added: 'With the bulky appendices I fear the volume will be large. Perhaps you can give me some idea as to what its retail price should be?'[25] By 29 September he was feeling the pressure: 'I am struggling hard to send you the last of my copy by a month from date. If this can be achieved I trust it will enable you to forward a portion or leaves of the volumes to Mr Horsburgh by say the second week in March, in time for our jubilee.' He even gave up the idea of an index. Optimism still lingered, however: after talking to Horsburgh, he had a thought about raising the print run to 1500, some of which he hoped would sell in Britain. Based on this, he asked the firm to retain 500 or 600 unbound copies until they heard from him. And, with first-author optimism, he wrote: 'Should however the first portion you send sell out quickly & there be an urgent quick demand for the rest I will, to save time, send you the cable word "Hocken" which will apprise you to send them by first opportunity.'[26]

A month later Hocken received the firm's sample reproduction of the 'Plan of the New Edinburgh Settlement' (1844), with which he was very pleased. So far everything was proceeding nicely. The portraits with names attached had been dispatched, and his runs of the *Nelson Examiner* and the photographs and negatives had been returned.[27] One final chapter and short introduction were required and these he promised 'in a few days'. True to his word, Hocken sent the last chapter and preface off on 1 November 1897. Relieved that there were no other obligations, he opened up to the publishers:

> I must express my regret for all the annoying trouble to which you must have been put, due to the distance between us. This was unavoidable & I have to thank you for your services under the unusual circumstances. For my part I have gained considerable experience in the preparation of a book for the press, & my next work will not be so problematic or so much trouble to either of us. I shall be happy to forward a draft whenever you inform me of the amount of my indebtedness. I need only repeat that I shall take it as a great favour if you could forward even a portion of the volumes by or before the 23rd of March – as possible. Mr Horsburgh will distribute them.[28]

Again he apologised for the lack of an index, feeling that a contents page would suffice.[29]

Perhaps by accident rather than good planning, copies of *Contributions* arrived almost to the day that Hocken had requested them. 'Gentlemen,' he wrote on 16 March 1898, 'The books arrived safely a few days ago by the "Ionic" & so far are selling rapidly. I hope this is also the case with you. I have to thank you for the handsome volume you have issued which has received praise on all hands.' This was despite mistakes in the last appendix and a few errors with some pictures. 'However complaint is now of no use & I must tell you that in having gained much assistance as a young author as will avail me in future volumes.' He enclosed a draft of £200 which, while not paying off the full debt, went a large way towards it. No precise figure is known for the cost of pre-press work, printing and binding, but presumably it was about £300 to £350, for some 1500 copies priced at 14s each. Pleased to learn that Edward Marston had enjoyed reading the book, Hocken enclosed the first review, which had appeared in the *Otago Daily Times* almost immediately the book was offered for sale.[30]

And of course he collected most of the reviews, pasting and filing them in his F&J Volume 10. Of the six local and 18 'British' reviews, only one was disparaging. The anonymous reviewer in the *Athenaeum* began his attack on

Hocken's use of Virgil's 'Forsan et haec olim meminisse juvabit' (Perhaps some day it will bring pleasure to remember even these things), calling it a 'hackneyed quotation'.[31] He then criticised the limited nature of the work and doubted that the 'details of events in themselves very trifling' would be attractive to English – 'we beg pardon, to the British reader'. The reviewer noted Hocken's intention to write more volumes. This fact explains the pre-press notification by Sampson Low, Marston & Co., who were interested in starting a series called 'Contributions to the early history of New Zealand'. Hocken's book was to be the first.[32]

Other reviewers were positive. The review in the *Otago Daily Times*, the first in New Zealand, was understandably the longest. It began: 'Dr Hocken's qualifications to write a history of New Zealand, especially that part of it called Otago, have long been known.' It praised Hocken's lucid, impartial narrative, and his effort in putting order to 'the tangled threads' of the province's history. Coverage was largely chronological, up to 1861, with the proviso 'that, whilst the facts of history are best written as they run, it may not be possible to accord them their just interpretation until long afterwards. Distance gives the best view of a landscape.'[33] Those who took part in the pageant of the early settlement would find the book's contents more interesting, but Hocken's 'judicious blending' of other historical matter would appeal to others. And his style was deemed a winner. It was charming, with 'chatty little divergences' interspersed throughout the narrative. Hocken's love of gossipy minutiae stood him in good stead. The review mentioned the jubilee celebrations as the prime catalyst for the book's appearance, and blamed a number of typographic errors on the rush to print. But the book was 'handsomely illustrated', and most of the illustrations were presented for the first time. The appendices were 'valuable records'.[34]

Other reviews repeated the above sentiments. Words and phrases such as 'diligent', 'fascinating', 'true genius of a historian', 'distinct', 'fresh material', 'valuable appendices', 'most absorbing interest', 'author draws upon his own experiences', 'valuable record', 'painstaking addition' and so on filled the reviews appearing in the *Evening Post*, the *Otago Witness*, the *New Zealand Herald*, the *Scotsman*, the *Westminster Gazette*, the *Publishers' Circular*, the *Leeds Mercury*, the *Manchester Guardian*, the *Pall Mall Gazette*, the *Colonial and Indian News*, the *Globe*, the *Glasgow Herald*, the *Journal of the Royal Colonial Institute*, the *Bookseller*, the *Home News*, the *Illustrated London News*, the *Field*, the *Daily News*, the *Saturday Review* and the *Speaker*.[35] The Scottish contingent was particularly pleased with the historical treatment of Otago and Dunedin (the 'Edinburgh of the South'), maintaining the book was 'a chapter in the history of Scotland' (*Glasgow Herald*) and, in particular, 'the record of an experiment in systematic colonisation' and 'a study of the Scotch colonist in a separate colony' (*Speaker*).

Local, personal responses were also positive. Fellow collector William Downie Stewart promptly wrote a letter to the editor, reinforcing Hocken's 'excellent literary style' and his 'judicial impartiality'. He concluded: 'Dr Hocken's book should prove of lasting interest not only to those early settlers who still survive, but also to all persons interested in the settlement of Otago, the circumstances connected with which were somewhat unique.'[36]

The publication was not perfect, as Hocken himself realised. On 15 March 1898 George Street resident F.W. Whiston conveyed a truism that must have pleased Hocken: 'The opportunity is given to few men to record the beginnings of a new country gathered from personal contact with the original pioneers, and you have made the very best use of yours.' He also noted 'one or two printer's errors', which he listed for any second edition.[37] In early April W.G. Filleul wrote from Nelson to express 'great interest & pleasure' in reading the book but again pointed out, and listed, 'one or two inaccuracies', this time concerning his relatives, the Valpys.[38] The Rev. William Gillies of Timaru was equally complimentary. He wrote in late April, thanking Hocken 'for the valuable & interesting volume you have written upon early Otago'; he had read it in one sitting.[39] Similarly, in early July 1898 William Martin from nearby Fairfield congratulated Hocken on a good read. He wondered how Hocken had managed to 'acumulate [sic] such a mass of facts and so to disentangle the skein and bring such order out of such confusion … All honor to the author for such patience – perseverance – and *Patriotism*.'[40]

There were comments from overseas. One of the first to read *Contributions*, 'with pleasure', was Edmund H.W. Bellairs who on 18 February 1898 wrote to James Buckland, Hocken's brother-in-law, via the publishers. Bellairs was the son of Captain Edmund Hooke Wilson Bellairs, who was associated with the Canterbury Association and who was mentioned on page 143 of *Contributions*. This letter brought a more direct correspondence with Hocken, which resulted in his securing a rich vein of historical materials. Bellairs' further comments must have settled Hocken's mind on the worthiness of the project: 'In conclusion, allow me to congratulate Dr Hocken on the high-minded tone of his book and let one say that that was the spirit that animated Gibbon Wakefield, my father and all the band that surrounded them.'[41]

Fiji and Samoa Bound

After the whirl of publication, Hocken needed some relaxation. In March 1898 he wrote to Mr Herton at the Dunedin branch of the Bank of New South Wales to inform him that he was going to take a Pacific trip. It was to be a five- to six-week venture, funded by an overdraft facility based on shares jointly owned with Bessie. The cost was roughly £1000.[42] A few days later he, Bessie, 14-year-old Gladys and Daniel Colquhoun left for Samoa and Fiji. In Wellington on 1 April they boarded the *Warrimoo*, a Canadian–Australian mail steamship, as saloon passengers.[43] Tucked in Hocken's pocket was a letter of introduction from James Mills, managing director of the Union Steam Ship Company in Dunedin, which no doubt facilitated smooth travel arrangements.

It is unclear why the Hockens went to Samoa and Fiji. Certainly the opportunity was there: mail and merchant ships plied back and forth from Wellington and Auckland.[44] Subconsciously, the prompt may have emanated from Percy Smith and the activities of the Polynesian Society. He and Hocken had certainly discussed in person and through letters the gathering of ethnographic information from the islands.[45] There was also fellow society member John Fraser, who had talked about compiling a Polynesian bibliography, and the recent exposure to Pacific Island customs and language, gleaned from the South Seas Court at the exhibition. And perhaps there was pressure from Bessie? Hocken owned a copy of the Burton Brothers' *The Camera in the Coral Islands: A series of photographs illustrating the scenery and the mode of life in the Fijis, the Navigator Islands (Samoa), the Friendly Islands (Tonga) … in June and July, 1884* [1884]. Bessie may have wanted to take photographs similar to those of the Burtons. She was certainly one of the 'three amateur photographers' he would later mention in his article about Fiji.[46] Gladys, a budding photographer, took seven photographs, now found in her 'Fiji and Samoa' album in her father's pictorial collection.[47]

Hocken certainly owned books that dealt with the South Sea Islands, including standard voyage and travel titles by Cook, Parkinson and Dumont d'Urville. He also owned a number of nineteenth-century publications such as the Rev. Michael Russell's *Polynesia* (1845), the Rev. Joseph Copeland's *Lecture on the New Hebrides* (1866), John Williams's *Narrative of Missionary Enterprises* (1867), F.J. Moss's *A Planter's Experience in Fiji* (1870). W.C. Gardenhire's *Fiji and the Fijians and Travels among the Cannibals* (1871) and John L. Kelly's *The South Sea Islands: Possibilities of trade with New Zealand* (1885).[48] This last title is packed full of maps and statistics that would have been very useful in preparation for the trip. Although it is not certain that Hocken used any of these titles, others contain annotations and sure proof that they were consulted before, during or after the trip.

Apia was the first port of call. No details exist of their stay except for the already mentioned visit to Robert Louis Stevenson's library through the kindness of Edwin Gurr. Fiji was next. Hocken had obviously read about the Fijian fire-walking ceremony that took place on Beqa Island, south of Suva. The ceremony, known as Na Vilavilairevo, was actually hot-stone walking, carried out by a small clan or family who lived on the west coast of the island. It had rarely been seen by Europeans, and Hocken made up his mind to see it for himself. He asked A.M. Duncan, a member of the Legislative Council of Fiji and agent at Suva of the Union Steam Ship Company, to make the necessary arrangements. Three days' notice was required to dig the pit, construct the oven and heat the stones to the right temperature. Duncan was successful: a few days later the Hockens, Colquhoun and Mr Vaughan, a local meteorologist, headed for the island.

Like true scientists in the field, both Hocken and Colquhoun obtained permission before the ceremony to check out the two participants, making sure there was no trickery.[49] Hocken examined their pulse, legs and feet, which were 'free from any apparent application'. He licked the feet of both men, finding their soles 'comparatively soft and flexible – by no means leathery and insensible'. He repeated this examination after the walk. When the men were walking over the hot stones, Colquhoun detected 'anxiety' in their faces; Hocken dismissed this notion. And the stones were hot. Hocken dangled a thermometer over them, using a large wooden stick. Before the solder melted and the thermometer was destroyed, it had registered 138.8°C.[50]

The event was not only a 'red letter' one for Hocken, but had a life of its own. On his return to Dunedin, eager to disseminate information on what he had seen, he promptly wrote up a talk about the ceremony and read it to Otago Institute members on 10 May 1898.[51] He then submitted it for printing in the *Transactions of the New Zealand Institute*, where it duly appeared in 1898. Folklorist Andrew Lang, already fascinated by such things, penned another article about July 1898, using Hocken's account. This was later reprinted in Lang's own *Magic and Religion* (1901) and referenced in S.P. Langley and Lang's 'The fire walk ceremony in Tahiti' in *Folklore* (December 1901). Hocken's description also got mention in Robert Fulton's later 'An account of the Fiji fire-walking ceremony, or Vilavilairevo, with a probable explanation of the mystery', which was read before the Otago Institute on 23 September 1902 and then published in the *Transactions of the New Zealand Institute* (Volume 35, 1902). The subject made good copy. In September 1898 Londoners walking along the Strand could view a red and black billboard headed 'A Fiji miracle', which advertised Lang's work.[52] Hocken relived the whole experience in Japan, where he arranged for the publication of his institute talk in the *Japan Daily Herald* of 19 October 1901.[53]

Hocken remained mystified by the experience, which he found inexplicable: 'The whole subject requires thorough scientific examination.' At one stage he asked Walter Sinclair Carew, one-time Resident Commissioner for Colo East and Stipendiary Magistrate for Rewa (Fiji), about it. Quoting one of the Fijian participants, Carew said: 'I can do it, but I do not know how it is done.' Hocken and Carew continued to correspond, and in time the latter gifted his collection of letters and documents to Hocken.[54] Many of the manuscripts, including certificates documenting Carew's official appointments in Fiji and correspondence relating to land claims in Fiji, were placed in Hocken's Variae volumes.[55] Printed items included two Malagasy language items, a dictionary (1875) and an 1845 grammar by David Griffiths. Hocken held the resident commissioner in high regard, as is clear in a note written just before he died, which also gave sound advice on preserving documents:

> Mr Walter Carew was by far the most able Fiji officer & faithfully trusted by the various Governors. There is much in connection with Fiji in

my collection which can presently be notated & availed of. I intended, had health spared to have had the whole of his correspondence bound (the only way of properly preserving documents). This should be done hereafter — also any collection of other letters which increase in value with time. T.M. Hocken, April 17/10.[56]

By early May 1898 the Hockens were back in Dunedin. One quirky by-product of his South Sea experience was evident when, during a talk to Otago Institute members, his friend William Benham mentioned marine worms. Hocken was able to tell the audience that earthworms found in Fiji appeared only twice a year and only for two days. He added that they were considered a local delicacy.[57] It was business as usual.

14
'For a Boxful of Such Rubbish I Should be Infinitely Obliged'

There was a waxing and waning in Hocken's letter writing over the years: individuals appeared, disappeared and then reappeared; topics re-emerged. On his return from Samoa and Fiji he faced a pile of letters that had accumulated at Atahapara. There were bills, payments and receipts for services rendered, gossipy letters from family and informative ones from his growing list of correspondents.

The Melbourne-based educator Edward E. Morris was one such correspondent. A trustee of the Melbourne University Library, Morris was an enthusiast about Cook, Banks and the fate of the *Endeavour*. In March 1896, after following Cook's tracks throughout New Zealand, Morris visited Hocken in Dunedin, where both men were 'closeted' for some days together. Cook was certainly on the agenda but so was philology.[1] Two years later on 28 May 1898 Morris typed out a letter, not only expressing interest in Hocken's recent trip to Fiji, but also reconnecting with an old passion: 'You think all that has to be said about the *Endeavour* Voyage has been said. Much new matter has come to light of late. Put together Wharton's Cook, Hooker's Banks, and the first volume part I of the Historical Records of New South Wales.' He asked Hocken to send 'any thing in the way of a pamphlet that you have printed about Hawkesworth &c'. And after a hint of another visit to New Zealand, Morris signed off with the hope that, armed with his own copy of Parkinson (1773) and Becket and de Hondt's printing of *A Journal of a Voyage round the World in His Majesty's Ship* Endeavour (1771), he would improve on Hawkesworth's account.[2] Hocken was also armed: he owned copies of Parkinson and the anonymous *Journal*, now attributed to James Magra. He responded by sending a pamphlet on Hawkesworth and a copy of the *Otago Daily Times* that carried a complimentary review of Morris's own work. A month later on 20 June Morris replied. The pamphlet not only helped to prove Morris's 'contention that Hawkesworth is not final for the present day', but prompted more questions for Hocken.[3]

On 11 August 1900 Morris was in touch again, sending Hocken a copy of his article 'Captain Cook's First Log in the Royal Navy', which had appeared in the *Cornhill Magazine*.[4] Morris was in a despondent mood, claiming that the article 'did not make any stir' because of the excitement of the South African War, 'when nothing went down that was not khaki'. Morris poured out his feelings: not only were his publishers dismissive of his voyages book, *Cook and his Companions*, but he felt that the 'British Public' had lost interest in Cook.[5] At least he was encouraging towards Hocken: 'I hope your history of New Zealand is prospering, and will meet a better fate.'[6] On 6 September Morris responded to Hocken's letter of 28 August (proof again of Hocken's quickness in reply) and thanked him for references to Captain Nathaniel Portlock. He was, however, perplexed: 'When do you think your book will be out? I cannot quite make out whether you are simply writing a Life of Cook, for which there is plenty of room, or whether it is a history of New Zealand.' The 'history' was Hocken's *The Early History of New Zealand*, that part which had been discarded from his *Contributions* and which would eventually appear in 1914. Although Morris's attention had wandered to Matthew Flinders, 'this second hero of Australian exploration', it did not stop him from posting through a copy of his 'Doctor John Hawkesworth, Friend of Dr Johnson and Historian of Captain Cook's First Voyage' (1899), which appeared in the *Gentleman's Magazine* for September 1900.[7] Hocken, or more probably Trimble, filed it in Pamphlet Volume 174, between a single sheet headed *Court of Directors of the NZ Company, 1 August 1849* and a fragment of a journal by the Rev. John Hobbs (1908).

Angus & Robertson

Another Australian connection was the firm of Angus & Robertson. As prominent booksellers-cum-publishers, they were well positioned to control much of the book traffic in late nineteenth-century Australasia. Hocken knew George Robertson personally and had dealings with the firm. However, apart from the presence of the firm's book label in some of his books, which does not by itself prove that they were bought directly from Angus & Roberston, there is very little documentation on transactions in Hocken's own collection or in the firm's archives at the State Library of New South Wales.

There are, however, a few glimpses. Sometime in early April 1899 Robertson sent Hocken a copy of John Thomas Bigge's 'Report of the Commissioner of Inquiry into the State of the Colony of New South Wales' (1822), which elicited a disappointed response that reflected Hocken's liking for associational and presentation copies: 'I am sorry you did not put my name in it as from yourself. But this you can do when next you visit Dunedin.' Hocken found Bigge's report interesting: 'I devoted the whole of yesterday to its perusal.' And, in the interests of completeness, he asked Robertson if he could send through the evidences and appendices that accompanied the work.[8]

Hocken liked completing sets. He owned the earlier volumes of G.B. Barton's *History of New South Wales from the Records* (1889–94) and secured the last volume from the firm about November 1896.[9] Sometimes he was more discriminating and on one occasion refused a book. After being sent the firm's publication of Henry and Annie Parkes' *An Emigrant's Home Letters* (1896), he returned it, claiming it was a 'singularly uninteresting & valueless little book'.[10] Remembering that the young, boastful, bookish Henry Parkes had been on the SS *Great Britain* with him in May 1861 may have coloured his decision.

Contact with the firm was not just over acquisitions. In May 1899, when Hocken informed Edmund Bellairs that he had turned down the Canterbury history because of personal priorities, it was not quite the full story. In late March, and no doubt spurred on by Robertson's visit to Dunedin, Hocken had agreed to proof a copy of the firm's forthcoming 'School History' on Australia and New Zealand, which was Arthur W. Jose's *A Short History of Australasia* (1899). After examining the Australian content, Hocken turned to the more familiar:

> The N.Z. portion does not satisfy me (so well) (& I agree with your second memorandum that the style wants improvement). I judge that the writer has derived much of his information from 'Grey's Life' by Rees, & Reeves' 'Aotearoa' both of which are in my opinion poor guides, the former especially. Many matters in the School History are quite debatable & others incorrect. Of course it was not possible for me to recast the whole. I think however it will do well.'[11]

Hocken also made passing reference to his intended letter to David Scott Mitchell and the collector's proposed conditions on gifting his collection. On 10 April he wrote to Robertson: 'Before getting your letter I had written a letter to Mr Mitchell addressed through you, but lazy as he seems to be it is not probable I shall get a reply.' Blaming his own slow reply on a couple of carbuncles on his arm, Hocken reiterated his opinion about the New Zealand component of the 'history': 'I hope you received my emendations to your School History. They were quite necessary. I think I said that it was quite evident from what source the writer had derived his information regarding N.Z. It was a glorification of Grey for one thing & other matters also were put in in a very biased style – quite wrong for a school history.'[12]

Another Australian contact at this time was Harington E. Wade, *Hansard* reporter of Kew, Melbourne. He was the son of the Rev. William Richard Wade, a CMS member sent out to superintend the press but who eventually went out into the field as a missionary. Harington Wade lent Hocken his father's 160-page journal for copying in June 1900. Although no doubt pleased with this gesture, Hocken surely did not admit to the son that 'much of it is not worth transcription'. He managed to squeeze the essence out of the journal and have it bound up with the 'Journal of John Wallis Barnicoat, February 1842 to October 1844'.[13]

Maori Language Materials and Karere Maori

As mentioned earlier, in late 1900 Hocken's 'Some account of the beginnings of literature in New Zealand', with its focus on early Maori language printing, appeared in the *Transactions of the New Zealand Institute*.[14] It was a ground-breaking article, read to members of the Otago Institute on 11 September 1900. Indeed, Hocken himself acknowledged there was little documentation on 'this interesting piece of history' and felt the results he 'gathered from all quarters' should be recorded.[15] Of course such an article demanded primary documents: 'It may here be stated that for some time I have been engaged in collecting and cataloguing not only these, but all publications whatsoever in the Maori language of which I have any acquaintance.'[16] A greater permanence was later achieved when he included a printed Maori publications component in his *Bibliography* (1909), the compilation of which, as he claimed in 1900 to the Napier-based collector Henry T. Hill, was 'very laborious but necessary & will be valuable'.[17]

Over the years William Colenso had given Hocken a number of early Maori language books including four catechisms, *Ko nga Katikihama e wa* (1833), a number of books from the Old Testament including part of Exodus, *Upoko 21* (1846), and a later printing of four catechisms (1842).[18] From Dean Jacobs Hocken had obtained Bishop Selwyn's copy of the third edition of the complete New Testament, *Ko te Kawenata Hou o to tato i Ariki te Kai Wakaora a Ihu Karaiti* (1842); from Bishop William Williams a copy of the fourth edition of the complete New Testament (1844); from Gilbert Mair, on 19 May 1886, a copy of Favell Lee Mortimer's *More about Jesus* (1885); and from the Rev. James Stack who, wanting to 'add to your valuable collection', sent Hocken on 28 October 1898 'a few books which I thought might interest you', including a Maori manuscript by Mohi Turei, an old clergyman resident at the East Cape, and a piece of an artillery shell from Gate Pa.[19] Hocken also obtained from an unknown donor on 30 March 1897 the scarce 'coarse paper' issue of Kendall's 1820 *A Grammar and Vocabulary of the Language of New Zealand*, which had once belonged to Bishop Selwyn and C.J. Abraham, Bishop of Wellington. This was Hocken's second copy. And in 1899 Hone Heke Ngapua, Member of the House of Representatives for Northern Maori, sent his whakapapa; Hocken duly noted that he was 'the grand-nephew of the first Hone Heke of war fame'.[20]

While he was slowly gathering the above Maori language material, Hocken constantly wished for more issues of *Te Karere o Nui Tireni*, New Zealand's first Maori-language newspaper, which was government sponsored and first published on 1 January 1842. In fact, he pestered his correspondents about the availability of copies in order to complete his holdings. For almost 20 years, the publication went through various changes: it was *Te Karere o Nui Tireni*, edited by George Clarke, Protector of Aborigines, until 15 January 1846; then it was *The Maori Messenger – Te Karere Maori*, edited from 4 January 1849 to 4 May 1854 by C.O.B. Davis (identified as such in the 3 January 1850 issue); then it was edited by Davis, David Burn and Walter Buller from 1 January 1855 to 28 February 1861; and finally it became *Te Karere Maori or Maori Messenger*, edited by Davis from 16 December 1861 to 28 September 1863.[21] The fact that it contained an English translation of the text made the newspaper all the more accessible to those without Maori.

Hocken liked going straight to the source. About April 1898 he wrote to William Scott Wilson, son of W.C. Wilson who, along with John Williamson, had printed the *New Zealander* and at times *Te Karere Maori*. Hocken pressed Wilson for holdings of the newspaper at the *New Zealand Herald* office. Initially, Wilson delivered skimpy details but, encouraged by Hocken to dig further, discovered more issues running from Number 2 (19 January 1849) to May 1854. Their holdings were by no means complete, and Wilson listed the missing numbers for Hocken.[22]

Thomas Cheeseman was another correspondent who fielded *Te Karere* queries from Hocken. There was an acknowledged respect between these two, though tarnished by the occasional firm word, especially over the debacle of the South Seas Exhibition. Hocken was astute enough to recognise that institutions like the Auckland Institute and Museum were excellent sources of materials, especially when it was likely that they held duplicate books, pamphlets and newspapers for possible disposal or exchange. He had contacted the institute years before on such matters and found that Cheeseman, embarking on his own institutional collecting, was predisposed towards a little give and take. A wish list, including those desired issues of *Te Karere Maori*, almost always accompanied each letter. Hocken made such lists regularly, revamping holdings when they were acquired and tailoring lists to the recipient. Just over two years after the correspondence with Wilson, Hocken repeated his plea to Cheeseman about duplicate *Te Karere Maori*:

> I am making a strong effort to complete my set & shall be very glad for even a few numbers. If you can I will give you a list of the desiderata. I know how your time is occupied but you might ask your assistant to look through the various holes & corners where such things accumulate & lie for years. I have many duplicates & might be able to exchange with you. With this view I have written to G.M. Main [author of *The Newspaper Press of Auckland*] & am writing to Dr [John] Kinder.[23]

Two weeks later, Hocken's frustrations were telling: 'I am so sorry that your duplicates are not noted & this I well know is because you have not the time yourself; year after year we discuss the matter & year after year it is left undone.' As a practical man who liked to get things done, Hocken mooted a solution, 'that you engage some intelligent competent fellow to go through & make a list of your duplicates & your requirements. For this labour I will *gladly pay*. Set him on at once & let us bring the matter to a head.' And he repeated his plea *again*, and noted that he would be 'heartily obliged if you will set your intelligent man to work at once'.[24] Cheeseman seemed oblivious to Hocken's entreaties and in October 1900 the collector wrote again, reiterating his willingness to pay any expenses and suggesting Cheeseman might let him have his small number of *Te Karere* issues 'in exchange for something else'.[25] There is no inkling of whether Hocken's suggestion was agreed to.

One particular transaction was completed quickly, however. On 13 August 1900 Hocken asked Cheeseman if he could 'lend for a day or two' Thomas Kendall's *A Korao no New Zealand*, an elementary Maori language primer printed by George Howe in Sydney in 1815. Hocken furthered his case for the loan by stating that he needed to see the book so that he could include its bibliographical details in his forthcoming institute paper.[26] This specific work is the only known surviving copy and is now housed in the Auckland War Memorial Institute Library. Cheeseman packaged it up and sent it south; it was in Dunedin for less than two weeks, returned by registered mail on 28 August.[27] Hocken was extremely pleased and grateful to get his hands on this 'necessary and praiseworthy attempt to open communications between the two races': 'You have always been very good in lending me things & I thoroughly appreciate it.'[28]

Another to whom Hocken appealed for issues of *Te Karere Maori* was Henry T. Hill, whom he had met in 1895 and who was an active member of that small band of early book and manuscript collectors in New Zealand.[29] To this enthusiast Hocken sent a full list of wants with a suggestion to pass it on to Donald McLean, 'who when here a few weeks ago said that he would look over his numbers & see if he could help me. This as well as yourself.'[30] Hill's lack of response was also unacceptable. On 16 May 1900 Hocken pressed him again, and a month later, more desperate, wrote once more: 'Surely you must be back by this time & so able to again look over my letters.' And of course he included his usual 'extras', adding queries about any spare copies of early Kororareka or Auckland newspapers and *Government Gazettes*. He signed off: 'Give me an exhaustive letter & oblige your envious friend T.M. Hocken.'[31]

Within two weeks, undoubtedly brow-beaten by Hocken's missives, Hill obliged by sending through a number of issues of *Te Karere Maori*. Hocken thanked him on 21 June 1900, mentioning other items he lacked and proudly listing some of his own treasures. He also touched on the New Zealand, Australian and Pacific holdings in the Grey Collection at Cape Town: 'I have two or three times moved in the direction of getting the collection here but with no result.' He had already exclaimed to Hill in a previous letter: 'What do Cape folk or the gentle Boer know of Maori!'[32] The notion of repatriating the Grey Collection in South Africa, especially the Maori language manuscripts, also consumed Alexander Turnbull's time. Happily, the first official exchange of this 'misplaced' material occurred in 1921.

Hocken also congratulated Hill on his effort to specialise in collecting Maori artefacts and language publications, adding that he, Hocken, was at the wrong end of the country. Although his trips north helped, he admitted that collecting was at times a lonely business. He appealed to Hill: 'I should very much like to have a long talk with you on all these most interesting matters. Can you not come down?' Envious of Hill's 'unexemplified opportunities', he admitted '*Here* there is no such chance.' Despite all this, Hocken maintained an air of importance, especially concerning his own collecting activities. 'I do believe if you saw my collection of literature you would say 'Here! Take Mine! Keep out of the vortex & help me to keep in it.'[33]

Hocken was thorough in his searches. The Rev. John Kinder, to whom Hocken wrote in August 1900, could not satisfy his request for 'any numbers of *Karere Maori*', but was more positive in other areas: two items sent included presentation copies of J.A. Wilson's *Missionary Life and Work in New Zealand* (1889) and John White's *Maori Superstitions* (1856). Kinder later presented Hocken with his *Remarks on the Report of the Commissioners on the General Synod* (1901).[34] Hocken also contacted 86-year-old Bishop Octavius Hadfield, known by Maori as Rangatira Pae (the mild white man). He replied in a shaky hand on 5 September 1900, apologising for his late reply and for not having any numbers of *Te Karere*. 'To tell the truth, when I ceased in my 80th year to hold office, & retired into private life seven years ago, I destroyed ordinances & pamphlets of which I had kept only for my own self, & which I was no longer likely to want.'[35] Hocken thought well enough of Hadfield's reply to file it in his named and famed F&J Volume 5.

George Clarke via John Webster

Hocken had first met John Webster in 1874. In the intervening 26 years correspondence was frequent, as were occasional visits. Hocken's 'Album 43: Ethnographic' contains photographs of Webster and his family outside his home in the Hokianga, presumably taken by Hocken or Bessie.[36] Hocken had asked the old settler to contribute display items to the 1889–90 exhibition and later asked if he could copy out passages from Webster's letters, to which the writer agreed, albeit advising discretion and judgment.[37] Their correspondence continued; typically, Hocken pressed for information on the early days and reminded Webster about posterity: 'Think this over: What will you finally do with this valuable collection. Not burn them merely.'[38]

Reading Webster's *Last Cruise of the Wanderer* on 6 June 1900 was a prompt for Hocken to send another letter: 'Have you any of the *Karere Maori*? ... Or do you know where I could get any? I am endeavouring to make a complete set & have the numbers moderately complete but still with many deficiencies.'[39] Throughout the two men's extensive correspondence there is no further mention of *Te Karere Maori*, but Hocken received far more interesting materials from one who was a key observer in the early history of the colony.

Hocken was certainly proud of what he had accumulated and said as much to Webster: 'You would be amazed to see my collection relating to N.Z. & Polynesia generally. Old portraits from Cook downwards to our Governors, politicians, & old settlers. Newspapers from 1840 onwards.' He also crowed about recent acquisitions: 'Quite recently [in December 1899] I received from Mrs [Eugenia] Shortland all her husbands' [sic] old journals &

other manuscripts & papers which I am now engaged in sorting & utilising.'[40] Edward Shortland had arrived in New Zealand in March 1841. He was private secretary to Governor Hobson, friend of William Martin and George Clarke, Protector of Aborigines, knew the Maori chief Te Rauparaha and was an assistant to Grey, editing the latter's *Polynesian Mythology*, published in 1885.[41] He was a key government interpreter in land claims inquiries, and through various overland journeys and familiarity with Maori customs and lore he wrote *The Southern Districts of New Zealand* (1851), *Traditions and Superstitions of the New Zealanders* (1854) and the later *Maori Religion and Mythology* (1882). The cache included Shortland's 'Journal Notes kept while in the Middle Island November 1843 and 4 to 21 January 1844', his 'Journal of an expedition through Waikato with Governor Hobson by Edward Shortland, Private Secretary. 9 May 1842' and a copy of David Monro's journal (c. 1844).[42] Hocken was right to exclaim to Webster: 'You can imagine what a splendid haul this is!'[43]

Despite an 'attack of La Grippe [flu]', Webster responded to questions about De Thierry from Hocken's 6 June 1900 letter, filling pages not about the eccentric baron but about the eccentric naval officer George 'Toby' Philpotts, who was a favourite with his men but disliked by the missionaries. According to Webster, Philpotts' last words were: 'I will shew these ___ missionaries I am not a coward!'[44] Hocken also broached the topic of old records: 'I don't know whether you are doing any burning, but if so anything so to be treated, if not of a private matter would be much valued ... I have gathered a host of information from documents & other papers that at my earnest entreaties have been spared from the flames. For a boxful of such *rubbish* I should be infinitely obliged.' And Hocken targeted specific items, pictures that he had seen when visiting the Hokianga: 'In what direction is your "Native Feast at Remuera" to go? I believe this is the only lithograph connected with N.Z. that I do not possess. No, there is one other, "View of Auckland" dedicated to Lord Stanley I think, about 1843 or /42. Then the portrait of your old friend Mr Brown is historical.'[45] In a calculated move, designed to soften the asking, Hocken enclosed with his July letter a copy of his *Contributions*. The Hocken and Webster correspondence continued, and both men later became involved in a number of publishing projects. Hocken certainly benefitted from the exchange, and even today these letters make excellent reading.

There was one other good result: through Webster, Hocken was introduced to George Clarke the younger, who was born at Parramatta, Sydney, in 1823 and moved with his parents to Kerikeri a year later. He mixed with Maori and gained a good grasp of the language. After schooling in Tasmania he returned to be taught at Henry Williams's mission school in Waimate. While his father was Protector of Aborigines under Hobson, the youngster was a clerk in the Native Section. He assisted Commissioner William Spain in some New Zealand Land Company claims, was an interpreter at the trial of Maketu

Wharetotara (also known as Wiremu Kingi Maketu) in March 1842 and in 1844 he represented Maori in the sale of the Otago block.[46] Clarke eventually became part of Sir George Grey's personal staff. In 1848, however, he turned his back on a bright future in officialdom and went to study in London, where he was ordained in 1851. He returned to Hobart where he became a minister of the Congregational Church, a member of the Royal Society of Tasmania and a co-founder of the University of Tasmania. He was also its first vice-chancellor and later chancellor. He died in Hobart on 10 March 1913. His extensive library was finally purchased by Angus & Robertson.[47] Clarke authored *Notes on Early Life in New Zealand* (1903) and wrote a small memoir about his good friend James Backhouse Walker, with whom Hocken was already acquainted.[48]

Hocken's correspondence with Clarke was similar to that with Webster. Although documents were sent back and forth, the two men mostly traded historical information and personal recollections of people and events from New Zealand's past. The correspondence was not one-sided. Hocken brought to the exchange, as he did with most, much accumulated knowledge on New Zealand's early history. In his own way he offered additional information, or filled gaps in the past that allowed a recipient such as Clarke to respond more fully. From all accounts, Hocken's knowledge base was appreciated, especially if it highlighted an ancestor's good name or went some way towards re-evaluating their place in history.

Hocken's letters to Clarke do not survive, but it is obvious that he raised the subject of the early missionaries in New Zealand. By about 1893 Clarke had written much of his *Notes on Early Life in New Zealand*, and although a good deal of its content was detailed in the letters, there were additional, often highly personal, asides. According to Clarke, William Williams was 'my guide philosopher and friend' who 'moulded my life', Hadfield 'carried me a little further' and William Yate 'affected me most of all'. Indeed, Clarke was Yate's 'pet boy'. Clarke described Yate as 'one of the family' at both Kerikeri and Waimate, and fondly remembered his voyage with him on the *Active* to Sydney when he was 'a small boy, with frill collar, and breeches buttoned outside the jacket'. Clarke even made slight reference to the disgrace surrounding Yate – he was dismissed from the CMS over alleged homosexual relationships – which was 'like the eruption of a volcano without the least hint or hearing of the catastrophe'. He added naively: 'I do not know to this day what his offence really was. But it was not entanglements with Maori women.' Clarke actually came upon Yate back in England when the latter was chaplain of the St John's Mariner Church in Dover. He described the experience to Hocken: 'I at once spotted my man. I drew him aside and told him who I was and trembling from head to foot he just poured out his heart in kindness.'[49]

Colonel Wakefield was 'kindly and considerate' and Clarke had 'no bitter thoughts about him at all'. And while not wanting to 'abuse the dead' he fired a salvo at Hocken's hero Edward Gibbon Wakefield, calling him 'personally malignant'. Of Edward Shortland Clarke wrote: 'What weeks and months I have spent on teaching him Maori, as I did Sir George Grey after him!' He was 'a most curious, intellectual and laborious student'.[50] Clarke was also perceptive about the role of interpreters who, through their presence and persuasive influence, carried the burden of care and responsibility between the two races. Many of the transactions that involved interpreters did not end in dispute.

Clarke obviously enjoyed recalling people and events: 'I wish I could lie on my back and shut my eyes and see the stuff …' He then asked Hocken: 'Is there any chance of you taking a trip round our way?'[51] The seed was planted and would bear fruit. Hocken's enquiries prompted Clarke to sift through his 'old papers' where, to his astonishment, he found a memorandum written the day before the trial of Maketu and a letter written from Robert Fitz-Roy to Clarke Sr. He was prepared to give these 'genuine relics' to Hocken. Clarke also included information on those 'staunch friends who shepherded' him through various trials and tribulations in his youth. All this was 'gossip of a very personal sort', but he had a receptive audience: 'I know you care about anything that can call up the New Zealand of the past, and any little light that I can throw back upon it I am quite ready to …'[52]

Clarke continued with his reminiscences, which included a small but vivid anecdote about Henry Williams:

> In the very early days the missionaries had an anniversary gathering which they called the 'Huihuinga'. All the missionaries and their belongings and adherents came to muster for the occasion. I remember one year the celebration was at Paihia. Old Archdeacon Henry Williams was an out and out British salt. On the hill, behind the settlement, he had mounted a few rusty cannonades, and of course on such an occasion he made them blaze out. It was a very wild outburst of 'Britannia rules the waves' but was a bit disastrous. Mair and Puckey, one or both of them had their fingers blown off, and carried the memories of their festival to their last days.

Clarke described Williams as 'brave, honest, chivalrous and true, but very adverse to all mincing ways. I think of him to the last with the greatest reverence and respect.' This was despite his frankness and unguarded responses, which often caused offence. Clarke recalled when Williams, at Port Nicholson, 'was so worried and disgusted with the insults and lies that the Company's agents heaped upon him that he said: "I wish I could take off my coat and call you out for your villainies."'[53]

Clarke also mentioned William Puckey and Robert Maunsell who, along with James Hamlin, were regarded as the three best Maori scholars of their day. Puckey he remembered as a true scholar who did not use 'pidgin Maori' when preaching, yet it was Maunsell, 'by far and away the best Maori linguist we ever had', who came in for high praise: 'What can I say of him except that

I love him.' He also wrote of Octavius Hadfield: every incident surrounding the latter's ordination at Paihia was 'photoed on my memory'.

For one who was always in 'my shell',[54] Clarke was extremely prolix. In a five-day period – from 28 November to 1 December 1900 – he sent Hocken three long letters. To Hocken's delight, Clarke realised the problems of distance and relented on the control of the original papers: 'I think the best thing I can do is to send you the relics of ancient correspondence just as they are ... if you care about keeping any of the originals that are at your service, only *send me back copies of them*. For the rest, post them back at your convenience.'[55] After informing Hocken that another packet of letters was on its way, Clarke continued the torrent, mainly about William Yate. Hocken was now part-time counsellor: 'But the memories of poor old Yate are crowding before me and I should like to discharge my mind. Whatever the faults I know he loved *me* greatly.'[56]

As Hocken sifted through all this information, one phrase written by Clarke would have surely registered with him: 'Remember I was on the spot.'[57] Such personal observations were of incalculable value, and the relationship that developed through this correspondence stood Hocken in good stead when he called on Clarke in Hobart in 1904.

15
A Welcome Break

By the end of 1900 Hocken was planning another overseas trip, this time to England and Japan, but there was much to be done first. In March 1901 he embarked on an excursion to Milford Sound with John Walker Fowler, a Southland farmer, and William Saunders, owner of the Otautau flour mill. In late May 1901 he was caught up in the festivities surrounding the Maori Carnival in aid of the Maori church at Puketeraki. Not only did this mean socialising with the likes of Bishop Nevill (who opened the carnival), Tame Parata and Augustus Hamilton, but it meant writing a 'lecturette' on 'The Maoris of the South Island', which was typically long, especially for the designated 'scanty limits of a quarter of an hour'. After touching on race migration, Abel Tasman, local tribal conflicts, moa sightings, acts of deforestation and Te Rauparaha, and reminding his listeners that 'those days were wild and lawless', Hocken made a telling Darwinian statement: 'It is right, perhaps, and in accordance with the principles of evolution and of the advancement of the human race, that those should possess the land who use it to the best advantage, even though this should involve dispossession of the original occupants.' He added: 'But this should be done with every consideration and sentiment of justice.'[1]

In late June 1901 the Duke and Duchess of Cornwall and York, the future George V and Queen Mary, visited Dunedin as part of a New Zealand (and empire) tour. On 25 June Hocken attended a celebratory dinner at the Fernhill Club, where he gave the duke a copy of his *Contributions* and his translation of the *Journal of Abel Tasman*.[2] In July he also attended the Agricultural Winter Show and an Arbor Day celebration where oaks were planted to commemorate the royal couple's visit.[3] During these proceedings Alice Karetai presented an illuminated address to the duke on behalf of the Maori of Otago. Hocken supplied the English text to the Maori original, which is filed in his F&J Volume 2.[4] There is no indication of how and why he was involved or who provided the Maori translation.

And finally, on 9 July 1901, one month before his departure, Hocken read to members of the Otago Institute his long article on early newspapers in New Zealand.[5] This had taken much time and effort. By utilising the samples he owned and marshalling the information supplied by other individuals, he documented in considerable detail rudimentary bibliographical data such as dates of first printing, issue formats and original pricing. It was an important first.

The report of this lecture in the *Otago Witness* of 17 July contained the initial public mention of his planned trip back to England. Some of his correspondents, such as *Taranaki News* editor Charles Keats Brown, Percy Smith and

Elsdon Best, were already privy to the news. Brown offered Hocken a letter of introduction to Sir Charles Wentworth Dilke, 'if you think it might be of service to you'.[6] Smith wrote, 'I envy you your researches at home in to our old history', and pressed Hocken for a contact address so that correspondence could continue.[7] Best asked if Hocken could search out publishers in London for his works on Maori mythology, religion and customs, and had some requests regarding the Japanese: 'How did they formerly dress their hair? What was their weaving like? Were sacred fires used? Any system of tapu? Were the voyagers in old times i.e. Pacific-wards?'[8] The newspaper article only hinted at the research Hocken planned to undertake, but regarded him as the best man to carry out the task.[9] There was also a passing reference to his being unwell, and hopes that his health would improve so that he could complete the proposed work.

Hocken was given a big send-off by friends and well-wishers at the Dunedin Club on 3 August; three days later the Otago Medical Association presented him with some Goertz field-glasses as a parting gift.[10] His friend Stanley Batchelor was to be locum at Atahapara.

England via Japan

The three Hockens and Sally Baker, daughter of the manager of the rectory at Otago Boys' High School, left Dunedin on 9 August. According to Gladys's diary entry, there was 'an enormous entourage' to see them off.[11] On their way to Sydney they passed through Wellington, which Gladys, a precocious 17-year-old, described as 'a dirty, windy hole and everything is dear – I never want to go there again'.[12]

Even though much of her diary of the 'world tour' is full of petulant schoolgirl observations – weather, men, everything is boring – its survival is extremely important on a number of levels. It reveals something of the family dynamics, documents their itinerary and mentions people Hocken met or events he attended, all of which had a bearing on his collecting.[13] To assist him in the latter he had a testimonial of introduction 'To All Universities and Libraries' from James Hector:

> This is to introduce and recommend to you my friend of 40 years standing Dr Hockin [sic] of Dunedin, a fellow of this University who is about to take a journey round the world and earn a well merited holiday from an arduous carreer [sic]. Dr Hockin is our foremost authority on everything that relates to the ancient lore of the Maori race & has in his possession the finest Polynesian Library & collection in existence.[14]

There were four other reasons for the trip: reconnecting with the Hocken and Buckland families in England; giving Gladys some 'finishing' at an overseas school; allowing Hocken to examine the resources in British institutions towards a planned publication on the early history of New Zealand; and fulfilling his intention to upgrade his medical qualifications by taking 'a doctor's degree' at a university in England, though he did not do this.[15]

On 29 August the Hockens finally left Sydney and reached Japan on 24 September.[16] Their first port of call was Nagasaki, where Hocken was struck by the beautiful and extensive harbour.[17] They stayed in Japan for some eight weeks, during which they travelled back and forth from Yokohama, Kobe and Tokyo, visiting museums, shops, temples and silk manufacturing outlets. Hocken of course had his own agenda and liked leaving the women to do their own thing.

In an interview given later in London, he expanded a little on why he travelled to Japan. Through his work on the New Zealand portion of Tasman's *Journal* he had noticed the reference to Maori twisting their hair after the manner of the Japanese.[18] This notion took root and he felt there might be a connection between the two races. With an opportunity to travel there he decided 'to find out all I could on the subject'.[19] On 2 October 1901 he left Bessie and Gladys 'until further notice' and travelled to Tokyo, which he called 'the city of magnificent distances'. The next day he called at the Anthropology Department of the Tokyo Imperial University (later the University of Tokyo) and met Tsuboi Shogoro, the department's first professor and co-founder of the Anthropological Society of Tokyo.[20] Hocken returned to the university on 12 October and admitted afterwards that he was forced to conclude that 'no indications existed of any connection whatever between the Maori people and the ancient Japanese race'.[21]

On 23 October he attended a function at the British Consulate that was attended by Sir Claude MacDonald, the new consul-general of the Empire of Japan. That same day Hocken packed for a four-day trip to Miyanoshita, in Hakone. By 31 October he was back at Yokohama and the family visited the grave of William Adams (Miura Anjin), a navigator and early English settler in Japan. With their departure date settled for 23 November, Hocken and Bessie travelled to Tokyo to attend a Chrysanthemum Garden Party on the emperor's birthday, leaving Gladys and her friend Sally in Yokohama. It was about this time that Gladys noted her father was coughing badly.

The Hockens arrived in Hong Kong on 27 November and left the next day for Singapore and Colombo, where they stayed five days. They reached Port Said on 30 December and took a train to Cairo. In Egypt for three months, they tried to see all they could: the many temples, the Cairo Museum and the Pyramids. Hocken travelled up the Nile twice, as far as Aswan. He also managed to collect a number of 'valuable old necklaces and scarabies [sic], carved stones and all sorts of odds and ends'. He was in his element, praising Cairo as 'a very fine city with splendid boulevards and reserves, beautiful gardens and terraces, and the magnificent houses and palaces of the upper classes'.[22] The family returned to Port Said and boarded the *Kawachi Maru* on

10 March for travel through the Mediterranean via Athens to Marseilles, then by train and ferry to England.

Arrival in England

In 1882 Hocken had stayed at 28 Euston Square. Twenty years later on 2 April 1902 he was back there and in 'a great surprise to both parties' he found the same landlady in residence. It was from this familiar base that he began his networking and collecting in earnest.

One person who featured regularly in Hocken's comings and goings in London was Major-General Horatio Gordon Robley, soldier, artist, collector of mokomokai (the preserved heads of Maori) and author of *Moko or Maori Tattooing* (1896), a book that Hocken owned. Robley made contact quickly, taking Hocken to lunch on 4 April. Six days later Robley invited him to attend a lecture on Japan; Hocken reciprocated by visiting Robley's Regent Street residence and 'Museum', which contained his growing collection of heads.[23] Hocken documented his thoughts on Robley's field of collecting: 'Not only is your collection unique, but it typifies a branch of savage art that is most interesting, and one which has now almost wholly disappeared.' Hocken was so enthusiastic about Robley's *Moko* that he initiated work on producing a second edition.[24] New blocks depicting various moko were crafted; Hocken made generous and full annotations to a draft copy, still in his library, but the project did not eventuate.

Founded as the Colonial Society in 1868 to promote social networks throughout the British Empire, the Royal Colonial Institute, as it became in 1882, had a valuable library and reading room at its Northumberland Avenue premises where members could congregate and discuss colonial matters. An agency that fostered such networking suited Hocken, and to solidify his involvement he was nominated on 11 June 1902 as a 'Non-Resident Fellow of the Royal Colonial Institute' by two members: S.W. Silver and vice-president Sir Frederick Young.[25] Hocken knew of Silver, who was a book collector of note; Young had a long association with the institute and was a strong advocate of the permanent union of the colonies. On the same day Hocken attended a lecture at the Japan Society's headquarters at 20 Hanover Square and expressed interest in joining the organisation, whose aims were dedicated to the enhancement of the British–Japanese relationship and the promotion of greater understanding between the two countries. Sometime before July 1902 he became a corresponding member, joining other members such as artists Walter Crane, Frank Brangwyn and Norman Lindsay. In 1906 Hocken was the only New Zealand-based member out of a membership tally of 1830.

Hocken made every effort to forge useful connections. Early in June he met Richard Garnett, past superintendent at the Reading Room of the British Museum, well-known antiquarian and author (as Hocken knew) of a biography on Edward Gibbon Wakefield. Garnett later wrote to Alice Mary Freeman, daughter of Edward Gibbon's brother Daniel Bell Wakefield – 'Decidedly the world is a small place' – and continued with a reference to the 'very agreeable, well-informed' Hocken, explaining the string of connections that had brought the two men together.[26] Two months later Garnett again praised Hocken's attributes to Freeman, calling him a 'highly intelligent man', and admitted that he had used Hocken's *Contributions* in his own work.[27]

June proved a busy month. Occasions Hocken attended ranged from a meeting with his nephew William at an ophthalmology gathering, a reception at the Duchess of Devonshire's home and a 'Colonial' function, where Premier Richard Seddon was present, to a social occasion at the Royal Geographical Society, a meeting at the Linnean Society and a gathering at the RCI (now Royal Commonwealth Society). Just before leaving for this last, Robley, who accompanied Hocken, gave Gladys a huia feather.

Gladys recorded her amazement that the aristocratic class such as 'Duchesses and Lords and Ladies get to hear of us' and thought (perhaps rightly) that it was through the office of William Pember Reeves, New Zealand's agent general. Even Hocken's relatives were mystified, especially when he returned from Reeves' office on 23 June with two invitations to the coronation at Westminster Abbey, an occasion later detailed in the *Evening Post* and read no doubt with envy by those back home.[28] According to Gladys there was some amusement during the preparations for the ceremony: 'mother's [court dress] fitted beautifully, but father's court suit was several sizes too large and he kept tripping over his sword …'[29]

By early July 1902 Hocken was preparing for a trip to Newcastle, while Bessie and her daughter were planning to go to Switzerland where Gladys would go to school. Before departure there was another round of engagements and Hocken made a point of contacting Charlotte Godley, wife of John Robert Godley, a prime mover in the Canterbury Association and the early settlement of Canterbury. In her eighties, Godley claimed 'I have lost my memory to a great extent!', but when Hocken called on her they talked of what she called 'ancient history' and she gave him a copy of her husband's *Letters from America* (1844). In this work Hocken noted: 'Mrs Godley died at Gloucester Terrace, London, on the 3rd Jany 1907, at 85. I saw much of her when in London in 1902–3 but she has ceased to take much interest in N.Z. affairs, & her memory was very imperfect'.[30] A letter from Charlotte Godley written on 24 September reached him at Newcastle. Having read through old letters and rediscovered documents pertinent to New Zealand, she enclosed a copy of a 'very clear statement of Association matters' and promised: 'if I see anything I think you might to know [sic] – I shall think of you'.[31] Back in London, his reply of 30 September generated another letter from her on 10 October 1902, although he did not read it until he returned from Europe: 'I have further considered the question of my husband's letters, & I have now decided to place a packet of them at your disposal.' Underestimating his diligence in such matters, she continued: 'I can hardly suppose that you will read them all, for some of them are very long & not easy to decipher.' If he were to publish them, she asked that he copy out the passages and let her see them, just in case they dealt with confidential matters. In the end, she trusted him: 'I will ask you to return the originals to me when you have done with them – there is no hurry about it.'³² Hocken actually copied out some 51 pages of letters and returned them. The copies now form part of the Canterbury Association Minutes and Letterbook, June 1851 – 28 January 1853.³³

On to Europe

On 8 October 1902 Hocken was in Lausanne, Switzerland, where he and Bessie consulted 'a famous Swiss specialist' about his throat.³⁴ On 13 October they left for Venice; a month later they were in Athens. According to Gladys, Bessie kept herself busy selecting photographs for 'A New Zealander on her travels' and 'Scenes in the Far East', photo-montages that appeared in the *Otago Witness* during 1903.³⁵ Gladys also reported that her father continued to suffer from a bad throat.³⁶ By 14 December they had left Athens and were heading towards Naples, and on 23 December they were in Rome. In January 1903 there was a small home-town reunion as Daniel Colquhoun and his wife, merchant and philanthropist David Theomin and his wife Dorothy and Isobel Cargill were all holidaying in Rome. Hocken occasionally escaped the socialising: in the first week of February he went book hunting and met a New Zealand priest called Buckley. By 25 February they were in Florence where they were reunited with the Colquhouns. By late February after visiting Pisa with General Robley and his sister, then Turin, the family arrived at Geneva where they stayed at another Hotel Suisse. (Gladys was complimentary about the Swiss and Switzerland.) In Geneva Hocken bought his copy of Louis Bouvier's *Flores des Alps* ([1882]), which, as Gladys noted, spurred him into action: he did 'a good deal of botanizing'. The family used Montreux, a Swiss resort town located on Lake Geneva, as a base for a brief period. This allowed time to organise piano and singing lessons for Gladys, and gave Bessie a chance to recover from what her daughter called 'slight internal disarrangement'. Hocken continued to botanise, travelling to Lyon to do some 'New Zealand research'. On 30 May they were in Paris. London (via Dieppe) was next, and the Hockens finally unpacked at 40 Kildare Terrace in Westbourne Grove, Bayswater, on 2 June 1903. This quietly placed semi-detached house was their London base until their return to Dunedin.

Return to London

Hocken's return to the city meant renewed activity, as Gladys noted: 'Father is very much occupied seeing old friends and doing research'.³⁷ Robley was again one of the first to call and both men went to a Linnean Society meeting on 4 June, where Hocken delivered a speech and encouraged Fellows to visit New Zealand, adding somewhat rashly that 'every facility for travelling at special rates to visit the celebrated scenery will be afforded by the New Zealand Government'.[38] He happily put himself forward as a contact for any prospective visitors.

There was a good deal more socialising, and Gladys turned 19. On her birthday it was announced that she would get an allowance of £4 per month, invested with the Post Office at 2.5 per cent. There was also the inevitable bundle of letters that had not been forwarded on. One was the Godley missive mentioned above. Another was from John Davies Gilbert Enys, who was instrumental in obtaining for Hocken a copy of the Cook portrait at Trinity House, Hull.[39] Enys's letter of 29 May 1903 carried the news that a 'good pile' of manuscripts and printed books owned by Edward Shortland had been posted to him, and that there were other items 'under offer' through Eugenia Shortland at Plymouth.[40] Hocken saw this as a unique opportunity to secure the materials Enys listed. Excluding obituaries, biographical sketches and advertising sheets for Shortland's own *Southern Districts of New Zealand* (1851), there are 25 separate Edward Shortland items in Trimble's *Catalogue* (1912), many of which are manuscripts. Hakena, the Hocken Library's archives and manuscripts database, contains 29 major manuscript items compiled or created by Shortland. These include documents that cover Maori mythology, tradition and customs, waiata and whakapapa (some contained in Shortland's *Maori Religion and Mythology* (1882)); various journals (the *Maketu Journal*, November 1842 to 8 August 1843, and *Coromandel and Kawhia*); accounts of travels, especially of the Middle [South] Island; inward and outward letterbooks (in English and Maori); and language primers, including botanical notes, general correspondence and a spread of Melanesian, Motu, Aboriginal and South African language manuscripts.[41] They comprise hundreds of hand-written sheets.

Hocken could combine these with his other Shortland materials, which he had received from Eugenia Shortland in December 1899. There was another item, perhaps secured earlier and from a more local source. This was Shortland's 'Collection of papers relating to Maori and the Maori language', which has a note attached by William Wildman, the Auckland bookseller, dated 12 December 1890.[42] Despite arrangement anomalies, the Shortland material forms a substantial component of Hocken's collection, especially with the unique manuscripts. Securing them all was a major coup, and he certainly recognised his good fortune. He followed up his thanks by corresponding with Eugenia Shortland and visiting her in Plymouth.[43]

About late June 1903 Hocken wrote to Mary Ford at Pencarrow, Cornwall. She was the widow of Richard Ford (1796–1858) traveller and author of *A Handbook for Travellers in Spain* (1845) and *Gatherings from Spain* (1846); and the sister of Sir William Molesworth (1810–1855), a director of the New Zealand Association (forerunner of the New Zealand Company) and for a short four-month term colonial secretary. His younger brother was Francis Alexander Molesworth, an early Wellington settler. Her reply on 6 July represented a nightmare for any collector: 'I regret exceedingly that I am unable to help you in the way of letters or papers on colonial subjects. In the great fire which occurred some years ago my dear brother Francis Alexander Molesworth's letters were burnt'.[44] She did, however, inform him that the Edward Gibbon Wakefield letters she once owned were now with Richard Garnett, whom Hocken had already met. Perhaps by way of compensation, she promised to ask the publisher John Murray to send through a copy of the speeches by her brother William. She also invited Hocken to Pencarrow. His reply was prompt, because she wrote back on 14 July asking for his recommendation of libraries in New Zealand that would take copies of her brother's *Speeches*.[45] Hocken not only listed four reputable libraries but added that he was actually reading the said work. Mary Ford responded on 18 August: 'Your expressions of reading my brother's most valuable & interesting speeches has greatly pleased his octogenarian sister.'[46] In mid-September Hocken finally made it to Cornwall, where she gave him another (his second) copy of *Selected Speeches of Sir William Molesworth* (1903), to which he added a note:

> Given to me by Mrs Ford, Sir Wm Molesworth's sister, of Pencarrow. I spent a day with her at Pencarrow in Aug. 1903. She was over 80 years of age but full of old reminiscences & good memory & was a thorough democrat. Referring to the well known portrait of her brother with long lank hair down the sides of his face she said that in youth he suffered from diseased neck-glands in the neighbourhood of his ear which left scars & these were covered by the growth of long hair.[47]

As a master of fostering such links, he sent her a copy of his *Contributions*, a photograph of Gladys (about which she was highly complimentary) and information on his gifting of his collection to Dunedin. A letter he received later carries a further note: 'a delightful old lady & a democrat of the best & truest type whilst of the bluest blood'.[48]

It was now two years since Hocken had left Dunedin, and although there was talk of planning a return journey home via the Trans-Siberian Railway, there was still much to do.[49] He was juggling numerous activities and his persistence bore fruit. August 1903 was a 'red-letter' month. Sometime after the 11th he received a letter from Sir William Lucius Selfe, third son of Henry Selfe Selfe, about 'a large box of M.S.S. chiefly connected with the Province of Canterbury N.Z. which were among my father's papers … I do not know whether they are likely to be of use to you, but they are quite at your disposal.' There was one proviso: '& return it to me when you have made what use you can of its contents'.[50] Three weeks later Selfe sent Hocken a postcard that allowed a little more latitude: 'Pray keep all the papers which you think will be of use to you & return the others and the box & photos at your leisure.'[51]

Much of what Hocken kept is filed in F&J Volume 6 and supplements his Canterbury Association material.[52] Gladys had a completely different view of these delights: 'Father had a huge box given to him the other day full of old New Zealand papers and what was our joy to see that nearly every envelope was smothered in rare old New Zealand stamps black with age! I think we are going to try and sell some.'[53]

16
The CMS, the Colonial Office and Home

As part of Hocken's search for documents pertaining to New Zealand's early history and development, he looked to the institutions involved: the Church Missionary Society and the Colonial Office. On his return from the Continent he began negotiations with both in earnest. Face-to-face contact was beneficial, but such bodies demanded formal letters. Judging from the CMS's response, Hocken's first letter had sought more than just permission to read records. On 12 August 1903 S.F. Purday, the Deputy Lay Secretary of the CMS, wrote thanking Hocken for his letter but refusing his suggestion of 'parting with the official letters' and 'portraits illustrating the early history of the Society'. The CMS was, however, happy to allow him 'full opportunities for examining New Zealand correspondence', although on the understanding 'that no letter or extracts from them are to be published without the consent of the Committee'.[1]

It was a good start that eventually paid dividends. Hocken found a wealth of historical letters as well as journals of Samuel Marsden and the missionaries who first worked in New Zealand. After much discussion he acquired the manuscripts, 'some of them all but illegible from the ravages of time, faded ink, poor writing requiring the interpretation of an expert, and other evident causes'. By 13 November 1903 they were in his hands.[2] They included two copies of Marsden's journal of his first visit to New Zealand, 1814–15; two copies of the journal of his second visit, 1819; two copies of the third visit journal, 1820; one copy of the journal of his fourth visit, 1823; Marsden's letters to the CMS, containing letters to various missionaries; and the correspondence of the Rev. John Butler, George Clarke and the Rev. George Clarke, the Rev. Richard Davis, William Hall, John King, Francis Hall and the Rev. Thomas Kendall, and copied works by the Rev. William Wade.[3] Gladys summarily dismissed this treasure trove as 'a whole load of old papers'.[4] Back in Dunedin Hocken had them bound into sturdy thick volumes. He also did not forget his debt and sent the society a cheque of £250.[5]

In 1882 Hocken had asked Francis Dillon Bell, the then-agent general, about the existence of the New Zealand Company records. After a cursory search and Bell's reply that they were no longer at the Colonial Office, Hocken had let the matter rest. Now, in London, he began the search again. Sometime in June 1903 he requested permission from the Colonial Office to view New Zealand Company records at the Public Record Office; they had been transferred there in June 1869. His request was successful, with permission to search and copy registered on 1 July 1903.[6] Thus began a prolonged undertaking, travelling regularly from Kildare Terrace (over Lord Hills Bridge) via rail to the Record Office. Although Gladys recorded that her father 'slaves there the whole day', his visits were sporadic, broken by social and search obligations elsewhere.⁷ On 17 August, for example, he was at Uxbridge visiting Angela J. Wakefield, who presented him with a copy of her grandson C.M. Wakefield's *Life of Thomas Attwood* (1885). She had married Daniel Bell Wakefield and was the daughter of the radical MP Attwood, as Hocken recorded in this privately published edition. At the end of the month the Hockens travelled to Liverpool and Edinburgh, where, as Gladys recorded rather caustically, there were 'more rapidly dying identities awaiting his coming'.⁸

Family obligations aside, Hocken continued his searches. While in Edinburgh he 'spent a day or two' with Admiral David Robertson-Macdonald, who had taken command of HMS *Hazard* at Kororareka in 1844. At their meeting Robertson-Macdonald gave Hocken a number of hand-written sheets titled 'An account of a fight at Matarai Gorge, 12 July 1844', which are now in Hocken's F&J Volume 2.⁹ Through his contact with Richard Garnett, Hocken arranged to have lunch with Mary Alice Freeman on 28 August, though she admitted to him in a letter dated 20 August that she would be a great disappointment as she was only six when she lived with Edward Gibbon Wakefield at Tinakori Road, Wellington.¹⁰ According to her reminiscences, Wakefield was a complete recluse in the last years of his life, and as she was devoted to him, she read him books. She had lent 'several touching letters' written by Edward Gibbon, and various business letters to Lord Lyttelton, to Jerningham Wakefield, who had lost them. When Edward Gibbon died all his papers went to Jerningham: 'what is most probable they have been destroyed'.¹¹ Regardless of this news Hocken surely enjoyed the occasion, especially given the historical connection and being privy to personal details about one of his heroes.

By 29 August Hocken was back in London, where he read Colonial Office Under-Secretary H. Bertram Cox's reply to his letter of 11 August, in which he had asked for 'further permission to see the papers of the Colonial Office which relate to New Zealand say for the first ten years of its existence as a Colony'. He had also made some comments on the state of the material:

> I should like to say that in going through these voluminous papers I find very many are absolutely useless, of no interest whatever, and simply accumulators of dirt and dust. Others again are of great interest but are massed together and docketed in such a way as to detract very greatly from their usefulness and availability. Under these circumstances I would suggest with great respect that steps be taken to put these papers into such order as would render them of public value. Should this suggestion meet with your approval I shall be very happy to place my services at your disposal, and purely as a labour of love. No one is more skilled in early New Zealand matter than myself. Upon them I have written, and am still engaged in writing, and my library on the subject and on colonization generally is probably the best in the world. I mention all this in no spirit of self-praise but as an earnest indication of my readiness to assist in a labour of so much importance.¹²

Cox's answer contained both good and bad news. Hocken was not allowed to see the material he had enquired about, but his offer to arrange the papers was gladly accepted. He was also allowed, at least initially, to retain a copy whenever there were duplicates. An inspection was necessary before any item was relinquished.[13]

Hocken began his search in the large Admiralty tomes, looking for any correspondence with Captain Cook and his companions connected to the three voyages to New Zealand. The meagre results made him turn to 'Company' documents.[14] His initial attempt at sorting faltered because other obligations intruded. Between 14 and 19 September he was in Devonshire 'hunting records'.[15] On 5 October Gladys found her 'father looking very well and working harder than ever at the Records Office among his papers. He has already gone through 40,000 letters.' There was also talk of returning to New Zealand, with 18 December mooted as departure day.[16] Although Bessie was unwell, she did manage to help transcribe documents for Hocken, particularly the 'Journal of Rev William Richard Wade' (June 1834 to September 1836) and the 'Journal of John Wallis Barnicoat' (February 1842 to October 1844). Inadvertently, this misdated joint transcription by husband and wife broke the Record Office rules, as recorded by Hocken:

> Just as I had completed the précis it was discovered that the contents were (or should have been) inviolably preserved from the public until a period of 50 years had elapsed ... How the oversight occurred I cannot say. Fortunately my work was completed when I was informed of the error. There is a vast amount of history condensed in these pages of great value and absolutely new. I must endeavour to fill the précis out so as to make it more intelligible.[17]

On 22 October 1903 Hocken finished his task of examining the papers and books of the New Zealand Company and told Cox: 'Though laborious and dirty the work was agreeable and very interesting and every assistance was rendered by the Officials of the Office. With the exception of vouchers, accounts, etc., I went through every document inserting the result with rough notes extending to about 60 double folio pages of a book supplied me for the purpose.' He also claimed there was 'a good proportion' of manuscript parcels and books 'fit for destruction', which he had marked for easy identification. Now he had a new proposal, this time encompassing all of the company's records, including the originals:

> Going through these the idea arose and developed that you would not perhaps offer any objection to presenting them to the Government of New Zealand by whom I am sure they would be warmly acknowledged and cared for. The papers are not those of the British Government but those of a private Company. Upon this suggestion, however, the Honourable W.P. Reeves, Agent General for the Colony will officially, and more fully address you.

He then chanced his arm on the duplicate and triplicate copies, adding: 'I should be very grateful if you would permit me to have those for my library which truly is the most extensive and unique on subjects connected with Polynesia.' He strengthened his proposal by adding: 'I should find great use for them and have them strongly bound so that in this way there would be another effective means of preserving much of the history of one of England's most interesting Colonies.'[18]

On 4 November the office responded, giving thanks for the work done and offering a glimmer of hope regarding his suggestion that 'papers should be handed over to the New Zealand Government and that you should be permitted to retain duplicate and triplicate copies'.[19] Perhaps this is why Gladys wrote: 'Father is in high feather just now.'[20] She also recorded that all the valuable documents would cost him £50. And in an entry that would have pleased Hocken, she wrote: 'Father's library is now as complete as it ever can be most probably.'

However, on 16 November 1903, Pember Reeves wrote to Hocken at Kildare Terrace stating that there was no precedent for the handing over of any documents. He dismissed Hocken's notion of obtaining duplicates and suggested employing agents to transcribe papers of interest, a practice undertaken by other colonies.[21] Two days later an official letter from the Colonial Office confirmed Reeves' decree and contained another body-blow: no duplicate or triplicate documents could be handed over. Indeed, those documents deemed 'not of sufficient value' were to be either destroyed or transferred to curators, trustees or other governors of a library in Great Britain or Ireland.[22]

Hocken's long reply of 23 November focused on those libraries in Great Britain that might take the records. He was adamant that no 'library … would covet for its shelves the transference of duplicate or triplicate copies of the New Zealand Company's despatches which are after all, but letters addressed to the Chairman and directors of a private company by its agent'. His request was unusual, not suited to the standing rule. He then made a plea based on his own undertakings: 'My application may I trust be considered specially well founded as I am preparing for publication a work of the very early history of New Zealand dealing with Tasman, Cook, the French, Samuel Marsden and his first missionaries and with the earliest colonization. It is evident that letters such as those now indicated would be of great help to me.'[23]

Further bad news arrived in mid-December from Cox: Hocken would not be given the duplicate and triplicate copies.[24] There was some small compensation, though: the opportunity to make public his endeavours, at least to readers back home. Interviewed by the London correspondent of the *Otago Witness*, he reported somewhat creatively on his labours: 'I have been hard at it for two years practically without a break, leaving my lodgings every morning at 9 o'clock and not getting back again until 7 in the evening!' He also revealed one of the main driving forces, the preparation of a second historical work to complement his *Contributions*. He was 'hunting up all the records of

New Zealand's early days of which I have been able to discover any trace'. He calculated these at 'fully 80,000 – EIGHTY THOUSAND! – letters, besides despatches and other documents. There were simply piles and piles of these.' He also reiterated his interest in Japan and repeated his success in meeting those people associated with New Zealand. As he stated somewhat irreverently: 'I managed to "rake up" several ancient people who were thought to have been dead for years, and each one proved "good for something" in the way of ancient lore.' The article appeared in the *Otago Witness* on 6 January 1904.[25]

In fact, the Colonial Office saga had a happy and profitable conclusion. After a change of rules in mid-February 1909, well over 34 classes of duplicate New Zealand Company records were to be presented to the New Zealand government or destroyed.[26] Hocken was again consulted, and it was decided to take them all. The records arrived in June 1909 and most, but not all, formed the basis of the archive collection at the Dominion Museum, now Te Papa, in Wellington. Hocken did not miss out totally. Through his friend Augustus Hamilton, the museum's director, he was given some duplicate copies.

The Chase Continues

Taking a break from print and old documents, Hocken became interested in the work of William Holmes, who after arriving in Lyttelton in 1851 began drawing pencil and ink sketches of Akaroa, Lyttelton and Canterbury. Sometime after June 1903 Hocken contacted someone in the British Museum – perhaps Richard Garnett – and arranged to have 12 sketches by Holmes 'lithographed at the British Museum' for himself. One image was not lithographed: Bessie went to the museum and copied Holmes's *The Canterbury Plains from the Heathcote River*. All 13 images are now part of the Hocken's Pictures Collection.[27]

There was one old chestnut: John Alexander Gilfillan's *View in a Native Village in NZ*, which he had been pursuing since his trip to England in 1882. Gladys recorded in her diary: 'Father is much taken up with an exciting hunt (which began 25 years ago) after the original picture of an old Maori Pa.'[28] Just before 6 October 1903 he sent the editors of the *Birmingham Weekly* and the *Daily Post* a plea for the whereabouts of this particular painting, commonly known as *Interior of a Native Village or Pa*, which had been exhibited in the New Zealand Court at the Great Exhibition of 1851 by Captain Frederick Moore, its one-time owner. Sometime after that it was lost. Amazingly, Hocken had three responses to his newspaper appeal, although the whereabouts of the original was not revealed. All three had lithographic copies; two were prepared to sell.[29] Hocken already owned his own rare coloured lithographic copy of the painting, which Sir George Grey had tried to buy from him for £10 in 1894.

Luck continued to follow Hocken on his Gilfillan quest, and his good fortune demands a chronological leap. In early 1906 he wrote to Augustus Hamilton congratulating him and the museum for securing John Gilfillan's sketchbook and mentioning his failure to find the pa painting. He also included an account of Gilfillan's life, which had been extracted from a notebook that contained references to Samuel Marsden and Thomas Kendall, for use in a future issue of the *Bulletin*.[30] During his northern trek of March 1906 Hocken met up with Hamilton in Wellington, and Gilfillan was again a topic of conversation. Among some friendly banter, Hocken made reference to another project, a publication entitled 'Collected papers', which would contain a much fuller account of Gilfillan, with known published extracts. This project, like his Marsden one, never came to fruition. On his return he found a letter waiting from Andrew Todd, manager of the Dunedin branch of New Zealand Loan & Mercantile Agency. It mentioned Gilfillan's *A Native Council at War* and communications with one James Grice of Melbourne, dated 15 May 1906.[31] Grice had informed Todd that a certain 'Doctor (resident of Dunedin) was returning here from England via Melbourne with his wife and daughter' and while there had seen Gilfillan's painting. The doctor had wanted to purchase it, but unfortunately it was not for sale. It was now available at the asking price of 'nothing less than 180 guineas'. Quite rightly, Todd guessed that Hocken was the unknown doctor. After letters to Grice, Hocken responded with a firm counter-offer that was accepted by telegram. He secured Gilfillan's painting for £105, which in 1906 was no mean sum; it also seems to be the largest individual amount that Hocken paid for any one item in his collection.[32]

The Royal Anthropological Institute

Hocken's networking also led to his becoming, on 10 November, an Ordinary Fellow of the Royal Anthropological Institute of Great Britain and Ireland. His nominators were James Edge-Partington, ethnographer, and Henry Balfour, curator of the Pitts Rivers Museum and the institute's president for 1903–04. The extent of Hocken's acquaintance with Balfour is not known, but a nominator had to have 'personal knowledge' of the candidate. Hocken certainly knew Edge-Partington, having corresponded with him from Dunedin. As an interested collector of Pacifica, Hocken owned a copy of Edge-Partington's privately produced *An Album of the Weapons, Tools, Ornaments, Articles of Dress of the Natives of the Pacific Islands* (1890). Indeed, he 'deconstructed' his own copy, breaking it up and compiling three large scrapbooks from it. Hocken even ignored Edge-Partington's original arrangement of the images and recreated his own, adding an index to the images of the islands within. He also owned Edge-Partington's *Third Series* (1898), which is of particular significance because, along with Turnbull, Chapman and Hamilton, Hocken is formally thanked in the preface as a private collector who placed parts of his collection at the author's disposal. Edge-Partington's work is doubly important because it carries one of the few definite prices Hocken paid for an item in his collection. A tipped-in prospectus describes the 'half morocco edition at £2 13s 6d plus postage at 6s 6d' with Hocken's brief note: '£3.0.0'. In his hand is also written, 'Messrs Palmer Howe, Booksellers & Publishers, 73, 75, 77 Princes St, Manchester' – presumably the firm from which he bought the book.

November and early December 1903 passed quickly. In between attending a talk on 13 November at the Anglo-Saxon Club honouring the Scout Movement founder Robert Baden-Powell (where Hocken was asked to speak), last-minute enquiries to John George Lambton, third Earl of Durham, and social calls to Viscount Cobham's residence at Hagley Hall, which resulted in acquiring two unidentified pamphlets, much of Hocken's energy was spent packing for the return trip home.[33] Gladys recorded that on 20 November the packers were in 'to cart away the loads of books father has amassed' and they continued up to 17 December.[34]

Heading Home

The Hockens left for Japan on 18 December on the *Hitachi Maru*. Hocken was still coughing badly, and he spent many days in bed. On 1 January 1904 they were back at Port Said and by 20 January had reached Singapore. The day before, Gladys had performed in a musical interlude on board; Hocken, now out of bed and perhaps reliving his SS *Great Britain* days, was 'Master of Ceremonies'.[35] On 4 February, the day the Japanese declared war on Russia, the family arrived back in Japan, staying at the Oriental Hotel, Kobe. They took quick visits to Kyoto and Osaka and returned to Kobe only to find the *Hitachi Maru* had been requisitioned for war duties. On 12 February they were back at Yokohama. Although this was their base, Hocken did travel to Tokyo, there meeting Homi Shirasawa, a Japanese botanist with expertise in dendrology, the science and study of wooded plants. He was given a copy of Shirasawa's *Iconographie des essences forestières du Japon* (1900) and dutifully recorded its acquisition on the title page. It was at this time that Hocken purchased one of the oldest books in his collection, the folio edition of Arnoldus Montanus's *Atlas Japannensis*, printed in London by Thomas Johnson in 1670. This large work covers subjects such as murder in Japan, Japanese baths, Japanese torture, wines and whaling. Again he recorded its acquisition on the title page: 'T.M. Hocken, Yokohama, March 1904'. He returned to Tokyo and the university on 23 March and according to Gladys 'enjoyed his time' there.[36]

By 1 April they had left Japan on the *Kosai Maru* and headed to Hong Kong, which they reached on 6 April. On 1 May, having travelled via Celebes, Timor, Darwin, Thursday Island, Cairns and Brisbane, they were back in Sydney. While Bessie and Gladys went on to Melbourne, Hocken stayed in Sydney 'hunting up the life of the Rev. Samuel Marsden'.[37] He finally met Frank M. Bladen, editor of the *Historical Records of New South Wales*, with whom he had corresponded back in 1896.[38] On 6 May Bladen presented Hocken with Volume VII of the *Historical Records*, the final book in the long series. Hocken was in Melbourne by 20 May, where he bought a Blüthner baby grand piano for Gladys, the shipment costing him £100. He then visited the University of Melbourne and called on old friends before travelling to Adelaide on 2 June. The visit to South Australia was prompted by an invitation from Chief Justice Sir Samuel Way, whom Hocken had first met back in 1901. Way not only relied on Hocken to secure him copies of the *Journal of the Polynesian Society*, but no doubt saw their bookish exchanges as a relief from busy judicial matters.[39] Way also gifted books to Hocken, including J.G. Reuther and the Rev. Carl Strehlow's *Testamenta Marra: Jesuni Christuni Ngantjani Jaura Ninaia Karitjimalkana Wonti Dieri Jaurani* (1897), the first translation of the New Testament into Diyari (an Aboriginal language), and *Galtjindamgamea-Pepa: Aranda – Wolambarinjaka* (1904), a translation into Aranda dialect of biblical selections, hymns, prayers and the Catechism of the Lutheran Churches.[40]

By 14 June the family were in Melbourne and by 23 June they were on the *Victoria*, heading to Hobart. On 28 June the Hockens visited the Rev. George Clarke, who, according to Gladys, was 'the oldest clergyman in Tasmania'.[41] Clarke gave Hocken a large number of pamphlets, including the second edition of the complete Anglican Book of Prayer in Maori, which once belonged to William Williams. Hocken recorded the presentation on its endpapers: 'T.M. Hocken from the Rev. George Clarke of Hobart, July 12 1904', with an additional note: 'This was one of the special presentation copies given to his friends by the Rev. (afterwards Bishop) William Williams on the final completion of the Maori Prayer Book in the translation of which Mr Williams had much to do ...'[42] In Tasmania Hocken was pushed somewhat reluctantly into talking to members of the local branch of the Royal Society.[43] Originally just a few remarks on the Forestry Department of Japan, his talk on 11 July expanded to 'Japan. Its People and Its Industries'.[44]

Back in Dunedin

On 16 July the Hockens left on the *Warimoo* and arrived in Bluff on 19 July. The next day they were back in Dunedin, where they were met by Harry, Janie and Hazel Buckland and Molly Neill.[45] Because Stanley Batchelor was still living at Atahapara, the Hockens took rooms at the Grand Hotel where, according to Gladys, 'the whole of Dunedin seemed to empty itself into this drawing room, the telephone was going all day, letters and telegrams poured in, newspaper reporters and custom officials hovered in the halls and passages. Father's progress up the streets resembled a triumphal procession. He was stopped every few feet of the way whenever he went in fact we have only seen him at meals since our return.'[46]

In late July 1904 Hocken gave an interview titled 'A three years' tour' to a reporter from the *Otago Witness*. In this he repeated his sentiments on the Japanese, who were 'most industrious, hospitable, and polite, and essentially patriotic, with a most ardent love for their country'.[47] In short, he was delighted with his stay there. As an admirable educator, he also offered to write more about Japan, giving greater particulars. This he never did.

Perhaps the most tangible reminders of Hocken's interest in Japan are the books that he acquired. In Trimble's catalogue there are 39 titles listed under the heading 'Japan'. There is the usual stock of English–Japanese dictionaries and grammars, which Hocken – or, perhaps more arguably, Bessie – would have used to gain some rudimentary language skills. There are the *Transactions of the Japan Society*, which he received as a society member, and also the Asiatic Society *Bulletins*, many from the Rev. Arthur Lloyd, a missionary and scholar who lived in Tokyo and whom Hocken had met there. In February 1905 Lloyd sent Hocken a privately produced copy of *Imperial Songs*, a translation of songs written by the Emperor and Empress of Japan. Lloyd wrote of this work: 'It is in truth a unique book, for never before have an Emperor or Empress of Japan vouchsafed to appear in a foreign literary garb.' Lloyd appealed to Hocken: 'I wonder if you could find me a few customers.'[48] There is also an entry simply titled 'Japanese books (17)', which remain unidentified.

Hocken's visit to the University of Tokyo also meant obtaining various university calendars and, because of his contacts there, works on archaeology, anthropology, forestation and botany feature. Owing to his interest in fire-walking, he had F. Arthur Jackson's Polynesian Society article on *Fire-walking in Fiji, Japan, India and Mauritius* (1899). He also owned Captain Matthew Perry's multi-volume *Narrative of the Expedition of an American Squadron to the China Seas and Japan* (1856); this is a seminal work. He also had an address to 'His Excellency Admiral Heihachiro Togo, Commander in Chief of His Imperial Majesty's Combined Naval Squadron' created in celebration of the victory of the Battle of Tsushima, fought on 27–28 May 1905. This, the last and most decisive sea battle of the Russo–Japanese War, signalled the eventual Treaty of Portsmouth, signed on 5 September 1905.[49] This particular item accompanies a photograph of a rather ornate silver casket with an image depicting a Maori whare, war canoe and warriors. Hocken's name is first listed on the address, along with 23 other signatories, including James Allen, George Fenwick, David Theomin and Frederic Truby King. The cover depicts an image of the rising sun.

On 30 November 1904 Hocken reconnected with his northern friend John Webster. 'After a long & most pleasant holiday of 3 years we have returned home, & once more I am amongst my favourite books & studies. I brought back with me a very great deal of interesting historical matter.' Somewhat morbidly, he closed the letter with: 'When our knowledge of things is getting so mature & valuable, & our own curiosity to see the continued development of scientific & other research so excited then we are extinguished.'[50]

17
'Marsden or Some Other Old Historical Subject'

In an interview with the *Otago Daily Times* in July 1904 Hocken gave details of his visits to Japan, Greece (Athens – 'very handsome'), Italy ('seeing Pisa … Vesuvius and Pompeii was not neglected'), Egypt, France ('gratified to see in the Salon pictures by Miss Hodgkins and Miss [Grace] Joel'), Switzerland and England, which included his foraging successes in the British Museum, the Public Record Office and the Church Missionary Society.[1] He made particular note of the letters and journals of Marsden and documents relating to the first missionaries. As news of his success spread, 87-year-old John Logan Campbell heard of Hocken's triumph through a number of telegrams. On 11 October the 'Father of Auckland' wrote saying that he had already dispatched a copy of his *The History of Maungakiekie* and another pamphlet that could be added to Hocken's 'already marvellous collection'.[2] About the same time Bishop William Leonard Williams had also heard of Hocken's 'successful raid' at the CMS in London. Acknowledging the 'successful haul of interesting manuscripts', Williams was somewhat bemused: 'I shall be curious to know how you managed it.' He added: 'It would indeed afford me great pleasure if I were able to pay you a visit, as you kindly suggest, for the purpose of inspecting your treasures …'[3]

North Again, 1905

Not one to let things rust, Hocken was soon off on another journey. He left Dunedin on 1 February 1905, and his trip to Auckland via Lyttelton, Wellington and New Plymouth took only 50 hours. Noticing 'everywhere signs of great progress', he remarked: 'What a difference in travel from my first visits to Auckland which took about 6 days!' He was, however, less than impressed with the Northern Club, which seemed to have 'entered on bad times.'[4] There were the usual social engagements. He called on Cheeseman at the Auckland Institute and Museum and was clearly struck by the new Maori exhibits, especially the whare from Taheke, Rotorua, which he had first seen when visiting the Hot Lakes in 1875. He considered the £100 that the museum paid for it a bargain. He also called on Edward Shillington at the Grey Collection in the Auckland Public Library.

By 7 February Hocken was in the Bay of Islands, where he thought the town of Russell was 'showing more signs of decay' and was 'sadly depressed and forlorn.' He met important locals and revisited old haunts. On 14 February Hocken and his friend Archdeacon Philip Walsh travelled to Mangonui (Doubtless Bay, or Lauriston) where they called on Thomas Trimnell, who had married Mary Serena Puckey, daughter of William Gilbert Puckey, a fluent Maori speaker and one of the best interpreters in the Far North. Emanating from their discussion was the fact that W.G. Puckey had translated John Bunyan's *Pilgrim's Progress* before H.T. Kemp's printed translation of 1854. Hocken also recorded that Puckey's version of 1836 was never published because Colenso got his hands on it and when asked for it was unable to find it.[5] Back at Russell he arranged for a boat to survey those places associated with Marsden and the early missionaries.

In Paihia, as in Russell, 'the glory ... has departed'. The old mission house had been pulled down and altered, and the promenade along the beach was reduced in width to make space for houses. The desecration had been through the orders of the Rev. Robert Burrows, remembered locally as 'Bob the Smasher' and whom Hocken termed 'an iconoclast'.

By 18 February he was at Waimate, where he stayed at the home of the Rev. George Clarke, which was then under the care of Clarke's daughter Sarah. While there, he would have certainly discussed meeting her brother in Hobart. She gave Hocken a number of historical letters belonging to her father which, even though they remain unidentified, added to the store of Clarke materials that he had secured from the CMS in London. He and Walsh then visited Okaihau and Ohae. The trenches were still visible at the old pa at Okaihau, and Hocken noted the dilapidated state of the church and the pa at Ohae; ferns were growing everywhere. It was 'most desolate' and 'going to dregs'. He also noted the further effects of time as he travelled the 35 km from Ohaeawai to Horeke. His somewhat despondent mood ended at Opiriri, where he arrived on 22 February to a 'warm welcome' at Webster's home.

One person he missed seeing was Robert Mair, son of Gilbert Mair. Hocken made amends by sending the younger Mair a copy of his work on Tasman as well as his paper on New Zealand newspapers. Mair's prompt reply must have struck Hocken with full force, for here was one who was steeped in New Zealand's early history. Although he had been only seven or eight at the time, Mair recalled seeing a stooped Marsden on his last visit to New Zealand, declined knowing about Darwin's visit in the *Beagle*, remembered seeing various ships such as the *Porpoise*, the *Terra* and *Erebus* and spoke of seeing Sir James Ross and Sir Joseph Hooker and of meeting Lady Franklin (who fell from her horse and had to be carried in a 'kauhoa' or Maori litter).[6]

When he got home Hocken gave an interview about his 'ramble in search of history', which appeared in the *Otago Witness* on 5 April 1905.[7]

Samuel Marsden

As early as the 1880s Hocken had begun his search for materials concerning the Rev. Samuel Marsden. Endless letter writing, persistence and good luck meant that he had amassed a strong collection about the 'great man', despite lapses brought about by the realities of his professional work, the pressures from other areas of collecting and the lack of availability of such materials, especially in Dunedin. Marsden was to remain a constant within his collecting field and he took every opportunity to follow leads, which often led to further search possibilities. While passing through Australia on his way home from England, he managed to write to some of Marsden's living relatives. For instance, he told Lizzie Betts what he was bringing back with him – '*all* your grandfather's old journals & a large number of his letters & other correspondence' – and sent her the photographs he had had taken of Farsley. 'So now what you must do is to apply to all your relatives & those who have anything of his in the shape of correspondence or manuscript &c & get them to let me have at least the loan of it. There is your cousin the clergyman at Cootamundra; I believe he has much.'[8]

Hocken was interested in Marsden's schooling, and even before leaving for England he had made enquiries at St John's College, Cambridge, in order to verify the missionary's attendance there.[9] While in England, he discovered that Marsden had entered Magdelene College on 24 June 1790 and 'may have migrated later on to St John's', where he took his degree. Hocken eventually found out that Marsden did not attend St John's.[10] Back in Dunedin, Hocken wrote to James Edwin Forty, headmaster at Hull Grammar, about Marsden's attendance at the school. Forty reported that all the registers and records of endowments were lost, and redirected Hocken's query to a local antiquarian called W.G.B. Page.[11] A man cut from the same cloth as Hocken, the enthusiastic Page sent five 'carefully copied' letters written between Marsden and William Wilberforce (another Hullarian) and extracts from Wilberforce's *Life*. With typical thoroughness, Hocken wrote to the editor of the well-known antiquarian journal *Notes & Queries*, asking for information about a portrait of Marsden. This query appeared in the issue of 19 May 1906.[12] Page not only offered to be a go-between, posting Hocken any replies, but was also prepared to sell a spare copy of a portrait of Marsden for 3s 6d, supply a photograph of Wilberforce and copy out extracts pertinent to Marsden from the *Christian Observer*.

In the chase for a print or photograph copy of Marsden, Hocken also contacted S. Woolly, who, through long-distance promptings, wrote to Bishop Samuel Edward Marsden, a grandson of Marsden.[13] The exchange brought its own reward: on 17 May 1906 the bishop wrote directly to Hocken on the understanding that 'you are kindly collecting material for a further account of my grandfather "The Apostle of NZ"'.[14] A later letter brought good news: a photograph was in the next mail.[15]

Bishop Marsden's passing comment verified what was known in local circles: the interview printed in the *Otago Daily Times* shortly after his arrival home noted: 'Dr Hocken intends to fully edit and publish these documents that have come into his possession.'[16] The goal was various articles on Marsden and his contemporaries and, more importantly, a biography of the man.

First, however, he had to make sense of what he owned, which, as he wrote to Cheeseman, was not easy: 'I am working away at Marsden very diligently, but the labour is great due to the mass of material.'[17] Giving lectures was one old familiar stand-by that gave him the opportunity to talk about his successful raid at the CMS, announce his Marsden project and marshal the material into a coherent format. During 1905 and 1906 he gave five lectures on Marsden and the early New Zealand mission. As usual, in the first lecture – given on 17 October and printed in the *Otago Daily Times* on Christmas Day 1905 – he enhanced his talk by laying 'the vast mass of material' before his listeners, 'most of which is entirely new and some of which extends back a century or more, and is full of interesting history, as may readily be conceived'. While enthusing his audience, he publicly thanked the CMS for their generosity in allowing these 'entombed journals and letters' to speak again. Through him these 'dilapidated' manuscripts – 'many of them were all but illegible from the ravages of time, faded ink, poor writing requiring the decipherment of an expert' – were to have 'a new dress, and to show how full they are of life and interest'. He also described the other Marsden materials obtained from Australia the previous year: 'They had been crumpled and thrust into an old corn-sack, a bottle of red ink having been then broken over them, and were then thrown into a coal or wood house, where hens, mice, spiders, and fungus abounded.' Here his preservation skills came to the fore: he had ironed them back into a reasonable condition.[18] In talking about his planned book, which was to be a 'Life' plus 'Journals', he looked to Frank M. Bladen's 'invaluable' *Historical Records of New South Wales* (1893) as a model.[19] It was to have a chronological approach, and he hoped that the government would assist with publication.[20]

He delivered the next four lectures on Marsden in quick succession; each was published in the *Otago Daily Times* and the *Otago Witness* by the end of January 1906.[21] The manuscripts needed much work; apart from deciphering the variant copies and their transcriptions, he made copious notes on place names, individuals, dates and events. Sheets containing this information are randomly dispersed throughout his collection.[22] Some are ephemeral, others a little more substantial, often carrying additional notes that helped Hocken formulate a fuller picture of his hero.

Hocken also renewed contact with Percy Smith, who, aside from his wide-ranging ethnographic and anthropological interests, also held his own on matters pertaining to Marsden. In replying promptly on 15 June 1906 to a query about the word 'Whetima' from Smith, Hocken said that this question had provided a break from bigger projects: 'I am working every day at Marsden or some other old historical subject.' There was progress, however, because he informed Smith that 'all but one of Marsden's journals are in type.' And because it was unlikely that Smith would visit Dunedin, Hocken contemplated another pilgrimage, a repeat of that accomplished in 1905: 'Next year we *must* take that trip which covers Marsden's footsteps in the Kaipara District.'[23]

On 5 December 1906 Smith informed Hocken that a pamphlet on Taranaki was on its way because 'I know you like to collect such things.' Smith also elaborated further on his plans for the proposed Marsden pilgrimage:

> I should like to leave it till – say, March, when it is not quite so warm in the north, for I am getting old, & very soon knock up. How would it do to see the few places about Auckland associated with him – such as 'Magoia' (Mokoia) at Panmure, then go up the Waitemata by steamer then to Kaipara & up the Wairoa – and across to Whangarei, which was his route, then to Kawakawa & Hokianga &c. It would be perhaps too far to go up the Thames, though it can be done quite easily now by train & on to Waihi, the goldfields, where his track launched off to Whangamata, or rather KatiKati.[24]

Hocken did go north the following year, but not with Smith. His travelling companion was his Dunedin colleague, Daniel Colquhoun. There was an attempt in 1907, but April, for Smith, was 'too late for our journey. The very heavy northern rains we have had for the last 3 weeks will have made the northern roads very bad.'[25] In another note that same year Smith wrote: 'I constantly think of our northern trip, but if it will suit you, let us leave it till March. I suffer from tender feet in this hot weather so much, that I could not at present do any walking.'[25]

As an interim measure, the now New Plymouth-based Smith offered his services to Hocken to establish the correctness of the Maori place names and individuals mentioned in Marsden's journals. Such assistance was invaluable. He also offered to facilitate the completion of a map showing those places associated with Marsden, maintaining that it 'should not be on too large a scale, otherwise they invariably rip.'[27] Hocken supplied a typescript of the original voyages for Smith's use, taking them to New Plymouth when he visited in March 1908. Some proof of their work together exists in the form of a sheet headed 'Answers to notes made when Hocken & I went through Marsden's journals', where a definite thoroughness is evident.[28] Hocken left the typescripts with Smith to complete the task, but by 6 August they were requested back. Smith replied: 'I have been keeping Marsden too long' and sent them promptly.

New Zealand's population was relatively small in the early 1900s and it was not surprising that individuals undertaking research in similar fields knew each other, corresponded and generally supported like-minded endeavours. An August 1907 letter from Bishop Williams was but one example, directed first to Smith and then passed to Hocken:

> I hear from my son Herbert that Dr Hocken is getting help from you in the matter of Maori names for his life of the Rev. S. Marsden. There is one name which is not easily deciphered from Mr. Marsden's spelling. That

is the name of the chief from whom he bought the site of the Mission station at Oihi (or Horshee, as Marsden gives it). He calls the chief 'Shodee o Gunna.' His name I am told was Te Uri-o-kana. I may mention also that Hongi's pa at Waimate which Marsden and Nicholas visited, and which Nicholas describes in his book, is called Okuratope. Mr John Clark took me to it some years ago. The earthworks were still standing though quite overgrown with brushwood. It is much nearer Waimate than Pukenui, and not very far from the house in which Miss Clarke lives.[29]

Smith, realising the importance of this information, spurred Hocken into action: 'The Bishop's note clears up two of Marsden's names about which there was much doubt. I would suggest you put in these names at once so they be not overlooked.'[30]

On 10 September 1908 a frustrated Hocken informed Smith that his efforts to get the maps produced by the Government Printing Office for his Marsden book had stalled. Even though he considered writing to Robert McNab, the minister responsible, his thoughts were that it was 'useless to ask them to print' the book, given his own experience of their staggered printing schedules, especially when parliament was sitting. He mentioned Whitcombe & Tombs as an alternative and asked Smith: 'Have you any idea as to what it would cost to get W & T to lithograph it?'[31] A note by Smith written three days earlier and crossing Hocken's letter revealed that there was a general impression that the government was going to print the Marsden book, even though McNab knew nothing about it. Smith was his buoyant self: 'I expect, however, they would make no difficulty about printing the map.'[32] Hocken finally received a map, but it was accompanied by Smith's criticism that it was far too detailed and that the 'proper thing would be to have had a map for each journey'. No doubt with costs in mind, Smith added, 'But that is out of the question.'[33]

Over this period, one project took much of Hocken's time. This was his *Bibliography*, which by 10 June 1909 was off his hands. As he told Smith: 'I must now settle down to Marsden for which I will be thankful.' He also told of a recent acquisition and the potential for more:

> Archdeacon Walsh spent a week with me on his way to Melbourne & we had a most delightful time together. I had a letter from him a few days ago enclosing some very old letters from Marsden given by Mrs King of Melbourne who is going to send me I hope a considerable collection of historical papers which belonged to her relative Governor King. This is a great find.[34]

Smith in fact knew about Walsh's visit: 'I heard from Arch. Walsh a few days ago from Melbourne in which he mentions the pleasant time he had with you.'[35] On 23 July 1909 Hocken wrote to Smith fulfilling a request about the 'discovery' of the Manukau, where Smith was still deciding who was first: Dumont d'Urville or Marsden. Hocken transcribed the information from the journals he owned, adding that the long account did 'not occur in the printed report of the "Missionary Register"'. The transcription led to an open declaration by Hocken: 'What a courageous, observant traveller he was!', a man who rejuvenated his efforts 'to get on with his life'.[36] Smith was enthusiastic about Hocken's efforts:

> Very many thanks for your note of the 23rd and the quick response to my request for an extract from Marsden's Journal, which is just what I wanted. I have quoted it word for word, and whilst depriving the distinguished Frenchman of the honour of the discovery of Manukau, have expressed my belief that he could not have been aware of Marsden's prior visit for he was the last man to deprive another of credit that was his.[37]

Six days later, on 3 August, Hocken reported to Smith that he had completed the full annotation of Marsden's third voyage and promised himself to finish 'them all by Sunday next' – and then get on to the 'Life' proper. He was, however, flummoxed by a few things and relied on Smith again for clarification: 'I am going through his routes with the map you marked for me for publication, but I find a very large number of the names of places and rivers not mentioned.' Hocken also sent through a copy of the map drawn by Tuki Tahua and Ngahuruhuru at Norfolk Island in 1793 for Smith to annotate and W.H. Skinner's 'drawing which he so kindly lent me & which my wife has most faithfully copied in Indian ink which I thought a superior mode of reproduction to pencil which so soon rubs out. Perhaps you will give it to Skinner to whom I am writing by this mail.'[38]

Smith's reply on 9 August 1909 offered Hocken an answer to the puzzle: 'About Marsden's mention of Mercury Bay & his supposed visit there. I am quite clear that he went to Katikati; not Mercury Bay. It was impossible he could have reached the latter place in time.'[39] Sadly, time was against Hocken. On 27 August 1909 he thanked Smith for the annotated map, which he had had framed. He also apologised for his tardy response: 'I should have written before but have been & indeed am so unwell as to prevent my doing much work or indeed taking an interest in anything.'[40] This was Hocken's last letter to Smith.

Hocken was a busy and productive collector, and it was natural that some undertakings were not finished. He did not complete his Marsden project although by all accounts much was done, especially the transcribing of most of the journals. His intention was certainly clear – he listed the 'Life and Journals of the Rev. Samuel Marsden' in his *Bibliography* under 'In Preparation'[41] – and his failure to complete it was an obvious disappointment. As Bessie wrote in 1910: 'He retained his mental faculties up to the last, giving instructions about everything connected with his books, & it was a source of great trouble to him that his life of Marsden should be unfinished & unpublished.'[42] After Hocken's death Bessie (and George Fenwick) endeavoured to advance the publication, advertising it under Hocken's name in the posthumous *Early History of New Zealand* (1914): '"The Life and Journals of the Rev. Samuel Marsden, Principal Chaplain of New South Wales, with Special Relation to the Mission at New Zealand" – Not published'. They also approached Canon Robert Woodthorpe of Selwyn College, Dunedin, to complete the task 'at his leisure'.[43] Unfortunately it was only in the 1930s, when John Rawson Elder took up the mantle, that publication was achieved. In the preface to *The Letters and Journals of Samuel Marsden*, Elder praised Hocken's efforts: 'No-one surpassed the late Dr Hocken of Dunedin, New Zealand, in his enthusiasm for Marsden and his work.' On completing his own book, Elder further acknowledged the debt to Hocken for his thoroughness in collecting: 'Almost every manuscript, newspaper, pamphlet, and printed book to which reference has been made in this volume is to be found in the Hocken Library …'[44] In this Hocken's dream was finally realised.

18
The Pinnacle

By 1887 Hocken had completed his draft 'Catalogue of books, pamphlets, maps, newspapers, prints, &c relating to New Zealand. In the Library of Dr T.M. Hocken of Dunedin, N.Z', and the following year he was proud enough to lend it to Walter Mantell in Wellington for perusal.[1] And just before exhibiting it as a supplement to his curio, book and map collections at the New Zealand and South Seas Exhibition of 1889–90, he showed the manuscript to shipowner and future Antarctic enthusiast Joseph Kinsey, who was visiting Dunedin from Christchurch. Not only was Kinsey struck with Hocken's physical book collection, but he made special mention of the 'catalogue' in an interview published in the *Star* on 7 October 1889.[2]

Hocken's first 'bibliographical' catalogue contains 1107 entries. Arranged chronologically, they carry very little descriptive matter apart from author, title, place and date of publication and format. Although the descriptions are sparse, the list represents an impressive array of books and manuscripts that Hocken had accumulated since the early 1860s. By 1887 it was no mere incidental gathering of books and papers but a collection that gave him an excellent base for his future work in the field of bibliography.

As bookman John Carter has observed, 'Probably few collectors are so methodical as to put themselves through any formal education for what is, after all, a fairly sophisticated pursuit. Few, on the other hand, even of the most happy-go-lucky, have not discovered at some point in their career the advantage they have gained from some sort of informal education, and perhaps wished they had had more of it earlier.'[3] Hocken did not have any formal bibliographical instruction and he would have no doubt discussed the intricacies of books and book collecting with fellow collectors Grey, Turnbull and Frederick Chapman, who were themselves self-schooled. His training in medicine certainly instilled method and the need for accuracy and documentation. And he read. As he embarked on his own slow and gradual bibliographical endeavours, which meant a move from mere listing to a more serious and scholarly undertaking, he looked to those local models on which he could base his work.

Predecessors in New Zealand

First, there was James Davidson Davis's posthumous *Contributions towards a Bibliography of New Zealand*, published in 1887. This was the first systematic attempt at recording printed materials concerning New Zealand, albeit with Davis's own acknowledgement of omissions – 'tons of Parliamentary Papers' and books published in Maori. It covered some 696 items, including pamphlets, books and a wide number of newspapers with their various issues, and was, according to him, 'the results of many months researches in Libraries, Catalogues, book-stalls, old books and newspapers'.[4] Arranged chronologically, it began with the 1739 two-volume French edition of Carl Friedrich Behrens's *Histoire de l'expédition de trois vaisseaux envoyés par la Compagnie des Indes Occidentales des Provinces Unies aux Terres Australes en MDCCXXI*. The entries in most cases were perfunctory, with simple title, author, place of publication and year, publisher (or printer) and bare essential format details. Davis's entry on Tasman's *Journal* made specific reference to the portion Hocken acquired in England in 1882, describing it as 'quite clean and fresh looking'. This suggests that the two men met not long afterwards, most likely in Dunedin. They certainly corresponded, as Davis acknowledged in his *Bibliography*: 'I am indebted to kind friends in all parts of the Colony, and particularly to Dr. Hocken, of Dunedin, who has courteously responded to each of my enquiries with that fullness of knowledge which places him above all other students of New Zealand history and literature.'

Davis's work was an important pioneering effort, but there were two other small debts to pay. The first was to Arthur Thomson's useful enumeration of 413 books, pamphlets, parliamentary papers, magazines and newspaper articles in the second volume of *The Story of New Zealand* (1859). The other was to the ground-breaking work of Sir George Grey and Wilhelm Bleek in *The Library of His Excellency Sir George Grey, K.C.B. Philology. Vol. II. Part IV New Zealand, the Chatham Islands and the Auckland Islands*, which was printed in Cape Town in 1859. Hocken owned both Thomson's *Story of New Zealand* and the Grey–Bleek catalogue.

No less interesting were the compilations by Edward Augustus Petherick and Charles Rooking Carter. Petherick was born to list. He 'collected, arranged and catalogued' some 600 items in the *Catalogue of a Collection of Books Illustrative of Discovery and Colonisation in Australasia. Now in the Possession of M. Larkin, J.P., South Melbourne* (1890), which Hocken acquired in 1891 from James Miller, a rope, twine and mat manufacturer in Melbourne.[5] Petherick also compiled two Francis Edwards catalogues (1898–99), started the quarterly *Colonial Book Circular and Bibliographical Record* (later the *Torch*) between 1887 and 1890, and published his *Library Presented to the Federated Colonies of Australia* in 1896, which described and summarised his 6500 books and pamphlets.[6] More important was Petherick's compilation of S.W. Silver's *Catalogue of the York Gate Geographical and Colonial Library* (1882) and the much larger *Catalogue of the York Gate Library Formed by S. William Silver* (1886), both of which Hocken owned.[7] Hocken made crosses and pencil marks against titles listed in the section of New Zealand-related items in the first volume. Both York Gate editions remain important bibliographical publications.

Carter was a Wellington builder, surveyor, politician and author, whose name is perpetuated in the Wairarapa town of Carterton (once 'Carterville') and the Carter Observatory in Wellington.[8] Over a six-year period he produced three catalogues that revealed not only the gradual growth in his collection but also the persistent disease of bibliomania. His first *Catalogue of Books on or Relating to New Zealand* (1887) listed 365 works (a total of 527 volumes) owned.[9] Although all the entries were brief, Carter did offer some interesting bibliographical information. For example, his entry on Dumont d'Urville's *Voyage autour du monde de la corvette l'*Astrolabe (1826–29) read: 'No library of New Zealand books can be said to be complete without this work. The second and third volumes are entirely devoted to New Zealand. Complete and clean copies are very scarce. After waiting a long time, I had to procure my copy through an agent in Paris. It is to be regretted that this work has not been translated into English.'[10] And of Robert FitzRoy's *Voyages of the* Adventure *and* Beagle (4 vols, 1839), he wrote: 'This work is one of the 100 volumes recommended by Sir John Lubbock as the best set of books for studious young men to read. It is getting scarce and dear. I was considered fortunate to get a copy for £5.'[11]

While in London in 1890 Carter amassed another 148 books that he detailed in his *Continuation Catalogue of Books Presented by C.R. Carter J.P., to the Wellington Museum and Colonial Institute, in the Year 1892* (1892). The format was exactly the same as the first catalogue: an alphabetical arrangement with occasional description. The *Second Continuation Catalogue of Books* followed in 1893, with some 242 works including newspapers, pamphlets and New Zealand Company books and papers listed. This catalogue carried a description of the book collector, with which Hocken would surely have agreed:

> But to return to book-collecting, I may say, that, after all, the life of a book-collector is not without its pleasures. It is true he has his sorrows and disappointments in mildly encountering and contending with rival book-collectors, and the crooked ways, and, in some cases, discreditable practices, of various dealers in the second-hand book-trade, and, also, at sometimes not finding what he is in search of; but he also has his joys and successes in, at last, obtaining the books he has long sought after; besides, I am happy to say, he has his compensations in leaving behind him literary treasures from which future generations may reap the full benefit.[12]

In the preface to his 1892 *Continuation Catalogue*, Carter proclaimed: 'My book collecting days are over.'[13] In the 1893 catalogue he retracted this statement: 'Perhaps my readers will now pardon me for saying, this is incorrect, for, I have been tempted with offers of "rare books" and could not resist buying them.' He continued: 'From this incident I am free to admit that there is a certain amount of fascination in searching for and purchasing rare books; which, when once commenced, is extremely difficult to discontinue.'[14] Sir George Grey, New Zealand's first collector, who understood the dilemma faced by those caught up in the world of books, had written to Carter: 'I thank you very much for your valuable Catalogue; but you have made an extraordinary mistake. You state – "I have now but to say that my book collecting days are over, and my work in this line is done." Alas, you do not know yourself, you will soon be at it again.'[15]

Hocken and Carter eventually met and corresponded briefly. They also exchanged material: Hocken gave Carter duplicate copies of the *New Zealand Journal* and the *Otago Journal*, while Carter presented Hocken with the three catalogues suitably marked: 'Dr Hockin [sic], Dunedin, New Zealand. With the author's kind regards, 1894'. Hocken also received from Carter information on Jerningham Wakefield's distressing later career – he was arrested for stealing flowers – and the duel between fellow Masons Isaac Featherston and William Wakefield.[16] Hocken used Carter's catalogues: there are pencil strokes against 296 entries in the first and a similar number throughout the other two volumes.[17]

The Australians

There was also an Australian contingent of collectors. In 1866 George Burnett Barton, lawyer, journalist and lecturer, compiled his *Literature of New South Wales* and *Poets and Prose Writers of New South Wales*, the first volumes of a bibliographical and critical character to be published in Australia. There is no evidence of use in Hocken's copy, but he surely noted Barton's words on the difficulties inherent in compiling a bibliography: 'It has not proved an easy matter to procure the necessary material ... Every one knows how rapidly these things are apt to disappear. Newspapers and magazines are thrown aside as soon as they are read. Books too often share the same fate.' Barton also recognised the intellectual component inherent in bibliographies, especially 'determining what works come within the limits of our literature'.[18]

Another compiler was Henry Field Gurner (1819–1883), Crown solicitor in Melbourne, who owned a large and valuable collection of books on the colonies and produced in 1878 his *Books on the Colonies and Colonial Publications*. Hocken did not own a copy, but he may have spied Grey's copy while on Kawau. He did, however, own Gurner's *Chronicle of Port Phillip* (1876).[19]

There was also the Hobart-based James Backhouse Walker, who in 1884 compiled an 11-page publication on books relating to Tasmania and sent it to Hocken in May 1889. By the time the gift arrived, Hocken was well into compiling his own 'bibliography'. Competition can be healthy, and Walker's sentiments perhaps gave Hocken impetus:

> I am glad to comply with your request, and send you a copy of my list of Tasmanian books. It was compiled for a History of Tasmania published here a year or two ago. You will see at a glance that it does not profess to completeness, but I hope some day to be able to produce a more respectable Bibliography of our island ... It will give me great pleasure to hear from you at any time you feel inclined to write, especially on subjects connected with Australian or New Zealand bibliography or history.[20]

There were also the library catalogues that Hocken amassed, ranging from the *Catalogue of the Zoological Library* in London (1887), the *Public Library of Victoria Catalogue* (1880) and the General Assembly Library of New Zealand catalogues (1885, 1897, supplement 1899) to the Auckland Public Library's catalogue (which included the Grey material), the Church of Otago Library catalogue (1861) and the Royal Society of Tasmania Library catalogue (1885).[21] Hocken also kept a few dealer catalogues such as *Books and Pamphlets relating to New Zealand* (1840), E. Dufossé's *Catalogues of Books for Sale* (c. 1894), and *Catalogue of Old, Rare and Curious Books* (Melbourne, 1906), but unfortunately those that he must have seen and read, such as from Sotheby's and Quaritch, have long since disappeared. The almost entire lack of these ephemeral publications in Hocken's collection is one marked difference from the Grey or Turnbull collections, where catalogues do exist to offer tangible evidence of when, and from whom, purchases were made.

All these book publications offered Hocken a full range of formats, descriptions and methods by which he could devise his own work – and documented the growing number of titles about New Zealand that he could include. Owning a copy of Charles Blackburn's *Hints on Catalogue Titles and on Index Entries* (1884) may have helped him to refine part of the process.

James Collier

On 19 July 1888 Hocken received a letter from Parliamentary Librarian James Collier (1846–1925), accompanied by 19 pamphlets. These were duplicate stock from the Parliamentary Library, which Hocken himself had selected when he was last in Wellington. The gift was conditional, however, as Collier wrote: 'You were kind enough to offer in exchange certain nos. lacking to the Library, of the Canterbury Papers, the New Zealand Cos. Reports, or the *Otago Journal*.'[22] Hocken no doubt honoured this obligation.

Hocken had already encountered the Scots-born student of classics and mathematics whose major claim to fame was his association with Herbert Spencer, the nineteenth-century English philosopher and author of *Descriptive Sociology*.[23] They first met in Wellington in 1885, the year Collier took up his post at the Parliamentary Library. By then both men had started their personal projects to document the printed literature on and about New Zealand. Hocken recalled the occasion in a 1906 letter: 'Learning some years ago that Mr Collier, the government librarian, was preparing a Bibliography of N.Z. Literature I called upon him during a visit to Wellington & explained to him what I had already done in the matter.'[24] And plans took shape, as Hocken described: '[Collier] was greatly pleased & suggested that we might carry out the work conjointly – he doing the pamphlets & I the books. To this I readily assented & with this view he visited Dunedin to inspect my work & make final conclusions.'[25] Collier called on Hocken sometime after 30 August 1888 and examined something more than a bare-bones list of books with titles, author and date authority. Indeed, as Hocken recalled, '[Collier] considered my work so extensive & careful that it would be unfair to group it with his own under our joint names, & that it should be issued separately & from this view he did not recede.' Gratified by Collier's judgement, Hocken also 'regretted this extremely for not only did Mr Collier's skill as a librarian far exceed mine, but the appearance of his Bibliography stamped his labours as being far superior to the diffident way in which he apparently estimated them – indeed his book is excellent, & for long I was deterred by this from taking further steps with regard to mine'.[26]

Collier's *The Literature Relating to New Zealand: A Bibliography* (1889) was produced by the government printer. In 175 pages he listed in chronological order some 1200 printed items on or about New Zealand. The first entry dealt with Abel Tasman's voyage to New Zealand in 1642 and, with the 1898 Muller facsimile not available to him, Collier chose an abridged Dutch account that was later translated and printed in James Burney's *Chronological History of the Voyages and Discoveries in the South Sea or Pacific Ocean* (1813). Collier's greater knowledge of languages, especially French and German, gave him access to some of the more obscure European references to New Zealand, such as the German translations of Crozet's *Nouveau voyage à la mer du sud* (1783) and a Weimar printing of J.L. Nicholas's *Narrative of a Voyage to New Zealand* (1817). Collier's introduction was very brief, acknowledging Thomson and Davis and containing a note explaining the use of the asterisk, a symbol that would feature again. After the book entries a classification section followed with an alphabetical section of authors (with dates of titles) followed by anonymous and pseudonymous publications.

Like Hocken, Collier was not an analytical bibliographer. He was not concerned with the book as a physical object: its history, its appearance and the influence of the manner of production on its text.[27] It was enough for him to document the basic detail of a book and, where necessary, extend the description to include contents and an occasional historical or literary flourish. As would be expected, there was a general lessening of description in the later years, when a greater number of publications appeared. Where possible, however, he continued the practice of grounding an item to another, or at least surrounding it with interesting data.

Some titles in Collier's *Bibliography* appeared tangential to New Zealand, for example, Louis Figuier's *The Human Race* (1872) and *Annual Record of Science and Industry for 1873* (1874). Their inclusion not only reflected something of Collier's wide knowledge and scholarship, but also his brave attempt to gather in as much as he could, given the resources and the time.[28] Bibliographies are doomed to be incomplete and very rarely satisfy every reader. Collier did a sterling job in compiling his work, and it remains a very good read. On the face of it, it is no wonder that Hocken deferred his own attempt.

Hocken's own copy of Collier's bibliography is well marked up. Not only does it contain Hocken's usual ownership indicators, but beside almost every entry there is the letter 'G' ('Got'). There are also his emendations to Collier's text. For example, on page 2 in the entry to John Harris's *Navigantium atque Itinerantium Bibliotheca* (1744) Hocken writes: 'This is complete ed. v[ide]. Callander Vol. II p. 355'; on page 3, in relation to Hawkesworth's *An Account of the Voyages* (1773), he corrected the pagination description from 'XIV' to 'XV' and adds 'not pp. 395 but from 411 to 719 in 1st ed.'; and on page 5, with Captain Cook's *A Voyage towards the South Pole* (1777), he is emphatic: 'Wrong. 2nd ed. Published in 1777 also. Has same title as 1st & 3rd & same pagination.' There are many more.

Slow but Steady Progress

Faced with the disappointment of not working with Collier on the bibliography, Hocken kept busy. One activity was his already-mentioned foray into Polynesian bibliography.[29] There were also his 'rambles in search of history' and the lectures he compiled and delivered. Two years after the AAAS conference, Hocken was back in harness. On 18 December 1893 Smith wrote: 'I am so glad to hear you are progressing with the Bibliography – it will be most valuable, and who so well able to do it as yourself? I will ask you to let me see it when I am in Dunedin – about middle of January I expect …'[30] This was the first mention of Hocken embarking on his bibliography again, and it was not the 'Polynesian' one Smith so desired. Three years later Hocken was well into it. In August 1896 he told Cheeseman: 'I have been working hard at what you suggest – or rather more – a bibliographical record (very much more than a mere bibliography) of all books & pamphlets relating to N.Z. … Already it is of great dimensions.' No doubt remembering Collier's enterprise and believing in the inherent importance of the project, Hocken added: 'The Govt. should publish it & I am waiting to see if the place of our present wretched rulers is to be taken by a better class of men who would undertake the publication. If by speaking about it you can aid it – do.'[31]

The compilation of any bibliography requires special skills and attributes. Essential for the task is determination, persistence, a continued focus and accuracy in all things, especially title transcription, capitalisation, punctuation and collation. Fundamental to the above is that the items are actually present (or seen) to verify the information recorded. As the American writer Henry Miller suggested:

> One must be possessed of a certain kind of madness, I feel to compile a bibliography … This is the work not only of a bibliophile but of a sleuth, a proof-reader, a hunter and God knows what else. To collect all the material amassed in this huge tome represents the labor of a prisoner tunneling his way out of jail over a period of months or years. One can only imagine what cunning and ingenuity it required to gather all this information.[32]

Mad or not, Hocken had these attributes and skills, and the drive and ambition to undertake such a project. This was despite other priorities and plans disrupting progress: the journey to England via Japan, the securing of the Marsden materials and the decision to produce the projected 'Journals and Life'. Undertaking one topic of research while dealing with another was a fairly typical approach, however, and Hocken was an excellent juggler.

When passing through Wellington in February 1906 armed with 'some important manuscript' (the bibliography), he called on John Mackay, the government printer, and they discussed printing it. To Hocken's delight, Mackay carried through his promise to raise the matter with acting Prime Minister William Hall-Jones. Not one to miss an opportunity, Hocken wrote to Hall-Jones directly: 'Following [Mackay's] suggestion I desire to lay before you fuller particulars, which I think are of an interesting kind.' He explained that the manuscript had been examined by 'competent persons' such as Augustus Hamilton, Judge Chapman, Percy Smith, Sir Robert Stout and Professor Morris of Melbourne, who had actually hinted that the Victorian government should publish it – 'But of course to this I could not listen.' He then offered Hall-Jones an 'open-door' inspection: 'Of course I should expect & desire that some thoroughly competent person should examine it on behalf of the Government. And it will give me great pleasure on the occasion of your next visit to Dunedin not only to show it to yourself but also other manuscripts & my extensive library which is without doubt the best in the world on N.Z. literature.'[33] Hall-Jones passed his response to Charles Wilson, the relatively new government librarian. It read: 'As Dr Hocken's work appears to be of some value I think it would be as well for the Librarian to see the manuscript. I understand the Doctor would be satisfied with 35 copies for his own use.' Hall-Jones then added the phrase eagerly sought by most authors: 'The cost of printing this work to be bourne [sic] by the Govt.' Colonial secretary Albert Pitt agreed.[34]

Enter the 'competent' Charles Wilson, the first chief librarian of the General Assembly Library. Oxford educated, he was a former editor of the Liberal *New Zealand Mail* and a Liberal MP, a book collector and later author of jaunty books entitled *Rambles in Bookland* (1922) and *New Rambles in Bookland* (1923). As a book enthusiast Wilson responded positively to the proposal: 'I have often heard of Dr Hocken's work, and of his bibliography. If it really merits the encomiums that have been passed upon it, I for one, as Librarian of what is really New Zealand's National Library, would be only too glad to hear that the Government had decided to print and publish it.' After disparaging remarks on the previous bibliographies (Collier – 'very imperfect'; Petherick – 'many good features … but confined'; Edwards – 'merely a trade list'), and somehow forgetting Davis's first attempt, Wilson continued:

> If Dr Hocken has done his work well, he has produced a bibliography, which will be welcomed by librarians all the world over … But I would not like to say, that the work is worth undertaking, unless I saw the

manuscript. I have not yet taken my yearly holiday and if you approve I would be glad to place a portion of it at the disposal of the Department, and personally examine the Manuscript on the spot I could then give a reliable report upon the whole matter. The incidental expenses for travelling, etc., would be comparatively trifling. Such an investigation would also be useful in affording an opportunity of ascertaining particulars of many publications that at present the Library lacks. To show how incomplete is our own Collection, I may mention, that I know of nearly 380 books and pamphlets, which we have not got, and very few of these are included in Collier's bibliography.

With an eye on improving the collection he looked after, Wilson also suggested that he could 'thoroughly inspect Dr Hocken's famous library of New Zealand books'. He continued: 'If ever Dr Hocken's library comes onto the market, I hope it will be secured by the Government, for the General Assembly Library. The Doctor has, I believe, hundreds of items, especially rare pamphlets, which we have not got …'[35]

Wilson finally visited Hocken in Dunedin in early June 1906 and inspected the library and the draft manuscript. Greatly impressed, he reported back to his superiors. His account of Hocken's library is one of the few that survive and offers a brief glimpse of the two bookmen enjoying the very private world of collecting. Significantly, too, Wilson gives a value to Hocken's collection.

Arriving in Dunedin on Monday night June 11 I waited upon Dr Hocken on the following morning and was most courteously received … I spent several hours each day from the Tuesday to the Saturday inclusive, in going through the manuscript, sheet by sheet, and was from the outset greatly impressed with the industry, patience, and perseverance and most scrupulous regard for accuracy which have been displayed by the Doctor. I compared many scores of entries with the originals of the volumes and pamphlets … in the bibliography. As you are doubtless aware, Dr Hocken possesses what is far and away the most comprehensive collection of works dealing with the early history and literature of this colony that is in existence … His library, which at a rough estimate, I would say, is worth at least from £6000 to £8000 (actual value in the open book market) consists of thousands of volumes of books, bound pamphlets, broadsheets and proclamations also valuable charts and illustrations, and has thus afforded the bibliographer opportunities, lacking in so many instances to previous workers … for personally comparing, checking, and correcting his entries by reference to first sources.

With Collier's work close at hand, Wilson commented on the increased number of entries, the additional identification of many pseudonyms and greater voyage details that Hocken had included. Cognisant that a well-written bibliography can be a good and useful read, Wilson claimed: 'Were it merely a dry-as-dust record of all that has been written and printed in or about the Colony of New Zealand there might be some reasonable objection to it being printed at the expense of the state. But it is much more.' This said, he cast his vote: 'The publication of such a record as that to which the Dr has devoted so many years of patient industry and careful research cannot fail ... to be of widespread interest and value. There is nothing like this work in print that in any way approaches it in practical value ...'[36]

Hall-Jones authorised the printing to proceed on 3 August 1906, even though Cabinet had given approval as early as 28 June.[37] Pre-empting these official decisions, Hocken's own networks began working overtime. On 15 June he declared to Smith: 'The Gov't has decided to print my bibliography & with this view sent down the Govt Librarian who yesterday inspected it & was, I am happy to say, loud in his appreciation & praises.'[38] Smith's reply arrived in December: 'I am delighted to hear the Govt is going to print your Bibliography – it is a very proper thing to do – and you are the proper man to do it. I congratulate you heartily on having such a congenial work on hand.'[39]

This did not end the intrusion from Wellington. In early December 1906 John Mackay visited Hocken to make final arrangements for the printing of the *Bibliography*. To facilitate progress, he took back to Wellington the first instalment of the manuscript, leaving Hocken with the other portions to tidy up. At this point, the government's commitment was made public, with notices appearing in various newspapers of the day.[40]

The actual printing and publishing of the bibliography took three years. This was because the Government Printing Office had other responsibilities, such as printing *Hansard*, the Parliamentary Papers, railway tickets, postage stamps and postal notes and statutes.[41] And there was competition: in 1908 the final portion of Robert McNab's *Historical Records of New Zealand* was going through the government presses, with only the index required for completion.

Hocken was keen to see his work appear but obviously underestimated the work involved. Mackay kept Hocken's zealousness in check by informing him it was in the queue for printing and stressed that 'copy is not yet all in the hands of the printer'.[42] This did not stop Hocken from complaining. 'I suppose,' he wrote to Augustus Hamilton, 'when the Session is over the printing of my bibliography will recommence. It is a great nuisance to me having it thus suspended as it interferes with other labours.'[43] Although he must have been aware of his own overcommitment to other projects, he grumbled to Smith: 'I have been seriously handicapped in my work [on Marsden] by the bibliography as the printer sends me down batches for correction &c in the most spasmodic manner & latterly, during the session of the House, nothing has been done further with it. Beside this the Maori section is wholly untouched.'[44]

Additions, Exchanges and Byways

Although Hocken was frustrated by the staggered schedule, the process unwittingly benefitted him. After all, he continued to gather in materials, either by purchase or gift. The new arrivals included a reprint of James Hawthorne's *A Dark Chapter from New Zealand History* (1905) in February 1906; a 10-page manuscript entitled 'Struggles of an early settler in the district around Lake Wakatipu' from Gertrude von Tunzelmann in late March 1906;[45] a copy of *The Unveiling of the Statue of Sir John Logan Campbell at Cornwall Park, 24 May 1906* (1906); and a presentation copy of Edwin Meredith's *Memoir of the Late George Meredith* (1897) sent on 24 July 1906. Other arrivals included the *New Zealand International Exhibition Fine Art Section Official Catalogue* (1906); Stuart Reid's *The Tickler: 100 Caricatures* (c. 1907), which contains a sketch of Hocken and Andrew Carnegie on page 15; a reference catalogue from Whitcombe & Tombs (1907); and Colenso's edition of the *New Testament* (1837, i.e. 1838), from Bishop Williams on 13 February 1907.[46] To register late arrivals, Hocken included an 11-page 'Addenda'.

As all these disparate items tumbled in, Hocken continued to field enquiries and gather more information. Sometimes this meant altering existing entries or creating new ones for previously unrecorded items. As he told Robley: 'I am working hard. incessantly writing at the Bibliography which the Govt is about to publish.'[47] At times his 'incessant literary work' was halted by illness.[48]

In the need to advance the work, Hocken also sent out prompts. On 25 April 1907 while writing to Hamilton, Hocken added: 'By the bye – for the Bibliography – when will your index of the Transactions be ready? I want to insert the notice. If you have a spare copy of your list of the Challenger' references I should be glad to have it. They are printing my Bibliography but sadly slowly I fear, as though I keep them well supplied with copy I get little in turn to correct.'[49] Other letters generated more pathways. James McKerrow, an explorer involved in surveying Otago and Southland, had heard that Hocken was not only writing another book, but desired 'anything I had written of my explorations in Otago which had already appeared in print'.[50] He no longer had any copies left of the account of the expedition but referred Hocken to his 'On the physical geography of the lake district of Otago', a more general paper written for the third volume of the *Transactions of the New Zealand Institute*. He also rewrote the narrative of his reconnaissance surveys during 1862 and 1863. 'If you can find anything in it, or in the printed matter I have referred to suit your purpose I shall be glad.' In March 1908 Hocken was in Wellington, returning home from a trip north devoted to travelling through 'Marsden country'. He gave an interview to an *Evening Post* reporter and was confident enough to claim that his *Bibliography* 'was shortly to be out of the hands of the printers'.[51] He also called on Mackay.

By May that year there was progress. In between dealing with presidential responsibilities of the Otago Institute, Hocken was fine-tuning his entries and, as he told Justice Chapman, had reached page 288.[52] Twenty-three days later he had completed another 62 pages, informing John Webster: 'I am doing a great deal of literary work & my *Bibliography of New Zealand Literature* is advancing to the 350th page. Your new book (*Reminiscences*) will appear in it as one of the last items.'[53] By 10 September Hocken was receiving more proofs, yet still he complained. From a distance, Smith could only offer encouragement: 'I am sorry to hear of the delay in printing the Bibliography – but now that the Session is over the Govt Printer will be able to give it more attention.'[54]

There was even a little pre-production promotion. The editor of the *Poverty Bay Herald* placed a notice of the forthcoming *Bibliography* – described as 'a work of great value to students and future historians' – between advertisements for Chamberlain's Colic, Cholera and Diarrhoea Remedy and Rheumo (a cure for rheumatism). Seven months later, a smaller notice in the same newspaper appeared between an 'Obtain a patent' notice and an advertisement for Phosphol, a cod liver oil mixture that made the body glow.[55]

By 10 June 1909 Hocken had finished the 'Introduction' (dated 1 June 1909) and was putting the final touches to entries and doing the necessary proofing. His prediction to Smith that it would appear within four weeks was very nearly correct.[56] On 16 July 1909 Hocken received the first bound copy for inspection from Mackay. All he had to do was give the word and the rest would follow.[57] Smith, Hocken's 'mid-wife', was one of the first to learn about it: 'Mackay sent me an advance copy of the bibliography & most respectable it looks in a nice brown binding. You will find 11 items of yours inserted & altogether I think you will find the work most useful as well as a monument of labour …' From New Plymouth Smith wrote: 'I am delighted to hear the Bibliography has got into its clothing. If you have a copy to spare, the Polynesian Library would be thankful for a copy – one.'[58]

The Bibliography

A Bibliography of the Literature Relating to New Zealand appeared in late July 1909 in a functional brown buckram cover, with gold-tooled title on the spine and three rectangular blind impressed rules on the back and front covers. Delicate fern engravings formed the pattern of the endpapers. At 632 pages, which included a five-page introduction, corrigenda and omissions and text, this solid, plain book retailed at 10s. The title page listed Hocken's full credentials and a Maori motto: 'He mahi nui rawa atu', which he translated as 'Truly, this is a very laborious deed'. But it had also been enjoyable: 'The end sought will be accomplished if the student derives as much satisfaction and advantage from the use of this bibliography as the author has derived pleasure from its preparation.'[59] He gave credit to work done by Thomson, Davis and

Collier, and to the more specialised (and relatively current) bibliographies by H.R. Mill on the Antarctic and Leonard Cockayne on the outlying islands of New Zealand.

The longest review of this 'indispensable volume' appeared in the *Otago Witness* on 18 August 1909. The anonymous reviewer praised what he called 'this veritable treasure-house of knowledge' and remarked on Hocken's ability to make the book a good read – to put 'muscle, flesh and nerve' into what could normally be a dry-as-dust tome. And, not for the first time, Hocken made history come alive with romance and adventure, which, to the reviewer's mind at least, meant that the 'imagination may brood'. And in order to achieve this, Hocken himself admitted deviations: 'A cursory inspection will show how frequently the author has strayed from the ordinary track of a bibliography. He has introduced many little sidelights, biographical references, dates, and other special points, and an attempt has been made to run throughout a thread of historical interest.' In short, it was not of the scientific bibliographical school. After a number of pertinent entry examples, the reviewer noted deficiencies and omissions.[60] Hocken himself had realised the enormity of the task: 'Whilst every effort has been made to make this record complete, it is probable that many items must have escaped enumeration.' He had also admitted his bias against 'versifiers' (he listed only some 200 poetry titles) and those publications 'of little moment'.[61] Despite these small faults, he was congratulated for producing a book that was 'absolutely indispensable' in 'any decently furnished library', and for contributing to the building blocks of a national character.

The *Evening Post* review three days later was much shorter, and after beginning with the same quote on the 'laborious deed', it proclaimed Hocken's effort 'well done'.[62] He was recognised as a specialist in New Zealand literature and given full credit for the 'painstaking care' of documenting the bibliography of printed Maori.[63] While omissions and a few errors were noted, the anonymous reviewer acknowledged that 'its chief value lies in its extensive, pertinent, and illuminating annotations'.

Four days later a review in the *Taranaki Herald*, again anonymous, began by stating that 'New Zealand has not wanted for historians, both general and local' and then mentioned the remarkable amount of literature produced in the country's short history. After calling up the ghosts of bibliographers past (Thomson, Davis and Collier), the reviewer welcomed Hocken's *Bibliography*, which filled the breach left since Collier's attempt in 1889. Hocken's suitability for the task was also unquestioned: 'There is probably no one in New Zealand better fitted for the work of compiling such a work as that under notice than Dr Hocken, whose literary bent is accompanied by a strong antiquarian spirit.' Omissions in the work were noted – 'it would be wonderful indeed had nothing escaped him' – and a second edition was mooted, a way in which to capture missing titles as well as keeping it up to date. Praise was given to the government printer for producing an excellent volume, with an index compiled by a Miss Castle in Wellington.[64] 'The student of New Zealand literature and history will acknowledge a deep indebtedness to the really wonderful industry and research of Dr Hocken.'[65]

Hocken was happy with the largely positive feedback. On 27 August 1909 he wrote to Smith: 'I have been pleased with the uniformly favourable notices – that is so far as I have seen them. The *Dominion* of Saturday the 14th was especially laudatory.'[66] And he would have enjoyed the review in the Melbourne *Argus*, where his 'most valuable work of reference' was 'much more than a mere catalogue as the notes and references introduced by the author supply a great deal of historical information that could only be obtained elsewhere at the expense of an immense amount of labour'. Not only did the reviewer welcome Hocken's detailing the contents of works by such as Melchisédech (or Melchisédec) Thévenot, Callander, the early French voyagers and Angas, but also the brief summaries of equally rare reports, gazettes and official papers. The usefulness of the publication would come into its own, especially given the increased trend of original research into colonial histories. It was heartily recommended to 'every well appointed library, public and private, throughout the empire'.[67]

There were also individual reader responses, especially from Hocken's fellow collectors. Horatio Robley was circumspect – 'I read the reviews on the Bibliography' – but the reclusive Alexander Turnbull was more forthcoming, in a letter to fellow collector Downie Stewart:

> Have you yet received Dr Hocken's *Bibliography*? It is now for sale & if you care for one I can forward it with great pleasure having a spare copy by me. I have not had time to examine the contents of it properly but I can see many entries of books not in my collection. The author deserves great credit for his work.
>
> My friend Mr Ewen is as busy as ever collecting & now he has Dr Hocken's book before him I feel sure he will not rest until he has got *all* the items mentioned in it![68]

A week later Turnbull told Stewart that C.A. Ewen, the manager of a Wellington insurance firm and a rival book collector, had studied the book since its publication 'to the exclusion of everything else – wife, family & business'. Turnbull added that there were compensations for this effort: Ewen had found some omissions, which had pleased him no end.[69]

There was, however, criticism. In a letter to Smith, Hocken revealed that Edward Tregear had written complaining that his dictionaries of the Mangarevan and Paumotan languages were not included. Although Hocken claimed they were not within the scope of the *Bibliography*, Tregear was still 'very sore & I am sorry'.[70] Even Augustus Hamilton was critical, although in a private capacity: 'Ewen told me that he had gone through 3 shelves in his Library with the Hocken Bibliography and had added 70 volumes from the 3 shelves. Of course Hocken would say that he considered that these were not necessary to be mentioned. It would have been much better if he had accepted the offer of co-operation which was made to him at the time that the printing was started.'[71]

Charles Wilson, who had recommended the printing of the *Bibliography*, reviewed it in the *New Zealand Times* under the pseudonym 'Liber'. Hocken's response highlights his no-nonsense combative approach to something that he felt passionately about. After thanking Wilson for his 'very kind' remarks, he takes him to task for the three instances where the librarian had criticised Hocken's note about a title. One is the 'fiction by Lancaster' – surely the stories of G.B. Lancaster, the pseudonym of author Edith Lyttleton – which Wilson has clearly not read: 'If you will do so I think you will agree with me that the stories are indeed "coarsely told" and that even a "pemmican" note should say so and so far mark a proper criticism.'

> It is plain too that you have not read *Wakefield's Adventures* [*in New Zealand* (1908)]. Anyone knowing the very early history of New Zealand would be thankful to see this book thoroughly annotated and edited ... Stout knows nothing whatever of those old times depicted by Wakefield and I can only suppose that Whitcombe and Tombs asked him to edit the book because of his *mana* and because of his being in recent days Wakefield's fellow-politician. I repeat that 'this important work has yet to be competently edited. Where is the discourtesy in this truth which as a competent bibliographer I was compelled to utter? McNab is doing most valuable and yeoman service and I am delighted that with his wealth and energy he has taken up this work. His 'Murihiku' is precisely as I have characterised it ... Your remark about being 'published by the State' is surely very pointless. Would you muzzle a work of this character? You do not notice what I consider a very important and certainly unique feature – the Maori bibliography. This is something absolutely new and of great interest ...[72]

The 'Ghost' of James Collier

And then there was James Collier, whose review of Hocken's *Bibliography* appeared in *The Citizen*, a Wellington periodical, on 29 October 1909. By way of introduction, journalist and editor Arthur Nelson Field wrote that the 'perfunctory' reviews so far would be balanced by Collier's, describing it as 'a review of the work of one expert by another'.[73] After acknowledging the work of others in the field, including European examples, Collier mentioned his own work, 'really the first bibliography of that [New Zealand's] literature', and after outlining the approach he had taken, he turned to Hocken:

The possessor of the completest collection of New Zealandiana in existence ... has resumed the never-to-be-finished task. All the leisure of a busy professional life has been lavished on the patriotic duty of fitting himself to be the bibliographer of New Zealand. In fulfilment of it he has gathered together from every source all the books, maps, charts, manuscripts, letters and curios that could throw light on the history of the colony. He has ransacked public libraries and private collections. He has interviewed every person in the Dominion of any importance ... Minute researches among the other *incunabula* of New Zealand have made of him an expert. A more highly qualified bibliographer could not be found.

Criticism followed, which began with a discussion on the scope of the work. There was the title similarity – Collier maintained his was the more correct, since it included publications relating to New Zealand only. Hocken's was a 'complete misnomer' because it took in books relating to New Zealand and *other* materials, whether or not there was any specific New Zealand association. As Collier exclaimed: 'We ask ourselves, as we turn the pages, what is sermon after sermon "doing in this galley?" And what are so many collections of verse doing here? Why should we have Mr Bevan-Brown's interesting tract on *Plato and Christianity*? Did the old Greek philosopher, perhaps, intend to found his new republic in the South Pacific?' Collier went further, attacking the inclusion of those works not on New Zealand written by authors who had written on New Zealand. Edward Gibbon Wakefield was but one candidate, and perhaps Collier was thinking of his *England and America* (1833). His eminently sensible suggestion was to refer to such works in notes. He also felt that Hocken had extended the brief when it came to the detailed contents offered, especially with the voyages material. He had pared down descriptions to those portions relating to New Zealand; Hocken expanded on the works of Dalrymple, Burney and Dumont d'Urville, even though only a small portion dealt with New Zealand.

Collier applauded the inclusion of the Maori section in the *Bibliography*, but was unhappy about Hocken's use of the notes. This was the second borrowing, which was entirely unattributed, and a volley of examples followed: 'I find no fault with his adopting from my note'; 'It is a small matter that he should take from me'; 'It is little that he should have extracted, after me'; 'It is a light thing that he should have transcribed the titles ... and used my very words'; 'Nor is it, perhaps, of much importance that he should have carried off bodily the notes ...' He continued: 'Dr Hocken has verbally appropriated, without a word of acknowledgement, my analysis of Lesson's work on the Polynesians, which it cost some labour to make.' Collier then suggested that Hocken should have indicated rightful authorship by inverted commas, for as they stand now, 'no one is to know that he had not even seen the erudite works he will seem to have analysed'. Hocken also used the asterisk to indicate those books he had not seen: this was another borrowing from Collier, which was again not acknowledged.

Criticism off his chest, Collier reverted to praising Hocken's work, which was to him 'truly remarkable for its exhaustiveness'. And while acknowledging those few omissions, he concluded: 'The careful collations of difficult works are beyond praise. Errors of any moment are non-existent.'[74]

On 28 February 1910, racked with pain and 'in a sadly crippled condition', Hocken wrote to Turnbull: 'I am very pleased that you derive so much assistance from my bibliography which I am quite sure is of great value.' He then started on Collier:

> I was somewhat annoyed & still more so as unable to answer from illness that odd & curious criticism of Collier's ... He took & gave in the same breath. A most jealous spirit seems to have pervaded him – very very different from the correspondence I had with him before even he commenced his bib. 25 years ago when I offered to work conjointly with him. Fortunately I kept this correspondence, not certainly with the least idea that it might ever prove useful but simply as a pleasant reminiscence of what an able man like himself might say on the whole subject.[75]

Unusually for one who prided himself on excellent networks, Hocken had thought that Collier was dead until the arrival of the latter's work on Sir George Grey. Hocken also took a swipe at that book, which 'while interesting appears to be to me unfinished & somewhat erratic. Still the book did not profess to be more than a sketch of some incidents in his life.'[76]

Hocken's *Bibliography* was the only reference tool for scholars of New Zealand literature and history for over 60 years. Even now it has an important position in New Zealand letters, holding bibliographical and scholarly value despite Graham Bagnall's six-volume *New Zealand National Bibliography to the Year 1960* (1969–80) and the onslaught of computerised systems such as the National Library-driven Te Puna database. Hocken himself recognised the inherent value of his own work and said so on many occasions. Indeed, for him it was a very personal reference tool. Even when ill, he went back into his collection and wrote notes in his books and manuscripts, cross-referencing to his own and other works.

In July 1909 Mackay, recognising the importance of what he had printed, congratulated Hocken on its completion and recognised the 'infinite amount of labour' that had been involved.[77] After Hocken's death, Turnbull remarked to Smith on the considerable personal sacrifices that a collector like Hocken took on 'without hope or wish for reward': 'only those who come after ... will know and acknowledge the extent of the services rendered'.[78] Hocken's *Bibliography* was not only a tangible and lasting result of his collecting; it was also the pinnacle of those efforts.

Interim Projects: Maning and Webster

By the time Charles Wilson visited Hocken in Dunedin in June 1906 the latter was beginning another project that needed his full attention. This was a new edition of Frederick Maning's *Old New Zealand: A Tale of the Good Old Times*. On 25 July 1906 long-time correspondent John Webster had heard the news, remarking that Hocken was the right man for the job: 'Messrs Whitcombe & Tombs ought to be proud to get your valuable services for no-one is more able than yourself to carrie [sic] out the work faithfully.'[79] Because Webster had been a good friend of Maning, Hocken harassed him in a friendly way for information.[80] Webster sent Maning's portrait, more gossip on Maning as 'Judge', his mastery of the Maori language, his love of practical jokes, family information, birth date verification (5 July 1811) and letters, in which Hocken rejoiced.[81] Webster also explained that he had once possessed a presentation copy of the first edition of *Old New Zealand* 'but lent it to a party in Auckland, who died, & it was lost & I could find no trace of it. This copy I am sending you, you will kindly return to me. You will find at the end several articles which I see no reason why they should not appear in the new edition.'[82] Hocken owned a second edition which contains an obituary pasted in, a note about Maning's death, and comment on the first edition: 'published in 1862 & appears in the Otago Colonists in parts commencing April 1st 1862'.[83]

Hocken had actually met Maning in Auckland about June 1881, calling on him at least three times at his lodgings in Princes Street. On one occasion Maning gave him a presentation copy of *Hinemoa: A love song* (1881), now bound in his Pamphlet Collection, Volume 5, Number 6. Hocken also observed that the old settler was 'very tall, above six feet', an incessant talker who gave him little opportunity to ask any questions. Hocken could only sit and listen. Whether the facts and stories communicated were true, false or exaggerated, they were grist to Hocken's mill and he duly documented them.[84]

Weary of the fame and success attached to *Old New Zealand*, Maning once wrote that he was tired of the intrusion of others, especially those who treated him 'as if I was a two legged book'.[85] He even told a friend of having to stave off 'Dr Hocking and all sorts of beggars'.[86] Unaware of this opinion, Hocken continued his effort in dressing Maning's works for a new reading public, hoping to follow the author's 'endeavour to call back some shadows of the past'.

> To such a man what glorious possibilities life in New Zealand must have held forth! Every whaler and trader brought back stories of that little known but lovely land, held by a splendid race of savage men, whose pastime was war, with whom to live was to be brave, and whose women were dark-eyed, soft-voiced, and affectionate. To all like him such was a call from the wild, nor did he seek to resist it.[87]

Another to whom Hocken appealed for information was J.W. Leys, director of the Brett Printing and Publishing Co. and at one time sub-editor of the *Daily Southern Cross*. Leys not only sent biographical data on Maning, but confirmed the bibliographical data on *Old New Zealand*: that the first edition was printed and published by Creighton & Scales of Auckland in early 1863, followed quickly by the second edition in the same year. A London edition published by Smith, Elder & Co. also appeared in 1863. And, like Webster, Leys offered the kind of gossip that always makes good copy:

> He had private means, and only acted as a Judge intermittently. Mackay says that the last time he was engaged with Maning on a case was at a Court – held at Taupo in bitterly cold weather. Maning always wrapped himself round with rugs while sitting in the Court, and spent the night over the fire sipping rum hot and spinning yarns. At parting, he remarked that the theological definition of hell was manifestly wrong; cold and not heat was the worst punishment that could be inflicted on man.[88]

In the early part of 1907 Maning's *Old New Zealand* was published, and the unnamed reviewer in the *Otago Witness* claimed this 'delightful book' was one of 'the happiest inspirations which the little publishing world of the antipodes has known'. Praising the 'gentle art' of introductions and the book's excellent 'get-up', the reviewer proclaimed the book would be forever known as 'The Hocken Edition'.[89] Hocken was delighted and hoped Webster felt the same: 'You would be pleased, doubtless, with the appearance of *Old New Zealand* and I hope you thought well of the introduction.'[90]

John Webster's Reminiscences

With seemingly little effort, Hocken leapt from Maning to Webster, embarking on another book project that helped him mark time during the printing of his *Bibliography*. On 24 April 1907 Hocken broached the subject with Webster: 'I am moreover so anxious to go through your journals and papers with you and see if we cannot get them put into shape for printing.' He wanted Webster's early reminiscences of Australia to 'see the light before you depart from us'.[91] It was not an effortless undertaking; when he visited Webster in the north, both took much pain over getting the contents right. By 29 April 1908 Hocken informed Webster that the book 'is now fairly under weigh', and as it was his initiative, he contacted George Whitcombe, imploring him for proofs for revision. Indeed, Hocken was so excited about it that he wanted another book from Webster covering the period through to Heke's War. 'I shall take infinite pleasure in cross-examining you and keeping you up as before until 11 o'clock at night! How delighted would your old friend Maning be.'[92]

In addition to providing progress reports on the book, Hocken also regaled Webster with information on recent acquisitions. While travelling back from Auckland he had discovered some 50 dirty, grimy charts of New Zealand executed by John Lort Stokes and Byron Drury from 1848 to 1854, two of which included charts of the Lower and Upper Hokianga.[93] Hocken also offered medical advice:

> I have little doubt but that you have yet a long time of fair health if you will be careful. By no means overdo yourself in working or walking. Remember what I said of your heart, that though it was free from disease you must not overdo it. It is a *muscle* like those of your legs and arms; these you may tire and even overdo and a night's rest will put them right, but not so with your heart. At your age you must not over tax it by too much physical exertion. This is absolutely important. Take plenty of walking on the level or doing a little in the garden, but not more.[94]

On 10 June 1908 Hocken informed Webster that the book was progressing well and that every other day he received 'a batch of proofs to correct & to divide into paragraphs, &c'. According to Hocken, 'it is extremely well printed in good type & reads very well'. In the anticipation of local sales, especially with its small New Zealand component, Hocken asked for illustrations. 'If you can have a few ready I shall know exactly where they should be inserted, so you need have no trouble on this score – leave that to me.' He also added that there should be a portrait of Webster and a short preface.

> The latter I would endeavour to write for you and as though written by yourself if you find that you cannot undertake it. But make an effort. Something like this – that these reminiscences appear at the earnest desire of your children & of your intimate friends, that you are quite conscious how incomplete they are from your failing memory & advanced years, & how much you regret they were not undertaken 25 years ago and so on & so on.

Hocken also suggested to Webster that he should add 'J.P. of Opononi, Hokianga' on the title page. And like the terrier that he was, his postscript to this long letter reiterated his suggestion on the introduction, which he was obviously keen to do himself: 'If you should wish me to write the introduction you might suggest any special lines or remarks. Of course I should write it as though written by yourself.'[95]

Reminiscences of an Old Settler in Australia and New Zealand by John Webster, 'J.P. of Opononi, Hokianga', was published by Whitcombe & Tombs in 1908. In his preface, Hocken reiterated the fact that there was little relevant to New Zealand and recorded for readers Webster's experiences in Australia, America (as a gold digger) and the Pacific, including his time on board the *Wanderer*, which was written up in 1858 as *The Last Cruise of the* Wanderer. Hocken also referred to Webster's 'hospitable home', which was the resort of governors and distinguished people when they visited the north. As a coda to publication Hocken received a letter from Webster in February 1909, wishing that 'writing letters had never been invented'. Since the publication of his book he had faced an influx of correspondents asking for signed copies. He had run out of his own copies and was forced to buy more from Whitcombe at 5s, and then get credited 3s 6d, less 10 per cent. After all this, Webster even mooted the idea of republishing *The Last Cruise of the Wanderer*, but that was an aberration: 'Prudence condemns it as I find it does not pay nor am I fitted for the work in my old age.'³⁵ Perhaps if Hocken had lived he might well have advanced this idea. As it was, he surely got great satisfaction from completing this project for Webster.

19
An Act of Patriotism

As mentioned earlier, Hocken's intention to gift his collection of books and manuscripts to the nation had been made public in the *Otago Daily Times* on 19 March 1897.[1] The announcement caused an immediate buzz, and local lobbying began over where his famed collection would actually reside. Coincidentally in April 1897 the Free Public Library Association pushed to commemorate the jubilee of Queen Victoria's reign by building a library, and there was a proposal to purchase the Colonial Bank Building at 'a moderate price' to serve as a public library and an art gallery. Further impetus for Hocken's gift and the desire to obtain the much-needed library came from R. Hudson, almost certainly Richard Hudson the successful biscuit and confectionery manufacturer, who offered £1000 towards the project if nine other citizens would subscribe a similar amount, or 19 others with the lesser sum of £500.[2]

After the initial reaction, however, the mention of Hocken's gift was forgotten, as he himself admitted to David Scott Mitchell in March 1898:

> When making my offer to the public I said that it was dependent on their housing and making provision for the due care of my collection. But so far I have been much disappointed, as with the exception of a little stir and few laudatory letters at first, nothing effective has been done. I thus begin to feel not only somewhat chagrined but also inclined to withdraw from my position, and to leave my library in the safekeeping of some trustee until in the fullness of time proper provision is made.[3]

As time passed Hocken was still flat about the lack of public response. About July 1906 he wrote to *Evening Star* editor Mark Cohen: 'Gradually, however, the matter died out, and I am not aware that steps of a satisfactory character have been undertaken with regard to it since.'[4]

One major reason for the inaction was that civic energies were directed towards the development of a library in Dunedin. The story of the protracted city-wide discussions, the efforts of Cohen, Robert Stout and clothing manufacturer Bendix Hallenstein and the gift of £10,000 by Andrew Carnegie towards the establishment of a Free Public Library that was finally opened on 2 December 1908 is admirably told in Mary Ronnie's *Freedom to Read: A centennial history of Dunedin Public Library* (2008).[5] Another reason was that Hocken himself was preoccupied. In April 1898 he travelled to Samoa and Fiji. In that same year he worked through the complexities of publishing his *Contributions*, and at the beginning of the new century he planned and undertook an extensive overseas trip. He also continued to collect, a gradual but sustained effort with an eye to documenting all of his printed books in his *Bibliography*.

In early 1899 Hocken received a boost in the guise of a visit from George Robertson. After the Australian bookseller left, Hocken wrote asking if he could pass on his enquiry to Henry Anderson about the gift conditions laid down by David Scott Mitchell. Anderson replied directly on 25 March 1899, calling Mitchell's library of 30,000 volumes a 'noble gift'. He tabulated the points laid down:

1. That they must be suitably housed in a separate wing of a new building to be erected at once by the Government for the National Library of this colony.
2. That this wing shall be always kept separate from the general collection and shall be known as the 'David Scott Mitchell Library'.
3. That admittance to it will not be absolutely free without restriction, as at present to the general Library; but will be by ticket issued by the Principal Librarian on recommendation from a respectable householder as is done in the British Museum.
4. That the Library Trustees shall be made into a Corporate body by Act of Parliament, in order to provide for their continuous succession.

Anderson added that Mitchell was prepared to endow the library 'very handsomely', not only because there was a need to collect more Australasian materials, but also because it enabled the trustees to use accumulated funds to purchase any large collection if and when one came up for sale. Anderson also noted that Mitchell had included no conditions about the administration of the library, nor on the appointment (future or otherwise) of the trustees.[6] All this matched what Mitchell himself told Hocken in a letter written a few days after Anderson had sent his letter (see Chapter 11).[7]

Announcing a gift is one thing; making it happen is quite another. In Hocken's case, it was the indefatigable and tireless Mark Cohen who brought matters to a head. He finally persuaded the Dunedin City Council to call for tenders to erect a building in Moray Place 'in accordance with the prize design of Messrs Crichton and M'Kay'.[8] On 2 May 1906 Cohen, as honorary secretary of the Public Library Association, wrote to Hocken, reminding him of 'the splendid offer you made to the City' and asking whether the planned building, with its Carnegie grant behind it, would suit his requirements. Aware of the realities of city council workings, the diplomatic Cohen offered a general commitment:

> I cannot, of course, say what accommodation the City Council will be prepared to furnish in the event of your deciding to hand over your unique library and art collection to the City, but I am quite satisfied that, in the event of your so deciding, the City Council will be only too pleased to do their part toward meeting your wishes, and will make the future home of the Hocken Library well worthy of its owner and a credit to our City … [9]

Cohen was astute enough to recognise the psyche of the collector. He also acknowledged that the collection was still being used as a research resource and that Hocken's initial announcement was made, in part, to stimulate the public into raising funds for the erection of a building that would house it.

As Percy Smith often claimed of Hocken, 'you generally answer so promptly', but in this instance he was like molasses, replying to Cohen's letter as late as 1 July.[10] While appreciating Cohen's concern for making the new library the home for his collection, Hocken was firm: 'But I cannot agree with you.'[11] He maintained that the proposed building was too small and unsuitable for his purposes and mentioned two other proposals that could be profitably considered. The first was the proposed art gallery, to which 'a considerable sum had already been subscribed'; the second, the Early Settlers' Association, with their land on Moray Place 'worth perhaps £15,000 or more'. Drawing on his recent and favourable impression of Auckland and its new library and art gallery, Hocken suggested 'combining in a common purse' to achieve the same for Dunedin. After reiterating his own feelings on his collection – 'of great value, monetarily worth many thousands, intrinsically unique and inestimable as connected with New Zealand history and to a degree with that of New South Wales' – and highlighting a few treasures, he offered an open invitation to 'a few thoroughly competent gentlemen' to examine the collection and report back. They would need to put aside one or two days to complete the examination. He was also adamant that something needed to happen:

> In conclusion, it cannot be reasonably expected that my offer can longer remain open for an indefinite period. I am thus compelled to say that if it be not complied within eighteen months from the date of this letter I shall have no alternative but to withdraw it and to make other arrangements regarding it. But, of course, my sincere desire is that it should remain in New Zealand, and preferably in Dunedin.[12]

On 23 July 1906 a meeting of representatives of the art gallery trustees and the Early Settlers' Association, including Hocken, discussed the practicalities of placing the collection within the planned art gallery and Early Settlers' building.[13] Almost immediately there were practical difficulties, especially over costs of maintenance and custodial staffing. When lawyer, company director and conservationist Alexander Bathgate asked for greater clarity about his views, Hocken replied that it was his 'intense desire' to keep the collection in Dunedin, that it must be thoroughly looked after and properly housed in every way. In a moment of prescience, Bathgate broached the 'practical solution' of applying to government for funds to complete the museum and house the collection there. At this stage Hocken was not 'for' the museum site, feeling that one single curator could not look after both artefacts and the library. He was also asked about the monetary value of the collection, to which he replied that, about 1890, the late Sir Walter Buller put the collection's worth at £10,000. It had been greatly added to since then and 'was now worth many more thousands of pounds'.

In response to further quizzing, Hocken reiterated his 'common purse' notion, favouring it not only because, as a 'colonial matter', it would attract a government grant, but because his collection contained 'a great deal of real art' – not just paintings, but old maps, charts and plans – which would sit well within a building that also housed an art gallery. On hearing this, Bathgate claimed that there had been no communication with the gallery on this matter and asked for clarification on space requirements. Hocken's 'quite the size of the Choral Hall' was an inadequate answer, while John Halliday Scott was more definite with '45 ft x 60 ft [13.7 x 18.3 m]'. Mayor George Lawrence maintained that 'there was plenty of space' and favoured the three agencies option because there would be comparatively little extra cost – and the Tourist Bureau could be in the same block. Some confusion followed over whether the Free Public Library was included, but Bathgate and Cohen then explained that the terms of Andrew Carnegie's agreement did not allow for such a collection as Hocken's to be in the public library. Cohen expanded privately on this subject to Robert McNab:

> We would have gladly taken charge of the collection in the new Public Library, but unfortunately the terms of the Carnegie grant prevent us from taking charge of anything but *books*, and Dr Hocken would not separate his books from his art treasures ... On principle I think the Government should assist, as Govts do elsewhere, in subsidising benefactions for the general good like Hocken's. For example, what did the Govt of NSW do the other day? Where Mr Mitchell, barrister, gave his valuable library to the State ... Now if the object appeals to you I don't mind taking a subscription from you ... The Dr will be delighted to show you his entire collections, if you will name a day ...[14]

Although by the end of the meeting there was a general agreement on approaching the premier for funds, the immediate result was the formation of yet another committee and the emergence of definite party divisions.

A week later another meeting was held, and Augustus Hamilton was present.[15] George Fenwick, one of Hocken's Musketeers, was unable to attend; his apologies included what may have been the first mention of a subscription fund for Hocken's collection organised through the *Otago Daily Times*. In fact, £1650 had already been collected. It was encouraging, but there was still the difficult decision on the best site. The mayor again opted for co-operation, hoping that 'during the consideration of these matters there would be no friction'. The Tourist Bureau was mentioned again because it would attract government funding and surmount the problem of supervision.

Indeed, to Mayor Lawrence it seemed that 'the Government would be the proper party to be the custodian of the collection'. Because of this 'national' status, he suggested that the government should subsidise what was collected on a pound-for-pound basis.

Throughout all these discussions Hocken tried to remain objective, feeling that the decision regarding the site should be left to the citizens. He did acknowledge the popularity of the railway site, however, knowing that for one person visiting the museum there would be 50 visiting the station, in the heart of the city. On mention of this option there was loud applause.[16]

Another of Hocken's Musketeers *was* present. Professor William Benham, curator at the Otago Museum, pushed for the museum, not only because it was open almost every day for visitors, but because, contrary to Hocken's statement, it 'was visited by a very large number of people, and all those interested in science or in history naturally went there for enquiries'. He admitted that the iron annexe was an 'eyesore' and that the museum needed upgrading. The solution was to build an addition that 'might be called the Hocken Wing, and the Hocken collection stored there – not merely stored there, but housed and looked after by people who are accustomed to look after treasures'. After further discussion, some of it heated, local MP James Allen weighed in with his opinion that the museum site was worthy of consideration. He did not like the idea of the Tourist Bureau, which to him was 'a sprat to catch a mackerel'. He also felt that the government should be approached for a subsidy, but control must remain with the citizens of Dunedin. Allen was also astute enough to recognise the real problem of the gift: 'the building was nothing compared to the large question of custody. Who was to look after the collection? Who was to pay for the possible necessary rebinding of a lot of these books, and so on?' This was at the heart of Hocken's own concern. After taking advice from Augustus Hamilton, Allen also revealed that the control, cataloguing and arrangement of the collection would take 'two years' hard work' to get it ready for use by anyone.

Amid this to-ing and fro-ing sat Dr Hocken. Again his thoughts were asked for. He reiterated his prime concerns towards the collection, repeated his liking for the railway site and stressed that he did not like the idea of the Tourist Bureau. He even felt that the museum site was worth consideration. He also repeated his invitation for some competent men to examine the collection. Finally an amended motion was put and accepted: 'That, in the opinion of this meeting, a committee should be appointed to inquire into the nature of the collection offered by Dr Hocken; the kind of building that would be necessary to house it, the custody of the same, and the annual cost of caring for it and keeping it in repair: the best site for the building.'

On 8 August 1906 a deputation called on Joseph Ward, the new premier, to ask for a government contribution of £1500 towards a building to house Hocken's collection. Cohen raised the idea of a pound-for-pound subsidy.

Ward, who knew something of Hocken's collection, felt that the people of Dunedin and Otago should find the money themselves, and that if this failed they could come back and renegotiate.[17] The deputation took a positive view of this outcome. The *Otago Daily Times* announced that 'in effect, the Premier may be said to have challenged Dunedin to manifest its earnestness in the matter', and proceeded to list those individuals who had already given money to the Hocken Fund. The subscription sum for the first 15 listed came to £1025 10s.[18]

By this time, however, Hocken was feeling the pressure. In a letter to his friend Chapman he said he felt like 'the lamb amongst wolves' when it came to the jostling by and divisions between all the parties, which now included the Otago University Museum. In a rare display of invective Hocken called Cohen 'a little troublesome – I had almost said *nasty*', especially in his push for the new triangle site near the railway, which he now regarded as highly unsuitable: 'Dust, smoke, noise & probably in 20 years not a desirable or even central position.' And Hocken wanted 'nothing to do with the Early Settlers''. He appealed to Chapman to sway the museum faction: 'Therefore I think a *strong* letter from you would have much weight & might give direction to the wavering forces. Address the "Times".'[19] The other two Musketeers, Fenwick and Benham, were also called upon to lend support.

Fenwick was doing his bit. The *Otago Daily Times* fund continued to grow, and by 22 August £2222 16s had been raised.[20] News of the fund had even spread to Australia, where the Melbourne *Argus* announced that the gift was 'really splendid' and that the Dunedin people had 'joyfully accepted' the offer and were now raising funds to erect a building to house it.[21] Hocken received a personal communication from Sir Samuel Way in Adelaide, who extolled the virtues of gifting a collection and all its subsequent benefits:

> Yours is a rare example of patriotism, and yet your generosity will be its own exceeding great reward. It would be wicked to submit to the hammer a collection like yours, which embodies the best work of your life. Your labour would be thrown away if the collection were distributed, because its value is so much enhanced by its completeness. You are setting an admirable example to other collectors, and you will enjoy the gratitude of your fellow citizens to whom you have so generously presented what has cost you so much in time, in pains, and in money. Besides, the future historians of Australasia will always have to make pilgrimage to Dunedin before their investigations into our early history can be complete.

Unaware of the machinations surrounding the gift, Way ended his letter: 'Our custom in Australia has been to get the Government to provide the means of housing gifts of this character. I am not sure that in New Zealand you have not found out a more excellent way, because the public have the opportunity of showing how they value your gift, by voluntarily supplying the funds for adequately preserving it.'²²

From Narrandera in New South Wales John Sutcliffe Horsfall wrote to Bessie welcoming the gift and hoping that the government would contribute to a building 'which will form an attraction for generations to come'. He did, however, express surprise that Hocken could actually part with books that he loved. Nevertheless, now that it was done, Horsfall maintained Hocken deserved 'a handsome monument, and I should think he will get one when he departs from this life, or perhaps before, but I hope the departure will be postponed for at least another thirty or forty years, because such men can ill be spared'.²³

Questions continued about the nature of the collection. Dunedin's townsfolk knew that Hocken was a book collector and a recognised authority on New Zealand's early history. Very few were privy to the full extent of his collection, however. Even his friends and acquaintances had difficulty in articulating the real importance of individual pieces and the collection in toto. Professor Benham was at a loss, knowing there were 'a certain number of books, maps and pictures', but ignorant of 'the exact number of each', while Councillor John Duthie's stab of 500 books and 300 pictures was well below the mark. On 1 August 1906 Fenwick, also uncomfortable about describing the collection, asked Hocken to give full particulars for the benefit of the public, including 'the value from an educational and historical standpoint of the literary and artistic treasures you have in the course of years, with such praiseworthy perseverance and at very great cost, gathered together'. Two days later Hocken responded, and both letters were promptly published in the *Otago Daily Times*.²⁴

His summation, a 'mere bald sketch or outline', was significant. It included descriptions of choice items that he felt were important, and it gave a good indication of what he owned at the time (with some quantifying attached). Hocken began with his newspapers, which he described as well bound and numbering 'perhaps 350 volumes'. Every district or province was represented, and they dated from the beginning of settlement in 1840 through to the 1860s. Many were now defunct: 'the Kororareka papers [*Bay of Islands Advertiser*], *Wellington Gazette, Spectator, Independent, Nelson Examiner*', and so on. Hocken also added that there were 'about 100 volumes of New South Wales, Tasmanian, and Victorian papers dating from the twenties'. As he well understood: 'Of course our earliest history is in these.'

Printed books were next. These numbered between 3000 and 4000, and most related to New Zealand, to colonisation, to Australasia, to voyages and explorations in the Southern Seas, to Cook and his companions, to the French, to the Wakefields and to 'old Blue Books, etc'. Pamphlets – 'very many being of great rarity and importance, and old' – followed, along with 'very complete' Maori literature, starting from the earliest publications by the missionaries.

Hocken did not give the quantity of pictures and illustrations he owned, but he called them 'legion', 'of great rarity and importance' and 'all of historic value'. He listed a few choice items, such as Angas's elephant folios of *New Zealanders Illustrated* (1847) and *South Australia Illustrated* and Edward Jerningham Wakefield's *Illustrations to 'Adventure in New Zealand'* (1845), then checked himself: 'But I must catalogue no further.'

Manuscripts followed, comprising documents by missionaries such as Marsden, old Canterbury and Otago records, Shortland's manuscripts and 'many letters of Governors Hobson, FitzRoy, and officials of their time, and of other New Zealand colonists, etc.' Finally, there were plans and maps, which included those emanating from the New Zealand Company, sketches of Maori pa and proclamations. After this brief summary, Hocken not only reissued the invitation for an examination by selected individuals, but reiterated his demands for the care of his collection:

> But it will be gathered from this sketch how certain it is that such a collection must be thoroughly cared for as well as housed. No mere caretaker would do, but someone of book knowledge and culture, and this must evidently be a sine qua non. Otherwise, however much I should regret it, my offer must be withdrawn. It is necessary to be thus plain spoken, as thereby misunderstanding is avoided at the very beginning.

Only one person took up the opportunity to examine the collection. This was Robert McNab, author of *Murihiku and the Southern Islands* (1907) and *Historical Records of New Zealand* (1908). As a collector of New Zealand materials himself, McNab certainly knew the value and scarcity of what he was looking at. His opinion was hyperbolic but fair: 'The mere mention that there are 3000 to 4000 books conveys no idea of the value even of that one department. Their value lies in the fact that they all relate to the colony of New Zealand and, taken together, constitute the largest and most complete collection in the world.' And then McNab struck at the heart and reality of the game – the chase.

> All printed books have originally many copies, and it may be argued that it only requires industry and a big purse to duplicate the collection. This is not so. My own personal experience justifies me in saying that the demand for these old works about the colony is so great that no length of life, no industry, and no purse could to-day enter into the market and duplicate the collection. The day of these things is past.

McNab also noted Hocken's predilection for annotating his books, adding 'special information about them of an extremely interesting and valuable kind'. Rather than castigating the collector for disfiguring his books, McNab saw real value in these notes, claiming that in time they would be appreciated.

He then turned his attention to Hocken's newspapers. Because of their ephemeral nature, he knew the reality of their precarious existence: 'More numerous in the first instance, a far larger proportion are forthwith destroyed.' He was obviously pleasantly surprised with what he saw: 'clean, well-kept, and complete copies of the earliest papers' and 'in splendid order'. Lastly he examined the manuscripts:

> Books come out with hundreds of copies, and many are preserved; newspapers come out in thousands, and few are preserved; manuscripts come out with but one copy, which, when once destroyed, can never be supplied. The manuscript makes the collection. The manuscript log of the *Mayflower* is in Parliament Buildings in Boston. The diplomacy of a nation brought it across from England; the army and the navy of the United States would now be called on, if necessary, to keep it there. Measured by the standards of value thus set up, the proposed gift to the City of Dunedin defies all assessment. There are manuscripts – all relating to New Zealand – of old explorers, of old divines, of old settlers, of old whalers, of old Governors, of old politicians, of old everybody who, when the colony was young, was young also, but who now, in the colony's maturer years, is almost forgotten.

He also touched on future usage of the collection, which he rightly predicted would increase and in areas and fields that he, the donor and the people of Dunedin could never imagine:

> When this collection is safely housed and open to the public, not only will the inspection of it be a source of pleasure to the citizens, but it will supply valuable information to the student of history. I doubt whether Dr Hocken realises what use the material will be put to by the student of future years. None of us realise it. We only know the growing demand for the material and the incorrect and misleading history which the want of the material foists upon the community.[25]

Two other authorities endorsed McNab's opinion. In a short letter Augustus Hamilton, who certainly knew something of the collection, targetted the 'unique and almost priceless collection of printed books and pictures and sketches' and 'an unrivalled collection of newspapers'. Rather than list items, he impressed upon his readers Hocken's 'unceasing labor' in bringing his collection to completion, and that the material within required 'special treatment'. Written before McNab's report was made public, Hamilton's letter also pointed out the need for an examination of the collection, which should be neither hurried or cursory.[26]

Frederick Revans Chapman was the other authority. Writing from Christchurch he not only underplayed his own experience and knowledge in the field but, like Hamilton, stressed similar aspects of Hocken's collection.

> I cannot profess to know all the details of Dr Hocken's library, but in a general way I know it well, having for more than thirty years been in the habit of exchanging views with Dr Hocken on the subject of the Early History of New Zealand. I need hardly say that it in most respects surpasses all other collections in New Zealand, and I think I ought to add in all respects. Beyond the mere collection, Dr Hocken's notes and memoranda in his books add greatly to their value. The collection of old newspapers is certainly one that could not be repeated.[27]

In another letter Chapman expanded on his association with Hocken's library — indeed, he felt that to some extent' he had helped to form it and was thus concerned about its future care and housing. He favoured the museum with its association with the university, and demanded that there be trustees and 'skilled custodians to make it available to the public'.[28]

Persistence Pays Off

Persistence can bring great results. In early September a small delegation met the premier in Wellington and discussed the government subsidy towards the housing of Hocken collection. This time the decision was favourable. Allen reported the good news to Hocken on 11 September 1906: 'I have just come away from a deputation to the Premier on the matter of your gift to the Colony, and you will be pleased to hear that he has promised to recommend cabinet to make a £ for £ vote up to £3,000 for all the money subscribed in Dunedin.' Allen also reported that Ward 'did not favour the Railway site and preferred the Museum site'. He continued with a few more construction cost details:

> If the Cabinet agree to this amount it will put us in the position of having some £6,000, and I know that Mr J.E. White, the City Councillor, has gone over the cost of constructing 75 feet of a new wing to the Museum, and estimates it at between £4,000 and £5,000. Assuming that the 75 feet costs £5,000, we shall then have £1,000 for equipment, and have a handsome addition to our Museum and a fire-proof building to keep your valuable collection in, a skilled and qualified gentleman to control and take charge ... I congratulate you upon this successful issue and hope that all the difficulties now are removed.[29]

It was all confirmed when the subscribers to the 'Hocken Library Fund' met on 17 September and passed the following motion: 'That this collection be housed in the Museum, and that a hearty thanks on behalf of the city and the colony be tendered to Dr Hocken for his patriotic action in making so magnificent and valuable a gift.'[30] Benham was congratulated for his courage, support and persistence in the crusade, with Daniel Colquhoun

– D'Artagnan to the Musketeers – adding his enthusiastic support. Colquhoun also added that the museum and the university 'hung together' to foster both learning and knowledge, and that it was appropriate that Hocken's collection resided within the sphere of both institutions. Hocken, asked to speak, admitted that his attitude had been 'a peculiar one', and yet if faced with it all again he would adopt the same. He also reaffirmed his neutrality, not wanting to dictate where his collection should be housed, and acknowledged that, though initially keen on the railway site with a building similar in style to the Auckland Gallery and Library, he had swung around to the museum option. The government subsidy had helped greatly towards this change. And he agreed with Benham's sentiments on the difficulty of giving a collection away, especially one that had been amassed over many years. He did, however, hark back to a disheartening experience in 1876 when he had visited the old Mechanics' Institute at Auckland and found newspapers – items now worth their weight in gold – lying about, tattered, dirty and uncared for. Adamant that this was not going to happen to his collection, and to ensure the building project advanced smoothly, he insisted upon the formation of a committee called the Hocken Library Trustees: two members named by him, two by the city council, two by the government and two by the subscribers. The trustees were John Roberts, H.E. Williams, Mark Cohen, J.E. White, William Burnett, George Fenwick, Professor Benham and John Ross. At their first meeting on Tuesday 18 December this group, entrusted with taking the Hocken building to completion, announced that the subscriber fund was £2555 4s 6d. With government money, the total was £5110 9s.

During all these protracted discussions there were detractors. When central government funding was first mooted, indignation arose in Christchurch, with editorials in the *Press* headed 'A Preposterous Request' and 'Dunedin's Strange Lapse from Virtue'.[31] An editorial from the Dunedin *Evening Star*, printed in the *Press*, reiterated Dunedin's positive response to the gift and promised that after all the discussion there would be success.[32] The *Otago Daily Times* also applauded the notion of government funding, especially when considering the Parliamentary Library in Wellington: 'It is only to members of Parliament, public officials, and a few privileged individuals in Wellington that the Parliamentary Library is open. With the Hocken collection, when it is secured – as we have no doubt it will be – it will be different: it will be accessible to the public, under proper safeguards, as freely as the Public Library and the Public Art Gallery will be. It will in truth be a collection held by the city "for the good of the people as a whole …"'[33]

An unknown wit penning the regular 'Dunedin Letter' in the *Tuapeka Times* was a little more cutting, though amusingly tongue-in-cheek:

> There is an element of bathos and humbug and cant about the whole business [the site controversy]. The general public as such are not interested in Dr Hocken's old newspapers and manuscripts and plans and maps. They

are the concern of the student, the casual visitor, and the curiosity monger, and why the citizens – or portion of them – should worry themselves about their housing, how they are housed, or where they are housed, would pass understanding were it not that one learns by experience how these agitations are worked.

The writer wanted to know two things: '1. What else would the owner do with his old lumber; 2. of what earthly use is it to Mr and Mrs Brown-Smith and the kids?'

> Their money is to be devoted, if possible, to the building of a new wing to the King-street collection of whale bones, moa skeletons, and the first necktie worn by the late J.G.S. Grant, of perfumed memory. Surely, surely, the indecision and vanity of an individual, plus the exuberant and unchecked vivacity and verbosity of the local press, have never been put to more peculiar uses with so amazing results.

And at one point 'Dunedin Letter' announced that the collection should go to Balclutha.[34]

Benham continued to lobby agencies for funds. By 6 February 1907 he received notification from the Dunedin city council that they would vote £200 per annum for two years towards the Hocken building.[35] Subscribers passed a resolution in early April 1907 that the City Council would hand over to the University Council any rights of actual custody; the latter would undertake the responsibility of the proper care of the collection for all time.[36] Benham actively lobbied individuals, especially through circulars. The following 'plea' is a sample of what many prominent citizens read when they opened their mail.

> Our worthy fellow citizen, Dr Hocken, has as you are no doubt aware, presented his valuable library, a collection of pictures, maps, etc concerning the early days of the colony, to the people of New Zealand with the proviso that the collection shall be preserved and exhibited in this Museum.

> By the energy of Mr Geo. Fenwick, of the *Otago Daily Times*, a fund was established for the purpose of erecting a building for the preservation of the Collection. This fund has amounts to £2603; we are desirous of bringing it up to at least £3000 in order to avail ourselves of the full amount of the subsidy promised by the Government. The 'Hocken Library Trustees' – appointed by the subscribers, the donor, the City and the Government – who have the matter in hand, are about to add a Wing to the existing Museum, to complete which, and to preserve its suitability, will require a sum greater than we hold at present.

It has been suggested to me that as you are interested in the Early History of the Colony, you might desire to aid in this effort to provide a building commensurate with the value of Dr Hocken's generous gift.[37]

There were the other campaigners. While the *Otago Daily Times* fund was accumulating a larger sum for the building, the *Evening Star* – despite 'a slight difference of opinion' with Fenwick's paper – generated its own 'Hocken Equipment Fund', aiming for £1000. Even the people of Clutha were targetted. Recognising that every little bit helps, 'the Hocken Fund' announced: '"Many mickles make a muckle," and the smallest contribution will be welcome.' Subscriptions from 1s upwards were requested.[38] Funds also came from dramatic enterprises, among them the 'delightful' play *Jane* performed in early May 1907.[39] Fenwick continued with his efforts, at one point receiving a draft for £20 from Douglas MacLean of the Royal Colonial Institute, England, along with the heartening words: 'I hope the efforts being made to procure sufficient funds for building will be successful. As New Zealand grows older such a collection as that of Dr Hocken's will be more and more prized by the people of New Zealand.'[40]

The Deed of Gift

With the University Council now in charge, Hocken obviously felt more comfortable about advancing to the next stage – legalising his gift. In early June he submitted the first draft of his deed of trust and waited for the reaction from the university's solicitors.[41] Although the document was passed at the August meeting, there was a brief hold-up when Councillor Downie Stewart suggested that the government or the city council should be approached to undertake the care and upkeep of the collection because the University Council did not have any legal right to expend money in that direction.[42] Hocken was 'amazed … to hear such difference of opinion amongst the local bodies regarding maintenance'. His rescuer on this particular occasion was the Rev. A. Cameron, who stated that such a responsibility was never likely to be a serious drain, and if and when the council faced hardship over upkeep, it would then approach others. Cameron suggested that it accept the gift heartily and agree to the deed drawn up by Hocken.

On 2 September 1907 the University Council sent through the legal documents concerning Hocken's deed of trust to the trustees for signing. It was unanimously agreed upon and signed that day. John A. Burnside was announced as architect for the Hocken wing, although acknowledgement was given to David Ross, the government-appointed architect for the original museum building.[43] The deed of trust carried the names of the trustees: John Roberts (merchant), Mark Cohen (journalist), Joseph Eli White (building contractor), William Burnett (sheep farmer), George Fenwick (journalist), Henry Edward Williams (insurance agent), John Ross (importer) and Professor of Biology William Blaxland Benham.[44] The fund raised for the building and the future care, preservation and maintenance of the collection was now £2776 14s, with the pound-for-pound government subsidy making a total of £5553 8s.

The erection of a new wing at the Otago University Museum was also documented in Part One of the deed; 'sufficient space on the second floor' was to be allotted to the collection, with proper and suitable cases and furnishings provided so that items could be displayed. Items that were 'particularly valuable' were to be safeguarded and kept under lock and key. Part Two announced Hocken's personal obligation. Once the building was completed he was to pass his collection to the University Council in trust. The trustees had their obligations: 'to permit the same to be used as a Library or Museum of information and reference by the general public of The Colony of New Zealand in perpetuity under and subject to the conditions and provisions hereinafter expressed'.

The collection was to be catalogued and arranged for reference and use by the general public, and open at all hours during the times the museum was open, without any fee or charge. The council was given permission to add to the collection, obtained either by purchase or donations, and was instructed to make suitable provision for the care and preservation of the collection; specifics noted were the repair or renewal of deteriorated or perished bindings. Insurance of the collection against loss or damage by fire was mandatory. And in a measure to combat further loss, defacement or injury and maintain the collection's integrity, the council was, under no circumstances whatsoever, to allow any material from the collection to be removed from the new wing.

Happily for the trustees, Hocken did allow small movement within their legal obligations. They could 'rescind or alter regulations' concerning when and how the collection was used, though a parenthetical clause of 'not being inconsistent with these presents' tempered any potential changes. Hocken also had to be happy with the plans for the building and all other particulars, such as cases and furnishings, before the funds were to be spent. Following similar arrangements with Samuel Pepys's Library at Magdelene College, Cambridge, a visitor was to be appointed to inspect the collection from time to time and report back to the trustees. The term of appointment for the visitor at the Hocken was five years. Fortunately, Hocken's deed did not include the 'threat' made by Pepys that if any books were lost or misused, his library would then move to Oxford. On 8 October 1907 Hocken received a letter from the chancellor of the University of Otago acknowledging his 'noble and generous gift'; it was all signed, sealed and delivered.[45]

The Library Building and Use

On 10 January 1908 Hocken, along with William Benham and John Burnside, examined and approved the plans of the new wing.[46] The frontage on King (now Great King) Street was to measure 14.3 m with a height of 10.3 m above the footpath, while the northern aspect measured 24.3 m with a height of 13.4 m above the land level. The new wing comprised a basement and two storeys. On the first floor a room measuring 12.1 x 7.6 m would house the library; the remaining space was devoted to a gallery displaying Hocken's pictures and prints. The total floor area measured 14.7 x 12.1 m. There were plans for proper lighting (skylights), prismatic glass windows (totara sills and frames) and a fibrous-plastered ceiling; the new structure was promised to be fireproof. The basement would be built of best 'fine axed' Port Chalmers stone, the two upper storeys of brick and cement and the floors and foundations were to be reinforced concrete. The timber used was to be free of sap, shakes, knots or other defects; the door to the library would be cedar. The exterior, finished in cement plaster, would be as 'architecturally ornate as funds permit'.[47] By March 1908 construction had begun, with slight modification to the original height measurements, and was predicted to finish seven months later.[48] Benham's end of year report for 1908 was no doubt a pleasure to write: the building was finished, and the fittings for the upper floor were being attended to. There was even a gas stove in the library to warm readers in the winter. Benham also reported that the trustees wanted a public opening, an occasion when the collection and building could be formally transferred to the University Council.[49]

The trustees were certain about what was required and a draft manuscript headed 'The Hocken Collection' reveals what they envisaged.[50] The final copy of these proposals was sent to the council. The spacing of the new wing was registered as above, with some give and take on the estimates from the architect. Almost all books in the library were to be exhibited in locked glass cases, either upright or flat, though some science books and those with no special historical value could – as in Sir George Grey's library – be displayed in unlocked cases and kept in the museum library with other books on natural history. Of course, Hocken's permission was required for this. There were to be tables and chairs for study and a light ladder to reach those books on higher shelves. The Hocken Picture Room, as it was called, had framed pictures around the walls, and unframed items of special interest in table cases.

The books were to be made available to any person who expressed a desire to consult them for a definite purpose of study: 'They should not be accessible to every merely curious & irresponsible individual.' Proper credentials were required beforehand: 'any well-known person' whose known investigations entitled special consideration; those who had a letter of introduction from any well-known resident in New Zealand; and those who had recommendations from two householders in Dunedin. Books were not to be removed from the library, although the trustees did acknowledge exceptional circumstances to those undertaking serious study. The keys to the bookcases were to be kept with the librarian, to whom all applications for permission to use the material were to be made. The opening hours were to be 2 to 4 pm daily (to 5 pm in summer), although those readers accredited could use the room from 9.30 am to 4 pm. An 'educated man' was requested from the University Council as an additional attendant, spending time at the University Library in the morning and at the Hocken Library in the afternoon. And, finally, the Picture Room was to be open at the same time as the museum: every weekday from 9.30 am till 4 pm (5 pm in summer), and on Sundays till 2 pm. A record of users was to be started.

As in any building project, there were compromises. There were also problems, some ongoing. Hocken wanted the best materials for his wing. Kauri shelving for the books was too expensive, and instead they would be made from 'well-seasoned Red Pine from the North Island, where it is stacked for some years before use'.[51] This passed the test. After viewing the new building in late October 1909, John Halliday Scott remarked to his daughters Marion and Helen:

> The Hocken Wing at the museum is at the north end of the main block. It is now almost ready to receive Dr Hocken's books ... There are two rooms on the second floor to be devoted to his collections, one a library, the other for pictures, portraits, plans etc. The bookcases are red pine and look very nice, and there is a most eloquent fireplace in the library. I suppose the transfer of the stuff will come off during next summer.[52]

John Burnside was doing his best. By 24 February 1909 he was ready to show Hocken the proposed fittings for the interior, but Hocken was too ill to attend and the meeting was postponed.[53] Eventually the tenders were settled, with Scott and Wilson getting the work for 16 Holland blinds (£9 8s 6d, including brass rod); David Scott for painting the walls but not the ceiling (£23 15s); and the Ormand Brothers for kalsomining the ceiling of the Lower Hall (£5 13s).[54] The surroundings of the new wing were also of concern. The footpath in King Street, the garden of shrubs and plants and the iron railings were successfully tendered for by A. & T. Burt but the trustees were not pleased with the outcome, calling the firm's attempt 'a very unsatisfactory piece of work'.[55]

In October 1909 problems arose with the work of painter-plasterer Orr Campbell. Plaster was peeling off the gallery wall, and even after repeated instructions, Campbell had taken little care with the new linoleum. Burnside, a man who obviously took pride in his work, reported to the trustees that the plaster work had to be redone.[56] The problem lingered: as late as December 1909 Burnside was 'at' Campbell about the necessary repainting.[57] Campbell was also responsible for cleaning and repolishing three pieces of cabinet work in which the drawers had split. Benham told Burnside: 'Let Mr Campbell understand that he will be held responsible.'[58] Campbell could perhaps afford any additional charges: by 8 February 1909 he had already been paid £2300.[59]

William Nees, the glazier, was also causing delays. In late December

1909 Benham wrote to Burnside that 'there is a hole made by Nees while working at the bookshelves which requires to be filled: I presume at their expense. Messrs Nees should be hurried up with the screens, and the glazing of the book cases and the keys for the same.' Benham was concerned that the transfer of the books would delay the opening now planned for 31 March 1910. Action was demanded: 'We are, of course, relying on you as Architect to urge the work forward, and I shall be glad to hear from you that steps have been taken in this direction.'[60]

Hocken still played his part. Keen to get his pictures and prints framed for the opening, he asked David Scott, the painter, for a quote on oak frames. Scott replied, giving various sizes: the largest was 76.2 x 50.8 cm at 6s; the smallest 30 x 25.4 cm at 2s 6d. There were limits: 'you cannot fit anything larger than 60 in x 40 in [152.4 x 101.6 cm] in light glass'.[61] Hocken was still working on this in September, as he reported to Charles Wilson: 'I am intently engaged in framing and describing the pictures &c & roughly cataloguing the books – another great labour.' He added his concern about the money running out: 'I wish some of your wealthy Wellington folks would give donations for a librarian. The whole of the £6000 has been spent in a museum wing & its fittings & no provision left for the due care of so important a collection.'[62]

Hocken reiterated his desire for the right man as librarian in a letter to Fenwick written in March 1910.

> The librarian of this institution should, indeed, be an archivist – a man of culture, a man with some predilections for historical research; in short, a man who would be more than a librarian in the ordinary sense of the term. He should have a thorough knowledge of the books, and be able to help students and scholars to investigate the numerous subjects that here have been slightly indicated.[63]

On 15 March 1910, approximately two weeks before the opening, William Heywood Trimble was offered the position of librarian for two years at £200 per annum.[64] His duties were to arrange and catalogue the books in the Hocken Library and prepare a catalogue of the collection for printing. Consideration was also given to a catalogue for Hocken's pictures. Trimble's hours of attendance were to be fixed by the trustees, who were keen to have him: 'I hope that you will be able to accept this appointment. I may tell you that all the Trustees were anxious that you would. The books are arriving now, so that the work could commence at once.'[65]

W. Heywood Trimble, as he liked to be called, was born on 21 January 1860 in Lancashire. In 1875 his family migrated to New Zealand and settled near Inglewood in Taranaki, where his father eventually became an MP.[66] Employed as a cadet in the Crown Lands Office, New Plymouth, young Trimble was eventually promoted and transferred to Christchurch. In 1881 his salary was £150 per annum. In July 1885 he married Henrietta Mary Rogers

Penn; their daughter Dorothy Heywood married John Wylie Stewart. Following Henrietta's death in 1897 Trimble married Annie Eliza Nelson on 9 May 1899 in Christchurch. After he was made redundant from the Public Works Department on 9 October 1909 he opened a bookshop in Dunedin's George Street, and later helped in Driver's Bookshop and Newbold's. Trimble amassed a significant collection of the works by and about American poet Walt Whitman, which his daughter donated to the Dunedin Public Library after his death in 1927. Trimble was not unknown to Hocken. In 1893 he saved 'a bundle of the wet papers' of New Plymouth's J.T. Wicksteed, transcribed them and gave Hocken a copy in 1908.[67] A year after this, on 11 September 1908, Trimble wrote to Hocken about two separate matters: the notion of the descendants of the Pilgrim Fathers reverting to the American Indian type and dying out; and a book on the *Bounty* and information on relics associated with Captain William Bligh, obtained through Trimble's brother-in-law Ernest Nutting, the great-grandson of the great navigator.[68] Trimble tantalised Hocken with the bullet Bligh used to weigh out his men's allowance of bread, the gourd from which the men drank their water and the compass by which they steered their 3618-mile course to Timor.

Fortunately a 'Journal of Librarian' survives that details Trimble's tasks leading up to the opening day.[69] He started work two days after receiving the offer from the trustees. On Thursday 17 March he began sorting out the newspapers, assisted by a boy called Phillips. The next day more books arrived, which Trimble promptly placed on shelves, helped this time by Benham and Phillips. The day was broken up by a call on Hocken. On 19 March more books appeared, and Benham was there again to assist. Phillips was charged with unpacking the great pile of *Sydney Morning Herald*s. Sunday allowed for a break, with work continuing on Monday with 'further loads rec'd'. The following days were taken up with sorting, and on 24 March some manuscripts arrived. During this time, one of Bessie's sisters called in. No work was done over the Easter break except for the Saturday, when Trimble wrote 'sorting just about completed'. On this occasion he had help from his wife. On 29 March, two days before the opening, Trimble completed the sorting and had a bevy of callers, including the public librarian from Gisborne and Evelyn Culverwell from Dunedin's Carnegie Library. The following day, in between some rearranging, Trimble had to deal with receiving a 'small load of etceteras', whatever they were.

The Official Opening

On 31 March 1910 the Governor, Lord Plunket, opened the new Hocken Wing. The ceremony took place in the lower room of the museum, which, as the *Otago Daily Times* reported, was 'prettily decorated with flags, the Union Jack being placed at the rear of the platform'.[70] Present were many Dunedin dignitaries, including William Downie Stewart, collectors and philanthropists

Willi Fels and David Theomin, and Benham. Premier Sir Joseph Ward was also present. Gladys was the only one of the Hocken family to attend.[71] Hocken's friend Judge Frederick Revans Chapman could not be there and sent a telegram: 'I congratulate you on having reached the point of dedicating your collection to the public – a noble and patriotic work. Such will have enduring result'.[72]

George Fenwick, chairman of the Hocken Library Trustees and perhaps Hocken's closest friend, began the proceedings by apologising for the fact that Hocken, 'the generous donor', was not present. He was too ill to attend the ceremony and see his collection of some 4300 printed books and pamphlets, photographs, maps, drawings, paintings and manuscripts in place. Nevertheless, Fenwick claimed that Hocken would 'rejoice with us at the fruition of his long-cherished hope that his great library should be installed in a public building for the use of the people'. Fenwick reminded his listeners of Hocken's remark back in the 1890s: 'It would be well to celebrate the jubilee of Otago by making a strong effort to get some fine building erected in which the archives of this settlement and many valuable and interesting things connected with its early history might be suitably housed.'[73] He then read Hocken's letter (see Appendix I) on how and why he collected his materials, the drive of collecting and an overview of the collection strengths. Mention was made of Hocken's collection of Japanese materials and his Maori artefacts (weapons, implements, ornaments, carvings and tattooed heads), destined specifically for the ethnographic department of the museum.[74]

Fenwick ended by summing up his friend, his words interrupted by regular applause:

> In that letter ... Dr Hocken has said everything that need be said to enable you to realise of what great value to New Zealand is the collection, which will be for all time associated with his name ... He has done more: for throughout it there is revealed that love of country and that entirely unselfish nature which have been characteristic of him during his long life in this community. He is the possessor in a high degree of that humanitarian spirit which, allied to the deep patriotism woven into every fibre of his nature, has endeared him to friends and caused him to be honored throughout the whole community.

Lord Plunket, who had written to Hocken expressing his regret that he could not be present, spoke of the 'excellent collection ... You have here practically the whole history of this Dominion'. Plunket then congratulated everyone present on this 'magnificent acquisition' and unveiled a marble tablet with the inscription:

> This wing was erected in 1908 by public subscription, aided by a subsidy from the Government, for the accommodation and preservation of the

generous gift to the people of New Zealand, made by Thomas Morland
Hocken, M.R.C.S., F.L.S., F.R.G.S., F.R. Anth. Inst.. etc consisting of
his books, pictures, and other documents relating to the early history of
Australasia especially New Zealand.[75]

Ward reiterated his own personal satisfaction in assisting the funding of
the Hocken building and securing a librarian. He also mentioned Hocken's
altruism, which will 'cause his name to be enthroned in the hearts not only of
the people of Dunedin, but of all who, in the future, will take an interest in the
old historical records and pictures he has presented to the people'. Although
it was 'a fine thing … for persons of means to make great benefactions in
their wills', someone who, 'during his lifetime, disinterestedly gives up a valuable
and hard-won treasure for the benefit of the community is worthy of
still higher praise'. He also pointed out that Hocken must have 'spent a little
fortune in binding and framing the works, apart from the labour and expense
he must have incurred in collecting'. He was certain that 'the memory of Dr
Hocken, who, I hope, will soon recover from his illness … will live in the
minds of our people for all time, and that his name will stand out as that of
one who did this noble deed during his lifetime'. Hocken's gift was then open
for inspection.

Of course not all the collection was fully ordered, and there was 'a tentative
arrangement' for the occasion; there would be a more detailed arrangement
when time permitted. This is certainly evident in Trimble's journal, where the
words 're-arranged' or 're-arranging' occur often. He was also obliged to write
his first report and deal with visitors: 'explained the library to 2 ladies from
New Plymouth and a Marist Brother' (1 April); 'callers – Mr Justice Chapman,
Mr Bathgate' (11 April); and 'showed two ladies (from Ch'church) over books'
(12 April). Trimble was also a dab hand at conservation, having to repair and
sew up the 'Auckland Provincial Records' (15 April) and House of Commons
papers (18 April).

Readers were given a glimpse of what was on show, albeit temporarily, in
'A Glance at the Books', which appeared in the *Otago Daily Times* on 1 April
1910. Hocken's pamphlets were described as the 'Heart of the Collection',
with 'reference to practically every subject under the sun'. Indeed, although
large – some 2800 pamphlets eventually bound into 218 volumes – it was by
no means comprehensive. Still, this 'library in miniature' represented a fine
start. There were the documents pertaining to the missionaries, synod histories
and records relating to the Roman Catholic faith abroad. There were
then the so-called 'literary' magazines, which included the *Otago Journal*, the
New Zealand Magazine, the *New Zealand Review*, *Chapman's Monthly Review*
and others. Hocken's Maori language collection also got a mention and was
lauded as complete, although it was not. The items had been saved, however,
and Hocken had made a brave effort in trying to document them in

his *Bibliography*. The legislative materials followed – acts and amendments of provincial and national governments, the Colonial Society reports, the New Zealand Company reports and the New Zealand *Hansard*. They were, said the report, 'dignified in their massiveness'. Then there were the Australian materials. In another 'cupboard' were New Zealand reference books, which included Hocken's Marsden material, arranged alphabetically 'pending final classification'. With this manuscript collection was the volume of letters addressed to Colonel Wakefield, dated 1840 to 1844, which was certainly Trimble's volume. Other 'cupboards' were taken up by Hocken's books on and about explorers. The article passed over those books that contained lithographed prints of early New Zealand to touch on relics, such as a rifle and bayonet found at the French stockade at Akaroa. Hocken's pictures, hung separately, proved very popular.

In conclusion, the writer recognised the immense value of Hocken's gift, and its legacy. 'Not in immediate years will these books be properly valued save by the few; but when New Zealand is as old in civilisation as Europe now is, then the record of these books will be as a gold mine to the historian and antiquarian.'[76]

The donor never saw his collection so housed, yet Hocken knew his personal obligations and the importance that such a gift can bring to a nation. It is no wonder that collectors are called patriots.

> This work has been to me a labour of love, and in it I have put into practice a sentiment I have always held: that it is the bounden duty of every citizen to do something for his State, in the welfare of which his own happiness and prosperity is very largely found. This feeling, I have long considered, should animate every member of the community – from the highest to the lowest, – for only in its increasing observance may a country expect a diminution of those troubles which often occur, and against which this feeling of patriotism and loyalty forms the best protection. A desire, then, to, in some measure, do something for the people among whom I have so long sojourned and the country in which I have so long resided has been the actuating motive in the formation of this collection which I have presented to the Dominion of New Zealand.[77]

20
The Hocken Legacy

On 7 June 1910, after reading the account of the ceremony on 31 March, Dublin-based Judge F.W. Pennefather wrote to Hocken with 'great pleasure' on his 'splendid gift' to the university. Trusting that his illness was 'nothing serious', Pennefather continued: 'May I say that I was specially glad that the gift was made to *the University*; it is a hopeful sight for the country when the University becomes the centre of all literary work; literature is too noble to be mixed up with politics, whether colonial or municipal …'[1] Hocken never read this letter. Attended by Dr Louis E. Barnett, he died of carcinoma of the oesophagus about 8 pm on Tuesday 17 May. He was 74 years old.

Banker and historian Thomas Hodgkin and his brother George had visited 'dear old Dr Hocken' in April 1909: 'He was in bed with a shawl round his head suffering from a severe cold but he was very friendly, seemed pleased to see us & sent affectionate messages to [their brother] Howard.'[2] In mid-December 1909 Hocken managed to travel to Rotorua, and in early February 1910 he and Bessie made a quick trip to Melbourne in the hope that doctors there could find out what was wrong with him. According to John Halliday Scott: 'I don't think he learned much more than he knew before. He is certainly not looking well, and he is worrying about getting his collections ready for shifting to their new quarters at the museum, in what is known as the Hocken Wing.'[3] A few days before Hocken's death Scott called to see him: despite talking 'quite cheerfully', his friend had 'shrunk away to nothing'.[4] On 16 May, and in what must have been a poignant moment, Hocken managed to sign, along side his wife's signature, a note reading: 'Please note that in future any cheques in my name will be signed as follows.' This declaration was positioned below his earliest extant writing, done back in 1842 and kept by his mother.

Hundreds attended the funeral, which was held at St Paul's Cathedral. Bessie received telegrams of condolence from Lord Plunket, Sir Joseph Ward, the Hon. Thomas Mackenzie, Sir Samuel Way, W.F. Massey, Sir Robert Stout, Alexander Turnbull and Downie Stewart. Hocken was buried in the Northern Cemetery, and the pallbearers were Drs Scott, Colquhoun, Barnett and Batchelor, George Fenwick and Horatio Massey, an Invercargill businessman and husband to Hocken's niece, Judith. Wreaths came from groups such as the University Council, the Otago branch of the Medical Association, the directors and staff of the *Otago Daily Times* and *Witness*, the Standard Insurance Company, the Otago Institute, the St Paul's Cathedral Committee, the Victoria League, the Canterbury Philosophical Society and Otago University medical students. The terms of Hocken's will (see Appendix II) revealed how many investments and shares he and Bessie had, including at one point shares in the

Kaitangata Railway and Coal Company; he had been a director in the Cromwell Gold Dredging Company, the Riverbank Gold Dredging Company and the Dunedin Peninsula and Ocean Beach Railway Company.[5] The value of his estate was said to be £26,000.[6] There was also his generosity towards community organisations. Although Bessie was the prime beneficiary, those who benefited from the sale of the shares included the University of Otago (some £10,000), the Anglican Diocese of Dunedin, the Maori Mission Board, the Salvation Army (equal shares between the Heriot Row Maternity Home, the Rescue Home at Caversham and the Children's Home in Middlemarch), the Dunedin Public Art Gallery and the Trinity Methodist Church. At one point, Hocken made provision in his will for

> income ... in payment of the Salary of a cultured librarian who will utilise his whole time in looking after and keeping in good order and from time to time as occasion shall require in cataloguing the Collection of Books Manuscripts Newspapers other documents Pictures Prints Photographs Drawings and other articles of a similar character in relation to the Early History of the Colony of New Zealand and the Australian Colonies given by me to the Public of the said Dominion of New Zealand now housed in the wing or addition to the Museum erected on the Otago University Museum Reserve ...'[7]

However, in a codicil added almost a year later he revoked this clause, hoping that the 'Citizens of Dunedin will raise sufficient funds to answer means of the ... yearly salary of a Cultured Librarian ...'[8] Unfortunately, this optimism was misplaced.

Council Matters

The days following the opening ceremony found the Hocken Wing still incomplete. Structural work, such as affixing battens near the stairways to create cupboards and further painting and distempering, was still required.[9] Hocken's Maori artefacts also needed housing, and suitable glass display cases had to be made. Tenders were called for and received from Herbert Haynes Co. Ltd (£92 15s), C. & W. Hayward (£130) and the troublesome William Nees who, within his costing of £92, included door locks and offered the option of red pine instead of kauri; the former cheaper by about £9.[10] Nees was successful. The cabinets and cases were to encroach on 'half the floor space' on the lower floor of the wing, allowing the public to see items such as mats, carvings and other objects, including 'a smoked Maori head' that Hocken had obtained from Robley.[11] Although this encroachment was not part of the original agreement, Benham, the force behind the initiative to display these artefacts, hoped that the University Council would agree to the move.[12] On 8 April 1910 he wrote asking for permission 'to utilise so much of the Lower Hall as is necessary for the adequate accommodation and exhibition of these Maori objects.' The council eventually agreed, as part of their responsibility towards the collection.[13]

Trimble as Hocken Librarian

Throughout all this, Trimble did his best as the public face of the Hocken Collection. He not only had to compile a catalogue of the collection, but further arrange it, make running repairs to items, dispatch book and pamphlet consignments to the binder, deal with incoming materials and show the collection off to visitors. Bessie recognised the importance of Trimble's role even before her husband died. In late March 1910 she sent the blocks that were used for illustrating Shortland's book on New Zealand and those used to illustrate the second edition of Robley's *Moko*, a work heavily annotated by Hocken.[14] Acknowledging that the latter was one of Hocken's unfinished projects, she wrote: 'My dear husband wishes it to be known that the blocks are in the collection so that if someone in the future should desire to bring out the fresh edition they could be used for the purpose.'[15]

Trimble's monthly reports are revealing. On 16 May 1910 he had made a 'fair start' on the catalogue, and informed the trustees that there were books and pamphlets requiring binding.[16] Hocken's gift motivated others to give books to the collection and, as a consequence, items poured in. Apart from a few early acquisitions such as Alexander Verner's *Clairvoyance* (probably his *Medical Hypnotism and Suggestion*), Joseph Taylor's *Principles of Absolute Philosophy*, *Cremation versus Earth-burial*, the *Rules of the Taranaki Philosophical Society* and two spiritualist pamphlets, there was 'a large mass of old newspapers' received from the estate of Mrs Christina Chapman, which needed sorting and arranging.[17] The library was 'very dirty', and there was no prospect of cleaning it until the Chapman papers were dealt with and a cache of Australian newspapers were removed from the floor.[18] On 17 June 1910 Trimble reported that he had sorted the Chapman newspapers and catalogued 80 volumes of Hocken's pamphlet collection, some 1046 pamphlets in total. His prediction was that he would finish the rest by mid-July. Classification was happening simultaneously, making the catalogue available for reference. Indeed, the collection was already being used, and according to Trimble, 'more people are interested in the "History of Australasia and of New Zealand in particular", than appears to be generally supposed'. With security a continuing issue, Trimble pointed out that all the presses now had locks, so that no one unauthorised could handle the books. He also asked if he could purchase 5000 more index cards to aid classification and cataloguing.[19]

A month later, Trimble expressed a new confidence. 'I have noted your instructions to have the loose pamphlets bound; but the receipt of many fresh ones has disturbed the arrangement of those I had ready for the binder; and I am leaving over the final division into volumes of convenient size until I am *certain* that there are no more to come in.' He continued: 'The Cataloguing of the books is so far advanced that I think the "No Admission" notice on the glass door may as well be removed. So far as the books are catalogued and classified they are easily referred to; and I am sufficiently intimate with most of the collection to be able to find almost any book that may be asked for.'[20] At this stage only 140 books had been catalogued and classified, and there were more items on the horizon. McNab had visited Trimble and suggested that, to keep the library up to date, the trustees apply to the Government Printer for all forthcoming government publications.

By December, 2640 volumes (presumably books) and 2865 pamphlets and miscellaneous papers had been classified and catalogued. Daniel Colquhoun donated a number of books on exploration in Egypt, and his and all other donations and acquisitions were reported in the newspaper for all to read. A severe storm that month resulted in water damage to the doors on the presses. Because they did not now shut properly, Trimble recommended that they be fixed immediately.[21]

On 5 June 1911 Trimble reported that he had 'completed the Card Catalogue of the Hocken Library', and had broken it down to 3817 bound books and newspapers, 145 volumes of pamphlets, 12 volumes of various papers and 11 volumes of 'Flotsam and Jetsam' – a total of 6958, which had been catalogued on 11,986 cards. Trimble was quick to say that there was much more that required binding, cataloguing and classifying: pamphlets, 'Variae' materials, periodicals and newspapers. There were also '10 parcels of Manuscripts which have not been examined.'[22] And because he had only started typing up the catalogue, many of them would not be in the printed version. A month later, he retracted this statement. Some of 160 volumes of uncatalogued material were deemed so important that he appealed to the trustees for £60 towards binding. Quite rightly, he felt 'the loss of interest on that amount would be trifling; and the gain to the Library would be very great'.[23] He was given £25 and the 'very plainest style' of binding was shared between binders Thompson (High Street) and Campbell (Moray Place). For Trimble, the 67 volumes represented another 2000 entries in the catalogue. He also tabulated the entire stock: 4137 bound volumes, 5025 contents of volumes of miscellaneous papers, 420 manuscripts catalogued, less 224 volumes of miscellaneous papers – total (incorrectly added) of 9338 (i.e. 9358). He had used 14,000 cards, and he valued the library at £20,000.[24] A bitter blow during all this was the death of his wife in July 1911.[25]

The catalogue still involved work. On 24 October he predicted that with 'scissors and paste' the draft would be ready for the printer by 11 November 1911. Owing to the entries of books that were now being bound, some of his past work was useless and would have to be redone. And then there was the proofing of the final copy: he was 'the proper person to correct them'. To this end, he suggested an extension of three months to his contract, finishing on 17 June 1912. This was accepted.[26]

The first portion of Trimble's draft copy was actually submitted for tender by Fenwick on 1 September 1911, with advice that more would follow. The specifications were: 'Type to be breviar, good quality of paper, weight 60 lbs, double-royal, number of copies 2,000; binding, buckram.'[27] The *Otago Daily Times* was the successful bidder, and 2000 copies were finally printed in October 1912, with a title page containing Trimble's name and a brief preface by William Downie Stewart. It did not incorporate any of the 429 pictures in Hocken's original collection; 36 years would pass before these were formally listed.

The effect among some book circles was immediate. Within two days of receiving a copy of the catalogue, Turnbull wrote to Downie Stewart: 'You can imagine with what interest I have been looking through the volume – looking through it without a tinge of envy – because though I am a greedy collector I have never been an envious one.' He praised the series of early missionary manuscripts: 'if the Library contained nothing else but these it would be in the front of all New Zealand Collections'. He was, however, astonished at the absence of many well-known works on New Zealand that he thought Hocken would surely own, since they were described. Despite the errors inherent in the work, it remained the first access point to most of Hocken's collections for users for many years.

Trimble liked his job. On 1 June 1912, 17 days before his contract ended, he appealed to George Fenwick for what was more than an extension: 'The last time I called upon you, you mentioned that £100 per year had been promised or provided for, I think, five years, to enable the recording work of the library to be continued. I then told you that I was willing to go on with the work, with reduced hours, for that salary, but I do not think that any final arrangement was made.' He also pointed out that his current work was sorting out newspapers and recording those important events reported in them, which 'Dr Hocken regarded ... as very important.'[28] The appeal did not work, and Trimble's final report was submitted nine days later.[29] Apart from reiterating figures already covered in previous reports and repeating the need to index the historical newspapers, Trimble mentioned Hocken's large collection of historical maps. Only 74 had been catalogued and many were still in rolls, unmounted.[30] The drawers in which some were housed were too narrow and needed replacement. Although an air of disappointment surrounded the report, Trimble was positive: 'The work of cataloguing this collection has been most fascinating. I think I may say that during my twenty-seven months' work in the library I have not spent a solitary dull hour ... The whole experience has resulted in my regarding Dr Hocken as one of the most industrious men I have ever met with.' And finally he made a prediction: 'Though not used very much at present, in a few years' time this Library will be recognised by scholars as a most valuable source of information; and is certain to be referred to very extensively.'[31]

Perhaps unbeknown to Trimble, there were moves afoot to keep him employed, and he may have had an inkling of the generosity of Bessie Hocken. She had agreed to give £100 annually for five years, the interest on this sum going towards the librarian's salary. There was also the money raised from the Endowment Fund, a city council grant of £25 and another £25 to be paid to the trustees for two years. A University Council meeting recommended using some of the interest accrued from these sums to employ Trimble again for another two years (from 17 June) and paying his salary 'per annum' as follows: £25 from the trustees, £24 from the Hocken Memorial Committee, £25 from the city council and £26 from the University Council. It also recommended using the other half of the interest to buy books for the collection and putting the interest on Bessie Hocken's generous gift towards the salary of the librarian.[32] It was also suggested that Trimble divide his time between the University Library and the Hocken Collection. Sadly, nothing came of these proposals, and from July to October 1912 he worked for no payment. On his last day, 31 October, Trimble spent time reading proofs of the catalogue, marking up a list for Alexander Bathgate, 'issuing cards for Mr Bathgate's books', recording Tasmanian papers, the *Australasian*, the *Southern Cross* and *Otago Gazette*s, arranging books received from A.F. McDonnell, replying to incoming letters and dealing with visitors.[33] On hearing that a young woman was to be employed to continue the newspaper indexing, he wrote to Benham from Lyttelton, suggesting that she contact him about the work.[34]

The Hocken Endowment Memorial Fund

There is often a double edge to any major bequest or gift. Securing Hocken's collection was a coup for Dunedin, but commitment was needed to look after it and enlarge it, as Hocken himself realised:

> In view of this gift being made to the Dominion, I feel that I might be quite justified in making this one request: that some persons who combine the possession of wealth, and who are imbued with those patriotic and public-spirited sentiments which I indicated in the early part of my letter, should take such steps as would result in the formation of a fund to adequately maintain the efficiency and usefulness of this collection which is about to be vested in the University Council. That body is unable to render financial aid, therefore outside assistance must be sought, and the fund, when established, given into the council's control.[35]

Robert McNab also recognised the need for ongoing funds:

> It must be understood that the collection cannot be kept even in its present condition, much less up to date, without the expenditure of a considerable sum of money. Students would come to this country to see the manuscripts alone, because of manuscripts there are no duplicates. The collection was worth thousands and thousands of pounds; it is amongst the

first collections in the world regarding Australasian historic literature; and it behoves the people of Dunedin to raise sufficient money to maintain it and keep it up to date.[36]

Because Hocken had deleted the 'income' provision from his will, and because the university 'was in such a chronic hard-up state' that it could not fully meet its obligations, the funding of the Hocken Library was soon proving problematic.[37] The Hocken Endowment (or Memorial) Fund was established in June 1910, with the aim of raising £6000 to provide for the salary of 'an intelligent librarian' and general maintenance of the collection. A prospectus was printed and sent out to individuals and institutions, including schools. The government was again approached for a pound-for-pound subsidy, with stress laid on the fact that Hocken's gift was to the Dominion and not just Dunedin. Sir Joseph Ward promised to put the proposal before the Cabinet for consideration, but on 3 September 1910 the *Evening Star* reported that 'the request is one that cannot be favourably entertained' and thus the fund-raising was left to Dunedin citizens and interested parties.[38]

Real and promised subscriptions did come in. No doubt because of Fenwick's association, the *Otago Daily Times* led the way with £50, followed by the same amount from Hallenstein Bros, P. Hayman and Co., J. Speight & Co., George Russell and two unknowns – 'Patriot' and 'Merchant'. With lesser amounts such as John Mee's 10s, F. Barkas's 5s, D. Patterson's 1 guinea and Dr Donald's 10s 6d, the total in mid-July had reached £624 14s 6d.[39] Annie E. Trimble's seven consecutive articles titled 'Raw material of history', which appeared in the *Evening Star* over October and November 1910, provided a boost. Covering 'The Hocken Library: A sketch of its contents', 'Pamphlets, deeds, and charts', 'Pictures and curios', 'Moko' and 'Mokomokai', she gave readers a real insight into the richness of Hocken's collection. She also recognised the process was a long-term one:

> All we have noticed has but touched the veriest surface. The depths are left still unexplored. An enormous mass of miscellaneous papers and manuscripts, perhaps the most valuable part of the collection, yet remains untouched, unbound, unclassified, and uncatalogued. Only when the whole is easy of access can the value of this magnificent gift be approximately estimated. The years will tell its worth.[40]

The desired amount of £6000 was never reached. To supplement the fund, Bessie sold duplicate items of the *New Zealand Gazette* still in her possession to Alexander Turnbull, duplicate newspapers to Downie Stewart and duplicate copies of the *Wellington Independent* to C.A. Ewen. Turnbull knew of the relatively poor response: 'I heard that the cash was not coming in fast & that not enough was likely to be collected to carry out the object for which the fund was started. Is this so?'[41] Robert McNab contributed by giving a public lecture on 'The early history of New Zealand' in the Art Gallery Hall on 3 August. The ticket sales of £18 8s 6d went to the fund, which by early September totalled £916 2s 4d.[42] In November a concerned Downie Stewart asked the city council, without success, for a supplement of £250 towards the museum and the Hocken Collection. Bessie also organised Maori and Pacific Island curios and artefacts to be sold through Park, Reynolds in September 1910, sold mere and greenstone chisels privately and sold to Augustus Hamilton and the museum the carved lizards (for £2) and other curios. All the proceeds were added to the fund.[43] She also asked Hamilton to value and dispose of additional curios: 'Does A. Turnbull buy Maori things I wonder?'[44] By 1913, £1495 had been collected; although a significant sum, it was not enough to meet the projected needs and future requirements of the Hocken Collection.[45]

When selling items to raise money Bessie often relied on the expertise of others to settle on a fair asking price. Given that the process was undoubtedly a sensitive one, she actually preferred the items to go back into the collection. It was certainly the easier option: 1913 and 1920 were key years of gifting books, sketches and artefacts. A hoeroa, a long weapon made from a whale's jaw-bone, was but one example. She had offered it to a collector for £60, but the deal fell through. To her, this item and others such as carved lintels, calabash rims, adzes, greenstone mere and even skirts and wedding dresses from Greece were better in the collection 'than knocking about the world'.[46] She also had a greenstone tiki that once belonged to the Maori wife of soldier, merchant and politician Isaac Newton Watt. On taking it to London to show General Robley, she decided to return it to the collection in Dunedin.[47] Quite rightly, 'by their gift to the Museum, further, of their large ethnographic collection, Dr and Mrs Hocken became the virtual founders of the Ethnographic Department of that institution'.[48] Print culture was not forgotten. Bessie sent through a copy of Stack's views of Auckland, and in October 1913 she discovered a 'box of Marsden papers – copies of his voyages' which were promptly dispatched to the library.[49] Family involvement did not end when she died in 1933. Gladys, living in Cape Town, continued to send items through, including a taiaha, a paddle-shaped cultivator and, later, family manuscripts.[50]

Despite the University Council's reluctance to spend any additional money on Hocken's gift, Benham had continued to push for greater financial commitment. As he wrote to James Allen, the university's chancellor, in August 1910: 'The Trustees think that the University Council should now definitely decide what annual sum they are prepared to set aside for the expenses of repairs and binding. It appears that a large number of pamphlets, which had Hocken lived would have been bound at his charge, will need binding in the course of a few months, when the librarian has examined and arranged them.'[51] On 30 August Allen replied that the building had not been handed over – 'not withstanding the Deed' – and that 'certain insurances' that had not been paid were the responsibility of the trustees, until such time as the building was handed over. 'I do not see how we can set aside any definite sum for repairs and binding, nor do I think it to be our duty to bind the pamphlets not already bound.' The Memorial Fund should pay for such work, including the librarian's salary.[52]

This situation continued into late September, even though Allen reluctantly agreed to provide funds for roller blinds to protect the Maori objects on display. 'I cannot take the responsibility of saying that it is a right charge to make against the University Council without knowing the position of the funds of the trustees.'[53] Although not wanting to commit further university funds, he was equally adamant about the spirit surrounding the gift: 'I am quite sure the Council will fulfil to the very utmost the responsibility that it took upon itself with regard to Dr Hocken's valuable gift. It goes without saying that they will do all in their power "to maintain the valuable and historic collection".'[54]

On 29 October 1910 a concerted effort by the trustees finally spelt out the situation to the University Council 'in the matter of the control of the Hocken Collection':

> That, according to the Deed of Gift, the Council is clearly under the obligation to take over the maintenance of the Hocken Collections in the Hocken Wing.
>
> It is true that there has been no ceremonial 'handing over' of the collections, nor is this deemed to be necessary.
>
> The books, pictures, etc have been open to the public for some months, and the Maori collection for some weeks. These are now under the care of the Curator of the Museum.
>
> As to balances of the Fund subscribed by the Public and the Government:
> – it will be used for the following purposes.
> 1. Salary of the Librarian
> 2. Cost of publication of a catalogue of the contents of the library
> 3. Any surplus will be handed over to the Endowment Fund now in course of collection
>
> The responsibility of the Trustees will cease when they have paid some outstanding accounts, for fitting up the Lower Hall of the Wing.[55]

The Hocken: Marching Forward

The fate of the Hocken Collection hung in the balance over the years that followed the official handover, and because it was tied integrally to financial support from the university, a brief overview is necessary. After Trimble came Beatrice Howes, who was part-time University Librarian and part-time Hocken Librarian. Henry Devenish Skinner, founding father of New Zealand anthropology, followed. In 1919 he was appointed librarian-in-charge of the

Hocken Library and also assistant curator at Otago Museum. Librarian until 1928, Skinner was given little or no funds to acquire books, and under his stewardship a decision was made to restrict new acquisitions to those published before 1901, leaving the Dunedin Public Library and their relatively newly acquired McNab Collection, officially handed over on 10 March 1914, to collect books after that period.[56] Hocken's *Bibliography* was thus the driving force for acquisitions, used to fill the gaps by buying books mentioned in it but not held within the collection.

Rachel Walker McDonald, who was the part-time librarian from 1926 to 1935, again had to deal with the shortfall of funds. Opening hours were restricted to Tuesday, Wednesday and Friday afternoons and, later, Saturday mornings. Despite this, McDonald was able to write in her annual report for 1926: 'upwards of eighty people, three-fourths of whom were students, have made use of the Library for periods ranging from a day to seven months'.[57]

Over the years, donations and acquisitions trickled in, with like attracting like. Items and collections received included watercolours by John Buchanan (1920s), the John Kinder collection of photographs and paintings (1922), letters from the Rev. Josiah Pratt of the CMS to Samuel Marsden, J.A. Gilfillan sketches, letters by Walter Buller (1934) and George Bayly's 1824–38 'Journal of Voyages' (1934). In 1936 'the most important single benefaction since Dr Hocken's foundation gift' arrived.[58] This was the bequest of Sir Frederick Chapman, which included books and a large run of pamphlets owned by Chapman and his father, Henry S. Chapman.

That same year Eric McCormick was appointed Hocken Librarian after a brief stint as acting librarian for Archie Dunningham at the Dunedin Public Library.[59] On £80 a year and part time, McCormick busied himself with the Hocken Collection, determined to make it more relevant to future users. The report written during his one-year tenure covered the scope of the collection, staffing, publications, cataloguing and collection emphasis. Because he was conscious that the library needed to buy more modern publications, the pre-1901 clause was revisited. McCormick was also dismayed at the lack of literary and foreign language publications. In later years, he wrote *The Fascinating Folly: Dr Hocken and his fellow collectors*, the seminal work on Grey, Turnbull and Hocken. Written as lectures to commemorate the jubilee of the Hocken Library and printed in 1961, this slim volume has stood the test of time. During McCormick's brief stay, full control of the library was moved from the museum to the university library.

In October 1935 the '*really* radical' John Harris was appointed University Librarian and took charge of the Hocken after McCormick's departure.[60] Harris was also hampered by the lack of funds, and the war years did not help: in 1946 there were only 41 readers and a fund of £53 that allowed for a paltry 111 items to be added. In 1948, perhaps owing to activities surrounding the Otago centenary, reader numbers rose to 132. That year, too, Harris left

THE NEW ZEALAND ADVERTISER,
AND
Bay of Islands Gazette.

No. 1.]   KORORARIKA, JUNE 15, 1840.   [Vol. I.

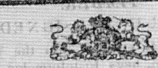

THE GAZETTE.
NEW ZEALAND.

NOTICE IS HEREBY GIVEN, that all communications from this Government inserted in the "NEW ZEALAND ADVERTISER AND BAY OF ISLANDS GAZETTE," are to be deemed official.

Given under my Hand at Government-House, Russell, this 12th day of June, in the year of our Lord 1840.
W. HOBSON,
LIEUT. GOVERNOR.

By His Excellency's Command,
(For the Colonial Secretary,)
JAS. STUART FREEMAN.

PROCLAMATION.

In the Name of Her Majesty VICTORIA, Queen of the United Kingdom of Great Britain and Ireland, By WILLIAM HOBSON, Esquire, a Captain in the Royal Navy, Lieutenant Governor of New Zealand.

WHEREAS I have it in Command from Her Majesty Queen VICTORIA, through Her principal Secretary of State for the Colonies, to assert the Sovereign Rights of Her Majesty over the Southern Islands of New Zealand, commonly called "The Middle Island," and "Stewart's Island;" and, also, the Island commonly called "The Northern Island," the same having been ceded in Sovereignty to Her Majesty.

Now, therefore, I, WILLIAM HOBSON, Lieutenant Governor of New Zealand, do hereby proclaim and declare to all men, that from and after the date of these Presents, the full Sovereignty of the Islands of New Zealand, extending from thirty-four Degrees thirty minutes North to forty-seven Degrees ten minutes South Latitude, and between one hundred and sixty-six Degrees five minutes to one hundred and seventy-nine Degrees of East Longitude, vests in Her Majesty Queen VICTORIA, her Heirs and Successors for ever.

Given under my Hand at Government-House, Russell, Bay of Islands, this twenty-first day of May, in the year of our Lord one thousand eight hundred and forty.

(Signed) WILLIAM HOBSON,
LIEUTENANT GOVERNOR.

By His Excellency's Command,
(Signed) WILLOUGHBY SHORTLAND,
Colonial Secretary.
GOD SAVE THE QUEEN!

PROCLAMATION.

In the Name of Her Majesty VICTORIA, Queen of the United Kingdom of Great Britain and Ireland, By WILLIAM HOBSON, Esquire, a Captain in the Royal Navy, Lieutenant Governor of New Zealand.

WHEREAS by a Treaty bearing date the fifth day of February, in the year of our Lord one thousand eight hundred and forty, made and executed by me, WILLIAM HOBSON, a Captain in the Royal Navy, Consul, and Lieutenant-Governor in New Zealand, vested for this purpose with full powers by Her Britannic Majesty, of the one part, and the Chiefs of the Confederation of the United Tribes of New Zealand, and the separate and independent Chiefs of New Zealand, not Members of the Confederation of the other; and further ratified and confirmed by the adherence of the Principal Chiefs of this Island of New Zealand, commonly called "The Northern Island," all Rights and Powers of Sovereignty over the said Northern Island were ceded to Her Majesty the Queen of Great Britain and Ireland, absolutely and without reservation.

Now, therefore, I, WILLIAM HOBSON, Lieutenant Governor of New Zealand, in the Name and on the Behalf of Her Majesty, do hereby Proclaim and Declare to all Men, that from and after the date of the above-mentioned Treaty, the full Sovereignty of the Northern Island of New Zealand, vests in Her Majesty Queen VICTORIA, Her Heirs and Successors for ever.

Given under my Hand at Government-House, Russell, Bay of Islands, this twenty-first day of May, in the year of our Lord one thousand eight hundred and forty.

(Signed) WILLIAM HOBSON,
LIEUTENANT GOVERNOR.

By His Excellency's Command,
(Signed) WILLOUGHBY SHORTLAND,
Colonial Secretary.
GOD SAVE THE QUEEN!

GOVERNMENT NOTICE.

Colonial Secretary's Office,
Russell, 9th June, 1840.

HIS EXCELLENCY THE LIEUTENANT GOVERNOR has been pleased to direct that notice of the following Appointments having been made under this Government from the dates set opposite the respective names, be published for general information:—

Major THOMAS BUNBURY, 80th Regiment, commanding Her Majesty's Troops in New Zealand, appointed a Magistrate of the Territory—30th March, 1840.

WILLOUGHBY SHORTLAND, Esquire, J.P., Acting Colonial Secretary and Registrar of Records—7th March, 1840.

FELTON MATHEW, Esquire, J.P., Surveyor General—1st January, 1840.

JOHN JOHNSON, Esquire, M.D., J.P., Colonial Surgeon—6th February, 1840.

WILLIAM DAVIES, Esquire, M.D., Surgeon, Health Officer—1st June, 1840.

WILLIAM CORNWALLIS SYMONDS, Esquire, Police Magistrate—17th March, 1840.

CHARLES BARRINGTON ROBINSON, Esquire, Police Magistrate—28th March, 1840.

MICHAEL MURPHY, Esquire, Police Magistrate—30th March, 1840.

H. D. SMART, Lieut. 28th Regiment, Magistrate of the Territory—1st January, 1840.

JAMES READY CLENDON, Esquire, Magistrate of the Territory—21st February 1840.

THOMAS BECKHAM, Esquire, Magistrate of the Territory—17th March, 1840.

Mr. WILLIAM MASON, Superintendent of Public Works—1st March, 1840.

Mr. CHARLES LOGIE, Colonial Storekeeper—15th January, 1840.

By His Excellency's Command,
(For the Colonial Secretary,)
JAS. STUART FREEMAN.

GOVERNMENT NOTICE.

Colonial Secretary's Office,
Russell, 29th May, 1840.

NOTICE is hereby given, that in the absence of WILLOUGHBY SHORTLAND, Esquire, Colonial Secretary, the duties of that Office will be performed by JAMES STUART FREEMAN, Esquire, who has been duly appointed to the charge of the Colonial Office, until the return of the former Gentleman to the Seat of Government.

By His Excellency's Command,
(For the Colonial Secretary,)
JAS. STUART FREEMAN.

GOVERNMENT NOTICE.

Colonial Secretary's Office,
Russell, 10th June, 1840.

MAIZE.

TENDERS will be received at this Office until twelve o'clock of Tuesday, the 30th instant, for the supply of "Three Hundred Bushels of Maize," to be delivered at this Station.

Parties tendering, or their Agents, are requested to attend at this Office on the day of opening the offers.

Security for the due fulfilment of the Contract will be required.

By His Excellency's Command,
(For the Colonial Secretary,)
JAS. STUART FREEMAN.

Sales by Auction.

To be Sold by Public Auction,
By W. Wilson,
At his Rooms on Thursday, 18th June, 1840, at 11 o'clock,

ONE case Navy blue prints
1 bale calico
6 Hhds. rum, 19 O. P.
4 Hhds.
4 ditto porter
Cross-cut saws
Spades
2 Tents.

ALSO,
Two Shares in the Kororarika Land Company.

Terms made known at time of Sale.

For Sale by Public Auction,
By W. Wilson,
At his Rooms, on Thursday, 18th June, at 12 o'clock,

ONE valuable black Horse, suited for saddle or harness.
Terms at time of sale.

PREVIOUS PAGE: Vol. 1 No. 1 (15 June 1840) of the *New Zealand Advertiser and Bay of Islands Gazette*, the country's second newspaper. Hocken was proud of his newspaper collection, and especially his copies of the *New Zealand Advertiser*. He showed this item, among others, to Otago Institute members in July 1901. *S14-081c, Hocken Collections, Uare Taoka o Hakena, University of Otago*

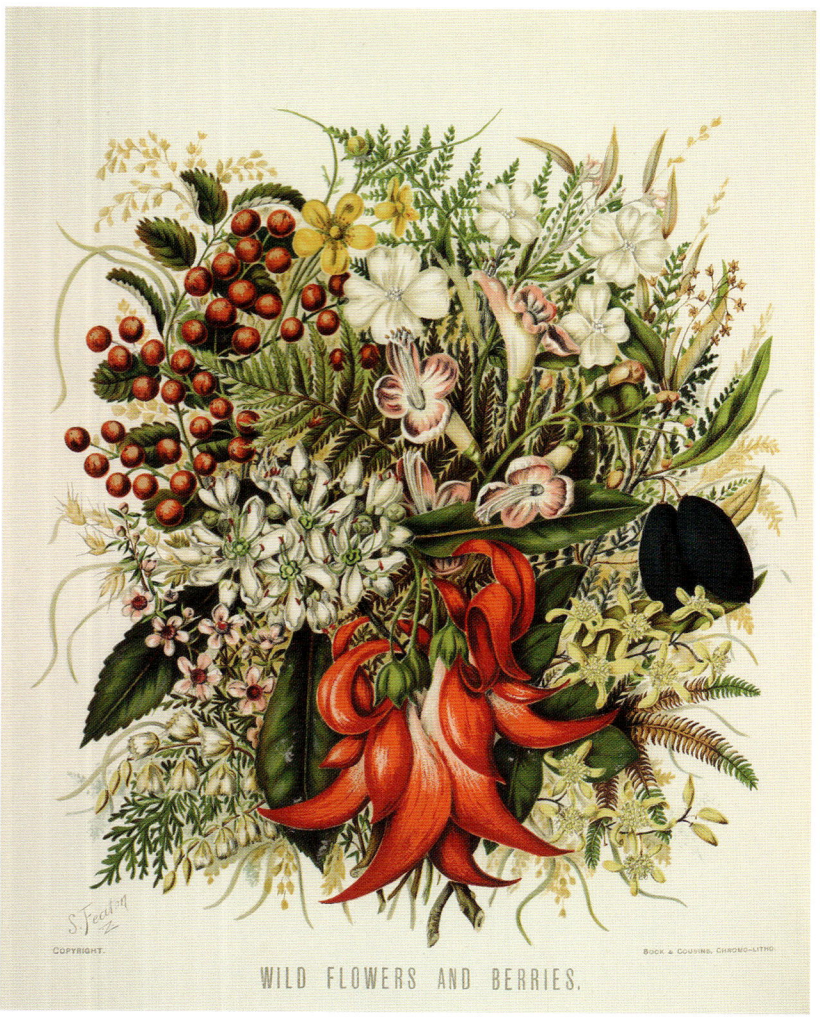

Edward Henry Featon and Sarah Featon *The Art Album of New Zealand Flora* (1889) was the first fully chromolithographic book to be published in New Zealand. Given his interest in botany, Hocken was delighted to secure this copy of 'Mrs Featon's Art Album', as it is more commonly known. *S14-081d, Hocken Collections, Uare Taoka o Hakena, University of Otago*

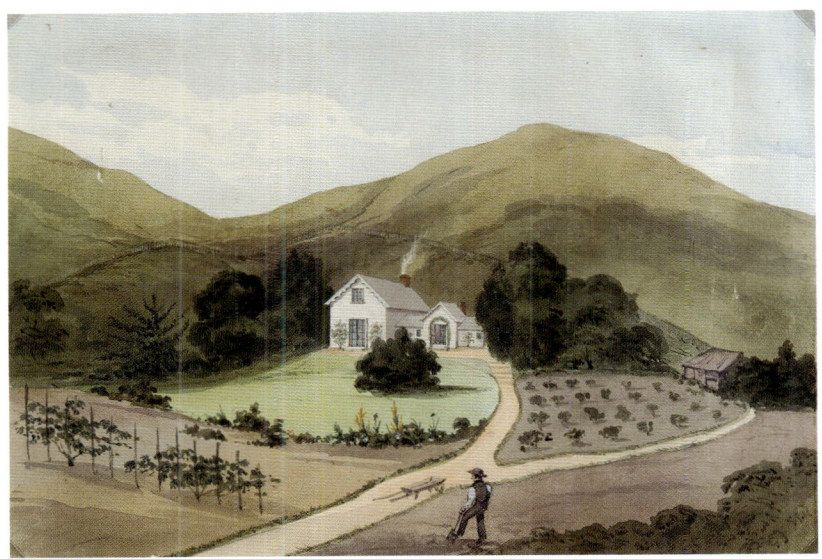

William Fox, *W. Fox's House, Nelson* (1848). Because Fox knew of Hocken's great interest in 'old New Zealand', he bequeathed 118 of his own pictures to the southern collector Hocken was inordinately proud of this collection.
4274-31, Hocken Collections, Uare Taoka o Hakena, University of Otago

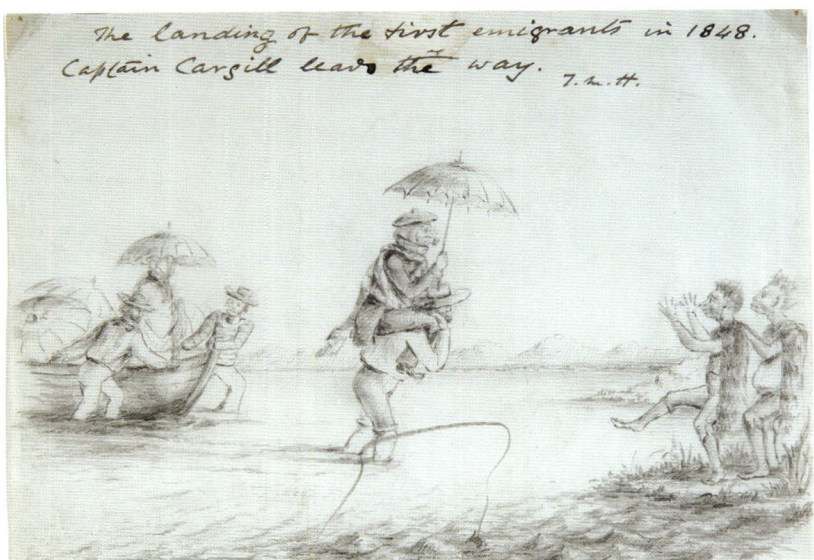

James Brown, 'The landing of the first emigrants in 1848' (1848). Perhaps the earliest of Dunedin's caricaturists, Brown put pen to paper to spoof old identities such as Captain Cargill and Walter Mantell. Hocken acquired some 48 of his pencil drawings. Knowing that time would eradicate their meaning, he has added his characteristic annotations. *7740, Hocken Collections, Uare Taoka o Hakena, University of Otago*

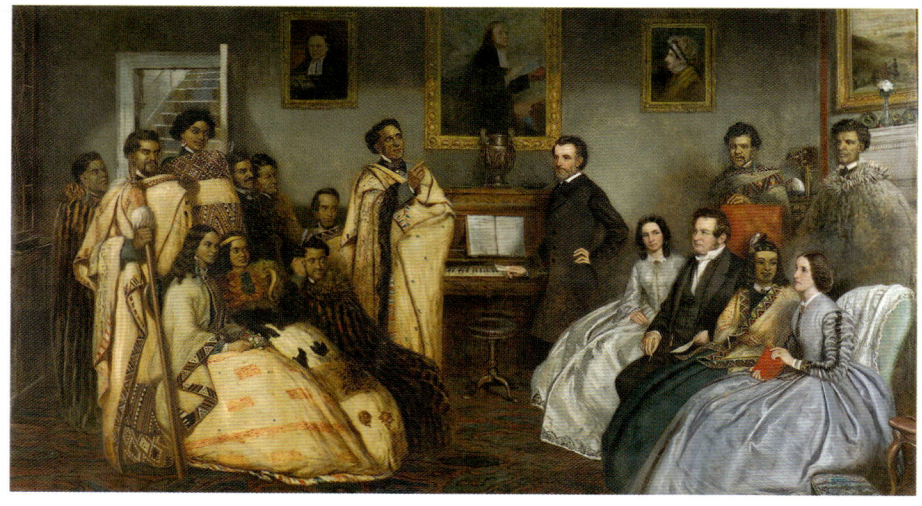

LIST OF BOOKS RELATING TO TASMANIA.

CALLANDER (JOHN).— Terra Australis Cognita: or, Voyages to the Terra Australis, or Southern Hemisphere, during the Sixteenth, Seventeenth, and Eighteenth Centuries. 3 vols. 8vo. Edinburgh, 1766-68
[The second volume contains portions of Tasman's Journal of the Discovery of Van Diemen's Land, New Zealand, &c. See also the Collections of Harris, De Brosses, Dalrymple, Burney, and others.]

COOK (CAPTAIN JAMES).—Voyage toward the South Pole and Round the World, performed in H.M.S. *Resolution* and *Adventure*, 1772-75, &c. 2 vols. 4to. London, 1777

MARION'S Voyage in the ships *Mascarin* and *Marquis de Castries*. Paris, 1783

COOK (CAPTAIN JAMES).—Voyage to the Pacific Ocean, &c., under the Direction of Captains Cook, Clerk, and Gore, in H.M.S. the *Resolution* and *Discovery*, 1776-80. 3 vols. 4to, and folio atlas. London, 1784

MORTIMER (LIEUT. G.)—Observations, &c., made during a Voyage in the Brig *Mercury*. London, 1791

BLIGH (LIEUT. WM.)—A Voyage to the South Sea, with a Narrative of the Mutiny of the *Bounty*. 4to. London, 1792

COLLINS (LIEUT.-COL. DAVID).—An Account of the English Colony in New South Wales, &c., &c., with an account of the Discovery of Bass Strait by Flinders & Bass. 2 vols. 4to. London, 1798-1802

LABILLARDIERE (JACQUES JULES).—Relation du Voyage à la Recherche de la Pérouse. 2 vols. 4to. and folio atlas Paris, 1800

LABILLARDIERE (J. J.)—Voyage in Search of La Pérouse 1791-94. 2 vols. 8vo. London, 1800

GRANT (LIEUT. JAMES).—Narrative of a Voyage of Discovery in the *Lady Nelson* in 1802. 4to. London, 1803

LABILLARDIERE (JACQUES JULES).—Novæ Hollandiæ Plantarum Specimen. 2 vols. 4to. Paris, 1804-6

TUCKEY (LIEUT. J. H.)—Account of a Voyage to establish a Colony at Port Phillip, in Bass Strait, in H.M.S. *Calcutta*, in the years 1802-4. 8vo. London, 1805

ROSSEL.—Voyage de D'Entrecasteaux, redigé par M. de Rossel. Paris, 1808

ABOVE: James Smetham, 'The New Zealand Chiefs in Wesley's House' (1863). Smetham was a fellow 'Grovian', who started at the school in 1832. Hocken bought this painting in 1887.
13395, Hocken Collections, Uare Taoka o Hakena, University of Otago

LEFT: In 1889, when Hocken was working on Abel Tasman's *Journal* and beginning his own bibliography, he was assisted by James Backhouse Walker, a Hobart-based solicitor also studying Tasman and compiling his own *List of Books Relating to Tasmania* (1884). This is a presentation copy, which carries Hocken's ink provenance stamp.
Pamphlet Vol. 63, No. 9: S14-524g, Hocken Collections, Uare Taoka o Hakena, University of Otago

JUDGE MANING.

Judge Maning, the author of "Old New Zealand," as most of our readers are aware, is suffering from a cancer, and lies at the point of death in London, whither he had been ordered by his medical advisers. The following is the concluding portion of a letter he writes to Mr Wickham, editor of the Auckland 'Free Lance':—

This is a miserable climate – dark, dismal, foggy, cold. Oh, how I do long to get back to that lovely country and climate where the sun shines and the country is so picturesque, to die amongst you all, my friends. It cannot be, however; I must linger out a certain space in pain, and remain in what is to me a foreign land. I have, however, met with a few friends here. Mr Jackson's brother, Dr Jackson, is a very fine fellow and very kind, and comes to see me. Mr S. Morrin visited me to-day; he is very ill, poor fellow, and cannot return soon. I also have been visited by Captain Daldy's brother; had a call from Mr Domett, our ancient Premier, whom I knew at Wellington; and many others are kind and ready to do me service.

I have nothing more to say but farewell. I have nothing more to do in this world but to die, as quietly as I can. The doctors say they can prevent me having too much pain. I may linger out several months, and so might have time to get a line or two from you, which would be a great pleasure.

I am sorry I am prevented from writing a book, an endeavor to make out some of the ancient history and migrations of the Maori race, of which I have got some very surprising glimpses. I can look at the prospect of death with equanimity, thank God, and hope I may do so to the end; it is the long pain I repine at. I have caught myself smiling more than once at the idea of the fuss we sometimes make about dying, seeing we all know we must die, and what an insignificant thing an individual man is on the earth, less than a mote in the sunbeam; though of mighty consequence to ourselves, as we feel too often for our peace. The priests tell us many tales; and we really know nothing of the future nor why all things exist, but I do believe in God—the sign is in our conscience—and that men were not made for an evil purpose or end, and that we may lie down having a trust and hope that a future state may be no harm to us, though few have earned much good. Remember me sincerely to Dr Pollen and all Auckland friends. I wish I could get back to die amongst you. Wield the 'Lance' in the cause of right and common sense—that is the best, though of course you must be with a party. Now, farewell, my dear sir; and farewell, beautiful New Zealand—would that I might rest there, but it cannot be.

T. M. Hocken.

Frederick Edward Maning was born July 5th 1811, died of cancer of the jaws at a private hospital in Fitzroy Sq. London, July 25, 1883. His remains were brought to New Zealand & interred at Auckland Dec 8, 1883.

Obituary of Frederick Maning (1811–1883) and a note by Hocken in 'Judge' Maning's *History of the War in the North of New Zealand* (1864). When the two men met in Auckland in 1881, Maning gave Hocken this copy, among other works. Hocken used some of the information in his edited version of Maning's *Old New Zealand* and *A History of the North of New Zealand*, which was published in 1907. Pamphlet Vol. 115, No. 1: S14-524f, Hocken Collections, Uare Taoka o Hakena, University of Otago

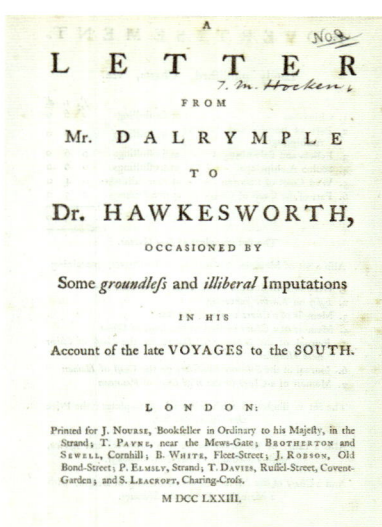

A Letter from Mr Dalrymple to Dr Hawkesworth, Occasioned by Some Groundless and Illiberal Imputations in his Account of the Late Voyages to the South (1773). Hocken was fortunate to secure one of Alexander Dalrymple's letters – in which he vented his anger on being rejected as the leader of the scientific expedition to observe the Transit of Venus in June 1769 and criticised John Hawkesworth's editorial account of Captain Cook's first voyage – first printed in 1773.
Pamphlet Vol. 13, No. 2: S14-524e, Hocken Collections, Uare Taoka o Hakena, University of Otago

BELOW: *The Province of Otago, in New Zealand: Its progress, present condition, resources and prospects* (1868). To assist future readers, Hocken identified the names of streets in early 'North Dunedin'. Pamphlet Vol. 91, No. 15: S14524c, Hocken Collections, Uare Taoka o Hakena, University of Otago

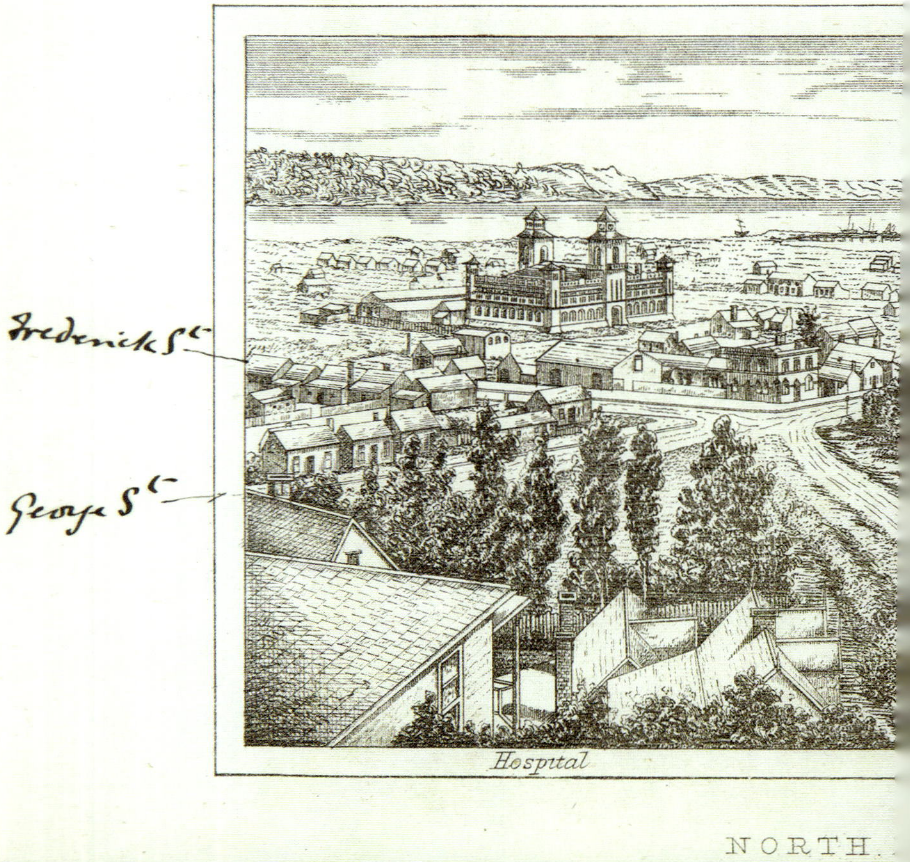

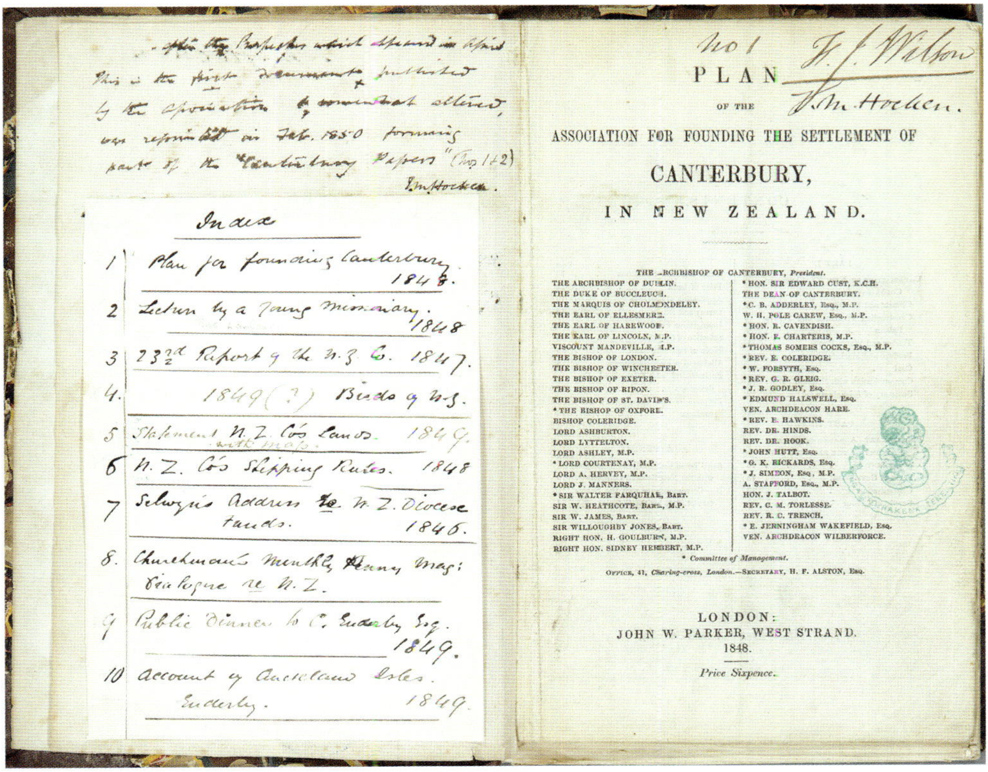

No 1 — W. J. Wilton — T. M. Hocken.

PLAN

OF THE

ASSOCIATION FOR FOUNDING THE SETTLEMENT OF

CANTERBURY,

IN NEW ZEALAND.

THE ARCHBISHOP OF CANTERBURY, *President.*

THE ARCHBISHOP OF DUBLIN.
THE DUKE OF BUCCLEUCH.
THE MARQUIS OF CHOLMONDELEY.
THE EARL OF ELLESMERE.
THE EARL OF HAREWOOD.
THE EARL OF LINCOLN, M.P.
VISCOUNT MANDEVILLE, M.P.
THE BISHOP OF LONDON.
THE BISHOP OF WINCHESTER.
THE BISHOP OF EXETER.
THE BISHOP OF RIPON.
THE BISHOP OF ST. DAVID'S.
* THE BISHOP OF OXFORD.
BISHOP COLERIDGE.
LORD ASHBURTON.
LORD LYTTELTON.
LORD ASHLEY, M.P.
* LORD COURTENAY, M.P.
LORD A. HERVEY, M.P.
LORD J. MANNERS.
* SIR WALTER FARQUHAR, BART.
SIR W. HEATHCOTE, BART., M.P.
SIR W. JAMES, BART.
SIR WILLOUGHBY JONES, BART.
RIGHT HON. H. GOULBURN, M.P.
RIGHT HON. SIDNEY HERBERT, M.P.
* HON. SIR EDWARD CUST, K.C.H.
THE DEAN OF CANTERBURY.
* C. B. ADDERLEY, Esq., M.P.
W. H. POLE CAREW, Esq., M.P.
* HON. R. CAVENDISH.
* HON. F. CHARTERIS, M.P.
* THOMAS SOMERS COCKS, Esq., M.P.
* REV. E. COLERIDGE.
* W. FORSYTH, Esq.
* REV. G. R. GLEIG.
* J. R. GODLEY, Esq.
* EDMUND HALSWELL, Esq.
VEN. ARCHDEACON HARE.
* REV. E. HAWKINS.
REV. DR. HINDS.
REV. DR. HOOK.
* JOHN HUTT, Esq.
* G. K. RICKARDS, Esq.
* J. SIMEON, Esq., M.P.
A. STAFFORD, Esq., M.P.
HON. J. TALBOT.
REV. C. M. TORLESSE.
REV. R. C. TRENCH.
* E. JERNINGHAM WAKEFIELD, Esq.
VEN. ARCHDEACON WILBERFORCE.

* *Committee of Management.*

OFFICE, 41, *Charing-cross, London.*—SECRETARY, H. F. ALSTON, Esq.

LONDON:
JOHN W. PARKER, WEST STRAND.
1848.

Price Sixpence.

Index

1 Plan for founding Canterbury. 1848.
2 Lecture by a Young Missionary. 1848
3 23½rd Report of the N.Z. Co. 1847.
4. 1849(?) Birds of N.Z.
5 Statement N.Z. Co's Lands with map. 1849.
6 N.Z. Co's Shipping Rules. 1848
7 Selwyn's Address to N.Z. Diocese funds. 1846.
8. Churchman's Monthly Penny Mag: Dialogue re N.Z.
9 Public Dinner to C. Enderby Esq. 1849.
10 Account of Auckland Isles. Enderby. 1849.

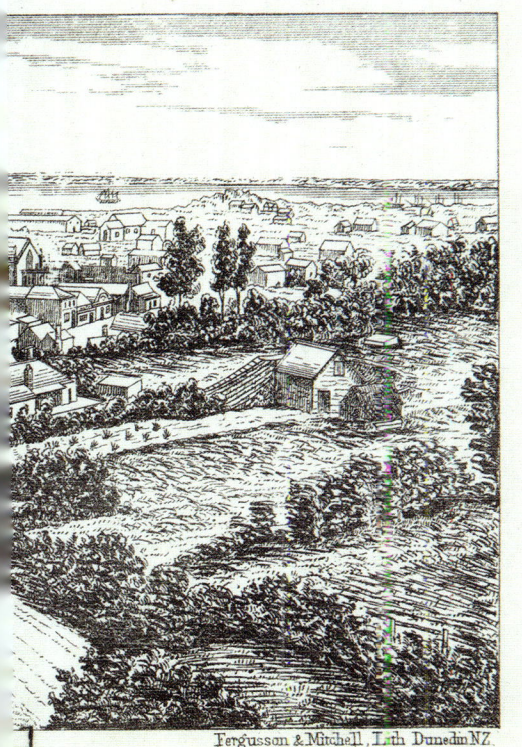

ABOVE: *Plan of the Association for Founding the Settlement of Canterbury in New Zealand* (1848). Determined to establish ownership of his books, Hocken usually signed his name three times in a single publication, often pasted in a bookplate or a green hei-tiki label and then used a specially designed hei-tiki stamp. He was also an inveterate scribbler, writing notes that helped to clarify specific points on the publication or its author.

Pamphlet Vol. 31, No. 1: S14-524d, Hocken Collections, Uare Taoka o Hakena, University of Otago

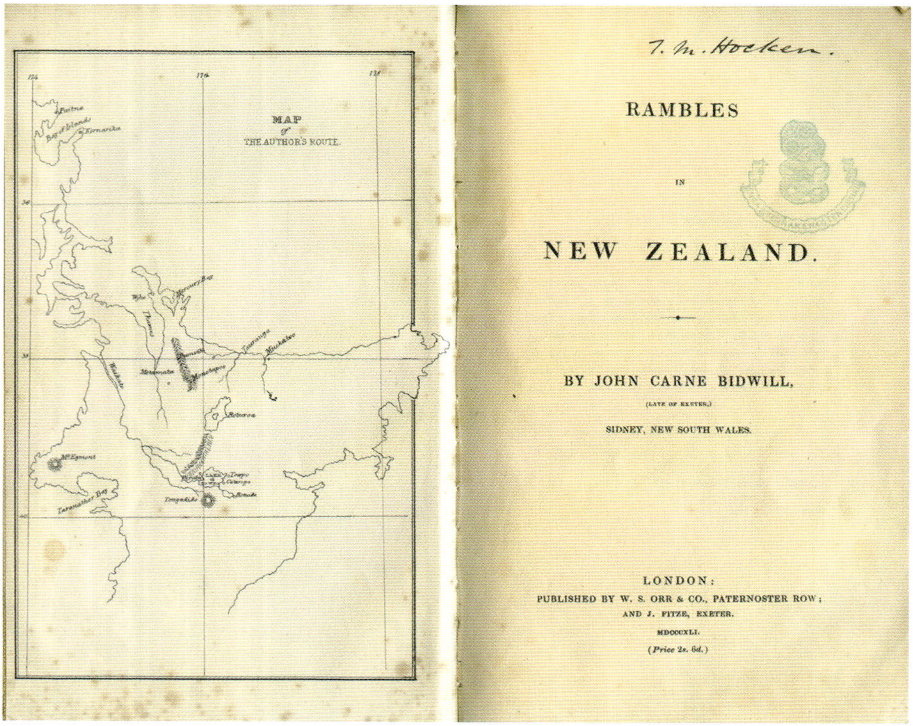

T. M. Hocken.

RAMBLES

IN

NEW ZEALAND.

BY JOHN CARNE BIDWILL,

(LATE OF EXETER,)

SIDNEY, NEW SOUTH WALES.

LONDON:

PUBLISHED BY W. S. ORR & CO., PATERNOSTER ROW;

AND J. FITZE, EXETER.

MDCCCXLI.

(Price 2s. 6d.)

Exeter-born botanist John Carne Bidwill, whose *Rambles in New Zealand* (London: W.S. Orr & Co.) was published in 1841, was the first Pakeha to climb Tongariro. His home-town acquaintances bought over 680 copies of this book, making this one, owned by Hocken, a very scarce work.

Pamphlet Vol. 100, No. 1: S14-524b, Hocken Collections, Uare Taoka o Hakena, University of Otago

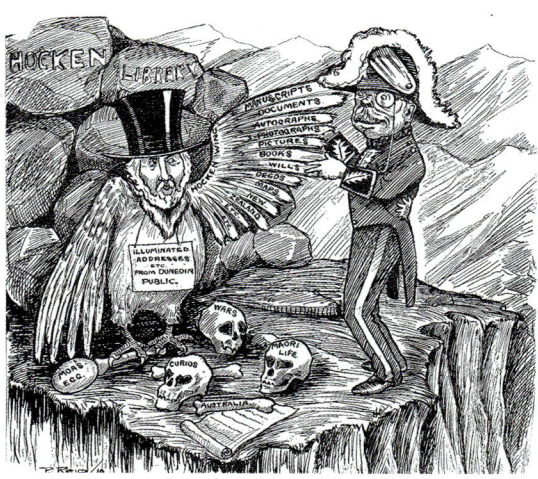

Only one TMH – 'A Rare Bird, rarely plumed, shedding rare gifts as he wings his way'. This P. Reid cartoon appeared in the *Magpie*, Dunedin, on 28 April 1910. *Private collection*

for Nigeria, and archivist and historian Frank Rogers was appointed University Librarian. He not only enjoyed increased funding but was able to secure the Hocken as an approved repository for Justice Department records. He also began collecting local authority records such as those of the Otago Education Board, and in February 1952 was instrumental in appointing Gloria van der Poots (later Strathern) as the first full-time professional librarian for the Hocken. Opening hours became full time, and that year 450 books were accessioned. Strathern had an assistant, Linda Rodda, who, along with Jean McGill, in 1948 created a 'Catalogue of Pictures in the Hocken Library', the first such listing. That year Rodda also compiled a 'Calendar of Dr. T. M. Hocken's Personal Letters and Documents Preserved in the Hocken Library, Otago University'. Both these works were indispensable for readers wanting access to Hocken's picture and manuscript collections. Of this period Stuart Strachan has aptly written: 'A new era had begun.'[61]

With greater publicity, exhibitions and an increased awareness and activity by members associated with the Hocken, its profile and use rose within the university and throughout New Zealand. Acquisitions now included post-1900 works, and in 1959 endowments amounted to £350. There were more donations too, including 10 Hoyte watercolours (some of which were reproduced for the 1969 university centenary), Lieutenant-Colonel Arthur Edward Williams's Taranaki War sketchbook, the papers of historian and ethnologist Herries Beattie and those of collector and researcher George Craig Thomson. The pictorial section of the Hocken received national recognition when the Sargood Trust gave £500 towards the purchase of paintings. On the heels of this were the gifts by artist Rodney Kennedy (1956 onwards) and writer Charles Brasch (1958 onwards), which dramatically altered the emphasis of the pictorial collection, pushing it away from a largely historical-based collection and towards a representative museum of New Zealand art. Their efforts resulted in further art donations by artist and teacher J.D. Charlton Edgar (1961 onward) and the family of Colin McCahon (1973). This new emphasis led to the appointment of a full-time curator of pictures.

It was the beginning of good times. University librarians Peter Havard-Williams (1957–61) and Jock McEldowney (1962–87) followed Rogers. During McEldowney's tenure, Michael Hitchings was employed as Hocken Librarian, enjoying a good 20 years in the position (1965–85). After his retirement, archivist Stuart Strachan was hired, for another long stint of 23 years (1985–2008), and on 7 April 2008 Sharon Dell, with experience at the Turnbull Library and later the Whanganui Regional Museum, began her work as Hocken Librarian.

During these years archive and manuscript collections expanded, so much so that a curator of manuscripts position was established. Map and photograph collections grew exponentially, gathered in by gift or purchase. Music and musical score collections also came into their own, as did literary manuscripts by purchase, donation and bequest from writers such as James K. Baxter and Janet Frame. The establishment of the Robert Burns and Frances Hodgkins fellowships, in 1958 and 1962 respectively, did much to raise the Hocken's (and the university's) profile, as well as encouraging further donations, gifts and endowments. Again Brasch showed his munificence by donating his personal papers, his *Landfall* archive, a portion of his residual estate and the rest of his paintings to the Hocken in 1973. The 461 paintings given by Brasch included works by McCahon, Toss Woollaston and Rita Angus. As Strachan has written, 'after Dr Hocken [Brasch] was, by far, the Library's most important benefactor'.[62] Donations and bequests from Frank and Molly M. Canaday (1974), C. Ernie R. Webber (1984), Bruce Godward (1991–92), the Hall-Jones family (1992) and numerous others have added considerably to the collection at the Hocken.[63] The Endowment Trust is used to purchase unpublished material; university library funds are used for acquiring published collections.

Physical relocation has also been necessary. Overcrowding at the Hocken Wing of the Otago Museum necessitated a move to the Ted McCoy-designed Richardson building on campus in 1979. And yet, even though the photograph and archive collections were redistributed to the old vehicle testing station on Leith Street in 1989, growth continued to outstrip proper housing and full services to ever-increasing numbers of users. In 1998 the Hocken Collections were again consolidated into one and moved to an old dairy factory on Anzac Avenue. Specially converted for the purpose, in 2007 this environmentally controlled area housed 240,000 published volumes, 8500 linear metres of archives, 13,500 sound recordings, 11,500 maps, over a million photographs and 14,000 pictures. There were dedicated staff in such areas as archives, published collections, serials, pictures and maps; by then they were dealing with an average of 12,000 visitors per year.[64] Collections grow, and in 2014 the university and the Hocken Collections Committee were already eyeing up the nearby Unipol building as a solution for much-needed space. (This was yet to be finalised at the time of writing.)

Adding to the Legacy

Hocken's publications reinforced his legacy. His *Contributions* (1898), with a title-page quote from Scottish poet Allan Cunningham: 'Much with hoary men/ He walked conversing, and sedately glad/ Heard stories which escaped historic pen'[65] has been described as 'the first genuine political history of southern New Zealand, written with a good grasp of the motivations involved, well-proportioned between detail and generality, peopled with three-dimensional humans, and written with verve and confidence'.[66] Despite some inaccuracies, it remains an excellent regional history, aided enormously by an as yet unpublished index compiled in 1938 by Joan Collis Wood. Hocken's *Bibliography* (1909) was by far the more important publication. Despite omissions and errors, A.H. Johnstone's *Supplement* (1927), the later improvements and greater scope of Bagnall's multi-volumed *New Zealand National Bibliography to the Year 1960* (1969–80) and the development of electronic national union catalogues (Te Puna), it remains a very useful reference book for librarians, book historians and book dealers. Indeed, an 'In Hocken' or 'Not in Hocken' reference still carries weight in many book dealer catalogues.

Although Hocken completed his Maning and Webster books, he had a strong desire to finish his 'Life of Marsden' and was troubled that he had been unable to do so. He had spent much time and effort on deciphering and transcribing the text, especially those parts relevant to Marsden's accounts of his missions to New Zealand. Bessie was determined to keep the Marsden flame burning. About June 1910 she succeeded in finding 'a cultured clergyman – a Marsden enthusiast' to finish it. This was Canon Robert Woodthorpe, chaplain of the Maori Mission and the Chatham Islands' Mission in the Diocese of Christchurch, and later warden of Selwyn College. She even prepared 'Notes for the Preface to Marsden's Journals', which were clearly based on Hocken's researches but also contained her addenda and written instructions: 'Mention Percy Smith, New Plymouth, as having rendered valuable aid in making map tracing M's routes through N.Z.' and 'Write to Minister for Railways ... for permission for Govt to get the maps reduced for print.'[67] Although there is no evidence of her making contact with any prospective publishers, in early June 1910 she hinted to Smith that the Society for Promoting Christian Knowledge (SPCK) in London would publish the book.[68] This did not happen. The commission was also obviously unrealistic, especially in the light of Woodthorpe's own activities and future appointments. Between 1913 and 1917 he was archdeacon of Oamaru, and he was also a lecturer in history and economics at the University of Otago until 1925. He eventually left for Sydney and died there in 1931, aged 70.[69]

In addition to the Marsden crusade, Bessie busied herself with the 'publication of the unprinted & other lectures on the early colonization of New Zealand'.[70] As with past publications, she mooted the idea that the government should print the work. She mentioned again the Minister for Railways, John A. Miller, and George Fenwick, who supplied a lengthy 'Memoir' of Hocken for the publication, albeit with some inaccuracies. Largely unedited and taken from the past newspaper copy, Hocken's *The Early History of New Zealand* appeared in 1914, printed in Wellington by the government printer.[71] Carrying a posed frontispiece photograph of Hocken, complete with greenstone mere and a cloak draped around one knee, it was another tangible reminder of his legacy.

Research and Publications

In 1912 T. Lindsay Buick, who later gave funds to the Hocken, used a portrait of Te Rauparaha as a frontispiece to his *An Old New Zealander* (1912), while James Cowan used a sketch of the fight at Moturoa for *The Adventures of Kimble Bent* (1912). Both illustrations were reproductions of originals held in Hocken's collection.[72] Robert McNab's *From Tasman to Marsden: A history of northern New Zealand from 1642 to 1818*, published in 1914, led the charge in trumpeting the collection: 'Of unpublished manuscripts relating to the Mission the largest collection in the world is in the Hocken Library in Dunedin, and it is to be hoped that at no distant date we may have these available for the general reader as well as the student.'[73] These three works signalled the beginning of the use of materials in the Hocken, but J.R. Elder's *The Letters and Journals of Samuel Marsden* made a greater impact. Published in 1932, it was a significant joint publication with printing firm Coulls Somerville Wilkie Ltd, publisher A.H. Reed (his first major publication) and the Otago University Council. Elder not only acknowledged his debt to Hocken's thoroughness in collecting, but also made the point that 'almost every manuscript, newspaper, pamphlet, and printed book to which reference has been made in this volume is to be found in the Hocken Library'. In addition, Elder relied heavily for illustrations on those Maori materials at the Otago Museum (largely from Hocken's bequest) and in the Hocken Collection. He was certainly conscious of the work done by Hocken and, no doubt to a lesser degree, by Canon Woodthorpe:

> The publication of letters and journals of Samuel Marsden under the auspices of the Council of the University of Otago is to be regarded, therefore, as the fulfilment by that body of a sacred trust imposed upon it by its acceptance of the custody of Dr Hocken's library. It is certain that no more fitting memorial than this could be erected to one with whom history was a passion and the elucidation of New Zealand history a patriotic duty.[74]

Elder's *Marsden's Lieutenants*, which quickly followed in 1934, established, according to Downie Stewart, 'a further instalment of the rich treasures to be found in the library bequeathed by the late Dr Hocken to the University of Otago'.[75] In this work on Thomas Kendall, William Hall, John King and others, Elder once again paid his due to Hocken: 'It is impossible to emphasize too much the indebtedness of New Zealand to the man whose enthusiasm for her early records resulted in the collection and preservation of so much invaluable material.'[76] The jacket of this book carries a note informing buyers that only a few copies of the *Letters* were still available: it was an important 'best-seller' for Reed and the University Council.

Fittingly, the Elder Collection was also destined for the Hocken. This extensive collection not only contains many of Hocken's Marsden typescripts, with many of his annotations and notes, but also Elder's own typescripts. There are also sundry books and pamphlets, all pertaining to Marsden and his fellow missionaries.[77] A lock of the missionary's hair is also present, secured through

Mary Allan, one of Marsden's descendants in Sydney, about 1933. No doubt Hocken would have been pleased with this relic and the sentiment conveyed by Allan: 'I thought as the Mitchell Library has a similar relic, one of N. Zealand's historical museums may care to have this piece; please return to above address if no use for same.'[78]

Over the years, many scholars and professional writers have used Hocken's collection to produce works that are themselves significant. This scholarly activity is the highest compliment, and is aptly summed up by Wilmarth Lewis, the American collector of Walpoliana: 'Collecting ... is a form of scholarship – exacting, imaginative, creative. Where, pray, would scholars be if there had been no collectors before them to bring together the books that make research possible? Collecting, libraries, publication, these three, and the first of these – without which the other two would not exist – is collecting.'[79]

Aside from those works mentioned above, other published titles emanating from research done using Hocken's collection include Robert McNab's two volumes of *Historical Records of New Zealand* (1908; 1914), his *Murihiku* (versions 1905; 1907; 1909) and *The Old Whaling Days: A history of southern New Zealand from 1830 to 1840* (1913); James Herries Beattie's works including *European Place-Names in Southern NZ* (1912); Robert Fulton's *Medical Practice in Otago & Southland* (1922); Basil Howard's *Rakiura: A History of Stewart Island* (1940); A.H. McLintock's *History of Otago* (1949) and *Port of Otago* (1951); A.H. Reed's *The Story of Early Dunedin* (1955); Sheila Natusch's *On the Edge of the Bush* (1976) and *The Cruise of the Acheron: Her Majesty's steam vessel on survey in New Zealand waters, 1848–51* (1978); Erik Olssen's *History of Otago* (1984); and Atholl Anderson's *The Welcome of Strangers: An ethnohistory of southern Maori A.D. 1650–1850* (1998). Others, some broader in scope, include James Hight and C.R. Straubel's *A History of Canterbury* (1957–1971); Angus Ross's *New Zealand Aspirations in the Pacific in the Nineteenth Century* (1964) and other works such as *They Built in Faith: A short history of Knox Church (1860–1976)* (1976); Judith Binney's *The Legacy of Guilt: A life of Thomas Kendall* (1968; 2005); William Parker Morrell's *The Anglican Church in New Zealand* (1973) and his other works on colonial government; Harry Morton's *The Wind Commands: Sailors and sailing ships in the Pacific* (1976); A.T. Yarwood's *Samuel Marsden: The great survivor* (1977); Tom Brooking's *And Captain of their Souls: An interpretative essay on the life and times of Captain William Cargill* (1984); Erik Olssen's *Building the New World: Work, politics and society in Caversham 1880s–1920s* (1995); *Sites of Gender: Women, men & modernity in southern Dunedin 1890–1939* (2003) edited by Barbara Brookes, Annabel Cooper and Robin Law, which used Hocken illustrations extensively; Anne Salmond's *Two Worlds: First meetings between Maori and Europeans, 1642–1772* (1991) and her other later works; and those scholarly publications and activities with a Maori focus, including Herbert W. Williams's *A Bibliography of Printed Maori to 1900* (1924; and supplement by Sommerville, 1947), Phillip Parkinson and Penny

Griffith's *Books in Maori* (2004), the use of the Edward Shortland papers and ongoing Waitangi Tribunal research.

Two recent publications are of note. *Ka Taoka Hakena: Treasures from the Hocken Collections* was edited by Stuart Strachan and Linda Tyler and published by Otago University Press in 2007 in time for the hundredth celebration of Hocken's signing of the deed of gift. Aside from highlighting other components of the Hocken Collections, this work displays in glorious colour a range of manuscripts, books, maps, sketches, paintings and photographs from what is designated Hocken's 'Original Collection'.

The other is *Gaining a Foothold: Historical records of Otago's eastern coast, 1770–1839*, edited by the late Ian Church and Paul Sorrell and published by the Friends of the Hocken in 2008 to commemorate the work of David McDonald, reference librarian at the Hocken from 1974 to 2000. Many of the documents on early European exploration, whaling, sealing, interaction between local Ngai Tahu, old land claims and settler reminiscences were sourced from Hocken's collection of manuscripts and printed books.

The list could be longer if it included unpublished theses (note Olga Fitchett's 'Dr Hocken and his work', a 1928 history honours thesis), smaller pamphlets, private genealogical research publications and articles that contain materials and sources (photographs, maps, sketches) from the collection. And of course, this discounts forthcoming work and all those publications that Hocken knowingly contributed to while he was alive, including works by Dean Jacobs, Professor Hutton, William Colenso, Sherwood Roberts, Alexander Bathgate and Percy Smith. His advice was free to scholars and researchers; he gave much.

The Hocken Name Perpetuated

Today 30,000 items from the Hocken Collections are used in the reading rooms each year, and 9000 people use the collections onsite. Of these a third are from the University of Otago and Otago Polytechnic, a third are independent researchers and academics from other universities and a third are family and local historians. There are some 2500 distant users. Over the last five years an average of 210 books, theses, exhibition display boards, websites and television programmes annually have used material from the Hocken Collections. On average, 55 items are lent to exhibitions each year, and an increasing number of people are able to use the collection online. For example, 1200 images from the pictorial collections are on the university library's Our Heritage website, and over 30,000 photographs are available on Hocken Snapshot.[80]

New positions have been established that not only allow staff to provide greater service and deal with increased usage of materials, especially by those researching family genealogies but also enable such twenty-first-century initiatives as digitisation and an enhanced web presence. The use of Hocken's material has increased year by year. Computerised cataloguing, dedicated websites, Facebook and blogs, printed inventories, publications, regular exhibitions and talks to school, and community and student groups raise awareness of the collection. Access has also improved, with full-week opening hours, a late night on Tuesday and a Saturday morning service.

By being at the 'Hocken', going through the process of reader registration and learning of the 'Hocken' rules (such as no bags, and pencils only), each reader by osmosis gains some notion of Hocken and his achievements. A permanent wall display reinforces this information. The calling up and use of a travel book such as Parkinson's *Journals of a Voyage to the South Seas* (1773) or a manuscript on emigration, is a talismanic experience, especially if the items carry Hocken's stamp of ownership: bookplates, signature, hei tiki and 'Hakena' labels.

Most of Hocken's printed books are filed with other printed books in the much larger Hocken Collections. At one stage – certainly around the centenary – there was talk of bringing all his books together as a discrete unit. This was not done. They are, however, easily recognised owing to his very determined effort to establish ownership. His printed Maori language books are filed separately along with other Maori language books, arranged numerically by the Williams *Bibliography* number. His 'Variae', 'Flotsam & Jetsam' and Pamphlets volumes are arranged numerically and filed separately from the printed books. His pictorial collection is filed with other materials but items are easily recognised, especially if they contain his notations. An electronic file titled 'Original' aids identification. Although most of Hocken's manuscripts have early MS numbers, and are thus kept together, some that have been unearthed more recently have necessitated later MS numbers. His maps are arranged by geographical location and so filed with others. And much of his 'Original' collection, especially those parts pertaining to the New Zealand Company and New Zealand Mission archives, is enhanced by a large microfilm library.

There are no schools named after Hocken, nor are there statues, like the two for Sir George Grey. There is, however, Hocken Street, a cul-de-sac in Kenmure, Dunedin, named about 1956.[81] There are numerous photographs of Hocken: lecturing, sitting with his daughter Gladys in the Atahapara study, seated on a chair, standing beside a large carved wooden slab, behind his microscope in his library and straight portrait shots. Many were taken by Bessie. There are numerous cartoon caricatures, such as those appearing in the *Press* on 3 October 1906, *Dunedin Punch* (September 1865), the *Tickler for Otago and Southland* and the *University of Otago Capping Magazine* (1907). And there are portraits of Hocken: a charcoal-on-paper sketch by Halliday Scott, and a pastel-on-paper portrait by Fanny Wimperis, which Bessie proclaimed was 'a really good piece of work'. This was hung in the Hocken Wing about August 1910.[82]

Atahapara has long disappeared, and the only reminder of it and Hocken's residence is a plaque outside the RSA building (now Arrow House) on Moray Place. Hocken's name, however, is perpetuated in other ways. There are Hocken Library Fellows within the university, who, unless under special circumstances, cannot exceed 15 in number. To commemorate the centenary in 2007, Dorothy Page, Erik Olssen, Roger Collins and Ian Farquhar were inducted as new Fellows. Ray Hargreaves and Gordon Parsonson are also Hocken Fellows, as was the late George Griffiths.

On 16 October 1991 a Friends of the Hocken Collections group was established which, as the website notes, 'promotes public awareness of, and support for, the various collections, services, and publications of the Hocken Collections'. Members also undertake various projects to enhance collection access, which have included paying for the microfilming of records of the Otago Provincial Council and Southland Provincial Council, and the purchase of a microfilm reader. A newsletter, suitably titled *F&J*, is produced three times a year to keep the friends, general readers and the wider community informed of recent activities and aspects of the Hocken; and a series of bulletins details aspects of the collections. As the *Evening Star* of 2 April 1910 noted, 'In some of the great schools of the Old World there is an annual festival or service entitled the "Commemoration of Benefactors". If, at some future time, Dunedin (or, indeed, New Zealand) were to hold a similar ceremony, the name of Thomas Morland Hocken would rank high on the list of benefactors to be honored.' Since their inception, the Friends have held a formal dinner annually on 2 September, the day of the signing of the deed of trust. There is often a dedicated theme, a guest speaker, and always a toast to the founding father of the library.

Exhibition catalogues, greeting cards and pictures from the collection, and reproductions of some of the paintings owned by Hocken, are sold, exchanged and dispersed nationally and internationally. There is also the annual Hocken Lecture, the first given by historian W.H. Oliver in 1969. Other lecturers have been A.G. Hocken, Sir Robert Jones, Brian Easton, Philip Temple, Lloyd Geering, C.K. Stead, Judith Binney, Peter Simpson and Helen Leach.

The True Spirit of the Collector

There was no particular trigger for Hocken's collecting, although it is certain that he had a strong historical sense. His salvaging of testimonials from Newcastle and Dublin and ship's newspapers compiled in 1860, when he was in his early twenties, represents the first flowering of his collecting instinct. This lifelong activity, fostered by a family environment that respected education and book learning, was carried out alongside the demands of a busy professional career and family commitments. His collecting was slow, gradual and continuous, and he was extremely fortunate to find areas of interest early in his life. That they concerned the history and development of his adopted home of Dunedin, and New Zealand, makes his collecting much more understandable: it perhaps helped to ground him and give him a sense of place. His collecting was certainly made easier because it was largely local and indigenous, posing fewer problems with distance than those faced by contemporaries such as Sir George Grey and Alexander Turnbull. He gave the materials he found value and saved them from destruction. This was truly visionary. He also had a strong sense of destiny, of making his mark, and followed the examples of Grey and Mitchell by placing his collection within the public domain. He would certainly have agreed with the remark of American book collector Henry Huntington that 'the ownership of a fine library is the surest and swiftest way to immortality'.[83]

A lack of invoices and letters to and from book dealers makes it difficult to ascertain buying trends and therefore any peak period of collecting for Hocken. It can be said with confidence, however, that his trip to England over 1901–04 was momentous: he not only secured the highly significant CMS and Colonial Office materials, but also enjoyed the pleasures of London, the centre of the book world. There he accumulated a great store of books and materials that was returned to his library in Dunedin.

George Fenwick wrote of Hocken's attributes and industry:

> He was imbued with the true spirit of the collector. Year by year he added new treasures to his library – rare papers, maps, periodicals, & manuscripts. He searched the world for anything that would find its proper place in such a collection. He realized that the history of New Zealand is involved with that of Australia at so many points that any collection confined to New Zealand publications would be inadequate for the purposes such a collection should have. Hence many of the early Australian periodicals & pamphlets were gathered by the industrious doctor … Only the student of history can fully realize that such a gift is more valuable than one of many thousands of pounds. Indeed, that its value cannot be represented in terms of money; and only the genuine collector can realize that such a gift involves a greater sacrifice to the giver than any monetary benefaction from a rich man's purse.[84]

Trimble was another who knew Hocken well, and was perhaps the first to work through his collection systematically. 'Dr Hocken's system of collecting,' he wrote, 'was very thorough. His historical instinct told him that every scrap of writing, or of printed papers has its value, however trifling, in the development of our civilisation.' Trimble also found it marvellous that 'the quantity of rubbish in his accumulation was very small indeed. When asking for people's old letters, or other waste papers, the Doctor claimed to be the only judge of what ought to be kept and what destroyed: he used to say – "*I can burn papers.*"'[85] For him, Hocken's collection was 'a monument of the memory of a benefactor to New Zealand: a man who tho' small in body, was great in intellect, heart and spirit'.

> We can think of him going and coming amongst us; living his life; thinking his thoughts; attending to his patients; writing papers, and books, and lectures, and letters on historical and other subjects; giving liberally of his time and means to countless public objects; taking an intellectual interest in most of the affairs of the Universe. And all thro' the years accumulating these books, and papers, and pictures, and maps, and manuscripts, the recorded history of his adopted country: and hoarding them away in his house as a bee accumulates honey in a hive. So that soon there being no more space available in his library, he was obliged to intrude his material into the bed-rooms; the space beneath the drawing-room sofas; the stable and its loft; and even the horse's manger. And when he felt that death was approaching, rather than contemplate the breaking-up of his Collection, he calmly handed it over to his fellow-citizens; and died before his treasures were fairly housed in their new quarters. When I think of his activities, Dr Hocken appears to be one of the busiest men of his time: and to him the well-worn quotation from *Hamlet* may be applied with singular fitness: He was a Man!/ Take him for all in all,/ I shall not look upon his like again.[86]

Trimble was right. There was only one Dr Hocken, and good fortune smiled gladly on this pocket-bantam who collected books and manuscripts on and about his adopted home, and then gave them selflessly away for use by others in the future.[87] He was certainly the right collector at the right time. As a nation, we would be much poorer without his having collected, and thus preserved, some of our earliest records. For his industry and his vision, future generations of New Zealanders will be forever in his debt. This is justly so.

Appendices

Appendix I

T.M. Hocken's Letter to his Friend George Fenwick
Reproduced Otago Daily Times, *1 April 1910*

Moray Place, Dunedin, March 31, 1910

Dear Mr Fenwick,
It is a matter of great grief to me that I am unable to be present on the occasion of the opening of this building, but a serious illness is the cause of my absence. I particularly regret this, as I had desired to give an account of many interesting little incidents which occurred in connection with the gathering together of this collection. This work has been to me a labour of love, and in it I have put into practice a sentiment I have always held: that it is the bounden duty of every citizen to do something for his State, in the welfare of which his own happiness and prosperity is very largely found. This feeling, I have long considered, should animate every member of the community – from the highest to the lowest – for only in its increasing observance may a country expect a diminution of those troubles which often occur, and against which this feeling of patriotism and loyalty forms the best protection. A desire, then, to, in some measure, do something for the people among whom I have so long sojourned and the country in which I have so long resided has been the actuating motive in the formation of this collection which I have presented to the Dominion of New Zealand.

In this connection with the pictures comprised in it I have been very careful to see that to each one of historical interest there is attached an adequate account of its scope and theme. The value of a picture in itself is but little if there is no full description of that to which it refers. With this description its educational value is vastly increased, and to attain this end I have, as will be noticed, endeavoured to describe the pictures and arrange them so that it will be easy for all – our young folk especially – to secure a good idea of the incidents of early colonisation; and from this basis they will, perhaps, be induced to enter upon a most interesting study for themselves. The collection begins with Tasman and passes on to Captain Cook, giving incidents about him and his companions; and then, after dealing with the intermediate events, reaches the thirties, when colonisation in the true sense of the word began.

Passing to the bound files of newspapers, there is a large collection of the old publications of early Sydney and Tasmania, as well as a very complete set of our own earliest papers. Many of these are unique, the copies here being the only ones extant. It has always struck me that a great feature which differentiated the early papers from those of the present day is the function they fulfilled of being true historical recorders, in that they simply and truly reflected the daily life of the people, with all its routine of dullness, dire wants, and severe struggles. That was a condition of things which, in the advance of colonisation, will never occur again: the adoption of steam and the initiation of electricity, with all their increased comforts and speed of conveyance, preclude the possibility. Another feature of note in these early papers is the manner in which they deal with other than parochial affairs. In them we find, very often, extracted leaders and articles from *The Times* and the *Morning Chronicle* dealing with the very great political changes and movements which were on foot at that time in England and the Continent. In this way we see that, though so far from the scene of action, this outer corner of the world still preserved a breadth of outlook which enabled it to take a keen and intelligent interest in affairs other than those of local moment.

In the papers of the New Zealand Company – all of which are here – there is ample material for research and inspiration in noticing the wonderful methods adopted by the members of the company – how they spared not money and shrank not from trouble in their determination to prosecute their aims and attain their ends.

In the section of books there is quite a complete collection of works relating to New Zealand. One very great feature, which will be more appreciated as time goes on, is the splendid collection of Maori bibliography. I have taken infinite pains to collect all the early literature published in the Maori tongue. There were many good men amongst our early colonists, such as Bishop Selwyn, Sir William Martin, and, later, Sir George Grey, as well as others, who took exceptional pains to raise the status of the Maoris, and one of their methods was to issue in the Native tongue little books and pamphlets designed to elevate the race. Patriotic and praiseworthy, indeed, were these men. Their work was excellent, and had it not been for the opposition which constantly met them from a large section, I am sorry to say, of our own countrymen, those wars between the natives and ourselves which so disfigure our early settlement would never have been fought. In addition to the work of these earnest men, there is a very complete collection of publications in Maori of the books of the Bible, the Testament, etc. The earliest portion of this was printed so far back as 1829, but the complete Bible was not finished till about 1860.

Then in the manuscripts there is much of great interest. They contain, for instance, the original journals of Samuel Marsden, the apostle of New Zealand, who was a great traveller and discoverer. He paid several visits to this country, and was often alone for weeks amongst the Natives, exposed alike to the weather and physical danger. The manuscripts of his experiences and his voyages are all here; also, there are the manuscripts of the early missionaries – Kendall, Hall, King, Kemp, George Clark, Colenso, Hamlin – and in these is contained a mass of history as yet untouched and unrealised. Further, there are numberless documents relating to the settlement of the provinces, especially of Otago and Canterbury, amongst them original letter-books and letters from various Governors of the early days. These letter-books as yet await full investigation – I have not been able to do it completely.

Though this collection is, of course, principally a gathering of printed books and documents relating to the history of New Zealand, I wish it to be understood that it is not entirely confined to this Dominion in its scope. For it will be seen that much of the material relates to the other colonies, and there is also a great collection of voyages of men who never came to New Zealand, so that students of travel in general may here find opportunity for work. Indeed, I view this building as a repository for the archives of history not only of New Zealand, but of the colonies generally, and that that might be accomplished I do hope that those who have in their possession valuable documents will see their way to present them to this library, where they will be most gratefully received and utilised. In the fullness of time it is my intention to present, further, a number of Japanese works of various kinds. In fact, there are numerous additions to be made, and among them I specially wish to mention an extensive collection of Maori weapons, implements, ornaments, and carvings, which will in time find a place with the library collection now housed in its new abode.

In conclusion, let me say that, generous as the Government and the public have been, yet full provision is by no means made for a proper librarian. The librarian of this institution should, indeed, be an archivist – a man of culture, a man with some predilections for historical research; in short, a man who would be more than a librarian in the ordinary sense of the term. He should have a thorough knowledge of the books, and be able to help students and scholars to investigate the numerous subjects that here have been slightly indicated. In view of this gift being made to the Dominion, I feel that I might be quite justified in making this one request: that some persons who combine the possession of wealth, and who are imbued with those patriotic and public-spirited sentiments which I indicated in the early part of my letter, should take such steps as would result in the formation of a fund to adequately maintain the efficiency and usefulness of this collection which is about to be vested in the University Council. That body is unable to render financial aid, therefore outside assistance must be sought, and the fund, when established, given into the council's control.

Last of all I have to thank in the very warmest fashion the present trustees for the efforts they have continually made and for the manner in which they have so thoroughly and capably brought about the successful issue of this afternoon's ceremony. I also desire to cordially thank his Excellency the Governor for having consented to open this building. My sincere thanks are also due to Dr Scott for his kindness in superintending the hanging of the pictures, a work which he has carried out with his usual artistic taste.

Now I say farewell, with a sincere expression of regard and the heartiest of wishes that the success which I hope will attend this auspicious occasion may continue to prevail in connection with the maintenance of the collections.

Yours very sincerely,
T.M. Hocken.

Appendix II

T.M. Hocken's Last Will and Testament

THIS IS THE LAST WILL AND TESTAMENT of me THOMAS MORLAND HOCKEN of Dunedin in the Provincial District of Otago in the Dominion of New Zealand Surgeon I REVOKE all Wills and Testamentary Dispositions heretofore made by me I BEQUEATH to my dear wife ELIZABETH MARY HOCKEN absolutely all the furniture plate pictures linen napery consumable stores and all personal property effects and things which shall at the time of my death be about or belonging to my then dwelling house I APPOINT my said wife Elizabeth Mary Hocken and John Halliday Scott of Dunedin *aforesaid Professor of Anatomy and Physiology Executors and Trustees hereof AND I DEVISE unto the said Elizabeth Mary Hocken and John Halliday Scott their heirs executors administrators and assigns all the real estate and I BEQUEATH to them their executors administrators and assigns all the personal estate of or to which I shall be seized possessed or entitled at my decease UPON TRUST to sell and convert into money my said estates or such parts thereof as shall be of a saleable or convertible nature and to get in the other parts thereof AND I DIRECT my trustees to hold the moneys to arise from such sale conversion and getting in upon the trusts and subject to the Declarations hereinafter contained that is to say:–

1. TO pay or retain all the expenses incident to the execution of the preceding trust and my funeral and testamentary expenses.
2. TO invest the surplus of the said moneys in manner hereinafter directed (which said moneys and investments are hereinafter referred to under the denomination of the said "trust fund".)
3. TO pay the annual income of the said trust fund to my wife during her life.
4. IMMEDIATELY after the decease or future marriage of my said wife as to as well the capital as the annual income of the said trust fund UPON TRUST as to my shares in the National Mortgage and Agency Company of New Zealand Limited my shares in The Otago Daily Times and Witness Company Limited my shares in the Union Bank of Australia Limited my shares in Brown Ewing and Company Limited my shares in The New Zealand Paper Mills Limited and my shares in The Knox Patent Improved Level Fresh Air Inlet Company Limited for my daughter GLADYS HOCKEN absolutely.
5.* AS to my shares in the National Insurance Company of New Zealand Limited my shares in The Westport Coal Company Limited my shares in The Standard Fire and Marine Insurance Company of New Zealand Limited and my shares in The Talisman Consolidated Gold Mining Company Limited UPON TRUST for "The T.M. Hocken University of Otago" AND I DECLARE that a receipt under the Seal of the University shall be a sufficient discharge to my trustees for the shares or moneys paid or transferred by my trustees to the University of Otago.
6. AS to my shares in The Dunedin Stock Exchange Proprietary Limited my shares in Whitcombe and Tombs Limited and my shares in the Mosgiel Woollen Company Limited UPON TRUST for The Dunedin Diocesan Trust Board to be held by the Board as a fund to provide out of the income thereof for the increase of the stipends of the poorer Anglican Clergy in the Diocese of Dunedin AND I DECLARE that the allocation of the said income shall in each year be made by the Bishop and Standing Committee for the time being of the said Diocese AND I DECLARE that a receipt under the Seal of The Dunedin Diocesan Trust Board shall be a sufficient discharge to my trustees for the shares or moneys paid or transferred by my trustees to The Dunedin Diocesan Trust Board for the purposes aforesaid.

7. AS to my shares in The Dunedin Fernhill Club Proprietary and my shares in The National Bank of New Zealand Limited UPON TRUST for The Dunedin Diocesan Trust Board IN TRUST to invest the same in any of the modes of investment hereby authorized and pay the income from time to time arising therefrom to The Maori Mission Board constituted under Canon VII Title B of the Code of Canons of the Church of the Province of New Zealand commonly called The Church of England to be distributed by the said Maori Mission Board in manner provided by the said Canon I DECLARE that if the said Maori Mission Board shall at any time cease to exist the said The Dunedin Diocesan Trust Board shall pay the said income to such person or persons as the General Synod of the said Church shall from time to time direct to be expended in the work of the said Church among the Maori population of New Zealand AND I FURTHER DECLARE that a receipt under the Seal of The Dunedin Diocesan Trust Board shall be a sufficient discharge to my trustees for the shares or moneys paid or transferred by my trustees to the said Board for the purposes aforesaid.

8. AS to my shares in The Port Chalmers Gas Company Limited my shares in Mason Struthers and Company Limited of Christchurch and my shares in the Junction Dredging Company Limited (a Company registered in the State of Victoria) UPON TRUST for the Salvation Army to be expended and laid out in equal shares between the Maternity Home in Heriot Row Dunedin aforesaid the Rescue Home at Caversham near Dunedin aforesaid and The Children's Home in Middlemarch in the Provincial District of Otago aforesaid AND I T. M. Hocken *DECLARE that if the Maternity House the Rescue Home and the Children's Home or any of them shall not be in existence at the time of my death or the death of my said wife the share bequeathed to any of such Homes as may not be in existence at the time of my death or at the death of my said wife shall be expended by the Salvation Army for General Social work in the Dominion of New Zealand AND I FURTHER DECLARE that a receipt under the hand of the Commanding Officer for the time being stationed at Dunedin aforesaid shall be a sufficient discharge to my trustees for the shares or moneys paid or transferred by my trustees to the Salvation Army for the purposes aforesaid.

9. AS to my shares in The Trustees Executors and Agency Company of New Zealand Limited my shares in The Taupari Coal Company Limited and my shares in Burnside Hydraulic Limited UPON TRUST for The Dunedin Public Art Society Registered AND I DECLARE that a receipt under the Seal of the Society shall be a sufficient discharge to my trustees for the shares or moneys paid or transferred by my trustees to the Dunedin Public Art Gallery Society Registered.

10. AS to my shares in The Dannevirke Gas Company Limited and my shares in The Phoenix Company Limited UPON TRUST for the Trinity Methodist Church Dunedin for the benefit in equal shares of the various Methodist Churches in Dunedin and Suburbs AND I DECLARE that the receipt of the Treasurer of the Trinity Methodist Church Dunedin shall be a sufficient discharge to my trustees for the shares or moneys paid or transferred by my trustees to the Trinity Methodist Church Dunedin aforesaid for the purpose aforesaid.

11. AS to my shares in Dalgety and Company Limited my shares in The Napier Gas Company Limited my shares in The Perpetual Trustees Estate and Agency Company of New Zealand Limited my shares in the Waihi Gold Mining Company Limited and the moneys to arise on the policy of Assurance on my life effected with the New Zealand Government Insurance Department UPON TRUST for The University of Otago to be held by The University of Otago IN TRUST to apply the income thereof in payment of the Salary of a

cultured librarian who will utilize his whole time in looking after and keeping in good order and from time to time as occasion *shall require in cataloguing the Collection of Books Manuscripts Newspapers other documents Pictures Prints Photographs Drawings and other articles of a similar character in relation to the Early History of the Colony of New Zealand and the Australian Colonies given by me to the Public of the said Dominion of New Zealand now housed in the wing or addition to the Museum erected on The Otago University Museum Reserve and which are now in the management and control of the University of Otago under a certain Trust Deed dated the Second day of September One thousand nine hundred and seven made between myself of the First part John Roberts C.M.G. of Dunedin aforesaid Merchant and Mark Cohen of the same place Journalist and Henry Edward Williams of the same place Insurance Agent and John Ross of the same place Importer and William Blaxland Benham of the same place Professor of Biology in the University of Otago of the Second Part and the University of Otago of the third part and in looking after and keeping in good order and from time to time cataloguing all other Books Manuscripts Newspapers documents Pictures Prints Photographs Drawings and other articles of a similar character as may be from time to time added to the said Collection.

12. IN case I shall at any time or times in my lifetime sell any share or shares which I have hereinbefore directed my trustees to stand possessed of on the trusts hereinbefore contained I DIRECT my trustees to appropriate out of the said trust fund such a sum or sums as shall represent the net price at which I sold any such share or shares as aforesaid and to stand possessed of such sum or sums upon the same trusts and subject to the same provisions hereinbefore declared of and concerning the share or shares so sold by me AND I FURTHER DIRECT my trustees in case my trustees in exercise of the power of sale hereinbefore contained shall at any time or times sell any of such share or shares to stand possessed of the net proceeds arising from any such sale or sales upon the same trusts and subject to the same provisions hereinbefore declared of and concerning the share or shares so sold by my trustees as aforesaid.

13.* I DIRECT my trustees from time to time when the Lease of the house and premises occupied by me in Moray Place Dunedin aforesaid shall expire during the life time of my said wife to take all proceedings and to do or concur in doing all things which may be necessary for the purpose of having the valuations referred to in such Lease duly made and of having a renewed Lease of such house and premises *offered for sale by auction and if requested by my said wife so to do to bid for and become the purchaser of any such renewed Lease either at the upset rent fixed on any such valuation or at an advanced rent AND I FURTHER DIRECT my trustees to permit and allow my said wife to occupy the said house and premises for such term and so long as she may desire without payment of rent to my trustees PROVIDED my said wife so long as she elects to occupy the said house and premises shall at her own expense keep the said house and premises in good and tenantable repair and duly insured against loss or damage by fire and shall pay the ground rent to the superior landlord the Property Tax the Rates Taxes and all other outgoings whatsoever imposed or charged on the said house and premises and shall observe and perform all the covenants and conditions in any such Lease contained and on the part of the Lessee to be observed and performed.

14. AS to the residue of my said estate I DIRECT my trustees to hold the same IN TRUST for my niece EMILY BENSTEAD and my nephew ERSCA HOCKEN in equal shares or if they or either of them shall die in my lifetime IN TRUST for their or her or his executors and administrators to be disposed of as part of their her or his personal estate.

15. I EMPOWER my trustees to sell my real estate by public auction or private contract together or in parcels subject to such terms and conditions as to title or evidence or commencement of title or time or mode of payment of the purchase money or indemnity against or apportionment of encumbrances or as to any other matters relating to the sale as my trustees shall judge expedient and to fix reserved biddings and buy in property offered for sale and vacate or vary contracts for sale and to resell as aforesaid without liability to answer for any consequential loss and generally to effect the sale and conversion of my said estates on such terms and in such manner as my trustees shall deem most advantageous.

16. I EMPOWER my trustees to postpone for such period as they shall judge expedient the sale conversion or getting in of my real and personal estates or any parts thereof respectively notwithstanding that the same may be of a wasting speculative or reversionary nature and during such period to manage and order all the affairs thereof as regards letting occupation cultivation repairs insurance against fire receipt of rents indulgences and allowances to tenants and all other matters.

17. I DECLARE that pending such sale calling in and conversion the whole income of property actually producing income shall as well during the first year after my decease as in subsequent years be deemed the annual income thereof applicable as such for the purpose of the said trust without regard to the amount of such income *or to the nature of the property and investments yielding T.M. Hocken the same and that as between the capital and income of my estate no apportionment of rents dividends or other periodical payments shall take place for or in respect of the period current at my decease.

18. I DIRECT that all investments of moneys to be made by my trustees shall be made in their names in or upon some one or more of the investments or securities following that is to say in securities in which trustees are authorized to invest trust moneys by an Act of the General Assembly of New Zealand and in or upon the bonds or debentures of any Local Authority or other Corporate Body authorized by any Act of the General Assembly of New Zealand to borrow money upon debentures or in or upon the shares and debentures of any Bank Public Company or Private Company at the time of the investments respectively paying a dividend on their ordinary shares AND I EMPOWER my trustees from time to time at their discretion to vary the investment or investments of my said trust moneys for any other or others of the kinds prescribed.

19. I DECLARE that my trustees shall have full discretionary power to permit any part of my personal estate which may at the time of my decease be invested in any species of investments yielding interest or income (other than shares in Gold Mining Companies) forming part of my residuary estate to remain in the same state of investment for such period or periods as my trustees shall think fit.

20. I DECLARE that the expression "my trustees" used by me in this my Will shall be construed as comprising and referring to the trustees or trustee for the time being of this my Will.
IN WITNESS whereof I have to this my last Will and Testament contained in this and the five preceding sheets of paper set my hand this twenty seventh day of April One thousand nine hundred and nine.
SIGNED by the said Thomas Morland Hocken as his last Will and Testament in the presence of us both present at the same time who at his request in his presence and in the presence of each other have hereunto subscribed our names as witnesses:

Spencer Brent
Solicitor Dunedin
T.S. Brent
Clerk to Haggitt Brent & Williams
Solicitors Dunedin

This is a Codicil to the last Will and Testament of me Thomas Morland Hocken which Will bears the date the twenty seventh day of April 1909.

1. I revoke Clause eleven of my said Will being confident that the Citizens of Dunedin will arise sufficient funds to answer by means of the income thereof the yearly salary of a Cultured Librarian to utilize the whole of his time in the manner mentioned in said Clause Eleven.
2. I revoke Clause fourteen of my said Will disposing of the residue of my estate.
3.** I bequeath to my friend Margaret Malcolm the sum of One hundred pounds to be paid to her as soon after my death as convenient.
4.** I bequeath to my Trustees the sum of (£1500) fifteen hundred pounds in Trust for my niece Emily Benstead and I bequeath to my Trustees the sum of one thousand pounds in Trust for my nephew Ersca Hocken I direct that if the said Ersca Hocken shall die in my lifetime my Trustees shall hold the sum of One thousand pounds bequeathed to him in Trust for the said Emily Benstead and I direct that until the said sums are paid they shall bear interest from my death at the rate of five pounds per centum per annum payable half yearly.
5. I bequeath all the residue of my estate to my Trustees including the said shares and policy money mentioned in Clause fourteen of my Will in Trust for my wife for life and after her death in Trust for my daughter Gladys Hocken.

Witnesses
    Spencer Brett
    Molly Neill

In witness where of I have hereunto set my hand this third day of April Thomas Morland Hocken One thousand nine hundred and ten
Signed by the said Thomas Morland Hocken as a Codicil to his last Will and Testament in the presence of us both present at the same time who at his request and in the presence of each other have hereunto subscribed our names as witnesses:

    Spencer Brent
    Solicitor Dunedin
    Molly Neill
    Spinster Dunedin

*   denotes marginal signatures T.M. Hocken, Spencer Brent and T.S. Brent
** denotes marginal signatures T.M. Hocken, Spencer Brent and Molly Neill

Appendix III

Selected Book-collecting Letters
Turnbull Letterbooks, Vol. I, pp. 388–89
Turnbull to Hocken, 9 May 1894

Dear Dr Hocken,
I have discovered a small parcel … Home. You will probably have most of them if not all however the titles are as follows:
1. Catechism of the Constitution of N.Z. by a member of a Provincial Council. Lyttelton, 1855. 12mo. Pamphlet. pp. 8.
2. Report of the Settlement of Nelson, N.Z. by Wm Fox. London, 1849.
3. Handbook of N.Z. & the Australian Continent by John Bright. London, 1841. pot. 8vo. pp. 210 (wants 2 pp. of addenda).
4. Hints to intending sheep farmers in N.Z. by F.A. Weld. Fourth edition, London, 1864. cr. 8vo. Pamphlet. pp. 40.
5. N.Z. & the N.Z. Coy. In answer to a pamphlet entitled How to Colonize by T. Heale. London, 1842. 8vo. Pamphlet. pp. 63.
6. N.Z. as a field for emigration by Rev. J. Berry. London, 1879. cr. 8vo. Pamphlet. pp. 40 with map.
7. Information relative to N.Z. for the use of Colonists. London, 1839. 8vo. Pamphlet. pp. 80 with map.
8. Memorial to his Grace the Secretary of State for the Colonies together with a vindication of the character of the missionaries & native Christians. London, 1861. 8vo. Pamphlet. pp. xi & 35.
9. Further Remarks on N.Z. affairs. London, 1861. 8vo. Pamphlet. pp. 30
10. The case of the war in N.Z. by E.H. Browne. Cambridge, 1860. 8vo. Pamphlet. pp. 51.

If there are any of the foregoing you have not got I shall be very happy to effect exchanges … number of pamphlets not in my collection.
    With kind regards I remain yours sincerely AHT

※ ※

Turnbull Letterbooks, Vol. III, p. 545
Turnbull to Mr Evans, 25 November 1897

Dear Mr Evans,
Here I have been on ecstasy of tiptoes and tenterhooks of tribulations (as my friend the Baboo would say) for ever so long thinking to regale myself on Mahan's 'Nelson' (ordered long ago to come post) and till now never a sign of it and numerous editions bred from the original one! I shall burst unless it arrives soon!
    Will you also keep an eye open for a work by Dr. T.M. Hocken on the early history of Otago, New Zealand, to be published by Low I think …

※ ※

Turnbull Letterbooks, transcript III, p. 689
Turnbull to Hocken, 5 May 1898

Dear Dr Hocken,
I trust you and Mrs Hocken had a comfortable journey to Dunedin and have been able to obtain plenty of uninterrupted sleep after all the voyaging you have gone through.
 By last mail I received from London a most valuable and interesting volume containing autograph and holograph letters from Capt Cook, Captain Carteret, King, Webber, Samwell, Solander. The volume contains the original log and Journal of Furneaux's voyage during his separation from Cook, the original report about the massacre of 'Adventure's [sic] boat's crew in Queen Charlotte Sound drawn up to Mr Burney and extracts from which appear in the printed voyage. There is likewise a letter from Brown the gunner's mate of 'Endeavour' giving an account of Capt. Cook's 'death at Owyhee'. Solander's letter, which is very long, is mainly about Omai. There are portraits too, of Cook, King and Carteret, the latter I have never seen before. I wish it had arrived previous to your visit. By the same mail I received that rare little pamphlet 'Popular Account of New Zealand' published in Glasgow in 1839. You probably have it, I have been on the lookout for the work for a long time.
 With kind regards, to Mrs Hocken and yourself, I remain,
  yours faithfully, Alex H. Turnbull

       *   *

Turnbull Letterbooks, Vol. III, p. 691
Turnbull to Edwin Gurr, Apia, Samoa, 10 May 1898

Dear Sir,
Dr. Hocken of Dunedin when giving me an account of his recent visit to Samoa mentioned your name in connection with his trip to Stevenson's house and said you were good enough to allow both him and his wife to select a few volumes from Stevenson's Library. Dr Hocken suggested that I should write to you, as I am anxious to secure a few souvenirs of Stevenson, and ask you to send me a few volumes. Will you do so? If you let me know what the cost will be I can remit you the money.
 I am also desirous of obtaining any newspapers, pamphlets, books, etc published in the Samoan language especially those issued in Samoa and if you can give me the names of any of them, with prices, and where they can be got I shall feel obliged.
 Yours faithfully AHT

       *   *

A.H. Turnbull, 1868–1918, Papers 0057-039
Hocken to Turnbull, 2 May 1899

Dear Mr Turnbull,
Going over my old newspapers – which has been an immense task, I find I have a great many duplicates of N.Z. Spectator, Wellington Independent, Nelson Examiner, Otago Witness, &c. They range from the forties upwards & are very fairly complete.

I do not specify them particularly as it is possible you may have some or may not want them. But if you do you could mention your requirements & we might effect exchanges or purchases. The newspapers I want are the old Kororareka ones (/40 to /43) & some of the early Southern Crosses. But you might let me know what you have, what you want, & what you think would be the value of these old records.

With our kind regards to you all,
Sincerely T.M. Hocken

P.S. I am also wanting some numbers of the 'N.Z. Gazette & Well. Spec' for 41, 42, 43, 44 – perhaps 15 in all. Of this paper I have many duplicates. Also want many of the earliest Auckland Papers – 'Herald' & Auck Gazette, 'Auck. Times', &c.

✳ ✳

Turnbull Letterbooks, Vol. IV, p. 170
Turnbull to Messrs Angus & Robertson, Sydney, 25 March 1899

Dear Sirs,
The box of books arrived here safely yesterday ... I am returning the above two books to you. Abstract report of the Geological Survey of N.Z. for 1869. price 10/-. The last page of this is defective, a bit being torn from it, and I think you should make a considerable reduction in the price. The work itself is marked 'Gratis' by Dr Hocken ...

✳ ✳

Turnbull Letterbooks, Vol. IV, p. 217
Turnbull to Dr Hocken, 30 May 1899

Dear Dr Hocken,
I am in receipt of your letter dated 24th inst enclosing list of the duplicate newspapers you possess and I am obliged to you for the trouble you have taken in compiling it but I was not prepared for so high a figure being put upon the papers and my idea of the value would be nearer £100 seeing that some of the sets are incomplete; but it is very difficult, without actually seeing them, to say what the value really is. Would it be possible for you to send me these duplicates to me here so that I might look through them. I paying freight both ways and insurance. I should then be better able to judge what to offer. It is not possible for me to get away from Wellington just now or I should do myself the pleasure of paying Dunedin a visit. If you do decide to send the newspapers up here I would guarantee to give you an answer within a week of their receipt.

Trusting that you will see your way to do this. I remain,
Yours sincerely, AHT.

✳ ✳

Turnbull Letterbooks, Vol. IV, p. 219
Turnbull to Dr Hocken [3 June 1899]
Dear Dr Hocken,
I am in receipt of your note dated 2nd inst. and am glad to learn that you will be sending the newspapers up for me to look at. Please let me know when you send the packages away from your house so that I may get insurance cover for them. I presume that you will ship them from Pt Chalmers by direct steamer to Wellington. I can quite understand the difficulty you have had in collecting these newspapers and their scarcity can partly be measured by the fact that I have so few – though of course I collected most of my N.Z. books in England.
    With kind regards to Mrs Hocken & yourself I remain yours sincerely AHT
p.s. There is an account of 'firewalking' at Rarotonga in last number of 'Polynesian Journal'.

✳ ✳

Turnbull Letterbooks, Vol. IV, p. 234
Turnbull to Hocken, 19 June 1899

Dear Dr. Hocken,
Your telegram reached me advising the dispatch of case of newspapers to hand and finally the case itself arrived at the house when I became all bustle – excitement. I have been carefully through the papers with the exception of 'The Illustrated N.Z. Herald' & 'Southern Cross' and enclosed you will find a list of those numbers missing & mutilated chiefly from the 'Independent', 'Spectator' or 'Nelson Examiner'. With regard to the list you sent up. The following years are missing: 'Spectator' 1856, 1858, 1863, 1864, 'Independent' 1855. I notice also that a good many supplements to 'Nelson Examiner', 'Spectator', 'Independent' are missing. Seeing how many numbers are missing & mutilated and I may say that I have not counted all the slight deficiencies in the text, I think that £200 is a fair price for the papers and if you will accept this I am prepared to send you a cheque for the amount, should you decide to take this I trust I may look to you to help me to fill in the missing parts from duplicates you have not yet looked over.
    'Otago Journal' – I do want No. 1 to complete my set – I also want sessions 2 & 23 of Proceedings of Wellington Provincial Council – Session 28 & after 34 of Proceedings of Provinc. Council of Otago and vols. 1, 2, 8, 13 & after 20 of Otago Provincial Gazette. I have very few Provincial votes & Proceedings of Southland, Nelson, Auckland. Of course these latter I look upon as distinct from the newspapers and will be very glad to pay for them. I wish I had some duplicates to exchange with you, so as to avoid the 'money' difficulty but you have everything in your library that I have in duplicate so there is no chance for me. My sister goes away in 'Waikare' for the South Sea Island trip and at present she is reading every available work in my collection bearing on the subject.
    With kind regards to Mrs Hocken & yourself, I remain,
      yours sincerely AHT
p.s. Was there a pamphlet printed giving an account of Capt. Jarvey's *Second* trial? I have the *first* trial.

✳ ✳

Turnbull Letterbooks, Vol. IV, p. 242
Turnbull to Hocken, 26 June 1899

Dear Dr Hocken,
I am in receipt of your letter dated 23rd inst. and I now have the pleasure to enclose cheque for £200 in payment of the newspapers you sent me. With regard to my list of missing and mutilated numbers; when I write – for example – 281–90 or 41–9, I mean that the numbers *from* 281 *to* 290 or *from* 41 *to* 49 are missing or mutilated, as the case may be. No I have not the 'scheme' nor the 'letter' you mention in your letter but if you can spare them I should like to add them to my collection. I am much obliged to you for your promise of the Otago Gazette & proceedings: of Nelson I possess nothing. I have never seen 'Otago Punch' nor have I any numbers of 'Dunedin Punch'. The 'Auckland Punch' I have one year of & some duplicate numbers – I think the latter at your service if you want them. Recently I purchased the 'remainder' at a sale, of a work called 'Jewlius Rex', a pamphlet published at Gisborne, lampooning Sir Julius Vogel & others. If you haven't got this can I send you a copy.
    With kind regards to Mrs Hocken & yourself I remain, yours sincerely, AHT
p.s. I have some duplicate numbers of Wellington Provinc. Council. Perhaps I can fill some of your vacancies!

※ ※

Turnbull Letterbooks, Vol. IV, p. 254
Turnbull to Hocken, 4 July 1899

Dear Dr Hocken,
I am in receipt of your two letters dated respectively the 28th and 30th June, likewise your telegram informing me of the despatch per 'Flora' of the second case of newspapers and of a parcel under care of Mr Cutten. The case must have missed the steamer as it was not on board when 'Flora' discharged her cargo here but no doubt it will arrive in due course. I thank you for your promise to look out for the numbers missing from my sets: I have already procured several locally and just the other day I secured 3 vols. – 2 of Independent for 1865 & 7, and one of a miscellaneous collection of Wellington Wanganui & Hawkes Bay papers, including the first numbers of 'N.Z. Times' – the first number of which was believed not to exist. I shall mind what you say regarding the 'Wellington Advertiser' caricatures and return them if they prove to be the same as those in my library. Statistics of Nelson & New Munster, the former I have but not the latter. Nor have I the view of Auckland by Hutchinson with key – you mention. The A.H. Turnbull figuring at Auckland must be my namesake as I have not been there for some months and he too is probably the happy possessor of the 'tall folio Shakespeare' because I do not aspire to such high game and *he* I know is an ardent book collector. There were two editions of Thevenot, as no doubt you know – one, the 8vo. published in 1681 *with* Tasman's map but no account of the voyage and the other in 1696 with the *account* but no *map* I have them both. I am sorry to say that I have no duplicates of 'Karere Maori'. No. 40 of N.Z. Spectator was not sent. Session 1 of Wellington Provinc. Council Votes & Proceedings I shall send you in due course of a day or so. It is the only duplicate I have of this set you want. Amongst some of my duplicates are the following and you are welcome to any or all of them:
1. Memoires touchant l'establissement d'une mission chretienne dans le troisième
    partie du monde appele la Terre Australe. Paris: 1 Vol. 1663 (wants the map)

2. Waka Maori of 1871. Vol. 1 & 2 others complete volumes I think.
How did you like Reeve's book 'Ao tea roa'? I thought it very good giving as it did a comprehensive view of N.Z. History. I have a good many of the old Maori publications including the 1835 Luke but I have not got the 1st 4to translation of the Bible nor have I any of the St. John's College publications. Great spouting & spluttering of politicians here just now in consequence of parliament sitting and the general election being so nigh members seem anxious to impress their constituencies, through the papers of the 'exuberance of their verbosity'.
    With kind regards to Mrs Hocken and yourself.
    Yours sincerely AHT.

✷ ✷

Turnbull Letterbooks, Vol. IV, p. 256
Turnbull to Hocken, 4 July 1899

Dear Dr Hocken,
Since writing my letter to you this morning I find that the Express Coy. have delivered the case of newspapers although they told me that it was not on board 'Flora'. The parcel however has not yet come to hand.
    Yours faithfully AHT
P.S. As I finished above my brother brought in your parcel which had been left at the office by Mr Cutten.

✷ ✷

Turnbull Letterbooks, Vol. IV, p. 261
Turnbull to Hocken, 6 July 1899

Dear Dr Hocken,
By this post I forward to you the Session 1 Wgtn: Prov. Council votes & Proceedings and I trust it will reach you safely. I received today from England Capt Mein Smith's map of Wellington dated 14th August 1840 & the sketch plan of the neighbourhood of Port Nicholson dated 4th January 1843. Have you got these? Do you happen to possess a duplicate of No. 2 Canterbury Papers *New Series*? J.G.S. Grant must be an extraordinary individual: I remember the late Mr Reynolds giving me a long account of him one Sunday.
    With kind regards I remain yours sincerely, AHT

✷ ✷

Turnbull Letterbooks, Vol. IV, p. 304
Turnbull to Hocken, 21 August 1899

Dear Dr Hocken,
I beg to acknowledge receipt of your letter dated 3rd inst. and I have not sent you a fresh list of my missing newspapers because two persons here have promised to give me some old numbers of 'Independent' & 'Spectator' and amongst them there may be some that I want. No, I did not know of the existence of 'New Zealand Examiner':

I hope you will be able to complete your set. By last mail I received a pamphlet called 'Abduction' giving a short account of Wakefield's run-away match with Miss Turner containing a portrait of the young lady. I suppose you have not a duplicate of Grey's 'Chants & Poems of the Maoris', the 1851 edition? I possess 2 copies of the 1853 edition but not the earlier. My sister will return to Wellington in a few days from her S. Sea trip: she saw the fire-walking ceremony but it was not a good display apparently and the arrangements were bad. I shall send you a list of the newspapers wanting to complete my sets as soon as my friends carry out their promises.

With kind regards to Mrs Hocken and yourself, I remain yours sincerely AHT

※ ※

Turnbull Letterbooks, Vol. IV, p. 432
Turnbull to Hocken, 10 April 1900

Dear Dr Hocken,
I am ashamed to look you in the face – even by means of a letter as it were, because I have not written to thank you for the view of Auckland, plan of Dunedin, and the other valuable papers you were good enough to send me by my sister. Everything reached me safely.

I have a catalogue of the late Mr Larnach's library to be sold at Dunedin this month by Park, Reynolds & Co. but it is an utterly useless document to anyone at a distance because no proper description is given of the books, the dates of publication in the greater number of instances are omitted as well as the edition and no indication is given as to 'condition'. There are one or two lots I may bid for 'on spec'. There has been nothing new, or rather old, added to my collection lately except some Milton pamphlets to fill some gaps in that series. I was very grieved that I could not manage to attend the opening of Nelson's carved whare at Whakarewarewa this month. I was invited but business prevented me going. The newspaper accounts of the ceremonies have been sent to me, and the photographs are promised later. The whole scene must have been a vivid one. I knew old Te Rangitahau, the celebrated tohunga who officiated. A friend of mine at Ohinemutu writes me under date 6th inst. That this old man died on the 5th in Tamata Kapua the carved house at Ohinemutu and the Maoris of the district ascribe his death to 'makatu'. Nelson having bewitched him! Just before his death he is said to have imparted to Nelson some very ancient Maori priest-lore. My sister is on the eve of arriving at San Francisco by this time and I look forward to hearing from her on Friday by the incoming 'Frisco mail.

With kind regards I remain yours sincerely AHT

※ ※

Turnbull to Hocken, 22 May 1900

Dear Dr Hocken,
It is very good indeed of you to let me have those pamphlets I named out of those purchased by you at Larnach's sale. I note too what you say about the Sydney trade list and proclamations. The sale must have been horribly mismanaged and the catalogue was without exception the worst one I have seen of a library containing so many books of colonial interest.

I have not yet collated the New Zealand and Southern Cross but from casually going through the files I gather that they are very incomplete. When I take them in hand I shall be pleased to let you know what duplicates I have. There are some I know of the Southern Cross for 1848. The Karere Maori too I have not yet gone properly through but up to No. 112 there is but 1 duplicate No. 66 or 67 but it is in so mutilated condition that it is scarcely worth having. You are welcome to it however. I have some duplicates I think of the 4to edition of the Messenger and I shall look them up for you. My set – so far as I have gone into it – is complete from No. 1 to 90 from then it runs consequentially to No. 112 but the numbers are in very bad condition from No. 112 until that publication of the 4to edition. I have no numbers nor have any after 1859 but as I said before I fancy that I possess some duplicates of the months between 1853 & 59.

With regard to J.G.S. Grant's productions I did have some duplicates of several but I have long ago exchanged them. My set of the Saturday Review is not complete – to make it requires Nos. 32, 34, 43, 49, 51, 56 & 18. The file ends with No. 100 on 21st Feb 1868. Were there any more issues of it after that date?

Bound up in the same volume are 2 months of Grant's Monthly Review nos. 1 & 2 (1864). Were any more published? The Hawke's Bay Herald & Hawke's Bay Times I have been collating from amongst Colenso's newspapers and find that there is a fine series of the former from 1857 to 1865. I require however several numbers including Nos. 1, 15, 16. Do you happen to possess duplicates? There are a good many duplicates of the Herald about the early sixties so if you lack numbers in your set let me know and perhaps I can find them amongst my duplicates. The H.B. Times is a very interesting publication.

I am now about to tackle Colenso's files of N.Z. Spectator (of which there are great numbers) & N.Z. Advertiser. There are a few numbers of The Echo, Stout's paper published in Dunedin. If there are any missing parts in your set of Spectator please let me know, because I might be able to find them.

With kind regards to Mrs Hocken and yourself. I remain,
Yours faithfully Alex. H. Turnbull

P.S. Enclosed note with final collation of Yate's Scripture Extracts.

'Collation of volume of scripture extracts, ets. seen through the press by Rev. Yate & printed at Sydney, New South Wales, in 1830[?]'.

Size 6" x 4" (actual size of page)
Size by signatures 12 mo.
My copy begins at page 5.
Kenehi (Genesis) pp. 5. double columns
Chapters 2 (part) or 3 (whole)
Matiu (8 Matthew) pp. 7–28. double columns
Chapters 1–9
1 Koriniti (1st Corinthians) pp. 41–51. double columns
Chapters 1–6
Page 52 is blank
Ko te inoinga i te ata (Morning Prayer) single column pp. 53–73
Ko te inoinga i te ahiahi (Evening Prayer) single column pp. 74–85
Ko nga ture o te Atua (The Commandments) single column pp. 86–88
1 Katikihama (1st Catechism) single column pp. 89–93
2 Katikahama (2nd Catechism) single columns pp. 94–100
Ko Nga Himene (Hymns) single columns pp. 101 (unpaginated) to 117 (19 Hymns)
Imprint at foot of page 117: – Printed by R. Mansfield for the executors of R. Howe. No watermark in paper. Pages 1–4 including title-page missing in my copy. An edition of 550 copies was printed. See Missionary Register for January 1831, p. 67.

* *

MS-0451-031
Hocken to Turnbull, 28 February 1910

My dear Turnbull,
I must not allow a second of your kind letters to pass unanswered though I am in a sadly crippled condition & do not know what the end may be. However I can & do still do some work though mostly in bed. I am very pleased that you derive so much assistance from my bibliography which I am quite sure is of great value. I was somewhat annoyed & still more so as unable to answer from illness that odd & curious criticism of Collier's in the – I forget what. He took & gave in the same breath. A most jealous spirit seems to have pervaded him – very very different from the correspondence I had with him before even he commenced his bib. 25 years ago when I offered to work conjointly with him. Fortunately I kept this correspondence, not certainly with the least idea that it might ever prove useful but simply as a pleasant reminiscence of what an able man like himself might say on the whole subject. His solar myth business – was on the ace of rejecting as it is now virtually valueless & disproved but at the time I was pushed for him to make further research & as the matter was of no great information I accepted his remarks.

I thought he was dead until at the last moment his 'Sir G. Grey' appeared which while interesting appears to be to me unfinished & somewhat erratic. Still the book did not profess to be more than a sketch of some incidents in his life. I hope in about 10 days to begin forwarding the collection to its final home. Still it is a great regret that I cannot superintend its proper distribution – especially the pictures. Few can understand this but you will most thoroughly. I was sorry indeed to pass twice through Wellington without seeing you. The first time I have ever done such a thing. But I was simply unable & had to remain on board. You know how much I should enjoy a long talk & browse with you. Let us hope that day may come again. I forbear to ask you questions.
Ever yours sincerely, my dear Turnbull,
T.M. Hocken.

* *

MS-0451-013/007 *Correspondence*
Anderson to Hocken, re Mitchel's endowment
Sydney, 25 March 1899

Dear Sir,
In accordance with the wish of Mr George Robertson of Angus and Robertson, I write to give you some particulars of the conditions made by Mr. D.S. Mitchell, in making his noble gift of his Library of 30,000 volumes to this Library:
He specifies:
1. That they must be suitably housed in a separate wing of a new building to be erected at once by the Government for the National Library of this colony.
2. That this wing shall be always kept separate from the general collection and shall be known as the 'David Scott Mitchell Library'.
3. That admittance to it will not be absolutely free without restriction, as at present to the general Library; but will be by ticket issued by the Principal Librarian on recommendation from a respectable householder as is done in the British Museum.

4.   That the Library Trustees shall be made into a Corporate body by Act of Parliament, in order to provide for their continuous succession.

Mr Mitchell intends to endow the Library very handsomely, to provide for the continuation of this Australasian collection, and will of course allow Trustees ample powers to accumulate the revenue from his endowment for any number of years in order that they may be able to buy any large collection that might be put under offer to them in future years. Mr Mitchell especially wishes it to be understood that he makes no condition about the administration of the Library or the appointment of men who are to deal with it in future.

He proposes to hand over 10,000 volumes as soon as we have the place adjacent to the present Library fitted up for their reception.

If I can give you any further information, please command me.
I remain,
Yours sincerely,
Henry Anderson

Notes

Abbreviations

ADB	*Australian Dictionary of Biography*
ACL	Auckland Central Library
AIM	Auckland Institute and Museum Library Collection
ATL	Alexander Turnbull Library
BiM	*Books in Maori, 1815–1900: An annotated bibliography*
BL	British Library
CMS	Church Missionary Society
DLB	*Dictionary of Literary Biography*
DNZB	Dictionary of New Zealand Biography
EHMSS	Early History, Maori and South Seas
EMH	Elizabeth Mary (Bessie) Hocken
F&J	Flotsam & Jetsam
GHD	Gladys Hocken's Diary
HC	Hocken Collections
HPC	Hocken Pamphlet Collection
JPS	*Journal of the Polynesian Society (Containing the Transactions and Proceedings of the Society)*
MONZ	Museum of New Zealand Te Papa Tongarewa
MS/MSS	manuscript/manuscripts
NE&NZC	*Nelson Examiner and New Zealand Chronicle*
ODT	*Otago Daily Times*
OW	*Otago Witness*
PRO	Public Records Office, London
SLNSW	State Library of New South Wales
TMH	Thomas Morland Hocken
W	*A Bibliography of Printed Maori to 1900*

Foreword

1. T.M. Hocken to Miss Betts, 16 October 1888. Betts Family Papers, Vol. I. Correspondence 1827–1910. ML A2563. State Library of New South Wales.

Introduction

1. A.H. Turnbull to Gilbert Mair, 12 July 1912, cited in E.H. McCormick, *Alexander Turnbull: His life his circle his collections* (Wellington: Alexander Turnbull Library, 1974), p. 240.
2. See *Journal of Polynesian Society (JPS)*, Vol. XVII (1908), prelims and p.50.
3. Percy Smith to Thomas Morland Hocken (TMH), 6 June 1908. MS-0451-028/003; Percy Smith to TMH, 7 August 1908. MS-0451-028/005. Hocken Collection (HC). By 21 October 1908 the fund had risen to £51. See Percy Smith to TMH, 21 October 1908. MS-0451-028/016. HC.
4. Isaac Selby, 'Memories of Maoriland', in Paul Peritas, *Hinemoa: The leap-year pantomime* (Melbourne: Tytherleigh Press, 1925), p. 76.
5. See A.G. Hocken, *Dr Hocken of Dunedin: A life*. (Oamaru: East Riding Press, 2008), pp. 6–7; Jim McCready, 'Some bookplates in the Hocken Collections', *Friends of the Hocken Collection Bulletin*, No. 52 (November 2005); and, for general coverage, Henry Bedingfeld and Peter Gwynn-Jones, *Heraldry* (Leicester: Magna Books, 1993). Thanks also to Gregor Macaulay, Dunedin.
6. My thanks to Ali Clarke for stumbling across this in Hocken's copy of Godfrey Charles Mundy's *Our Antipodes, or, Residence and Rambles in the Australian Colonies* (1852).
7. Werner Muensterberger, *Collecting: An unruly passion: Psychological perspectives* (Princeton, NJ: Princeton University Press, 1994), p. 4.
8. Cited in Fred Lerner, *The Story of Libraries* (New York: Continuum, 1998), p. 99.
9. J.H. Aumblin, University of Otago, to TMH, 2 August 1902. In 'Variae' 31, No. 12. HC.
10. Augustus Hamilton, 'Presidential address', Wellington Philosophical Society, 5 May 1909, pp. 1–6; Hocken Pamphlet Collection (HPC), Vol. 162, No. 17.
11. TMH to Elsdon Best, 13 September 1901, cited in MS-0451-015/010. HC.
12. F.A. Bett to Pat Lawlor, 29 September 1952; 27 March 1953. MSS 77-067-2/7. Alexander Turnbull Library (ATL).

Chapter 1: Childhood and Schooling

1. Cited in Introduction in Andrew Jenkins, *Stamford on Old Picture Postcards* (Nottingham: Reflections of a Bygone Age, 2002). Notably, *Middlemarch* (1994), *Pride and Prejudice* (as the village of Meryton), *The Golden Bowl* (2000) and *The Da Vinci Code* (2006).
2. *Minutes of the Methodist Conferences*, Vol. VII (London: [Thomas Cordeaux], 1838), p. 569.
3. Details of Circuit Records at Lincolnshire Archives, in particular Meth B Stamford/12/1, Circuit Steward's Account Book 1805–1836 (Meth B/ Grimsby/13/1), and Quarterly Meeting Grimsby Accounts 1838–1872 (Meth B/ Grimsby/13/2). Thanks to James Stevenson and Carol Tasker, Lincolnshire Archives, Lincoln.
4. Cited in A.G. Hocken, *Dr T.M. Hocken 1836–1910: A gentleman of his time* (Dunedin: Hocken Library, University of Otago, 1989), p. 6.
5. Cited in Obituary, Joshua Hocken, *Methodist Magazine* 76, No. 2 (London: G. Whitfield, 1853), p. 868. See also Hocken Family Tree, Misc-MS-1453; Hocken–Buckland Family Tree. Misc-MS-0614. HC.
6. Ibid. Cited also in A.G. Hocken (1989), p. 6.

7   Joshua Hocken, *A Brief History of the Wesleyan Methodism, in the Grimsby Circuit, including References to the Horncastle, Boston, Barton, Louth, Spilsby, Alford, and Rasen Circuits* (London: Sold by John Mason, 14 City Road and 66 Paternoster Row; Printed and sold by W. Skelton in Grimsby, 1839), p. 47; see also Misc-MS-0614. HC.
8   Copy of Hocken–Richardson marriage certificate, MS-1184/002. A copy of marriage licence, dated 15 August 1828, and signed by William Marsden, MS-1184-004. HC. The 1851 Windle Census registers both as aged 52.
9   Gladys Le Francois, Fish Hoek Collection (FHC). Copy now at Pictorial Collection, HC.
10 Lancaster Priory, City of Lancaster, Gravestone inscriptions in St Mary's Churchyard: 221.
11 Hocken Family Tree, Misc-MS-1453; Misc-MS-0614. HC. And A.G. Hocken (2008), pp. vi–vii.
12 Joseph Taylor, 28 October 1814, cited in Rupert E. Davies, A.R. George and E.G. Rupp (eds), *A History of the Methodist Church in Great Britain*, Vol. IV (London: Epworth Press, 1988), p. 346.
13 Thomas Percival Bunting, *The Life of Jabez Bunting*, Vol. II (London: T. Woolmer, 1887), fn 81.
14 Ibid., p. 161.
15 See *Minutes of the Methodist Conferences*, Vol. VII (1838). pp. 16, 121, 243.
16 Anne Hocken, 1861 Census, St Peter Port, Guernsey. RG 9/4380, fo. 36r.
17 Circuit timetables, in Skelton Posters and Bills Collection, Reel 1 (30 December 1836 to 31 December 1839) and Reel II (13 January to 29 December 1836). Grimsby Public Library, Grimsby.
18 Copy of TMH's baptism record, No. 81, p. 11. MS-1184/004. HC. PRO Reference No. RG4 1639 x/k5334, 10.
19 Davies, George and Rupp (eds), *A History of the Methodist Church in Great Britain*, Vol. II (1978), p. 108.
20 Ibid., Thomas Carlyle, cited p. 109.
21 TMH's First Specimen of Writing, 1842. MS-1184. HC.
22 *Rules to be Observed in the Sunday School, Great Coates* [1836]. In Skelton Posters and Bills Collection, Reel 1 (30 December 1836 to 31 December 1839) and Reel II (13 January to 29 December 1836). Grimsby Public Library, Grimsby.
23 Cited in Luke Tyerman's 'Life and times of the Rev. John Wesley', in Davies, George and Rupp (eds), *A History of the Methodist Church in Great Britain*, Vol. II (1978), p. 98.
24 Joshua Hocken, *A Brief History* (1839), p. [iii].
25 Joshua Hocken to the Rev. Jabez Bunting, 10 August 1840. Joshua Hocken. Correspondence with the Methodists. Misc-MS-1300 (reproduction copies). Acquired from John Rylands by A.G. Hocken, 1979. Photographed copies at MS 1184/001. HC. Thanks to Peter Nockles, Suzanne Fagan and Dominic Whitehead, John Rylands Library, University of Manchester.
26 Presumably TMH's older brothers James and Joshua were at boarding school.
27 Joshua Hocken to Jabez Bunting, 10 August 1840.
28 Joshua Hocken, Oldham St Chapel, to Dr Leppington, Great Grimsby, Lincolnshire, 29 July 1841. Joshua Hocken. Correspondence with the Methodists. Misc-MS-1300 (reproduction copies). HC.
29 *Minutes of Several Conversations at the … Yearly Conference*, Vol. 10 (London: 1844), p. 21 for 1844; Joshua Hocken, Norwich, to the Rev. J.C. Pengelly, 66 Albany Street, Regent's Park, London, 30 March 1844. Joshua Hocken, Correspondence with the Methodists. Misc-MS-1300 (reproduction copies). HC.

30 John Wesley, 'Letters', cited in *A History of the Methodist Church in Great Britain*, Vol. II, (1978), p. 98.
31 Jabez Bunting, notes entitled 'Best means of preparing missionaries for the work', June 1820. Cited in Bunting, *Life of Jabez Bunting*, Vol. II (1887), pp. 174–76.
32 Maria Webb to TMH, 3 August 1905. MS-0451-022/009; Henry Bull, Methodist Church of Australasia, to TMH, 15 December 1909. MS-0451-030/007. HC.
33 Kingswood School was a parallel school to Woodhouse Grove, each under the control of the Wesleyan Methodist Conference. Separate entities from 1812 to 1875, they were finally amalgamated even though some 200 miles apart. For details on Woodhouse, see J.T. Slugg, *Woodhouse Grove School: Memorials and reminiscences* (London: Published for the Author, T. Woolmer, 1885), *Woodhouse Grove School: Reminiscences, 1812–83* (Bradford: Printed and published for the Centenary Celebration Committee, 1912), H.W. Starkey, *A Short History of Woodhouse Grove School 1812–1912* (1912), and F.C. Pritchard, *The Story of Woodhouse Grove School* (Bradford, England: Woodhouse Grove School, 1978). Thanks to Beverley Osborne, Friends of Woodhouse Grove School, for supplying the relevant portions of Starkey. See also Rupert E. Davies, *Methodism* (Petersborough: Epworth Press, 1985), p. 78.
34 This changed in 1852 when the entrance age was raised to nine, the leaving age to 15.
35 From John Wesley's *Plain Account of Kingswood School* in his *Works* (New York: J. Emory & B. Waugh, 1831), p. 336; Pritchard, p. 58.
36 Slugg, p. 187.
37 See Joseph Strachan, cited in Slugg.
38 Pritchard states: 'Many of their pupils came from cultured homes in that their parents, though poor, were well-read.' Gas was first suggested in 1846 and by November 1849 tenders were sent out to build a gas plant. Cited in Pritchard, p. 128.
39 Pritchard is a little less certain about the uniform, although he does mention leather caps replacing the more expensive sealskin caps, p. 66.
40 Slugg, p. 126.
41 W.M. Shaw, cited in Starkey, p. 26.
42 Joseph Strachan, cited in Slugg, p. 138. There is an excellent overview of 'the Division of Time and Labour' at Woodhouse Grove c. 1829 in Pritchard, p. 73.
43 Cited in Pritchard, p. 64.
44 Ibid., p. 73.
45 Slugg, p. 127.
46 A fold-out plan in Slugg, opposite p. 32.
47 George Fenwick claims 300–400 students in his 'Papers relating to a memoir and bibliography of Dr T.M. Hocken', October 1911 (MS-0453/012. HC), while Pritchard gives 140 in his Appendix II (121 boarders; 19 dayboys), p. 384.
48 Fenwick, ibid. Thanks to G. Hugh Knowles, Old Grovian Association, for suggesting Priestley as the barrister. Personal correspondence, 1 February 2010.
49 Cited in Inga Bryden (ed.), *The Pre-Raphaelites: Writings and sources*, Vol. II (London: Routledge/Thoemmes Press, 1988), p. 44; TMH to W.N. Jenkins, 16 September 1909. MS-0214. HC.

Chapter 2: Surgeon and Sailor

1. *Minutes of Several Conversations at the ... Yearly Conference*, Vol. 10 (London: 1844), p. 478 for 1847.
2. 1851 Census: Windle. PRO Ref. H.O. 107-2195, p. 73; p. 547.
3. Cited in M. Jeanne Peterson, *The Medical Profession in Mid-Victorian London* (Berkeley, California: University of California Press, 1978), p. 69.
4. Cited in Peterson, pp. 43, 70–71.
5. *Regulations to be Observed by Students Intending to Qualify Themselves to Practise as Apothecaries in England and Wales 1843* (London: Printed by Gilbert & Rivington, 1843), p. 10. HPC, Vol. 164, No. 1.
6. Rayne began his medical career as an apprentice to a Mr Leighton in Newcastle, his home-town, and then was fortunate to be dresser to Mr Baird. He spent five years at University College, London, serving as dresser to surgeons Mr Cooper and Mr Liston. The latter encouraged Rayne to attend him at operations in his private practice. Rayne also spent time in various hospitals in Paris and married his first wife Ann Le Bontillies in December 1842. He married his second wife, Mary Lomax or Mary Arnold, in December 1875. His third wife was Annie Frances Walton. Rayne died in Winchester on 10 August 1887. See 'Infirmary, Newcastle on Tyne', *Newcastle Courant*, 7 January 1853; 'Septimus William Rayne to the governors of the Newcastle Upon Tyne, Northumberland & Durham Infirmary, 21 October 1854', in *Newcastle Courant*, 3 November 1854; and 'Death of Dr Rayne' in *Newcastle Journal*, 11 August 1887. Thanks to Derek Tree, Newcastle Public Library.
7. Joshua Hocken to the Rev. J. Rattenbury, 10 May 1853. Joshua Hocken. Correspondence with the Methodists. Misc-MS-1300 (reproduction copies). HC.
8. Death certificate of Joshua Hocken. MS-1184/003. Died Friar St, Lancaster, 26 May 1853, aged 54 years. Cause: Diseased Mitra valves; Congestion of lungs 2 months; Anasurca 2 weeks certified. Attended by Thomas Hargreaves; dated 28 May 1853. His will – under Joshua Hocken, Wesleyan Minister of Norwich – is logged at PROB 11/2177 (23 August 1853), Prerogative Court of Canterbury and Related Probate Jurisdictions, Vol. 13 Quire Numbers 601–650.
9. Obituary, *Methodist Magazine* 76, 2 (1853), p. 868.
10. Cited in Jeff Smith, 'The making of a diocese 1851–1882', in Robert Colls and Bill Lancaster (eds), *Newcastle upon Tyne: A modern history* (Chichester: Phillimore & Co., 2001), p. 105. Newcastle became a city in 1882.
11. See Smith.
12. TMH's note in J.G.S. Grant's *A Tale of Horror* (1874) 'Grant's account of his wife who was a Miss Richardson formerly of Newcastle on Tyne, afterwards of Melbourne where Grant married her.' In HPC, Vol. 90: No. 47: J.G.S. Grant – Delphic Oracle & Pamphlets. HC.
13. Peterson, p. 9.
14. As detailed in *Newcastle-upon-Tyne College of Practical Science. Medical Department Session 1852–53* in Dennis Embleton, Papers 16/2/1. University Archive. Robinson Library, University of Newcastle.
15. Cited in John Fife, *Inaugural Address Delivered at the Opening of the Newcastle-Upon-Tyne College of Practical Science, 1 October 1851* (Newcastle: M. and M.W. Lambert, 1851), p. [3]
16. 'Surgical instruments'. *Medical Students Guide Containing the Latest Regulations of all the Licensing Medical Corporations of Great Britain and Ireland* (Dublin: Fannin and Co., [1855]). p. 161.
17. *Medical Directory and General Medical Register for Ireland 1859* (London: John Churchill, [1859]), p. 245.

18   Lambert Hepenstal Ormsby, *Medical History of the Meath Hospital and County Dublin Infirmary*, 2nd edn (Dublin: Fannin & Co., 1892), p. 288.
19   *Medical Directory and General Medical Register for Ireland 1859*, p. 231.
20   *The Lancet*, 7 May 1859, p. 472.
21   *The Lancet*, 21 May 1859, p. 524; *British Medical Journal*, 28 May 1859, p. 437.
22   George Fenwick, 'Paper relating to a memoir and bibliography of Dr T.M. Hocken, October 1911'. MS-0453/012. HC.
23   Overleaf on testimonial document for TMH on SS *Great Britain*, 1 May 1861. MS-0451-002/006. HC.
24   Colin Macdonald, 'FitzGerald, Sir Thomas Naghten (1838–1908)', *Australian Dictionary of Biography (ADB)*, Vol. 4 (Melbourne: Melbourne University Press, 1972), pp. 180–81.
25   *Instructions to the Surgeons-Superintendent Appointed by the Court of Directors to the Emigrant Ships of the New Zealand Company*, 9 November 1841. F&J 3: 14. HC.
26   Ibid. Additionally, 'Surgeons were required to submit official logs of their voyage to colonial authorities on arrival. After scrutiny, logs were forwarded to London (Colonial Office) for auditing by the Emigration Commission. Surgeons were also required to submit a summary report of their voyage. These were retained in the colony.' Robin Haines, *Life and Death in the Age of Sail: The passage to Australia* (Sydney: University of New South Wales Press, 2006), p. 28. Unfortunately surgeon's reports for Victoria have not survived.
27   Although passed much later, 1885 legislation stated that a bona fide doctor must be appointed to every ship with more than 50 passengers and an anticipated voyage time exceeding 80 days under sail or 45 with steam, or if the total complement (crew and passengers) was greater than 300. Cited in Helen Woolcock, *Rights of Passage: Emigration to Australia in the nineteenth century* (London: Tavistock Publications, 1986), pp. 115–16.
28   Inserted as an NB on *Instructions to the Surgeons-Superintendent*.
29   Edward Ledwich, Testimonial, 6 April 1859. MS-0451-001/012. See also MS-0451-001/001; Thomas P. Mason, Testimonial, [April 1859]. MS-0451-001/012. See also MS-0451-001/011. HC.
30   William Stokes, Testimonial, 27 July 1859. MS-0451-001/012. See also MS-0451-001/007. HC.
31   Peterson, pp. 122–23.
32   Star October 1859, *White Star* log, BT 98/6257. PRO, London. See also Captain's Logs PRO ADM 51 Reels 1762–64, 1550–71, 2900, 5712–21, 5736–78 and Surgeon's Logs PRO ADM 101 Reels 3187–3216; MT 32 Reel 3181.
33   C. Fox Smith, *There Was a Ship: Chapters from the history of sail* (London: Methuen, 1929), p. 19.
34   Ibid., p. 30.
35   *Argus*, 21 January 1860, p. 4.
36   Cited in Adrian Ball, *Is Yours an SS* Great Britain *Family?* (Hampshire: Kenneth Mason Publications, 1988), p. 5.
37   Cited in Haines, p. 263.
38   Cited in David Frith, *The Trailblazers: The first English cricket tour of Australia 1861–62* (Cheshire, England: Boundary Books, 1999), p. 50.
39   Gladys Le François, Fish Hoek, Cape Town, 29 June 1970. F&J 5; Loose newspaper cuttings from *Argus* (Cape Town) on the SS *Great Britain*. F&J 5.
40   Crew List, Voyage 20, SS *Great Britain*, departing Liverpool, 17 February 1861. AJCP Microfilm 2347.
41   David Adams (ed.), *The Letters of Rachel Henning* (Sydney: Angus & Robertson, 1966), pp. 60, 51.
42   *Great Britain Magazine and Weekly Screw*. SS Great Britain Archives, Bristol.

43 Ibid., p. 3.
44 Typescript of 'The *Great Britain* magazine (Excerpts)', beginning 16 March 1861. American Society of Mechanical Engineers, *An International Historic Engineering Landmark: SS* Great Britain, *1843 Bristol, England* (New York, 25 September 1984).
45 *The Lancet*, 4 December 1858, p. 586.
46 *Great Britain Magazine and Weekly Screw*, pp. 5–6. No exact Horace quote conforms to TMH's usage. It may be referring to Horace, *Odes* 1.1 lines 15 to 17: '… luctantem Icariis fluctibus Africum mercator metuens otium et oppidi laudat rura sui, mox reficit rates quassas indocilis pauperiem pati …' (The merchant, fearing the South-West wind wrestling the Icarian Sea praises leisure and the fields of his own town, soon he repairs his broken ships untrained to endure poverty.)
47 TMH, 'Treatment of sea-sickness', *The Lancet*, 5 October 1861, p. 337.
48 *Great Britain Magazine and Weekly Screw*, pp. 22–23.
49 Typescript of 'The *Great Britain* magazine (Excerpts)', beginning 16 March 1861.
50 Testimonial for TMH on SS *Great Britain*, 1 May 1861. MS-0451-002/006. HC. Signatures include D. Mooney, C. Golden, Robert Payne, George Reid, G. Osborne.
51 Clara Aspinall, *Three Years in Melbourne* (London: Booth, 1862), p. 241.
52 See Aspinall (ibid) and 'The history of our ship', typescript. Misc-MS-0516. HC.
53 Aspinall (ibid), p. 250.
54 Diary of Charles Albert Chomley. MS 11000: 2494/13. State Library of Victoria, Melbourne. Chomley was born in Ireland on 25 December 1840 and drowned in Switzerland, 1 June 1862, while sailing on Lake Neufchatel. His father was the Rev. Francis Chomley, rector and rural dean of Wicklow, Ireland.
55 Brooke and Antonia Jones would appear on board again on a passage home to Liverpool in 1865. Brooke was alleged to have absconded with some £30,000 and police searched the ship for it before leaving Melbourne. The couple were hidden aboard by one of the ship's officers and travelled to Liverpool openly, giving theatrical performances. Charges were later dropped. In 1866 on another trip out to Melbourne, Brooke and Jones were drowned when the ship *London* went down in the Bay of Biscay. Cited in Ball, *Is Yours an SS Great Britain Family?* p. 12. For further insight, see Marion Diamond, 'Henry Parkes and the strong-minded women', *Australian Journal of Politics and History*, Vol. 138, No. 2 (August 1992), pp. 152–62.
56 Aspinall (1862), pp. 254–56. See also A.W. Martin (ed.), *Letters from Menie: Sir Henry Parkes and his daughter* (Melbourne: Melbourne University Press, 1983), especially pp. 20–23. TMH later rejected Parkes' *An Emigrant's Home Letters* (1896) as uninteresting.
57 Aspinall (1862), pp. 252–63
58 Ibid., pp. 293–94, 265.
59 Clara Aspinall, 'Miss Aspinall's Diary, Melbourne to Liverpool May–August 1861'. Part of Chomley Family Papers, MS 11000, Box 3416/9. State Library of Victoria, Melbourne.
60 Charles Albert Chomley: 'Full true and particular account of the voyage of the good steam ship *Great Britain* from Melbourne to Liverpool … 30 May–3 August, 1861. SS Great Britain Archive.
61 [TMH], *Great Britain Gazette*, No. 1, 6 July 1861, p. 2.
62 See Misc-MS-0516. HC.
63 Aspinall (1862), p. 272.

64 See Diary of Charles Albert Chomley. MS 11000: 2494/13. State Library of Victoria, Melbourne.
65 'Miss Aspinall's Diary'.
66 Aspinall (1862), pp. 63–64
67 Cecelia [Clara Aspinall], Correspondence, 5 July 1861, *Great Britain Gazette* (6 July 1861), p. 3.
68 Aspinall (1862), p. 264.
69 Ibid., p. 265. Her diary entry for Tuesday 11 June conveys the same message: 'The doctor then came to see me – he having once told me he had a morbid love of danger. I was not so alarmed when he said in a tragical voice "Once let us touch an iceberg & we shall not be three minutes above water."'
70 Figures from Frith, p. 53.
71 See *The Cabinet,* No. 1 (November 1861), p. 7. AJCP Reel M855. National Library of Australia, Canberra.
72 Helen Roland, Log, Journals, Notes 1853–1861. MS 2758. Ms Branch, National Library of Australia, Canberra.
73 'Accidents', *The Cabinet*, No. 2 (8 December 1861), p. 19; see Frith, p. 53.
74 Heathfield Harman Stephenson (1833–1896). In Heathfield Harman Stephenson Papers and Books, Entry 437, AJCP Reel M855, with acknowledgement to National Library of Australia and SLNSW. Permission to reproduce from H.S. Healy, London. See also William Caffyn, *Seventy-One Not Out: The reminiscences of William Caffyn,* edited by 'Mid-on' (Edinburgh: William Blackwood, 1889), p. 173; Frith, ch. 5.
75 *The Cabinet*, No. 1 (November 1861), p. [2]. AJCP Reel M855.
76 See Roland, MS 2758. *The Vestiges of Creation* was published anonymously in 1844. Forty years later authorship was tracked to Scottish publisher Robert Chambers.
77 Letter of Adam Sedgwick to Charles Lyell, 9 April 1845, in *The Life and Letters of the Rev. Adam Sedgwick*, Vol. 2 (Cambridge: Cambridge University Press, 1890), p. 84.
78 Roland, MS 2758. See also John Reid, 'Journey on SS *Great Britain*, October 1861'. NZMS, p. 763. Sir George Grey Special Collections, Auckland Central Library (ACL).
79 'Address', *The Cabinet*, No. 1, p. 1.
80 Ibid.; 'Pat Moloney to his darlin' Mary', p. 8.
81 John Gray, 'Our captain's letter', *The Cabinet*, No. 2, p. 11. In Heathfield Harman Stephenson Papers and Books, AJCP M855.
82 Morland Hocken, 'Dr Hocken's report: To the Editor of the Cabinet', *The Cabinet*, No. 2, p. 22.
83 Frith, p. 55.
84 *The Cabinet* (reprinted 1862), pp. 36–38.
85 Ibid., pp. 25, 35.
86 G.H. Wayte (ed.), *'Great Britain' Miscellany*. (Melbourne: Mason & Firth, 1862), p. 1.
87 *'Great Britain' Miscellany*, p. 138.
88 Ibid., p. 15.
89 Cited in Frith, p. 58.
90 Roland, MS 2758.
91 'Our last', *Great Britain Magazine and Weekly Screw* (1861). This last article is signed by TMH.
92 T.M. Hocken, 1 May 1861. MS-0451-002/006. HC.

Chapter 3: Early Beginnings in Dunedin

1. Robert Valpy Fulton, cited in Erik Olssen, *The History of Otago* (Dunedin: John McIndoe, 1984), p. 56.
2. Cited in Tom Field and Erik Olssen, *Relics of the Goldfields: Central Otago* (Dunedin: John McIndoe, 1976), p. 3.
3. John Blair, *Lays of the Old Identities* (Dunedin: Wheeler, 1889), pp. 34–35. Presentation copy to TMH from Blair.
4. TMH, cited in 'Old Dunedin', *The Cyclopedia of New Zealand*, Vol. 4. Otago and Southland Provincial Districts (Wellington: Cyclopedia Co., 1905), p. 71.
5. Sigismund Wekey, *New Zealand: Otago as it is, its goldmines and natural resources: Handbook* (Melbourne: F.F. Bailliere, 1862), pp. 41, 42.
6. Julius Vogel arrived in October 1861. He later acquired shares in the *Otago Witness* (*OW*), and then started (along with Cutten) the *Otago Daily Times* (*ODT*), which first appeared on 15 November 1861.
7. See A.H. McLintock, *The Port of Otago* (Christchurch: Whitcombe & Tombs, 1951), p. 46; Wekey, p. 68.
8. McLintock (1951), pp. 45–47.
9. Wekey, p. 72.
10. *ODT*, 27 March 1862 and cited in A.H. McLintock, *The History of Otago: The origins and growth of a Wakefield class settlement* (Christchurch: Capper Press reprint, 1975), p. 474, fn. 2.
11. 'Report of the Dunedin Sanitary Commission', *Province of Otago: Votes and proceedings of the Provincial Council*. Session XX (1865), cited in A.G. Hocken, *Dr T.M. Hocken 1836–1910: A gentleman of his time* (Dunedin: Hocken Library, University of Otago, 1989), fn. 46, p. 45.
12. McLintock (1975), p. 473, fn. 3.
13. Wekey, p. 70.
14. *OW*, 2 February 1862, p 1; *ODT*, 19 February 1862, p. 6.
15. See A.C. Strode's letter of certification, 26 February 1862. F&J 2: 60. HC.
16. *ODT*, 24 February 1862, p. 3.
17. 'Medical', *ODT*, 13 November 1862, p. 7.
18. See James Beattie, 'W.L. Lindsay, Scottish environmentalism and the "improvement" of nineteenth century New Zealand' in Tony Ballantyne and Judith A. Bennett (eds), *Landscape/Community: Perspectives from New Zealand*. (Dunedin: Otago University Press, 2005), pp. 43–56.
19. Annotation by TMH in William Lauder Lindsay's *Observations on New Zealand Lichens* (1866) and *Contributions to New Zealand Botany* (1868). HC.
20. *ODT*, 18 December 1862, p. 4.
21. Annotation by TMH in W. Lauder Lindsay's *Observations on New Zealand Lichens* (1866) and *Contributions to New Zealand Botany* (1868). HC.
22. Cited in Beattie (p. 46) but from Lindsay's *On the Toot Plant and Poison of New Zealand* (London, 1865) and extracted from *British and Foreign Medico-Chirurgical Review and Quarterly Journal of Practical Medicine and Surgery*, 71 (July 1865), n.p.
23. See Alec Lindsay Poole, 'Tutu', in A.H. McLintock (ed.), *An Encyclopaedia of New Zealand* (Wellington: Government Printer, 1966), p. 465; Te Ara – The Encyclopedia of New Zealand: www.TeAra.govt.nz/1966/T/Tutu/en; and J.M. Graham and M.E.A. Cartridge, 'Tutu poisoning in dogs', *New Zealand Veterinary Journal* (1961), p. 45. As early as December 1848, William Cargill published Dr Robert Ramsay's warning about tutu in the *Otago News*, 13 December 1848, p. 1.
24. *OW*, 22 February 1862, p. 5.
25. See *ODT*, 18 December 1862, p. 4. There is no antidote. When, in the early 1900s, a team of physiologists, including Frank Fitchett and John Malcolm, experimented on how the tutin poison affected its victim, TMH provided the

26 Warrant of appointment for the district of Dunedin, signed by Sir George Grey, Alfred Domett and James H. Cranford, 12 January 1863. 'Variae' 21, No. 17. HC; see also *Daily Telegraph*, 6 February 1863; *OW*, 14 February 1863, p. 5; *OW*, 31 March 1898, p. 27. For much of this chapter on TMH's position as coroner I am indebted to A.G. Hocken's *Dr Hocken of Dunedin: A life* (Oamaru: East Riding Press, 2008).
27 Robert Valpy Fulton, *Medical Practice in Otago and Southland in the Early Days* (Dunedin: Otago Daily Times and Witness Newspapers, 1922), p. 225.
28 TMH, cited in Fulton, p. 226.
29 Cited in A.G. Hocken (2008), p. 22.
30 See the brief report in the *Daily Telegraph*, 17 April 1863, p. 2, and Pamela Wood's excellent *Dirt: Filth and decay in a new world arcadia* (Auckland: Auckland University Press, 2005). See 'Variae' 4: No. 28 for copy of Sir George Grey's authority granting the post of Naval Brigade surgeon, 9 March 1865; 'Appointment', see *Otago Provincial Gazette*, 24 May 1865, IX, p. 126; resignation, *Saturday Advertiser* (Supplement), 30 July 1881, p. 7; see authority document for TMH as surgeon in the New Zealand Defence Forces, 17 April 1885. F&J 5: 131.
31 See 'Trials, notable' in *An Encyclopedia of New Zealand*, Vol. 3, pp. 447–48.
32 Jarvey's letter is addressed and dated 'Dunedin Gaol, 3 March 1865'. HPC, Vol. 44, No. 2.
33 TMH's note in *Trial of Captain Jarvey on a Charge of Poisoning his Wife* (1865), in HPC, Vol. 44, No. 2.
34 Ibid. TMH repeats the word 'atrocious' in his *Bibliography* entry, p. 241.
35 See 'Trials, notable' in *An Encyclopedia of New Zealand*, Vol. 3, pp. 448–49.
36 *Full Report of the Trial of Thomas Hall for the Murder of Captain Henry Cain* (1887). HPC, Vol. 44, No. 11.
37 'Church of England Bazaar and Industrial Exhibition', *ODT*, 20 December 1862, p. 3 and 'Report of the Committee of the Industrial Exhibition', *ODT*, 30 December 1862, p. 5.
38 First meeting 8 August 1860, as cited in *OW*, 11 August 1860. J.W. Hayward and A.E. Russell, *The Lodge of Otago No. 844, E.C. Centennial History 1860–1960* (Dunedin: The Budget Ltd, [1960]), p. 13.
39 Robert Booth, *The Lodge of Otago No. 844 E.C. Register of Members: 1860–1993* ([Dunedin: Booth, 1994]).
40 Ibid. The Household Census, *ODT*, 23 April 1863, p. 6 lists TMH's 'place of abode' as Princes Street.
41 *ODT*, 29 May 1863, p. 4.
42 Cited in Booth (1994).
43 Cited in W.P. Morrell, *The Dunedin Club 1858–1975: A new short history* (Dunedin: Dunedin Club, 1976), p. 55.
44 On one occasion TMH protested about the construction of a porch, which still exists. Cited in Morrell (1976), p. 25.
45 Ibid., p. 27.
46 *Sixth Annual Report* (1868) – Report of Honorary Surgeons for year 1868, signed by Frederick Richardson and TMH, 27 January 1869. HPC, Vol. 98, No. 5.
47 *Ninth Annual Report* (1871), p. 6. HPC, Vol. 98.
48 *Benevolent Inst. Reports* 1864–1896 – 33 pamphlets. The Second Annual Report … of the Benevolent Institution, Dunedin (1865). HPC, Vol. 98.

TMH's note opposite: 'The first report was not separately printed. It appears on the *ODT* of [20.6.1863].' In addition, 'For meeting vide "Colonist" May 24th, 1862'.
49 HPC, Vol. 49: General collection of 28 pamphlets, including George Bennett's *Acclimatisation* (1862) and other annual reports.
50 'Mss proposal to form a group to the re-annexation of the Province of Otago, Riverton, 5 March 1869. Held at Mr Daniels's house', 5 March 1869. F&J 2: 64. HC.
51 Fulton, p. 233.
52 *ODT*, 9 January 1864, p. 4.
53 Amusements, *ODT*, 8 January 1864, p. 3.
54 Fulton, p. 242.
55 Ibid., p. 236.
56 *ODT*, 7 June 1864, p. 4.
57 Fulton, p. 239.
58 TMH gives the boy's name as Charles Davis, yet his father was one George Cooroa, as named in the *ODT*, 17 November, 1865, p. 4.
59 'To make known the medicinal properties of certain trees', November 1865. MS-0451-003/003. HC.
60 TMH's note on J.F. Riemenschneider's 'On Maori habits of life'. MS-0303. HC.
61 J.F. Riemenschneider to TMH, 9 November 1864. MS-0451-003/002. HC.
62 TMH, F&J 9: 45.
63 Cited in McLintock (1975), p. 477.
64 *New Zealand Gazette*, 12 September 1863. Cited in F&J 11: 17.
65 'The New Zealand Exhibition at Otago', *Colonist*, 7 October 1864, p. 3.
66 Anna Blackman, 'First NZ Exhibition 1865', Hocken Library Blog, posted 16 June 2011; John Stacpoole, *William Mason: The first New Zealand architect* (Auckland: Auckland University Press, 1971), p. 74.
67 R.D.J. Collins, 'Caveat Lector: Notes on some exhibition catalogues', *Bulletin of New Zealand Art History* 16 (1995), pp. 21–27 (22).
68 *OW*, 18 February 1865, p. 1.
69 TMH's annotation in John Gully, *New Zealand Scenery* (Dunedin: Henry Wise, 1877).
70 Ibid.
71 F&J 11.
72 *Official Catalogue of the New Zealand Exhibition, 1865* (Dunedin: Printed for the Commissioners by Mills, Dick & Co., 1865), Section III, No. 680, p. 56.
73 Ibid., 'Miscellaneous Exhibits', Class 36B, No. 1055, p. 77.
74 *Reports and Awards of the Jurors and Appendix for the New Zealand Exhibition* (Dunedin: Printed for the Commissioners, 1865), p. 335. See also Strathern, 'Thomas Morland Hocken' in *An Encyclopaedia of New Zealand*, Vol. II, pp. 93–94.
75 Charles R. Thatcher, *Thatcher's Otago Songster* (Dunedin: Joseph Mackay, 1865), p. 21. Julius Vogel's contribution was 'On ancient and modern music and use of the Jew's Harp'; J.G.S. Grant's contribution was 'On the vanity of Otago's rulers'. Thatcher produced a number of songbooks such as *Dunedin Songster* (1862), *Invercargill Minstrel* [1864] and *Auckland Songster* (1864). These scarce items are bound with TMH's copies of the anonymously written *Jewlius Rex and Men of His Time: A burlesque poem* (Gisborne, 1876), and *Grimshaw, Bagshaw & Bradshaw's Comic Guide to Dunedin* (1869). The latter contains an advertisement for TMH's services and, despite the inaccurate use of the initials 'M.D.', it does confirm his sense of humour: 'Medical Officer: TMH, M.D. Life rate the lowest in the colony'. See HPC, Vol. 86, No. 3, p. 34. This

'humorous yet highly useful companion to strangers visiting Dunedin' was actually by Robert Percy Whitworth.
76 Dr F.A. Bett to Pat Lawlor, 29 September 1952. MSS 77-067-2/7. ATL.
77 TMH annotated the cartoon, giving his name and Hunter's to those depicted.
78 The building was demolished in 1933. 'Otago News Letter', 16 February 1867', cited in Hardwicke Knight and Niel Wales, *Buildings of Dunedin: An illustrated architectural guide to New Zealand's Victorian city* (Dunedin: John McIndoe, 1988).
79 TMH, 'New Zealand notes'. MS-0037, p. 63. HC. Jones – 'a little man with a characteristic draught-board waistcoat', cited in Olssen (1984), p. 68.
80 A note on *Sold Again and Got No Money*, a lithograph by James Brown (1819–1877) dated about 1865. Hocken Original Pictorial Collection.
81 TMH, 'New Zealand notes'. MS-0037, p. 63. HC.
82 Ibid. For the pyrotechnic 'Siege of Duppel' see *ODT*, 9 December 1864, p. 4.
83 TMH, 'New Zealand notes'. MS-0037, p. 48.
84 Ibid., p. 59.
85 Thomas Redmayne, *Royal Hotel, Dunedin*. Drawn 1876 from photo taken in 1858. Hocken Original Pictorial Collection. Au R318.

Chapter 4: Home and Garden

1 St John's Anglican Church (Waikouaiti) Marriage register, No. 50. MS-1869/001. HC.
2 Death certificate, 31 December 1881. Births, Deaths & Marriages, Folio 1881/1766; Ref: 7/0102218. Julia died after suffering from jaundice for 10 days and exhaustion for one day. Kind thanks to Katherine Milburn, Hocken Library.
3 Ruby Neill, 'The Hocken family', part of a recorded interview with Dr A.G. Hocken, 24 February 1960. Hocken Library Archives, MS-2847/62. See also A.G. Hocken, (1989), pp. 25, 28. Kind thanks to Susan Irvine for finding the Neill interview.
4 Cited in Fleur Snedden, *King of the Castle: A biography of William Larnach* (Auckland: David Bateman, 1997), p. 130. Like TMH's daughter, Eliza Larnach's baby was called Gladys.
5 Julia Hocken to Donald Larnach, 4 December 1880. Cited in Snedden (1997), p. 141.
6 Death notice, *OW*, 10 December 1881, p. 17.
7 The name change from MacAndrew to Burlington Street occurred in 1916. For information on Hardy see *The Cyclopedia of New Zealand*, Vol. 4. Otago and Southland Provincial Districts (Christchurch: Cyclopedia Co., 1905), pp. 383–84; Michael Findlay, 'Henry Frederick Hardy' in Jane Thomson (ed.), *Southern People: A dictionary of Otago Southland biography* (Dunedin: Longacre Press/Dunedin City Council, 1998), pp. 211–12; and Hardwicke Knight and Niel Wales, *Buildings of Dunedin: An illustrated architectural guide to New Zealand's Victorian city* (Dunedin: John McIndoe, 1988), pp. 12–118 (113).
8 'Minor Offences', *ODT*, 26 May 1869, p. 3.
9 *House of Representatives: Electoral district of the City of Dunedin: Roll of persons qualified to vote, 1870–71*. Also correspondence with and thanks to archivists Alison Breese and Chris Scott, Dunedin City Council, 26 October 2010.
10 Robert Valpy Fulton, *Medical Practice in Otago and Southland in the Early Days* (Dunedin: Otago Daily Times and Witness Newspapers, 1922), p. 243.
11 TMH to Thomas Cheeseman, 18 May 1891; 7 September 1891. Auckland Institute and Museum Library Collection (AIM). Perhaps *Meryta lucida*, which is a species of plant in the Araliaceae (ivy) family.
12 Dunedin City Council Building Permit 3357, 1916; 469 Moray Place, DCC Archives. Rate Book Vol. 83a 1920–22, Block XV, section 6. No. 163 Drainage

Plan, DCC Archives. There are no building plans before 1901. 1903 Reference Dunedin Drainage & Sewerage Board Drainage Plan S 103a, DCC Archives.
13   Interior of Dr Hocken's house, Augustus Hamilton No. 192. MONZ Collection.
14   Dr Hocken in his library. Album 43, Original Pictorial Collection.
15   Mary Isabella Lee, *The Not So Poor: An autobiography* (ed. Annabel Cooper), (Auckland: Auckland University Press, 1992), pp. 87–88.
16   Mark Twain, *Following the Equator: A journey around the world* Vol. 1 (New Jersey: Ecco Press, 1992), ch. XXX, pp. 246–48.
17   Annie Trimble, 'A collector's sacrifice: An interview with Dr Hocken', *Evening Star*, 1 February 1908, pp. 39–41.
18   Cited in Rewa Glenn [Marguerite Maude Johnson], *The Botanical Explorers of New Zealand* (Wellington: A.H. & A.W. Reed, 1950), p. 78.
19   Cited in Glenn, pp. 100–05; and Rex Wright-St Clair. 'Monro, David', from DNZB: www.TeAra.govt.nz/en/biographies/1m48/monro-david
20   W.H. Trimble, *Catalogue of the Hocken Library* (Dunedin: Otago Daily Times and Witness Newspapers Co., 1912), pp. 248–52.
21   Justice Ward, 'Inaugural address' to the Otago Institute. 24 August 1869 in *Transactions and Proceedings of the New Zealand Institute 1869*, Vol. II (Wellington: James Hughes, April 1870), pp. 425–26.
22   Alfred Eccles, 'Address', 2 November 1869. Ibid., p. 429.
23   John C. Ross, 'Thomas Morland Hocken', in *Nineteenth-Century British Book-Collectors and Bibliographers, Dictionary of Literary Biography*, Vol. 184 (1997), pp. 227–34 (229).
24   A.T. Thomson to TMH, 27 November 1871. '21 Important Letters, 1867–96'. MS-0084. HC. There are actually 23 letters in this volume.
25   *ODT*, 9 March 1870, p. 2.
26   Samuel Marsden Correspondence, Letter 9. MS-0055, MS-0056. HC.
27   'Paper prepared at home from New Zealand flax, December 1866'. See sheet at MS-0451-003/005. HC.
28   TMH, Transcript of 'Travel diary', 1885. Misc-MS-1730. HC.
29   Thanks to John Adams. Auckland.
30   Thomas Ralph to TMH, 9 December 1885. MS-0451-004/015. HC.
31   Ibid.
32   Now in Special Collections, these titles carry the familiar museum stamp with a pencil note reading: 'Presented by Dr Hocken in 1900.'
33   See A.W. Pollard, 'Book-collecting', *Encyclopedia Britannica* (1911), pp. 221–25 (224).
34   John White, *Maori Customs and Superstitions* (1861) in 'Variae' 2: No. 5.
35   W.L. Williams, 'Maori names of plants', copied from Archdeacon W.L. Williams's Private Notes. MS-0037a. HC. The collation is dated H.W. Williams, 14 February 1907, so TMH received it sometime after this date.
36   W.L. Williams to TMH, 17 October 1904. F&J 5: 181A. HC.
37   W.L. Williams, 'Maori names of plants', MS-0037a, p. 31, 89. HC.
38   See Berggren Papers MS-Papers 1002, ATL. Thanks also to the late David Galloway and his paper, 'The Swedish connection in New Zealand lichenology, 1769–2004', *Symb. Bot. Upsala*, Vol. 34, No. 1 (2004), pp. 63–85.
39   Berggren's diary (translated). MS-Papers-1002:2. ATL
40   A.G. Bagnall, 'Sven Berggren in New Zealand', Section I, *Turnbull Library Record*, Vol. 3, No. 1 (1970), pp. 29–42 (33).
41   Sven Berggren, *On New Zealand Hepaticæ* (Lund: Printed by E. Malmström, 1898), pp. 46–47.
42   TMH to Berggren, Monday [July 1874], Dunedin. Berggren Papers, MS-Papers 1002:7. ATL.

43 Cited in A.G. Bagnall, 'Sven Berggren in New Zealand', Section II: Tauranga and Rotorua, *Turnbull Library Record*, Vol. 3, No. 3 (1970), pp. 143–51 (150–51).
44 Sven Berggren to TMH, 5 February 1875. F&J 5: 112. HC.

Chapter 5: A Fondness for Anything New Zealand

1 Thomas Carlyle, *On Heroes, Hero-Worship and the Heroic in History* (London: Routledge, [1905]), p. 267.
2 TMH, *Contributions to the Early History of New Zealand [Settlement of Otago]* (London: Sampson Low, Marston & Co., 1898), p. [vii].
3 TMH, *The Early History of New Zealand: Being a series of lectures delivered before the Otago Institute; Also a Lecturette on the Maoris of the South Island* (Wellington: Mackay, Government Printer, 1914), p. 20.
4 Stuart Strachan, 'Not quite half a loaf: Dr Hocken and the "patriation" of the New Zealand Company Archives', draft paper, October 2005.
5 TMH, *ODT*, 12 July 1870, p. 3.
6 His coroner duties kept him busy. In 1873 he became medical adviser to Otago Girls' High School, and in 1876 he was instrumental in establishing a Medical Association in Dunedin; he was first president of the Otago branch. See TMH's F&J 11: 84. See also *ODT*, 17 September 1868, p. 2; *Otago Girls' High School Jubilee Magazine 1871–1921*, 40; *Evening Star*, 28 August 1873, p. 3.
7 Frederick John Knox to TMH, secretary of the Otago Institute, 25 November 1870. F&J 2: 65.
8 A newspaper scrapbook compiled by TMH. MS-2469/001.
9 TMH, 'The hot springs of New Zealand', *Saturday Advertiser*, 1 September 1877, p. 11.
10 TMH, 'The hot springs', 'Variae' 23: No. 27.
11 Ibid.
12 J.C. Beaglehole, *The Life of Captain James Cook* (London: Adam & Charles Black, 1974), p. 699.
13 *ODT*, 1 September 1880. Supplement, p. 1.
14 Two thousand were struck in base metal (copper and brass) and just over 100 in silver. The silver medals did not accompany Cook on his voyages, but appear to have been distributed in England. Two were struck in 24-carat gold. Cited by John Hope, Captain Cook Study Unit, 2006. See J.C. Beaglehole (ed.), *The Journals of Captain James Cook on his Voyages of Discovery: Vol 2: The voyage of the Resolution and Adventure 1772–1775* (Cambridge: Cambridge University Press/Hakluyt Society, 1961), p. 16. The 'Thomson' medal was found by Mrs Hunter at Murdering Beach (now Whareakeake), near the north head of Otago Harbour in 1863; it was gifted to the Otago Museum in 1925. Incidentally, TMH later secured the even rarer silver medal, which was certainly one of the medals described in a surviving invoice to TMH from W.S. Lincoln & Son, numismatists and antiquaries operating in New Oxford Street, London. Invoiced February 1906, these 'two medals of Cook and Banks' cost him £3 11s. See Trimble, *Catalogue of the Hocken Library Dunedin* (1912), pp. 44, 508. See W.S. Lincoln & Son to TMH, 19 February 1906. MS-Papers-0451-023/003. The silver medal is listed under the entry of Cook in the *Catalogue*, while Trimble's subject listing gives the bronze and a silver medal.
15 TMH, 'The early history of New Zealand: I', *ODT*, 1 September 1880. Supplement, p. 1.
16 H. Ling Roth's *Crozet's Voyage to Tasmania, New Zealand, the Ladrone Island* (1891). See TMH's copy with review from the *ODT*, 21 November 1891. KX C, HC.
17 TMH, *Early History* (1914), p. 6. See his 'The early history of New Zealand: I', *ODT*, 1 September 1880. Supplement, p. 1.

18   TMH's copy lacks the 'Right Honourable Lords of the Admiralty' dedication, which was withdrawn after objections to a spurious endorsement of an unauthorised publication. To make it complete, TMH copied Thomas Becket's letter dated 28 September 1771 to the Lords of the Admiralty and Messrs Banks and Dr Solander and tipped it in at the front. Hordern House, *Captain James Cook & His Pacific Legacy Catalogue* (Sydney: Hordern House, 2007), Entry 3. See also J.C. Beaglehole, *Journals* (1961), pp. 131–32; M.K. Beddie (ed.), *Bibliography of Captain James Cook R.N., F.R.S., Circumnavigator*, 2nd edn (Sydney [Council of SLNSW], 1970), p. 693. See also HPC, Vol. 15, No. 1; and A.G. Bagnall, *New Zealand National Bibliography*, Vol. 1 (Wellington: Government Printer, 1969–80), 3324 and C1430.

19   James Rattray paid the English-based B.S. Marks to execute an exact facsimile (including the elaborate frame) for £105. James Rattray to TMH, 5 July 1880. MS-0451-003/013. HC See TMH, 'The early history of New Zealand: I', *ODT*, 1 September 1880, Supplement, p. 1; *Saturday Advertiser*, 4, 11 September, pp. 13, 9. TMH also received feedback in the *Saturday Advertiser*, 18 September 1880, p. 13. See also TMH's *Early History* (1914), p. 5.

20   TMH, *Early History* (1914), p. 17; see also TMH's 'The early history of New Zealand: I'.

21   *Lyttleton Times*, 16 March 1908. Cutting in MS-0177/043. HC; TMH to Percy Smith, 10 June 1909. Polynesian Society Papers, MS-Papers-1187-263-13. ATL.

22   TMH, *Early History* (1914), pp. 17–18; see also 'The early history of New Zealand: I'.

23   TMH, 'The early New Zealand missions', *ODT*, 28 December 1905, 4 January 1906, 11 January 1906, 18 January 1906.

24   TMH, lecture II, *ODT*, 28 December 1905.

25   TMH, 'The early history of New Zealand: II', *Otago Daily News*, 18 September 1880, Supplement, p.1.

26   Tuhawaiki, 'Declaration of ownership of Robuka [sic] Island, 28 March 1840. MS-0808/B. HC.

27   TMH, 'The early history of New Zealand: III', *ODT*, 13 September 1884, Supplement, p.1; TMH, *Early History* (1914), p. 35; Wakefield, cited in TMH, *Early History* (1914), p. 37.

28   For information on Wakefield see Miles Fairburn, 'Wakefield, Edward Gibbon', from DNZB: www.TeAra.govt.nz/en/biographies/1w4/wakefield-edward-gibbon; and Philip Temple's *A Sort of Conscience: The Wakefields* (Auckland: Auckland University Press, 2003).

29   H.S. Chapman, cited in Temple, pp. 536–37. H.S. Chapman to father, 19 August 1847. qMS 0419. ATL.

30   TMH, *Early History* (1914), p. 36.

31   TMH, in lecture delivered to Otago Institute, 9 September 1896. and in *Early History* (1914), p. 253.

32   For E.M. Chaffers's chart, see Stuart Strachan and Linda Tyler (eds), *Ka Taoka Hakena: Treasures from the Hocken Collections* (Dunedin: Otago University Press, 2007), p. 126.

33   Newspaper scrapbook compiled by Hocken. MS-2469/001. Pasted above fuller coverage of TMH's 'The early history of New Zealand: IV', in *ODT*, 26 September 1885, Supplement, p. 1.

34   For the prints see *Catalogue of Pictures in the Hocken Library*, compiled by Jean McGill and Linda Rodda (Dunedin: Otago University Library, 1948), pp. 13, 29. See also 'Dr TMH's original collection', printout from the Hocken Library Pictorial Collection database.

35   TMH, 'The early history of New Zealand: IV', *ODT*, 26 September 1885, Supplement, p. 1.

36 For Merrett, see McGill and Rodda (1948), pp. 10, 39; see also 'Dr TMH's original collection'.
37 TMH, *Early History* (1914), p. 90.
38 McGill and Rodda (1948), p. 57; see also 'Dr TMH's original collection'.
39 TMH, 'The early history of New Zealand: I', *ODT*, 1 September 1880, Supplement, p. 1. See also TMH, *Early History* (1914), p. [1].
40 TMH, 'The early history of New Zealand: II', *Otago Daily News*, 18 September 1880, Supplement, p. 1.
41 TMH, 'Early history of New Zealand: The Otago settlement', *ODT*, 13 August 1887, Supplement, p. 1.
42 Ibid.
43 TMH, 'Early history of Otago', *ODT*, 24 September 1887, Supplement, p. 1.
44 Ibid. See Samuel Hodgkinson to TMH, 9 November 1886. MS-0451-005/003. HC.
45 TMH, 'Early history of Otago', *ODT*, 24 September 1887, p. 2.
46 Newspaper scrapbook compiled by TMH. MS-2469/001.
47 Those printed included 'Notes on the derelict ship in Facile Harbour, Dusky Sound', Vol. 22 (1887), pp. 422–28; 'Some account of the earliest literature and maps relating to New Zealand', Vol. 27 (1894), pp. 616–34; 'Tasman and his journal', Vol. 28 (1895), pp. 117–40; 'An account of the Fiji fire ceremony', Vol. 31 (1898), pp. 667–72; 'Some account of the beginnings of literature in New Zealand: Part I, the Maori section', Vol. 33 (1900), pp. 472–90; 'Some account of the beginnings of literature in New Zealand: Part II, the English newspapers', Vol. 48 (1901), pp. 99–114; and 'Early visits of the French to New Zealand', Vol. 40 (1907), pp. 5–8. Those not published in full included 'The etymology of the word "Penguin"', delivered in June 1895 and tenuously based on historical evidence of the derivation of the word from the Celtic *pen* (head) and *gwen* (white) (Notice under Second Meeting, 11th June 1895, *Transactions*, Vol. 28 (1895), p. 756); 'On a piece of Aztec statuary representing the sacrifice of a human victim', which was read on 11 August 1896 and initiated when TMH acquired a copy of an Aztec statue found by Mr Watson of Gisborne in an old Aztec mine at Te Oro, Mexico (see TMH to Thomas Cheeseman, 6 August 1896. MA 95/38/5 Correspondence Letterbook 1890–97. AIM. See D.178 'Cast of Statuette', Otago Museum. Thanks to Scott Reeves, Registrar, Otago Museum, for the TMH artefact inventory); 'Relics of the old native population on the Upper Molyneux', where TMH detailed old Maori encampments along the Clyde–Alexandra Road; and 'Notes on New Zealand earthworms', where he was co-presenter with Professor William Blaxland Benham and G.M. Thomson. On the latter occasion he displayed a preserved specimen of the Palolo, a Fijian marine worm (Otago Institute meeting, 9 August 1898, *Transactions*, Vol. 31 (1898), p. 738 and 743). In 1898 he exhibited a photograph of a curious nest found on the Rock and Pillar Range, with one suggestion from the floor that it was an old nest from the great extinct eagle *Harpagornis*, and later he exhibited a number of Maori weapons and implements, giving the history of some of the rarer specimens (Note, *Transactions*, Vol. 31 (1898), p. 737; Otago Institute meeting, 9 August 1898, *Transactions*, Vol. 31 (1898), p. 738).
48 TMH, 'Notes on a derelict ship' under 'Otago Institute', *OW*, 15 June 1887, p. 4. This work is repeated in the *Transactions*, Vol. 22 (1887), pp. 422–28.
49 William Docherty to TMH, 8 May 1880. MS-0451-003/012. HC; E.E. Morris to TMH, 28 May, 20 June 1898. MS-0451-012/006 and 007. See also letters in '21 Important Letters, 1867–96': Richard Henry to TMH, 28 July 1895. MS-0084/14; 30 November 1898. MS-0084/17; Captain John Fairchild to TMH, 5 April 1887. MS-0084/007. HC. See also reference in Robert

McNab, *Historical Records of New Zealand*, Vol. 1 (Wellington: John McKay, 1908), p. 204; and Ray Parkin, *H.M. Bark* Endeavour: *Her place in Australian history* (Melbourne: Miegunyah Press, 2006).
50 TMH, 'Notes on a derelict ship' (1887), p. 4.
51 See TMH's F&J 9: 30: 'The Madagascar mystery – wreck of the Madagascar at Facile Harbour'. For the fate of Cook's barque *Endeavour*, see www.captaincooksociety.com. According to various opinions, the ship either ended up as a hulk in the Thames or as one of the scuttled vessels in Narragansett Bay, Newport Harbour. Providence, New England. See also Beaglehole, (1974), p. 129.
52 TMH, 'Earliest literature and maps', *Transactions*, Vol. 27 (1894), pp. 616–34.
53 There had been condensed Dutch and English versions, many of the latter included in the numerous voyage books. Valentyn gave an extended account in 1726, adding in important maps. A copy of the journal came into possession of Sir Joseph Banks, and the translation emanating from that (by the Rev. C.G. Woide) formed much of what was published in Burney's *History of Discovery in the South Sea* (1814). See James Backhouse Walker, The *Discovery of Van Diemen's Land in 1642* (Tasmania: Government Printer, 1891), p. 128.
54 TMH, 'Earliest literature and maps', *Transactions*, Vol. 27 (1894), pp. 616–34 (621); p. 633.
55 TMH, 'Some account of the beginnings of literature in New Zealand: Part I, the Maori section', *Transactions*, Vol. 33 (1900), p. 484.
56 Ibid., p. 476.
57 TMH, 'Some account of the beginnings of literature in New Zealand: Part II, the English newspapers' *Transactions* (1901), p. 99.
58 Ibid., pp. 103 104–05.
59 TMH, 'Early visits of the French to New Zealand', *Transactions*, Vol. 40 (1907), p. 142.
60 TMH's set is incomplete, lacking the *Philologie* volume and the hydrographical atlas. See TMH, *Bibliography* (1909), p. 47. See also Bagnall, *National Bibliography*, Part I, A–M: 1687. Armand de Saint-Ferriol, son of Armand de Sibeud de Saint-Ferriol and brother of Louis de Sibeud, Comte de Saint-Ferriol. For book sale dispersal see *Catalogue des livres rares et curieux, anciens et modernes, principalement sur les voyages, provenant de la bibliothèque de feu M. Armand de Saint-Ferriol, dont la vente aux enchères publiques aura lieu le 5 décembre 1881*, Grenoble, Librairie A. Ravanat, 1881. Thanks to Jerry Morris and Michael Laird for information on Saint-Ferriol.
61 TMH, 'Early visits of the French', *Transactions*, Vol. 40 (1907), p. 143.
62 William Craig, letter to the editor, *ODT*, 22 August 1887, p. 4.
63 Editorial, *ODT*, 23 August 1887, p. 2.
64 *New Zealand Herald*, 12 November 1887, Supplement, p. 1. See TMH's scrapbook of newspaper cuttings. MS-2469/001.
65 Proceedings of *Transactions*, Vol. 21 (1888), 522.

Chapter 6: Cultivating Contacts
1 TMH, *Early History* (1914), p. 22.
2 Oliver Arthur Gillespie, Harper', in A.H. McLintock (ed.) *An Encyclopedia of New Zealand*, Vol. I (Wellington: Government Printer, 1966), pp. 910–11. See also W.J. Stack, *Through Canterbury and Otago with Bishop Harper in 1859–60* (Akaroa: Akaroa Mail, 1906).
3 '21 Important Letters, 1876–96'. MS-0084. HC.
4 HPC, Vol. 79, No. 11; Vol. 149, No. 29; Bagnall, *National Bibliography*, 1441. Most of the pieces in *Literary Foundlings* have no attribution. TMH has identified some, including: 'A tale I heard in the bush' by J.E. Fitzgerald;

	'Reminiscences of 1857' by Canon George Cotterill; 'A real ghost story' by the Rev. James Stack.
5	See Barbara Griffiths, *Life of Henry John Chitty Harper* (Timaru, 1956); Colin Brown, Marie Peters and Jane Teal (eds), *Shaping a Colonial Church: Bishop Harper and the Anglican Diocese of Christchurch 1856–1890* (Christchurch: Canterbury University Press, 2006).
6	Herbert W. Williams, *A Bibliography of Printed Maori to 1900* (Wellington: Dominion Museum, 1924), p. 167 (W); Phillip Parkinson and Penny Griffith, *Books in Maori, 1815–1900: An annotated bibliography* (Auckland: Reed, 2004), 352 (*BiM*); W103: *BiM* 196.
7	Information written by TMH in *The Murder of the Rev. C.S. Volkner* (1865). See HPC, Vol. 54, No. 14. Thanks to Phillip Parkinson, Wellington, for confirming synod dates.
8	Cited in Frances Porter, 'Williams, William', from DNZB: www.TeAra.govt.nz/en/biographies/1w26/williams-william
9	See Hocken's copy W434: *BiM* 716.
10	See HPC, Vol. 24, No. 2; Vol. 135, No. 1; Vol. 151, No. 22; see TMH's F&J 6: 8. MS copy of letter from Richard Hill, Sydney, to Rev. William Williams, Paihia, 31 January 1835; No. 9: MS letter from W. Williams, Waimate, to Rev. W. Jowett, Church Missionary House, Salisbury Square, London, 6 January 1835. Hill died unexpectedly the following year.
11	F&J 1: 98. Copies of three letters from Bishop Selwyn to Archdeacon Henry Williams, 20 April, 5 May, 8 May 1852; a copy of letters from H. Williams to Bishop Selwyn, 22 April 1852; and a copy of a letter from Marianne Williams to Samuel Williams, [May 1852?].
12	In F&J 6: 10. Henry Williams, Paihia, to Dandeson Coates, CMS, London, 26 August 1836.
13	HPC, Vol. 41.
14	W.L. Williams to TMH, 12 June 1891. The letter was pasted in 'Notes on the Maori-Polynesian comparative dictionary of Mr E. Tregear, by A.S. Atkinson; being a paper read before the Nelson Philosophical Society, April 11th, May 16th and Dec. 12th, 1892' (1893), but cannot now be located.
15	Report of the Third Meeting, Australasian Association for the Advancement of Science (AAAS), Christchurch, January 1891. Other 'Anthropology' members included A.W. Howitt of Melbourne as president, W.B.D. Mantell as vice-president and Augustus Hamilton. Other 'Philology' members included the Rev. S. Ella, the Rev W. Wyatt Gill and the Rev J.W. Stack. See p. xxiii of *Third Report*, 1891, for details on the 'Philology' section.
16	TMH, *Bibliography* (1909), p. 419.
17	W.L. Williams to TMH, 31 August 1893. '21 Important Letters, 1867–96'. MS-0084/012. HC.
18	W.L. Williams to TMH, 8 May 1894. F&J 5: 157. HC.
19	Ibid. Perhaps Bagnall, *National Bibliography*, 1220.
20	W.L. Williams to TMH, 24 August 1894. MS-0451-009/007. HC.
21	W.L. Williams to TMH, 13 February 1907. MS-0451-025/004; Hymns, c. 1860: W212; *BiM* 501; 1870: W322; *BiM* 740; Almanac, 1846: W120; *BiM* S201/1845); First Lessons: W351; *BiM* 593; Morals: W483; *BiM* 806.
22	See TMH's 'Variae' 19; W967; *BiM* S41.
23	TMH, *Bibliography* (1909), p. 289.
24	For further details on Davis see Alan Ward, 'Davis, Charles Oliver Bond', from DNZB: www.TeAra.govt.nz–biographies/1d3/davis-charles-oliver-bond
25	C.O.B. Davis to TMH, 5 January 1876. MS-0451-003/008. HC.
26	HPC, Vol. 8: 'Travels 1841–1872', No. 1 (of 11 pamphlets).
27	C.O.B. Davis to TMH, 28 October 1876. MS-0451-003/009. HC.

28 TMH's note at the end of Davis's *The Renowned Chief of Kawiti* (Auckland, 1855): HPC, Vol. 13, No. 7. HC.
29 C.O.B. Davis to TMH, 28 October 1876. MS-0451-003/009. HC.
30 C.O.B. Davis to TMH, 8 December 1885. MS-0451-004/014. HC.
31 C.O.B. Davis to TMH, 28 October 1885. MS-0451-004/012. HC.
32 'The seal of the Maori King Potatau', 1862? MS-1460 HC.
33 H.B. Morton, cited in Alan Ward, 'Davis, Charles Oliver Bond', from DNZB. See also D.M. Stafford, *The Founding Years of Rotorua: A history of events to 1900* (Rotorua: Ray Richards/Rotorua District Council, 1986).
34 William Mason, Queenstown, to TMH, 5 February 1836. F&J 5: 128. HC.
35 HPC, Vol. 134. See Bagnall, *National Bibliography*, 1546; 1551; 1548 (especially Williams's note on attribution); 1552. Davis's notes on tiki at MS-0451-034/002. See W.H. Trimble, *Catalogue of the Hocken Library Dunedin* (Dunedin: Otago Daily Times and Witness Newspapers Co., 1912), pp. 51–52 for full listing of Davis material, some of which is unidentified.
36 C.O.B. Davis to TMH, 16 September 1886. F&J 5: 129. HC.
37 HPC, Vol. 18, No. 13. Titi: design in the centre of the forehead; kauwae: chin patterns for men with facial tattoos; puhoro: scroll pattern adorning rafters of a house or bow of a canoe; whakairo: to carve, ornament with a pattern, sculpt. Davis was wrong in his opinion. Thanks to Roger Blackley, Victoria University of Wellington.
38 M.P.K. Sorrenson. 'Mantell, Walter Baldock Durrant', from DNZB: www.TeAra.govt.nz/en/biographies/1m11/mantell-walter-baldock-durrant
39 TMH to W.B.D. Mantell, 14 February 1876. No. 2465/76/18/2/76, MONZ Archives MU 000094/3/4. Thanks to Jennifer Twist.
40 Mantell's note to Gore on the letter from TMH to W.B.D. Mantell, 14 February 1876. No. 2465/76/18/2/76, MONZ Archives MU 000094/3/4. Richard Benjamin Gore (1840–1904), at one time Hector's clerk and then employed at the Colonial Museum and Geological Gallery. Thanks to John Yaldwyn, editor, with Juliet Hobbs, of *My Dear Hector: Letters from Joseph Dalton Hooker to James Hector 1862–1893*. MONZ Technical Report 31 (Wellington: MONZ, December 1998).
41 F.W. Hutton to W.B.D. Mantell, 22 March 1876. No. 2497/76/27/3/76, MONZ Archives MU 000094/3/4.
42 TMH, 'Travel diary', 1888. Misc-MS-1730. HC.
43 TMH, 'Travel diary', 1889. Misc-MS-1730. HC.
44 TMH, 'Travel diary', 1895. Misc-MS-1730. HC.
45 TMH, 'New Zealand notes', p. 81. MS-0037. HC.
46 At the third meeting of the AAAS in Christchurch in January 1891, TMH became a member of the Anthropology section, with A.W. Howitt of Melbourne as president, W.B.D. Mantell as vice-president, Edward Tregear and Augustus Hamilton.
47 W.B.D. Mantell to TMH, 17 February 1890. MS-1570-001/003. HC.
48 W.B.D. Mantell to TMH, 4 April 1892. MS-0451-007/018. HC.
49 W.B.D. Mantell to TMH, 20 May 1892. F&J 5: 182. HC.
50 HPC, Vol. 15, Nos 3, 4.
51 HPC, Vol. 52, No. 9.
52 'Variae' 4: No. 14.
53 HPC, Vol. 65, No. 2.
54 HPC, Vol. 93, No. 1.
55 HPC, Vol. 141, Nos 2, 4.
56 HPC, Vol. 167, No. 4.
57 HPC, Vol. 133.
58 W.B.D. Mantell to TMH, 9 March [1894]. MS-0451-009/001. HC.

59   F&J 5: 66.
60   J.F.H. Wohlers Collection. MS Papers 1410. ATL
61   TMH, 'Travel diary', 1879. Transcript of TMH's journal of his holiday trips to various parts of the North Island and to Christchurch. Misc-MS-1730. HC.
62   Ibid.
63   See H.F. von Haast, *The Life and Times of Sir Julius von Haast* (Wellington: H.F. von Haast, 1948), p. 5.
64   TMH to Dr Haast, 7 February 1880. Berggren Papers, MS-Papers 1002-7. ATL.
65   TMH, 'Travel diary', 1879. See HPC, Vol. 11 'Almanacs' 1844–59.
66   TMH, 'Some account of the beginnings of literature in New Zealand: Part II, the English newspapers', *Transactions* (1901), pp. 101–02.
67   See Kathleen A. Coleridge. 'Revans, Samuel', from DNZB: www.TeAra.govt.nz/en/biographies/1r5/revans-samuel
68   TMH, 'Travel diary', 1879.
69   'Death of Samuel Revans', *Wairarapa Standard*, 16 July 1888. F&J 4: 134.
70   TMH, 'Travel diary', 1879.
71   Ibid. Ellen Turner, whom Wakefield 'kidnapped' in 1826. See Philip Temple, *A Sort of Conscience: The Wakefields* (Auckland: Auckland University Press, 2003).
72   TMH, 'Travel diary', 1879. White's belief is evident in his *Ancient History*, where he relates a diverse number of tribal narratives of canoe migrations; no one dominates. Thanks to Michael Reilly, University of Otago, correspondence, August 2006.
73   Ibid.
74   Ibid.
75   Gerard Reid, 'Chapman, George Thomson', from DNZB: www.TeAra.govt.nz/en/biographies/2c16/chapman-george-thomson
76   TMH, 'Travel diary', 1879.
77   See J.R. Elder (ed), *The Letters and Journals of Samuel Marsden 1765–1838* (Dunedin: Coulls Somerville Wilkie and A.H. Reed for the Otago University Council, 1932), p. 93.
78   'Conversation between TMH and William and George (Edwin) Palmer, Otokia, 12 July 1879'. Notes loose in F&J 4: between 132 and 133. TMH eventually typed the notes up in August 1900.
79   See *ODT*, 13 August 1887, p. 5.

Chapter 7: Good Fortune, Dr Hocken, FLS

1   Charles Heaphy to TMH, 29 January 1881. MS-0451-004/001. HC.
2   TMH, 'Travel diary', 1881. Misc-MS-1730. HC.
3   See Stuart Strachan and Linda Tyler (eds), *Ka Taoka Hakena: Treasures from the Hocken Collections* (Dunedin: Otago University Press, 2007), pp. 178–79.
4   See Peter J. Vangioni (compiler), *Canterbury Society of Arts First Annual Exhibition (18 Jan.–12 Feb. 1881)* (Christchurch: Robert McDougall Art Gallery, 2000). Peele's *Christchurch in 1852* was No. 102; Temple's *Early Settlers* was No. 52.
5   Heaphy would leave Wellington in June in bad health and die in Brisbane in early August. See Michael Fitzgerald, 'Heaphy, Charles', from DNZB: www.TeAra.govt.nz/en/biographies/1h14/heaphy-charles. See also Iain Sharp's *Heaphy* (Auckland: Auckland University Press, 2008).
6   Specifically 'Early history and customs of the New Zealanders', *Nelson Examiner and New Zealand Chronicle (NE&NZC)*, 28 June 1851, p. 76; 'Origin of the New Zealanders', *NE&NZC*, 12 July 1851, p. 84.
7   TMH, 'Travel diary', 1881. Misc-MS-1730. HC. The copy of this legend has yet to be traced. Cf Ariki-mai-tai on the South Taranaki Coast (ref: John

White, *Ancient History of the Maori* (Wellington: Government Printer, 1887–90), Vol. II, p. 163), and 'Kahui-maunga at Patea', in *JPS*, Vol. 16, No. 4 (1907) pp. 189–206.
8 See Geoffrey Blake-Palmer, 'Sir Frederic Truby King' in A.H. McLintock (ed.), *An Encyclopedia of New Zealand*, Vol. 2 (Wellington: Government Printer, 1966), pp. 221–23.
9 Isaac Newton Watt to Thomas King, 2 February 1881 F&J 5: 118. Charles Flinders Hursthouse, *The Incorporation of Britain's Colonial with her Home Empire* [1866]. See HPC, Vol. 12, No. 13. For further information on Watt see Margot Fry, *Tom's Letters: The private world of Thomas King, Victorian gentleman* (Wellington: Victoria University Press, 2001), p. 78.
10 See history-nz.org/parihaka.html
11 See Hazel Riseborough, *Days of Darkness: Taranaki 1878–1884* (Wellington: Allen & Unwin, 1989) p. 141.
12 TMH to Sir George Grey, 24 January 1881. Grey Correspondence, GL:NZ H29 (1). Sir George Grey Special Collections, ACL; see also *OW*, 5 March 1881, p. 10.
13 Ibid., 24 January 1881.
14 Sir George Grey to TMH, 20 April 1881. MS-0451-004/002. HC.
15 The address is in the Darwin Archive at Cambridge University Library, DAR 229: 80 (ref. S 12733). It is owned by English Heritage, the body responsible for Down House, Charles Darwin's home in Kent. Thanks to Rosemary Clarkson, Cambridge, England.
16 Charles Darwin to TMH, 21 February 1881. F&J 5: 119. HC. See also the minutes of the Otago Institute, 1869–2006. ARC 0036. HC.
17 TMH to the Justice Department, 27 February and 22 December 1882. J1:82/2617, Archives New Zealand, Wellington. Cited in A.G. Hocken, *Dr Hocken of Dunedin: A life* (Oamaru: East Riding Press 2008), p. 29.
18 'Dinner to Dr Hocken', *OW*, 25 March 1882, p. 24.
19 Report by TMH, *OW*, 10 March 1883, p. 22.
20 TMH, *Bibliography* (1909), p. 130.
21 Annotation in TMH's copy of Angas's *New Zealanders Illustrated*. It was available to subscribers at 1 guinea. See Bagnall, *National Bibliography*, 114a and 114.
22 Note J.E. Traue's words: 'Even today [1991], the serious collector of non-New Zealand books will need to look outside New Zealand if he or she is to go beyond a very basic collection. The resources for serious connoisseur-collecting are not in New Zealand, have never been and are never likely to be.' J.E. Traue, *Committed to Print: Selected essays in praise of the common culture of the book* (Wellington: Victoria University Press, 1991), p. 35.
23 P. 2, Quaritch MS. Add 64222 (of MS Add. 64132-64, 217) Alphabetical Listing of Titles and Authors. British Library (BL). On p. 62 G.M. Thomson is mentioned with a two-volume illustrated edition by Scott of John Bunyan's *Pilgrim's Progress* (1840), and on p. 176, Alexander Turnbull's purchase of *Castiglione the Courtier* (1561) for either £4 10s or £6 6s.
24 c. 12 June 1882, p. 519, 'New Zealand', Quaritch MS. Add. 64222. BL.
25 'Asia, Africa, Australia' ledger for 1899. Quaritch MS. Add. 64221. BL.
26 As reported in *West Coast Times*, 22 August 1882, p. 2.
27 F.D. Bell to TMH, 6 January [1882?], MS-0451-033/001. HC.
28 F.D. Bell, 7 Westminster Chambers, London, to TMH, 8 August 1882. MS-0451-004/003. HC.
29 TMH, *Contributions* (1898), p. 67.
30 W.H. and Clara Hocken, 1881 Census, Newington. RG11/541/fo 75v; Joshua Hocken, 1851 Census, Liverpool. HO107/2321/fo 1v; Joshua Jr and Isabella

	Hocken, 1861 Census, Liverpool. RG 9/2686/fo 64v; Joshua and Isabella Hocken, 1881 Census, Liverpool. RG 11/3610/fo 63v; Joshua and Isabella Hocken, 1891 Census, Liverpool. RG 12/ 2907/fo 15r; Joshua and Isabella Hocken, 1901 Census, Liverpool. RG 13/ 3413/fo 140v. In 1901, Joshua (69) and Isabella (68) were still living at 31 Old Hall Street, Liverpool. Isabella was blind, which may explain two domestic servants: Norah Giles (41) and Florence Davies (15).
31	See F&J 6: 43 and 45. 'The most famous person from Farsley was Samuel Marsden, who was born in 1764 in the Bagley district, and later moved to Turners Fold, which adjoined Farsley Town Street. The Fold was demolished in 1923 and in 1934 a monument, appropriately incorporating a sheep's head, was erected on the site, which is now a small garden known as Sheepshead Park next to the New Inn.': http://mysite.wanadoo-members.co.uk/Farsley
32	Hatton was vicar from 1877 to 1892. Thanks to the Rev. John H. Walker (Vicar of Calverley since 1995) and Michele Walker, Calverley Vicarage. Private email correspondence, 17 April 2008.
33	TMH to Miss Betts, 16 October 1888. Betts Family Papers, Vol. I. Correspondence 1827–1910. ML A2563. State Library of New South Wales (SLNSW).
34	Petherick: Census 1881. RG 11/0615/59, fo. 17.
35	Cited in C.A. Burmester's entry on Petherick, *ADB*, Vol. 2, pp. 236–37.
36	E.A. Petherick, Obituary of S.W. Silver in *Geographical Journal*, Vol. 25, No. 4 (April 1905), pp. 465–66; 1881 Census. RG 11/137 fo. 15r.
37	S.W. Silver to TMH, [16 December 1903]. MS-0451-018/016. HC.
38	Copy 1: HPC, Vol. 13, No. 3; Copy 2: HPC, Vol. 15, No. 7. In No. 49 TMH wrote: 'This is a reprint by E.A. Petherick (who gave me this No.). Mr P. was connected with the publishing firm of Robertsons of Melbourne & took a keen interest in Australasia literature. He compiled the York Gate Catalogue for W. Silver.' Silver's York Gate Collection is now part of the Royal Geographical Society Collection at the State Library of South Australia, Adelaide.
39	See *New Zealand Journal of Science*, Vol. 1, No. 8 (March 1883), p. 391. HC; for Petherick materials see HPC Vol. 106.
40	Turnbull's nominators were W. Carruthers, E.G. Baker, J.B. Carruthers and G. Murray. Thanks to Gina Douglas and Lynda Brooks at Linnean Society, London.
41	TMH to the Treasurer, Linnean Society, 20 March 1886. Linnean Society Archives, London.
42	Otago Institute [derelict ship] in *ODT*, 15 June 1887, p. 4.
43	Captain F. Moore to TMH, 15 January 1883. MS-0451-004/006. HC.

Chapter 8: In Her Own Right

1	St John's Church, Invercargill. Marriage Register No. 3. Entry 195, 24 July 1883. HL; see also *OW*, 28 July 1883.
2	Cited in A.G. Hocken, *Dr T.M. Hocken 1836–1910: A gentleman of his time* (Dunedin: Hocken Library, University of Otago, 1989), p. 30.
3	TMH to Elizabeth Mary Hocken (EMH), 5 October 1890. MS-1258-001/015. HC.
4	Cited in Annette Facer, 'Elizabeth Hocken' in Charlotte Macdonald, Merimeri Penfold and Bridget Williams (eds), *The Book of New Zealand Women: Ko Kui Ma Te Kaupapa* (Wellington: Bridget Williams Books, 1991), p. 300.
5	*The New Zealander*, 16 December 1848, p. 4; see also Nancy M. Buckland, 'The Bucklands: A continuation of C.M. Gordon's story and a revision of the Buckland and Taylor trees'. Typescript, 1975. Sir George Grey Special

	Collections, ACL; see also C.M. Gordon, *The Taylors and Bucklands: Early Auckland pioneer families*, 2nd edn (Auckland: Pelorus Press, 1969).
6	Eric Beer and Alwyn Gascoigne, *Plough of the Pakeha* ([Cambridge]: Cambridge Independent, 1975), p. 68; Buckland Deeds Reference: IF 934 F2.17.1204. Cambridge Museum. Thanks to Michael Jeans, Cambridge, New Zealand.
7	Cambridge Museum website; Beer and Gascoigne (1975), p. 106; J.C. Firth, *Nation Making: A story of New Zealand savagism v. civilization* (London: Longmans, Green, & Co., 1890), p. 82.
8	Pre-nuptial agreement between TMH and E.M. Buckland, 23 July 1883. Cook & Allan Papers, Box 4. UN-003. HC.
9	'A sad occurrence: Decease of Mrs W. Buckland', *Daily Southern Cross*, 6 September 1871, p. 5. Thanks to David Verran, ACL.
10	EMH to TMH, May 1890. MS-1258-004/002. HC.
11	C.R. Allen. 'A few notes on Hocken' in Correspondence relating to Walter Empson Burdon. Randal Matthews 1896–1965. Papers. MS-85-109-2/05. ATL.
12	*OW*, 19 April 1894, p. 46; *OW*, 16 September 1897, p. 43.
13	*OW*, 13 August 1896, p. 43.
14	*OW*, 6 August 1896. p. 43. Banjo Paterson, 'Clancy of the Overflow', first published in the Australian *Bulletin*, 21 December 1889.
15	*OW*, 23 May 1889, p. 22; *OW*, 11 October 1894, p. 3.
16	*OW*, 12 January 1893, p. 33.
17	*OW*, 17 May 1905, p. 18; 15 August 1906, p. 78; 9 December 1908, p. 86.
18	Second Annual Report, 19 May 1909. HPC, Vol. 179, no 19. HC.
19	*OW*, 13 March 1887, p. 9.
20	TMH to EMH, 2 September 1894. MS-1258-001/024. HC.
21	Dr Hector, Auckland, to EMH, 13 July 1901. MS 1258-004/009; John Halliday Scott to his daughters Marion and Helen, 16 May 1909. MS-2673/001. HC.
22	'Alice's letters to her readers', *OW*, 1 June 1893, p. 45.
23	A.G. Hocken (1989), p. 52.
24	TMH to EMH, 22 January 1889. MS-1258-001/004. HC. She was also unwell when C.O.B. Davis visited in 1886.
25	Ruby Neill, typescript memoirs, 24 February 1960. MS-2847/62. HC. Thanks to Susan Irvine for pointing this manuscript out to me.
26	Sir George Arney to Bessie Buckland, 18 December [1860s]. F&J 5: 114. HC; C.O.B. Davis to EMH, 22 July 1886. MS-1258-004/001. HC; Thomas Pratt to EMH, 6 May 1895. MS-1258-004/004. HC; Samuel Tarratt Nevill to EMH, 6 July 1910. F&J 5 193. HC; EMH to Dr Benham, [n.d.]. MS-0451-032/008. HC; EMH to Stephenson Percy Smith, 4 June 1910 and 25 June 1913. Polynesian Society MS-Papers-1187-263. ATL; L.O. Beal, Sydney to EMH, 23 August 1895. MS-1258-004/005; G.W. Pogson, Tasmania, to EMH, Yokohama, 1 September 1901. MS-1258-004/010. HC; John Horsfall to EMH, 17 August 1906. MS-0451-024/004. HC. On Pogson, Gladys made the note: 'G.W. Pogson – an old family friend – bachelor – devoted to mother & father. He died shortly after this letter in Tasmania. He gave me my 2 copies of "Alice in Wonderland' & "Through the Looking Glass".'
27	James Backhouse Walker Papers, 'Walker's trip through New Zealand 25 February to 24 March 1898'. W9/C3/38. University of Tasmania, Hobart.
28	TMH to EMH, 28 June 1892. MS-1258-001/019. HC.
29	TMH to EMH, 19 February 1894. MS-1258-001/020. HC.
30	The couple had joint or personal investments in the Australian Leather Rubber Co., Melbourne, the Bank of New South Wales, property (some 70

	acres) at Catlin's Estuary, the Taranaki New Zealand Oil Wells Company, the Old Jubilee Gold Mine and the Junction North Broken Hill Mine. For EMH's involvement in stocks and shares see MS-0451-037. HC.
31	HPC, Vol. 43 contains 25 'Manufacturers' pamphlets.
32	Cited in A.G. Hocken (1989), p. 32.
33	C.R. Allen. 'A few notes on Hocken' in Correspondence relating to Walter Empson Burdon. Randal Matthews 1896–1965. Papers. MS-85-109-2/05. ATL.
34	John Halliday Scott to Marion and Helen Scott, 31 July 1910. MS-2673/002. HC.
35	EMH to Gladys Hocken, January 1907. MS-1258-004-001. HC.
36	HPC, Vol. 150, No. 11; signed E.M. Hocken.
37	See TMH to EMH, 24 January 1888. MS-1258-001/002; EMH to Gladys Hocken, [January 1907]. MS-1258-004-011. HC.
38	Percy Smith to TMH, 4 December 1893. MS-0451-008/006. HC.
39	Percy Smith to TMH, 25 January 1894. Tipped in George Windsor Earl's *The Eastern Seas* (1837). This work carries TMH's FLS printed bookplate, preliminary paged signature and the embossed arms on p. 35.
40	TMH to EMH, 2 September 1894. MS-1258-001/024. HC.
41	TMH, Dunedin, to EMH, c/- Mrs Hull, Moeraki, 3 September 1894. MS-1258-001/025. HC.
42	TMH, 'Abel Tasman and his journal', Art XV, *Transactions*, Vol. 28 (1895), pp. 117–40.
43	Annie Trimble, 'A collector's sacrifice: An interview with Dr Hocken', *Evening Star*, 1 February 1908, pp. 39–41.
44	C.A. de Fleurieu to TMH, 14 August 1906. MS-0451-024/002. See also C.A. de Fleurieu to TMH, 27 August 1906. MS-0451-024/006; C.A. de Fleurieu to TMH, 1 November 1907. MS-0451-025/013; C.A. de Fleurieu to TMH, 21 May 1908. MS-0451-027/009; C.A. de Fleurieu to TMH, 31 October 1908. MS-0451-028/020; and C.A. de Fleurieu to TMH 28 May 1909. MS-0451-029/010. HC.
45	*New Testament* in Maori (W233), copy 2. HC.
46	'Alice's letter to her readers', *OW*, 16 June 1892, p. 41.
47	*Early History Society of Otago Conversazione, Friday 17 April 1885* – No. 7 in Pamphlet Vol. 173; *Dresden Pianoforte Co. City Hall's Grand Tableaux Concert 2 July [1891?]*, at 29/31 Princes St. 'Variae' 3: No. 44; 'New Cathedral Building Fund', 1910. HPC, Vol. 151, No. 1. HC.
48	EMH to Gladys Hocken, [January 1907]. MS-1258-004-011. HC.
49	TMH to EMH, 24 January 1888. MS-1258-001/002. HC.
50	TMH to EMH, 27 January 1889. MS-1258-001. HC.
51	TMH to EMH, 29 March 1889. MS-1258-001/007. HC.
52	TMH to EMH, 25 May 1890. MS-1258-001/016. HC.
53	EMH to TMH, May 1890. MS-1258-004/002. HC.
54	*Otago Art Society 32nd Annual Exhibition Catalogue* (1908). HPC, Vol. 172. HC. See also Annette Facer, 'Elizabeth Hocken' in *The Book of New Zealand Women*, pp. 300–01; *OW*, 13 April 1899, p. 21.
55	Art Society notice, *OW*, 16 November 1888, p. 16; 27 February 1890, p. 17; 26 November 1891, p. 33; 15 December 1892, p. 33; 26 November 1896, p. 53; 24 November 1898, p. 61; 21 November 1906, p. 15; 11 December 1907, p. 13.
56	*OW*, 15 December 1892, p. 33.
57	*OW*, 16 November 1904, p. 87.
58	TMH supplied dimensions and plan of house: '29½ x 20 x 8 ft. Lined throughout partly with 6 x ⅝ Scotch & 8 x ¾ red pine T & G; 7½ ft high

inside. Shingle roof. Cemetery about ⅝ of an acre. Gravestones of Sydney sandstone.'
59 See Stuart Strachan and Linda Tyler (eds), *Ka Taoka Hakena: Treasures from the Hocken Collections* (Dunedin: Otago University Press, 2007), p. 218; see also Album 45. Original Pictorial Collection. HC.
60 'Arrested Attention', neg. 45/1/a; 76.277; 'Old Mission Station, Waikouaiti', c/n E6099/11; 696.01770; TMH and Gladys, c/n 45/1/b; 76.279. Originals D5d Hi to Hz, Box 146. HC.
61 *OW*, 26 April 1894, p. 3-; 13 May 1897, p. 59.
62 *OW*, 5 December 1900, p. 46; 5 August 1903, p. 42; 4 March 1903, p. 39.
63 Richard Henry, Resolution Island, to EMH, 5 May 1900. MS-1258-004/006. HC.
64 TMH to EMH, 2 September 1894. MS-1258-001-024. HC.
65 TMH to George Fenwick, 26 March 1910. Typed letter. MS-0451-031/003. HC.
66 TMH to Thomas Cheeseman, 18 April 1879. Cheeseman Correspondence Letterbook, Pre-1900. MA 95/40. AIM.
67 TMH to [Thomas Cheeseman], 30 March 1889. Ibid.
68 TMH to Thomas Cheeseman, 17 April 1905. Ibid.
69 Hocken, *Contributions* (1898), p. 125.
70 Hocken's fourth lecture on Otago Settlement, 9 October 1888. MS-0453/003. HC. Three of 36 foolscap pages of hand-written lecture by EMH; also Journals of Rev. William Richard Wade, John Wallis Barnicoat, Captain John Jermyn Symonds, Major Cyprian Bridges and Colonel Charles Stapp. MS-0051. HC.
71 Dedication note in MS-1258-001/028. HC.

Chapter 9: A Reputation Established

1 William Craig, Invercargill, to the editor, *ODT*, 22 August [1887]; Editorial, 'The early history of New Zealand', *OW*, 26 August 1887, p. 11. See newspaper scrapbook compiled by TMH. MS-2469/001. HC.
2 George Augustus Sala to TMH, 30 September 1885. F&J 5: 125. HC.
3 Thomas Moore Philson to TMH, 18 February 1884. MS-0451-004/007; Henry Jacobs to TMH, 30 April 1887. F&J 5: 130. HC. See also Judith Binney's 'Whatever happened to poor Mr Yate?', *New Zealand Journal of History*, Vol. 9, No. 2 (1975), pp. 111–25.
4 Henry Jacobs to TMH, 17 May 1887. MS-0451-005/005. HC.
5 Agnes J. Burns to TMH, 15 September 1880. MS-0451-003/015. HC.
6 C.W. Holgate, *An Account of the Chief Libraries of New Zealand* (London: Dryden Press, 1886), pp. 37–39.
7 James Cowan, 'Famous New Zealanders, No. 43 John Webster' in *New Zealand Railways Magazine*, Vol. 11, No. 7 (1 October 1936).
8 John Webster, c/- Northern Club, to TMH, 21 February 1874. No. 13, in '21 Important Letters 1867–96'. MS-0084. HC.
9 TMH, 'New Zealand notes', p. 21. MS-0037. HC. See Stuart Strachan and Linda Tyler (eds), *Ka Taoka Hakena: Treasures from the Hocken Collections* (Dunedin: Otago University Press, 2007), p. 128.
10 'Variae' 30: No. 1. The first piece is about a Roman colonist to Great Britain written by C.D.R. Ward, the second Robert Pharazyn's reply to the review of Jones's *Travels to Scotland* (1847); the third a review of Jones's *Travels to Scotland* by Sir William Fox; the fourth is 'Young New Zealand' composed and written by Catherine Waitt; the fifth a 'Song of Early Winter' composed and written by Catherine Waitt; and the sixth, H. Elliott's 'A Legend of Cloud Land, written by Mrs Featherston'.

11 'History of the first bell in Dunedin situated on a church reserve afterwards named "Bell Hill"'. MS-0451-015/009. HC. See also TMH's *Contributions* (1898), p. 102.
12 Letterbook of Charles Henry Kettle, Chief Surveyor. MS-0083. HC.
13 Robert Henry Wynyard, Journal and Letters. MS-0087. HC.
14 Third to fifth lectures, September 1884, September 1885 and September 1886. Only the *New Zealand Gazette*, Chaffers' *Sketch*, the *New Zealand Journal* and Raoul's work are listed in the draft catalogue of 1887.
15 TMH, 'Travel diary', 1885. Misc-MS-1730. HC.
16 TMH's note on p. [3]: 'this manuscript was given to me in 1885'. MS-0030. HC.
17 TMH does not mention Ralph's formation of the 'Microscopical Society' in Melbourne, and his scientific publishing with works such as *Opuscata Ominae Botanica Thomae Johnsoni* (1847), *Elementary Botany for Beginners* (1849) and *Icones Carpologiae* [Legiminoae], 1849. Thanks to John Adam, Auckland.
18 J.M. Philson to TMH, 18 February 1884. MS-0451-004/007. HC.
19 See TMH's compiled newspaper scrapbook for his 'Early pictorial illustrations of New Zealand', in *New Zealand Educational and Literary Monthly Journal*, 14 June 1884. MS-2469/001.
20 Ibid., [p. 1]: opening sentence.
21 E.H. McCormick, *Letters and Art in New Zealand* (Wellington: Department of Internal Affairs, 1940), p. 27.
22 Charles Heaphy, *View of Nelson Haven, in Tasman's Gulf, New Zealand; including a part of the site of the intended town of Nelson*. On stone by T. Allom from a drawing made in November 1841 by C. Heaphy, draftsman to the New Zealand Company. Tinted lithograph, Du H434; *Nelson from the Gaol* (1859), D H434. HC.
23 TMH's copy: George Duppa, *Part of the New Plymouth Settlement in the District of Taranake, New Zealand. Mount Egmont 30 miles distant*. Lithograph by T. Allom from a drawing taken on board the ship *Brougham* by George Duppa Esq. Published for the New Zealand Company by Smith, Elder & Co., London. 1841. F D941; Mrs Hocken's copy: *Part of the New Plymouth settlement, in the district of Taranaki, New Zealand. Shewing the range of houses recently built by the natives, in anticipation of the arrival of emigrants. Mount Egmont 30 miles distant*. T. Allom lithograph. Printed by C. Hullmandel. n.d. A D941.
24 TMH's note on the top of his copy of 'Early pictorial illustrations of New Zealand' in his scrapbook. MS-2469/001. HC.
25 Edmund Norman, *Town of Lyttelton*, Maclure, Macdonald & Macgregor lithograph, London. *Lyttelton*. Published by Martin G. Heywood. 1852. B N842; *Lyttelton, Port of Victoria*, Maclure, Macdonald & Macgregor lithograph, London.
26 TMH's newspaper scrapbook notation. MS-2469/001.
27 Cited in Gladstone's letter to Bernard Quaritch, 9 September 1896, in Quaritch's *Contributions Towards a Dictionary of English Book Collectors* (London: Bernard Quaritch, 1892–98; New York: Burt Franklin, reprint, 1968), Part VIII, December 1896.
28 J.F.H. Wohlers to TMH, 8 May 1884. No. 4. '21 Important Letters, 1867–96'. MS-0084. HC.
29 J.F.H. Wohlers to TMH, 30 September 1884. F&J 5: 123. HC.
30 J.F.H. Wohlers to TMH, 17 November 1884. MS-2399. HC.
31 Samuel Hodgkinson to TMH, 9 November 1886. MS-0451-005/003. HC.
32 Ibid. For Hursthouse's letters on colonisation (1866), see TMH, *Bibliography* (1909), p. 244.

33	*Sketch of the Rural District of New Edinburgh* drawn by Frederick Tuckett, 1844. HmapHm 880/1844/a, HC. See Samuel Hodgkinson to TMH, 9 November 1886. MS-0451-005/003. HC.
34	TMH, *Contributions* (1898), Appendix B: Letter from Mr Tuckett to Dr Hodgkinson, 16 August 1844, pp. 226–29.
35	TMH, *Early History* (1914), Chapter VIII, p. 147.
36	Ibid.
37	TMH, *Contributions* (1898), Appendix A: Mr Tuckett's Diary, pp. 203–25.
38	TMH, *Early History* (1914), Chapter VIII, p. 147.
39	F.F. Tuckett to TMH, 25 October 1887. MS-0451-005/011. HC.
40	F.F. Tuckett to TMH, 28 July 1888. MS-0451-006/005. HC.
41	Ibid.
42	J.W. Barnicoat, Wellington, to TMH, 11 June 1885. MS-1570-001. HC.
43	J.W. Barnicoat to TMH, 22 August 1887. No. 8, '21 Important Letters, 1867–96'. MS-0084. HC.
44	'Journal of John Wallis Barnicoat', February 1842 to October 1844. MS-0051. HC.
45	TMH, *Early History* (1914), p. 148.
46	Tuckett obituary, etc. See MS-2589. HC.
47	'Early History Society', *ODT*, 19 April 1884, pp. 1, 2.
48	Minute Books, Early History Society of Otago. MS-0097. HC.
49	'The Early History Society of Otago', HPC, Vol. 173, No. 7. See also 'Early Historical Society of Otago, Constitution and Bye-laws' (1884) Article III. HPC, Vol. 166, No. 20. HC.
50	Alfred R. Chetham Strode to TMH, 11 September 1884. MS-0451-004/010. HC. See also TMH's 'New Zealand notes', p. 10 (MS-0037) on his contacting Strode about issues of the *New Zealand Journal*.
51	Minute books, Early History Society of Otago. MS-0097. HC.
52	'Catalogue of books, pamphlets, maps, newspapers, prints &c relating to New Zealand. In the library of Dr T.M. Hocken of Dunedin, N.Z.' [1887]. MS-0044. Cited in TMH, 'Travel diary', 1888. Misc-MS-1730. HC.
53	TMH's three-volume *Terra Australis Cognita* (Edinburgh, 1766–68) repeats the usual ingredients: bookplate (scripted) in all volumes, signatures, and the embossed coat of arms on p. 35. The name of one previous owner is scrawled on the title page: 'Carnock'.
54	TMH's de Brosses's *Histoire des navigations aux Terra Australes* (1756) has the book label: 'Sevend chez Bachelier Libraire, Quai des Augustins, No. 55 Paris'. His Rochon has a ripped book label 'de Piltan Libraire, Rue de St Peres, 22, Paris'. TMH's Thévenot contains the bookplate of Thomas William Evans, his printed 'F.L.S.' bookplate and title-page signature; Duperrey's *Atlas* has TMH's printed 'F.L.S.' bookplate and signature on the title page.
55	TMH, 'Travel diary', 1885. Misc-MS 1730. HC
56	George Sisson Cooper's *Journal of an Overland Expedition from Auckland to Taranaki* (1851). See note 15 in Alex Frame, *Grey and Iwikau: A journey into custom* (Wellington: Victoria University Press, 2002), pp. 78–79.
57	TMH, 'Travel diary', 1885. Misc-MS-1730. HC.
58	Bishop Hadfield to TMH, 5 September 1900. F&J 5: 173. HC. At some time TMH obtained a manuscript testimonial from Octavius Hadfield and Richard Taylor to Bishop Selwyn 11 December 1851, sanctioning Samuel Williams's candidacy into priesthood. F&J 6: 19. HC.
59	Drew's collection formed the basis of the Whanganui Regional Museum Collection established in 1895. See Kaye Noble, 'Drew, Samuel Henry', from DNZB: www.TeAra.govt.nz/en/biographies/2d18/drew-samuel-henry
60	TMH, 'Travel diary', 3 April 1888. Misc-MS-1730. HC.

61   See frontispiece to A.T. Yarwood, *Samuel Marsden: The great survivor* (Melbourne: Melbourne University Press, 1977).
62   TMH, 'Travel diary', 3 April 1888. Misc-MS-1730. HC.
63   TMH to Lizzie Betts, 11 July 1889. Betts Family Papers, Vol. I. Correspondence 1827–1910. ML A2563. SLNSW.
64   Rev. Robert Maunsell to TMH, Monday [1882?]. Letter tipped in R. Maunsell, *Grammar of the New Zealand Language*, 2nd edn, Auckland (1862). HC.
65   Edward Markham, transcript of *New Zealand, or Recollections of It* (ed. E.H. McCormick). MS-0085. HC. The original is in the Alexander Turnbull Library, Wellington.
66   'Variae' 23: No. 12. HC.
67   HPC, Vol. 186, Nos 4 and 5.
68   Robert Maunsell to TMH, 3 October 1888, Auckland. Tipped in Rev. A.W. Murray, *The Bible in the Pacific* (London: Nisbet, 1888). HC.
69   Robert Maunsell to TMH, 12 October 1886. MS-0451-005/002. HC.
70   Giselle M. Byrnes, 'Smith, Stephenson Percy', from DNZB: www.TeAra. govt.nz/en/biographies/2s33/smith-stephenson-percy
71   S. Percy Smith to TMH, 9 October 1887, tipped in *The Kermadec Islands* (1887) in HPC, Vol. 47. HC.
72   See 'Variae' 1. HC.

Chapter 10: 'A Very Big Affair Indeed'

1   Newspaper cuttings, F&J 11: 5–18. HC.
2   HPC, Vol. 161.
3   One thousand and fifty gentlemen subscribed the sum of £15,689 for the purpose of holding the exhibition. Cited in D. Harris Hastings, *Official Record of the New Zealand and South Seas Exhibition. Held at Dunedin, 1889–90* (Wellington: Government Printer, 1891), p. 23.
4   Ibid., p. 12. For committee information see pp. 1–8. Items from Australia also received some compensation with a freighted double journey at a single journey rate on the same shipping line.
5   Ibid., p. 338.
6   TMH, Minute book for New Zealand Exhibition 1889–90 (Early History, Maori & South Seas Section (EHMSS)) meeting of 24 April 1889. MS-101. HC.
7   TMH, 'The Exhibition' and newspapers clipping, Minutes EHMSS. MS-101. HC; see *ODT*, 26 April 1889, p. 3.
8   TMH, Minute book for New Zealand Exhibition 1889–90 and Letterbooks of the EHMSS Committee. MS-101, and MS-0335 to MS-0354. HC.
9   Octavius Harwood to TMH, 8 February 1889. MS-0451-006/009. HC.
10   Hastings, p. 238.
11   Twopeny to Devore, 29 May 1889. New Zealand Exhibition 2nd Letterbook 7.2.89 to 14.7.89, p. 698. MS-338. HC.
12   Hastings, p. 229.
13   D.H. Hastings to TMH, 4 April 1889. New Zealand Exhibition 2nd Letterbook 7.2.89 to 14.7.89, p. 339. MS-338. HC.
14   Minutes: EHMSS, 7th meeting, 5 June 1889. MS-101. HC.
15   TMH to John Webster, 4 June 1889. Letters: TMH to John Webster, 1889–1908. NZ MS 4/16. Sir George Grey Special Collections, ACL.
16   Ibid.
17   Hastings, p. 246.
18   TMH to John Webster, 22 May 1890. NZ MS 4/16. Sir George Grey Special Collections, ACL.

19   TMH to John Webster, 4 June 1889.
20   Hastings, p. 225.
21   Ibid., p. 229.
22   See Linda Tyler's entry on Smetham in Stuart Strachan and Linda Tyler (eds), *Ka Taoka Hakena: Treasures from the Hocken Collections* (Dunedin: Otago University Press, 2007), pp. 178–79.
23   'Matters relating to Smetham's picture' [copied from the papers of W.N. Jenkins by Miss B. Howes]. MS-0214. HC; George Olver, London, to TMH, 23 December 1887. In William John Phillipps Papers, MS-Papers-1222. ATL.
24   Ibid., 'Matters relating'.
25   TMH, 'New Zealand notes', p. 31. MS-0037. HC.
26   Sarah Smetham to TMH, 12 April 1899. No. 18 in '21 Important Letters, 1867–96'. MS-0084. HC.
27   TMH to W.N. Jenkins, 16 September 1909. MS-0214. HC.
28   James Backhouse Walker to TMH, 28 May 1889. Letter tipped in Walker's compilation *List of Books Relating to Tasmania* (1884), in HPC, Vol. 63.
29   Minutes EHMSS, 10th meeting, 17 July 1889. MS-101. HC.
30   Minutes EHMSS, 13th meeting. MS-101. HC.
31   Minutes EHMSS, 15th meeting: 28 August. MS-101. HC.
32   TMH to Sir George Grey, 7 September 1889. GL:NZ H29(5). Sir George Grey Special Collections. ACL.
33   The original *God of Harvest* was given to Grey by the Arawa tribe. The one sent was a cast.
34   TMH to Thomas Cheeseman, 6 November 1889. AIM.
35   Hastings, p. 240.
36   Minutes EHMSS, 25th meeting, 8 November. MS-101. HC.
37   See Hastings for structure details.
38   Cited in J.H. Scott and W.M. Hodgkins, 'The Exhibition Art Gallery', in *Catalogue of the New Zealand and South Seas Exhibition* (Dunedin, 1890), p. 248. Cited in Linda Tyler's 'Art for Empire: Paintings in the British Art Exhibit' in John Masefield Thomson's *Farewell Colonialism: The New Zealand International Exhibition Christchurch, 1906–07* (Palmerston North: Dunmore Press, 1998), ch. 8.
39   'Fine Arts Court', Hastings, p. 252.
40   17 December 1889, Richard Combe Miller, *Round the World in Five Months: A diary October 1889 to March 1890*. For private circulation only. ([Dartford: Printed by J. Snowden, 1891?]), pp. 22–23.
41   TMH, 'Introduction' in a reprint of *Early History, Maori, and South Seas Court Catalogue* (1889–1890), pp. 150–157 (156).
42   Ibid.
43   Minutes EHMSS. MS-101. HC.
44   TMH, 'Introduction', *Early History, Maori, and South Seas Court Catalogue*, p. 157.
45   Based on figures from Eccles, Palethorpe, New Zealand yearbooks, exhibition catalogues and other publications. Cited in Thomson, p. 29; Hastings, p. 338; 'Dunedin', *North Otago Times*, 20 February 1890, p. 2.
46   HPC, Vol. 77: NZ & SS Exhibition 1889–90: 8 pamphlets; see also F&J 7: 7, for *New Zealand Jubilee and Exhibition Chronicle*.
47   HPC, Vol. 94, No. 2; TMH actually owned three copies of Joubert's *Proposed New Zealand Exhibition in London*: see HPC, Vol. 49, No. 21; Vol. 77, No. 8; Vol. 93, No. 5.
48   TMH to John Webster, 22 May 1890. NZ MS 4/16. Sir George Grey Special Collections, ACL.
49   Hastings, p. 267.

50 Minutes EHMSS, 31st meeting (and last) of the EHMSS, 2 October 1890. MS-101. HC.
51 TMH to Thomas Cheeseman, 10 May 1890. AIM. Farquhar was charged with establishing insurance amounts and had to list all the exhibits, their value, when and from whom they were received. At the 29th meeting of 14 January 1890, the total insurance figure of £5500 was set.
52 TMH to Thomas Cheeseman, 20 June 1890. AIM.
53 Ibid., Davie cited.
54 TMH to Thomas Cheeseman, 7 July 1890. AIM.
55 Thomas Ritchie to TMH, 30 June 1891. MS-0451-007/009. HC.
56 TMH, 'A Maori house for Dunedin', *ODT*, 21 May 1890, p. 3.
57 Karaitiana Takamoana died on 24 February 1879.
58 TMH's annotations on 'A Maori house for Dunedin' in F&J 9: 51. HC.
59 Note written on a letter from D.H. Hastings to TMH, 4 December 1890. MS-0451-006/021. HC.

Chapter 11: Bibliographic Connections

1 Henry Anderson's 'David Scott Mitchell: Some reminiscences.' ML A 1830, p. 43. SLNSW. See also: A *Grand Obsession: The DS Mitchell story* ([Sydney]: SLNSW, 2007); Brian H. Fletcher, *Magnificent Obsession: The story of the Mitchell Library, Sydney*. ([Sydney]: Allen & Unwin/SLNSW, 2007). *Father Damien: An open letter to the Reverend Dr. Hyde of Honolulu* was privately printed in Sydney in March 1890 in an edition of 25 copies. Many were sent out as presentation copies, but obviously not to Mitchell.
2 Cited in A.H. Spencer, *The Hill of Content: Books, art, music, people* (Sydney: Angus & Robertson, 1959), p. 84.
3 Isobel Strong, 'Vailima Table-talk: Robert Louis Stevenson in his home life', *Scribner's Magazine*, Vol. 19, No. 5 (May 1896), pp. 531–47 (537).
4 Robert Louis Stevenson to Sidney Colvin, February 1893, in *Works* (Edinburgh: Constable, 1897), Vol. 24, letter 27, p. 238.
5 Cited in a letter from Edward Shillington to Grey, 26 June 1895. GNZ MSS 124(23). Sir George Grey Special Collections, ACL. The set, edition number 852, cost £12 10s.
6 Robert Louis Stevenson, [1893], F&J 5: 135. HC.
7 A.H. Turnbull to Edwin Gurr, 10 May 1898. Turnbull Letterbook 1891–1900, Vol. III: 691. qMS-2050-2052. ATL.
8 Political biographies on Grey include: Edmund Bohan, *To Be a Hero: A biography of Sir George Grey* (Auckland: HarperCollins, 1998); James Rutherford, *Sir George Grey, K.C.B.: A study in colonial government* (London: Cassell, 1961); James Collier, *Sir George Grey: Governor, high commissioner, and premier: An historical biography* (Christchurch: Whitcombe & Tombs, 1909); George C. Henderson, *Sir George Grey: A pioneer of empire in southern lands* (London: Dent, 1907); James Milne, *The Romance of a Pro-consul* (1899); William Lee and Lily Rees, *The Life and Times of Sir George Grey, K.C.B.* (Auckland: H. Brett, 1892).
9 Grey to Richard Owen, 3 November 1848. Sherborn Autographs, Vol. IX 'Politics and professions', BL. MS.Add. 42,583, f.127.
10 Wilhelm Bleek, *Manuscripts and Incunables, Vol. III, Part I* (London: Trübner, 1862) and *Early Printed Books, Vol. IV, Part I: England* (Cape Town: J.C. Juta, 1867).
11 Cited in C. Pama (ed.), *The South African Library: Its history, collections and librarians 1818–1968* ([Cape Town]; Published for the trustees of the South African Library by A.A. Balkema, 1968), pp. 11–12; and Donald Jackson Kerr, *Amassing Treasures for All Times: Sir George Grey, colonial bookman and collector* (Delaware: Oak Knoll Press; Dunedin: Otago University Press, 2006), pp. 161–62.
12 Christopher de Hamel, in Margaret M. Manion, Vera F. Vines and Christopher

de Hamel, *Medieval and Renaissance Manuscripts in New Zealand Collections* (Melbourne: Thames & Hudson, 1989), p. 41.

13 Grey referred to Bohn, Boone and Quaritch in response to a library survey conducted by Clifford Holgate. Grey to Clifford Holgate, 13 June 1886. GL:H36 (3). Sir George Grey Special Collections, ACL. The results were published in Holgate's *An Account of the Chief Libraries of New Zealand* (1886).

14 E.H. McCormick, *The Fascinating Folly: Dr Hocken and his fellow collectors* (Dunedin: University of Otago Press, 1961); E.H. McCormick, *Alexander Turnbull: His life his circle his collections* (Wellington: Alexander Turnbull Library, 1974); John C. Ross, 'Alexander H. Turnbull' in *Nineteenth-Century British Book-Collectors and Bibliographers: Dictionary of literary biography*, Vol. 184 (Detroit: Bruccoli Clark Layman Book, 1997), pp. 427–34.

15 Cited in McCormick, *Alexander Turnbull* (1974), p. 69.

16 Ibid., p. 74.

17 Ibid., p. 71.

18 Ibid., p. 75.

19 Ibid., p. 89.

20 Turnbull had other bookplates devised, as did his brother, Robert Thornburn Turnbull. See Penelope Griffith, 'Alexander Turnbull's bookplates', *Turnbull Library Record*, Vol. XII, No. 2 (October 1979).

21 A.H. Turnbull to Robert Turnbull, 9 December 1891. Cited in McCormick (1974), p. 100.

22 Cited in Ross, 'Alexander H. Turnbull' (1997), p. 430.

23 Robert McNab to A.H. Turnbull, 24 June 1914. Cited in McCormick (1974), p. 101.

24 Cited in Ross (1997), p. 433.

25 Robert McNab, *ODT*, 10 March 1914, p. 2. At the same time, McNab acknowledged the Hocken Library and even though use was somewhat restricted, he hoped the presence of two collections would one day result in the formation of a chair of Australasian and Pacific Studies.

26 Bertram Stevens, cited in Anne Robertson, *Treasures of the State Library of New South Wales: The Australiana Collections* (Sydney: Collins Publishers/SLNSW, 1988), p. 3.

27 Ibid., p. 13.

28 DSM to Rose Scott. 19 July 1868. ML ZA1437, pp. 79b–82. See also Suzanne Mourot with Paulette Jones, *The Great South Land: Treasures of the Mitchell and Dixson Libraries and Dixson Galleries* ([Sydney]: Sun, 1979).

29 Frederick Wymark, in James Tyrrell, *Old Books, Old Friends, Old Sydney* (Sydney; Angus & Robertson, 1952), p. 83. See also Frederick Wymark–David Scott Mitchell, c. 1939. Typescript of reminiscences. ML, SLNSW.

30 Ibid., Wymark (c. 1939), p. 19.

31 Cited in Robertson *Treasures of the State Library of New South Wales* (1988), p. 14; cited in Spencer, *The Hill of Content* (1959), p. 79.

32 See Fletcher, *Magnificent Obsession* (2007).

33 See Dixson Correspondence and Papers, and Dixson family biographical file. Dixson Library, SLNSW. See also *Sir William Dixson: A passion for collecting* ([Sydney]: SLNSW, 2013).

34 Spencer, p. 140.

35 Dixson, cited in Robertson, p. 112.

36 Typescript letter from Grey to TMH, 28 October 1880, bound in at front of 'Historical narrative of an attempt to form a settlement in New Zealand' by Charles, Baron de Thierry. qMS-2013. ATL.

37 Grey to TMH, 10 November 1885. F&J 5: 126. HC.

38 Ibid., 10 November 1885.

39   See TMH, *Bibliography* (1909), p. 176.
40   TMH to Grey, 7 December 1885. GL:NZ H29(2). Sir George Grey Special Collections, ACL. See HPC, Vol. 25, No. 5.
41   TMH to Grey, 7 June 1888. GL:NZ H29(3). Sir George Grey Special Collections, ACL.
42   Robert FitzRoy, *Remarks on New Zealand* (1846), in HPC Vol. 41. HC. The signature 'M. Williams' is on the title page. See TMH, *Bibliography* (1909), p. 127 for limitation details.
43   TMH to Grey, 19 September 1888. GL: NZ H29 (4). Sir George Grey Special Collections, ACL.
44   TMH to Grey, 7 September 1889. GL:NZ H29 (5). Sir George Grey Special Collections, ACL.
45   Cited by McCormick (1974), p. 122.
46   A.H. Turnbull, cited by Margaret Scott to E.H. McCormick, 27 August 1970. See McCormick (1974), p. 207.
47   A.H. Turnbull to Robert Turnbull, 22 February 1894. Turnbull Letterbook Vol. I: 1891–1900: 358. qMS-2050-2052. ATL.
48   A.H. Turnbull to William Brown, 2 November 1893. Turnbull Letterbook Vol. I: 335. ATL.
49   A.H. Turnbull to TMH, 9 May 1894. Turnbull Letterbook, Vol. I: 388–89. ATL.
50   A.H. Turnbull to Mr Evans, 25 November 1897. Turnbull Letterbook Vol. III: 545. ATL.
51   TMH to A.H. Turnbull, 2 May 1899. A.H. Turnbull, 1868–1918. Papers 0057-039. ATL
52   A.H. Turnbull to TMH, 30 May 1899. Turnbull Letterbook, 1891–1900. Vol. IV: 217. qMS-2050-2052. ATL.
53   A.H. Turnbull to TMH, [3 June 1899]. Turnbull Letterbook Vol. IV: 219. ATL.
54   A.H. Turnbull to TMH, 19 June 1899. Turnbull Letterbook Vol. IV: 234. ATL.
55   A.H. Turnbull to TMH, 26 June 1899. Turnbull Letterbook Vol. IV: 242. ATL.
56   Ibid.
57   A.H. Turnbull to TMH, 4 July 1899. Turnbull Letterbook Vol. IV: 254. ATL.
58   Downie Stewart, Hocken, Turnbull Correspondence, 7 October, 28 December 1908; 11 January, 12 August, 18 September 1909. MS-0985-002/221. HC. See also McCormick (1974), p. 223.
59   A.H. Turnbull to TMH, 21 August 1899. Turnbull Letterbook Vol. IV: 304. ATL.
60   A.H. Turnbull to TMH, 10 April 1900. Turnbull Letterbook Vol. IV: 432. ATL.
61   See 'Interesting sale of books', *ODT*, 30 April 1900, p. 3. Thanks to Anthony Tedeschi for the transcript.
62   See the marked *Catalogue of Magnificent & Extensive Library … of Late Hon. W.J.M. Larnach* (Dunedin: Park, Reynolds & Co., April 1900) in the Hocken Collection; p. 14, item 571 (Z 988.L37 CB26). There are annotations within, but they are not in TMH's hand.
63   A.H. Turnbull to TMH, 10 April 1900. Turnbull Letterbook Vol. IV: 432. ATL.
64   A.H. Turnbull to TMH, 22 May 1900. MS-0451-014/002. HC.
65   Ibid.
66   Herbert W. Williams, *A Bibliography of Printed Maori to 1900* (Wellington: Dominion Museum, 1924), 337, 340, 361, 371 and 372. For details on the two mentioned papers, see *BiM*, S13 and S15.
67   A.H. Turnbull to TMH, 5 April 1909. HL. MS-0451-029/008. HC.
68   Cited in McCormick (1974), p. 247.
69   Cited in McCormick (1974), p. 224, 12 and 19 August 1909.
70   TMH to A.H. Turnbull, 28 February 1910. MS-0451-031/002. HC.
71   McCormick (1974), p. 225. 8 January and 28 February 1910.

72   A.H. Turnbull, 2 April, 3 May 1910, cited in McCormick (1974), p. 225.
73   A.H. Turnbull to EMH, 3 August 1910. See McCormick (1974), p. 226.
74   D.S. Mitchell to TMH, 8 April 1899. F&J 5: 165. HC.
75   Ibid.
76   Ibid.; Henry Anderson to TMH, 25 March 1899. MS-0451-013/007.HC.
77   TMH to Angus & Robertson, 8 October 1899. MS-Papers-0763. Reproductions from MSS 1116. ML, SLNSW.
78   HPC, Vol. 166.

Chapter 12: The Fieldwork Continues

1   'Auckland, February 15', *North Otago Times*, 16 February 1897, p. 3.
2   TMH, 'Historical notes' MS-0027; 'New Zealand notes' MS-0037. HC.
3   FHC Family Archives, HC, and cited in A.G. Hocken (2008), p. 154.
4   As registered in TMH's draft catalogue, c. 1887. MS-0044. HC.
5   Percy Smith's mother, Hannah, was a Hursthouse and the family had been encouraged to emigrate to New Zealand by her brother, Charles.
6   Percy Smith to TMH, 24 September 1890, tipped in 'Travels', HPC, Vol. 20, No. 2. HC.
7   Percy Smith to TMH, 13 July 1892. MS-0451-007/020. HC.
8   John White to TMH, 3 November 1890 (MS-0451-006/020) and 9 January 1891 (F&J 5: 144). On the final letter TMH received he wrote: 'White's last letter. He died suddenly of heart disease on Jany 13/91 on his way to Whakatane. It refers to his papers prepared for the Association for the Advancement of Science at the Christchurch meeting, 1891. T.M. Hocken.'
9   Cited in Hugh Stringer 'Shand, Alexander', from DNZB: www.TeAra.govt.nz/mi/biographies/2s16/shand-alexander
10 Alexander Shand to TMH, 11 April and 8 July 1891. MS-0451-007/005 and 010. HC.
11 Percy Smith to TMH, 2 February 1891. MS-0451-007/002. HC.
12 TMH to Percy Smith, 9 February 1891. Polynesian Society Papers, MS-Papers-1187-263-7. ATL.
13 Percy Smith to TMH, 16 February 1891. MS-0451-007/025. HC.
14 See TMH's Report of the first meeting of the Australasian Association for the Advancement of Science (August–September 1888), Sydney, New South Wales, and other issues, including Vol. III, third meeting in Christchurch, January 1891. HPC Vol. 73.
15 Percy Smith to TMH, 16 February 1891. MS-0451-007/025. HC.
16 Percy Smith to TMH, 2 March 1891. MS-0451-007/003. HC.
17 TMH to Percy Smith, 15 June 1906. MS-0451-023/012. HC. Refer Rachel Barrowman, in Stuart Strachan and Linda Tyler (eds), *Ka Taoka Hakena: Treasures from the Hocken Collections* (Dunedin: Otago University Press, 2007), p. 13. See HPC, Vol. 186 for further evidence of TMH's membership of the Polynesian Society.
18 Percy Smith to TMH, 13 July 1892. MS-0451-007/020. HC.
19 Percy Smith to TMH, 15 November 1892. MS-0451-007/024. HC. Turton's work on deeds, initially suppressed because it was seen as a resource to upset or overturn land title ownership, continues to be a much-used and important work in libraries.
20 Ibid. The manuscript is unidentified.
21 TMH to Percy Smith, 1 June 1893. Polynesian Society Papers, MS-Papers-1187-263-9. ATL. See Williams 14; *BiM* 21: *Sheets of Syllables and Works for Teaching Infant Classes to Read* [Sydney, 1834]. TMH also had a review of William Marshall's *Two Visits*, which appeared in the *Colonist*, Sydney, 6 and 13 October 1836.

22   Percy Smith to TMH, 18 December 1893. MS-0451-008/007. HC.
23   Edward Charles Stirling to TMH, 22 January 1891. MS-0451-007/001. HC.
24   James Miller & Co. [Rope, Twine, Mats and Matting Manufacturers], Baring Chambers, Market Street, [Melbourne], to TMH, 11 May 1891. MS-0451-007/006. HC.
25   TMH, 'Travel diary', 10 February 1894. Misc-MS-1730. HC.
26   TMH to Thomas Cheeseman, 18 May 1891. MA 95/38/5 Correspondence Letterbook 1890-1897. AIM.
27   TMH to Thomas Cheeseman, 8 July 1891. MA 95/38/5 Correspondence Letterbook 1890–1897. AIM.
28   TMH to Thomas Cheeseman, 7 September 1891. MA 95/38/5 Correspondence Letterbook 1890–1897. AIM.
29   John Fraser to TMH, 11 May 1891. Letter tipped in *Some Folk Songs and Myths from Samoa*, translated by the Revs T. Powell and G. Pratt (Royal Society of NSW, 5 November 1890, 1 July 1891), HPC, Vol. 62, No. 5: 'Ethnology'. HC.
30   John Fraser to TMH, 11 May 1891.
31   Letter from Bishop Samuel Tarratt Nevill to TMH, 16 March 1892, tipped into Nevill's *On the Establishment of Cathedrals* (1886), bound at HPC, Vol. 78, No. 19. HC.
32   Thomas Godfrey Hammond to TMH, 21 July 1892. MS-0451-007/022. HC.
33   Rev. W.G. Lawes to TMH, 13 February 1893. MS-0451-008/001. HC.
34   G. Gerard Shaw, Parkside, South Australia to TMH, 14 August 1891. 'Variae' 31: No. 1. HC.
35   TMH owned Augustus Hamilton's article on New Zealand tokens which appeared in the Colonial Museum *Bulletin* No. 1, 1905 (1906), pp. 52–56, and incorporated it in his 'Variae' 27: No. 20. HC.
36   See TMH's 'Variae' 24 for typescript list. HC.
37   G. Gerard Shaw, Parkside, South Australia to TMH, 14 August 1891. 'Variae' 31: No. 1. HC.
38   [TMH], 'Manuscript notes relating to G.B. Shaw's watercolour of Dunedin, 1851', 'Variae' 31; G. Gerard Shaw to TMH, 27 August 1898. 'Variae' 31. HC.
39   *The Otago Jubilee Industrial Exhibition Official Catalogue* (1898). HPC, Vol. 148, No. 4. HC.
40   For more on the promissory notes, see Strachan and Tyler, p. 37; also Misc-MS-1535/1-3. HC. The tattoo was certainly that of Hone Tuhawaiki, 'Declaration of ownership of Robucka [sic] Island, 28 March 1840'. MS-0808/B. HC. See Strachan and Tyler, p. 34.
41   H.T. Kemp to TMH, 29 July 1893. MS-1570-001/004. HC.
42   W.L. Williams to TMH, 31 August 1893. MS-0084/12. HC.
43   William Webster, Kohu Kohu, Hokianga, to H.T. Kemp, 28 August 1893. No. 11 in '21 Important Letters, 1867–1896'. MS-0084. HC.
44   Alithea Symonds to TMH, 28 May 1894. MS-0451-009/006. HC.
45   James Heberley to TMH, 22 July 1896. MS-0451-010/007. HC. The Heberley story was a long time coming; in 2002 descendant Heather Heberley produced *Last of the Whalers: Charlie Heberley's story* (Auckland: Cape Catley, 2002).
46   John Richardson Selwyn to TMH, 27 August 1894; F&J 5: 147. HC.
47   Albert Allom to TMH, 10 November 1896. MS-0451-010/015. HC.
48   Albert Allom to TMH, 27 November 1896. MS-0451-010/016. HC.
49   Richard Henry to TMH, 28 December 1896. MS-0451-010/017 HC; Richard Henry to TMH, 30 November 1898. MS-0084/17. HC.
50   Percy Smith to TMH, 24 May 1895. MS-0451-009/012. HC.
51   See HPC, Vol. 114. It was presented to TMH by Smith in December 1904.

52 Paddy Gilroy to TMH, 19 May 1896. MS-0451-010/002. HC.
53 TMH, 'New Zealand notes'. MS-0037, p. 70. HC.
54 See HPC, Vol. 186. HC.
55 William B. Taylor, Town Clerk, Dunedin, to TMH, 27 May 1896. F&J 2: 68. HC.
56 See Register of Hocken items at the Otago Museum. Kind thanks to Scott Reeves, Otago Museum for supplying this document.
57 TMH, 'Travel diary', 1895. Misc-MS-1730. HC.
58 Turanga became Gisborne. See Michael Spedding, *The Turanganui River* (2006). An 1895 'Travel diary of the late Dr T.M. Hocken' and the half-plate images of the late Augustus Hamilton are at MONZ.
59 Cf the photograph of Hori from HPC, Vol. 15, No. 9. HC.
60 TMH, *Bibliography* (1909), p. 114.
61 See HPC, Vol. 15, No. 9 HC.
62 Printed broadside, 'Variae' 24, No. 28; Barnet poster: F&J 13: 17. HC.
63 TMH, 'Some account of the earliest explorations in New Zealand'. MONZ Archive MU 000155/001/0027.
64 Ibid., p. 2.
65 TMH and G. Fenwick, *A Holiday Trip to the Catlins District (via Willsher Bay)* (Dunedin: Otago Daily Times, 1892), p. 3.
66 TMH, 'Abel Tasman', Art XV, *Transactions*, Vol. 28 (1895), pp. 117–40.
67 Cf TMH, 'Some account of the earliest literature and maps relating to New Zealand', *Transactions*, Vol. 27 (1894), pp. 616–34 (621), where Bessie appeared as an anonymous but 'valued co-adjudicator'.
68 James Backhouse Walker to TMH, 10 January 1896. This letter is tipped in TMH's own copy of his *Abel Tasman and His Journal* (1895).
69 J.E. Heeres to TMH, 7 March 1896. Letter tipped in TMH's copy of *Abel Janszoon Tasman's Journal* (Amsterdam: Müller, 1898). HC.
70 Note tipped in *Abel Janszoon Tasman's Journal* (1898). HC. The work contains TMH's 'F.L.S.' printed bookplate.
71 Edward E. Morris to James Backhouse Walker, 20 May 1898. James Backhouse Walker Papers W9/C1/7 (34). University of Tasmania, Hobart.

Chapter 13: A Gift, a 'Literary Venture' and the South Seas

1 Christmas Number, *OW*, 19 December 1895. F&J 7: 12. HC.
2 Christmas Number, *OW*, 17 December 1896. F&J 7: 14. HC.
3 See W167; *BiM* 352.
4 'Old Maori drawings by Tooi and Teeteeree', *OW*, 29 April 1897, p. 53. See 'Tui and Titiri. Drawings 1818' in *Real Gold: Treasures of Auckland City Libraries* (Auckland: Auckland City Libraries and the Auckland Library Heritage Trust by Auckland University Press, 2007), pp. 118–19.
5 'Observance of anniversary day', *ODT*, 19 March 1897, p. 3.
6 Ibid.; see also 'A munificent offer', *OW*, 25 March 1897, p. 19.
7 Sighted in an uncatalogued letterbook headed 'Books bought in America by John D. Enys' as part of the Auckland Library Archives; see also 'Local & general', *OW*, 13 May 1897, p. 55.
8 'A munificent offer', *OW*, 25 March 1897, p. 19.
9 'Dr Hocken's library', *OW*, 25 March 1897, p. 19.
10 Letterbook to 'New Zealand and South Seas Exhibition', Dunedin. MS-104. HC.
11 Thanks to Simon Eliot, Centre for Manuscript and Print Studies, University of London; Jane Wickenden, Historic Collections Library, Institute of Naval Medicine & Historical Books Collection, Royal College of Physicians London; and John Eggeling, via Exlibris and Sharp e-groups.

12   TMH to James Horsburgh, 10 June 1895. Letterbook to 'New Zealand and South Seas Exhibition', Dunedin. MS-104. pp. 157–59. HC.
13   Ibid.
14   TMH to Messrs Sampson Low, Marston & Co., 20 January 1897. Letterbook to 'New Zealand and South Seas Exhibition', Dunedin. MS-104. HC.
15   TMH to Messrs Sampson Low, Marston & Co., 17 March 1897.
16   Ibid.
17   TMH to Messrs Sampson Low, Marston & Co., 14 April 1897, p. 186.
18   TMH to Messrs Sampson Low, Marston & Co., 26 April 1897, p. 187.
19   TMH to Messrs Sampson Low, Marston & Co., 28 May 1897, p. 188 and verso.
20   TMH to Messrs Sampson Low, Marston & Co., 9 June 1897, p. 190.
21   TMH to Messrs Sampson Low, Marston & Co., 13 July 1897, p. 194 and verso.
22   TMH to Messrs Sampson Low, Marston & Co., 31 August 1897, p. 196.
23   TMH to Messrs Sampson Low, Marston & Co., 18 September 1897, p. 197 and verso.
24   TMH, *Contributions* (1898), p. 286.
25   TMH to Messrs Sampson Low, Marston & Co., 18 September 1897, pp. 197–98.
26   TMH to Messrs Sampson Low, Marston & Co., 29 September 1897, p. 199.
27   TMH to Messrs Sampson Low, Marston & Co., 27 October 1897, p. 202.
28   TMH to Messrs Sampson Low, Marston & Co., 1 November 1897, p. 200.
29   A typescript index for TMH's *Contributions* was compiled by Joan Collis Wood in 1938.
30   TMH to Messrs Sampson Low, Marston & Co., 16 March 1898, p. 203.
31   Review, *The Athenaeum* [1898]. The quote, also rendered as 'Maybe some day you will rejoice to recall even this', is what Aeneas tells his exhausted, shipwrecked followers in *The Aeneid*, Book I.
32   Pre-publication notice on TMH's *Contributions* in the *Evening Post*, 10 March 1898, p. 2.
33   Review, *ODT*, 12 March 1898, p. 2.; TMH, *Contributions* (1898), p. 2.
34   Various hand-written drafts and extracts that form part of TMH's *Contributions* are extant in the Hocken Collection. They are briefly 'Chapter XVI', MS-1570/002; an extract of 'Lay Association of the Free Church of Scotland', MS-0439/171; Monro's Notes, MS-2462/008; Extract of Tuckett's journal, MS-2462/003; and a comment by Kettle on Dunedin, MS-0439/047. HC.
35   *Evening Post*, 26 March 1898, p. 2; *OW*, 17 March 1898, p. 54; *New Zealand Herald*, 2 April 1898; *Scotsman*, January 1898; *Westminster Gazette*, 29 January 1898; *Publishers Circular*, 19 February 1898; *Leeds Mercury*, 21 February 1898; *Manchester Guardian*, 24 February 1898; *Pall Mall Gazette*, 25 February 1898; *Colonial and Indian News*, 26 February 1898; *Globe*, 28 February 1898; *Glasgow Herald*, 3 March 1898; *Journal of the Royal Colonial Institute*, March 1898; *Bookseller*, March 1898; *Home News*, 11 March 1898; *Illustrated London News*, 12 March 1898; *The Field*, 19 March 1898; *Daily News*, 24 March 1898; *Saturday Review*, 26 March 1898; and *The Speaker*, 3 September 1898.
36   William Downie Stewart, 'Dr Hocken's history. To the editor', *ODT*, 17 March 1898, p. 6.
37   F.W. Whiston to TMH, 15 March 1898. MS-1258-003/003. HC.
38   W.G. Filleul to TMH, 5 April 1898. F&J 5: 160. HC.
39   William Gillies to TMH, 29 April 1898. MS-1258-003/004. HC.
40   William Martin to TMH, 6 July 1898. MS-0451-012/008. HC.
41   Edmund H.W. Bellairs to James Buckland, London, 18 February 1898. MS-0451-012/001. HC.

42   TMH to Herton, Bank of New South Wales, 25 March 1898. MS-104, p. 204. HC.
43   *Evening Post*, 31 March 1898, p. 4.
44   See *Union Steam Ship Company Travel Guide*, 1898. AG 292 12/1/21. HC.
45   Percy Smith to TMH, 9 October 1887, tipped in *The Kermadec Islands* (1887). HPC, Vol. 47. HC.
46   TMH, 'An account of the Fiji fire ceremony', *Transactions*, Vol. 31 (1898), pp. 667–72 (669).
47   The photographs are: 'House at Mission Station, Navalon' (p. 31); 'Four boys in bush, Suva, Fiji' (p. 32); 'Three Indian coolies at a Nausari plantation sugar house' (p. 35); 'Wesleyan Mission Station, Navaloa, Fiji' (p. 36); 'Wesleyan Mission Station, Navaloa' (p. 40); 'Three kids in Nausari street' (p. 41); and 'Landing place, Navaloa' (p. 42). Gladys Hocken's Album 39, 'Fiji, Samoa, Solomon Islands', 1895. HC.
48   Moss: HPC, Vol. 5, No. 5. Of him TMH wrote: '[Moss] previously of Dunedin, afterwards British Resident at Rarotonga, author of school history of NZ & Atolls & Islands in the S Sea.' Also: 'Mr Moss was in 1862 a merchant in Dunedin & a politician. After his return from Fiji he resided in Auckland for many years & in 1891 was appointed British Resident at Rarotonga'; Gardenhire: HPC, Vol. 62; and Kelly: HPC, Vol. 66, No. 10.
49   TMH and Colquhoun were not the first to put the participants through such an examination. Glanvill Corney, Chief Medical Officer of Fiji, accompanied the Thurston party and examined those who walked through the fire. See J.W. Lindt, 'The fire ordeal of Beqa, Fiji Islands', in *Transaction of the Royal Anthropological Society*, June 1894.
50   TMH, 'An account of the Fiji fire ceremony', p. 671.
51   See 'Fire ceremony at Fiji', *OW*, 19 May 1898, p. 9.
52   As reported in 'Anglo-Colonial notes', *OW*, 15 September 1898, p. 24.
53   'The Fiji fire ceremony', *Japan Daily Herald*, 19 October 1901. See F&J 10: 180–81. HC.
54   Carew Papers, MS-0105. HC.
55   See 'Variae' 18 ('Fiji and Rarotonga') and 30. HC.
56   TMH, uncatalogued note, April 17/10. Carew Papers, MS-0105/03. HC.
57   'Otago Institute', *ODT*, 14 July 1898, p. 3.

Chapter 14: 'For a Boxful of such Rubbish I Should be Infinitely Obliged'

1   TMH to W.H.S. Roberts, 22 March 1896. In Edward E. Morris Papers. MSS 551. Mitchell Library, SLNSW. See Edward Morris, 'On the tracks of Captain Cook', Article LXII *Transactions*, 33 (1900), pp. 499–514. See also entry on Morris in Perceval Serle, *ADB*, Vol. II, p. 161.
2   Edward E. Morris to TMH, 28 May 1898. MS-0451-012/006. HC.
3   Edward E. Morris to TMH, 20 June 1898. MS-0451-012/007. HC
4   Edward E. Morris to TMH, 11 August 1900. Ibid.
5   Ibid. Cf this note on Cook: 'By the 1820s the fashion for collecting South Seas ethnography had all but disappeared, and the spate of publications honouring Cook's voyages had virtually come to an end.' Entry describing 'Cloth Manufactured from the bark of trees by the natives of Otaheite brought over by Captain Cook', in *Hordern House Catalogue* 2006 (Sydney, 2006), inside cover.
6   Edward E. Morris to TMH, 11 August 1900. MS-0451-014/007. HC.
7   Edward E. Morris to TMH, 6 September 1900. MS-0451-014/010 HC. See Ellis's *Doctor John Hawkesworth* (n.d.) at HPC, Vol. 174, No 3. HC.

8   TMH to George Robertson, 10 April 1899. Angus & Robertson Archives, 1824, 1848, 1858–1933 Z ML MSS 314 , pp. 36–38. SLNSW.
9   TMH to George Robertson, 11 November 1896. Ibid.
10 Ibid.
11 TMH to George Robertson, 27 March 1899. Ibid.
12 TMH to George Robertson, 10 April 1899. Ibid.
13 Journal of Rev. William Richard Wade, June 1834 to September 1836, bound with 'Journal of John Wallis Barnicoat, February 1842 to October 1844'. MS-0051. HC.
14 TMH, 'Some account of the beginnings of literature in New Zealand: Part I, the Maori section' in *Transactions*, Vol. 33 (1900), pp. 472–90.
15 Ibid., p. 477.
16 Ibid., p. 484.
17 TMH to H.T. Hill, [May 1900]. H.T. Hill Correspondence, 1900–1902. MS 0172-005. ATL. See 'Maori bibliography' in TMH's *Bibliography* (1909), pp. 499–547.
18 See *W*10, *BiM* 18; *W*122, *BiM* 260; and *W*76, *BiM* 108 respectively.
19 See *W*72, *BiM* 104; *W*103, *BiM* 196; and *W*696, *BiM* 1134 respectively. For Stack, see F&J 5: 162; Stack to TMH, 28 October 1898. MS-0451-012/015. HC.
20 Misc-MS-0084. HC.
21 The bibliographical complexities of this publication, including the subsequent later publication, *Te Manuhiri Tuarangi and Maori Intelligencer* (1861), is detailed, with further references to works by scholars, in *BiM*, S1 (pp. 744–46), S3 (pp. 746–48), S5 (pp. 749–51), S11 (pp. 755–56), and S12 (pp. 757–58).
22 William Scott Wilson to TMH, 7 April 1898. MS-0451-012/003; W.S. Wilson to TMH, 3 January 1900. MS-0451-014/001. HC.
23 TMH to Thomas Cheeseman, 13 August 1900. Post-1900 correspondence from MA 95/40 Cheeseman Correspondence. AIM.
24 TMH to Thomas Cheeseman, 28 August 1900. Ibid.
25 TMH to Thomas Cheeseman, 27 October 1900. Ibid.
26 TMH to Thomas Cheeseman, 13 August 1900. Ibid.
27 TMH to Thomas Cheeseman, 28 August 1900. Ibid.
28 TMH, 'Some account of the beginnings of literature in New Zealand', *Transactions*, p. 473; TMH to Thomas Cheeseman, 28 August 1900. Post-1900 correspondence from MA 95/40 Cheeseman Correspondence. AIM.
29 Kay Morris Matthews, 'Hill, Henry', from DNZB: www.TeAra.govt.nz/en/biographies/2h36/hill-henry. There is a good example of networking in Alexander Turnbull's letter to Hill, 3 May 1900: 'On September 1st Mr Yate together with his assistant, "James Smith" printed off on their press a few hymns in Maori. I have not been able to find anyone who possesses a copy of this publication, but I have written to Dr Hocken to ask him if he has one in his library …' Cited in H.T. Hill Papers. MS-0172-004. ATL.
30 TMH to H.T. Hill, [May 1900]. H.T. Hill Papers. MS-0172-004. ATL.
31 TMH to H.T. Hill, 12 June 1900. H.T. Hill Correspondence, 1900–1902. MS-0172-005. ATL.
32 TMH to H.T. Hill, 16 May 1900. H.T. Hill Papers. MS-0172-004. ATL.
33 TMH to H.T. Hill, 21 June 1900. H.T. Hill Correspondence, 1900–1902. MS 0172-005. ATL.
34 See HPC, Vols 95, 117 and 151 respectively.
35 Bishop Octavius Hadfield, to TMH, 5 September 1900. F&J 5: 173. HC.
36 Album 43, Original Pictorial Collection. HC.
37 TMH to John Webster, 1 June 1890. Typescript of NZMS 4/16 (3). Sir George Grey Special Collections, ACL.
38 Ibid.

39 TMH to John Webster, 6 June 1900. Typescript of NZMS 4/16 (4). Sir George Grey Special Collections, ACL.
40 Ibid.
41 Atholl Anderson, 'Shortland, Edward', from DNZB: www.TeAra.govt.nz/en/biographies/1s11/shortland-edward
42 See 'Variae' 31: Nos 4, 6 and 7; and later acquisitions in Shortland Papers. MS-0024. HC.
43 TMH to John Webster, 6 June 1900. Typescript of NZMS 4/16. Sir George Grey Special Collections, ACL.
44 John Webster to TMH, 22 June 1900. MS-0084/21. HC.
45 TMH to John Webster 10 July 1900. Typescript of NZMS 4/16. Sir George Grey Special Collections, ACL.
46 On 7 March 1842 Maketu Wharetotara (also known as Wiremu Kingi Maketu), the 17-year-old son of the Ngapuhi chief Ruhe of Waimate, was the first person to be judicially executed in New Zealand.
47 B.R. Mee, 'The Reverend George Clarke'. BA Hons thesis, University of Tasmania, 1965, p. 43.
48 George Clarke Papers, 28/114-136. State Library of Tasmania, Hobart.
49 Clarke reiterated his sentiment towards Yate in a later letter to TMH, 28 November 1900. MS-0451-014/016. HC.
50 George Clarke to TMH, 2 October 1900. MS-0451-014/012. HC.
51 Ibid.
52 George Clarke to TMH, 23 October 1900. MS-0451-014/012. HC. Although Clarke sent these items to TMH, there is no indication of their existence in his collection.
53 George Clarke to TMH, 26 October 1900. MS-0451-014/014. HC.
54 Ibid.
55 George Clarke to TMH, 28 November 1900. MS-0451-014/015. HC.
56 George Clarke to TMH, 29 November 1900. MS-0451-014/016. HC.
57 George Clarke to TMH, 1 December 1900. MS-0451-014. HC.

Chapter 15: A Welcome Break

1 TMH, 'The Maoris of the South Island: A lecturette by Dr Hocken at the recent Maori carnival', *OW*, 12 June 1901, p. 70.
2 'Duke and Duchess visit', *OW*, 3 July, 1901, p. 27.
3 See 'Winter Show', *OW*, 3 July 1901, p. 26; 'Commemorating the royal visit', *OW*, 24 July 1901, p. 11 At the latter, TMH was joined by James Rattray, Julius Hyman and T. Wright.
4 TMH, English text for 'Illuminated address', June 1901. F&J 2: 66. HC. It reads: 'To the Great Chief George, son of Edward, the King of England. Salutations to you both! We, Ngaitahu, Ngatimamoe, & Waitaha, tribes of Te Wai Pounamu, welcome you to these shores, for you are the grand-son of the great Queen who was a just woman & the loving mother of Her Maori people. Christianity & Her rule came together & have dwelt amongst us since. The love & loyalty we always bore her have passed to the King Edward, your father. We ask you to take this message to him from us. You must not forget us but again return to us from across the seas. Great is our love for you both. That is all. Farewell.'
5 TMH, 'The beginnings of literature in New Zealand: Part II: The English Section – Newspapers', *Transactions*, Vol. 34 (1901), Article VI, pp. 99–114.
6 Charles Keats Brown to TMH, 28 July 1901. MS-1570-001/007. HC
7 Percy Smith to TMH, 19 January 1901. MS-0451-015/001. HC. Smith also thanks TMH for his cheque, certainly his subscription to the Polynesian Society.

8   Elsdon Best to TMH, 2 May 1901. F&J 5: 176. HC.
9   Cited in 'Otago Institute', *OW*, 17 July 1901, p. 14. See also *Transactions*, Vol. 34 (1901), p. 584.
10 'Local and general', *OW*, 14 August 1901, p. 54; see also F&J 10: 87. HC.
11 GHD, August 1901 to September 1904. Entry for 9 August. Extracts taken from a transcript of the original in the Fish Hoek Archives, Cape Town, South Africa. Kind thanks to A.G. Hocken for making this copy available.
12 GHD, 9 August 1901.
13 It also covers the period when Gladys met her future husband, Alan Le François, on board the *Kawachi Maru*.
14 TMH, F&J 5: 177. HC.
15 Dr Garnett to Mrs Freeman, 22 August 1902 qMS-0057. Allom Collection of E.G. Wakefield Papers, 11F, Letters from Dr Garnett to Mrs Freeman, 23 January 1902 to 22 August 1902. ATL.
16 See also 'Dr Hocken on tour', F&J 43: 3. Thanks to Ian Farquhar, and to Captain Masaharu Akamine, NYK Maritime Museum, Yokohama (correspondence 15 August 2009), who supplied references to Shigetoshi Kizu's *A 100 Years' History of the Ships Nippon Yusen Kaisha* (1984).
17 TMH, 'A three years' tour: A chat with Dr Hocken', *OW*, 27 July 1904, p. 81.
18 See TMH, 'Abel Tasman', *Transactions,* Vol. 28 (1895), p. 131.
19 'Dr Hocken's tour', London, April 11, *OW*, 21 May 1902, p. 45.
20 Reference to Tsuboi Shogoro in Shinji Yamashita, Joseph Bosco and J.S. Eades (eds), *The Making of Anthropology in East and Southeast Asia* (New York: Berghahn Books, 2004); see also Joseph M. Kitagawa, *On Understanding Japanese Religion* (Princeton: Princeton University Press, 1987), p. 15.
21 'Dr Hocken's tour', London, April 11, in *OW*, 21 May 1902, p. 45; see also 'A three years' tour: A chat with Dr Hocken', *OW*, 27 July 1904, p. 81.
22 'A three years' tour: A chat with Dr Hocken', *OW*, 27 July 1904, p. 81.
23 See Timothy Walker, 'Robley: Te Ropere 1840–1930'. Vols I and II, MA thesis, Auckland University, 1985.
24 Cited in Horatio Robley, 'Relics of the historical art of the Maori', *OW*, 23 December 1902, p. 57.
25 Announcement of Hocken's election to the Royal Colonial Institute, 11 June 1902. HPC, Vol. 175, No. 8. The entrance fee was £3 1s. The institute became the Royal Commonwealth Society in 1958.
26 Dr Garnett to Mrs Freeman, 9 June 1902. qMS-0057. Allom Collection of E.G. Wakefield Papers, 11F, Letters from Dr Garnett to Mrs Freeman, 23 January 1902 to 22 August 1902. ATL.
27 Dr Garnett to Mrs Freeman, 22 August 1902. Ibid.
28 Cited in 'Personal notes from London', *Evening Post*, 19 September 1902, p. 6.
29 GHD, 23 June 1902.
30 Charlotte Godley to TMH, July 3 [1902]. Letter tipped in TMH's copy of John Robert Godley, *Letters from America*, 2 vols (London: John Murray, 1844). Note: 'Charlotte Godley exercised in her own sphere an important and beneficial influence on the early developments of society in the settlement, and after her departure she continued to maintain a keen interest in New Zealand affairs. She outlived her husband by 45 years and died in her house at Gloucester Place, London, on 3 January 1907.'
31 Charlotte Godley to TMH, 24 September [1902]. MS-0451-016/005. HC.
32 Charlotte Godley to TMH, 10 October [1902]. MS-0451-016/007. HC.
33 Canterbury Association Minutes and Letterbook, June 1851–28 January 1853. MS-0094. Other correspondents include General Chapman and, of course, Charlotte Godley.

34 GHD, 7–8 October 1902.
35 See Bessie Hocken's 'A New Zealander on her travels', *OW*, 5 August 1903, p. 42; 'Scenes in the Far East', *OW*, 4 March 1903, p. 39.
36 GHD, 2 December 1902.
37 Ibid., 10 June 1903.
38 General Minute Book No. 12 1898–1906, Linnean Society, London. Thanks to Lynda Brooks.
39 John D.G. Enys to TMH 30 October 1904. F&J 5: 185. HC.
40 John D.G. Enys to TMH 29 May [1903]. MS-0451-017/003. HC.
41 Hakena (Archives and Manuscripts Catalogue) details the following manuscripts as: MSS-0001: 'Maori manuscript No. 1, mythology & traditions'. 100 pp; MSS-0002: 'Maori manuscript No. 2, traditions – superstition', 100 pp+; MSS-0003: 'Maori manuscript No. 3, miscellaneous notes on Maori history and customs', 46 pp; MSS-0004: 'Maori manuscript No. 4, waiata – whakatauki, etc, miscellaneous' c. 1886. 112 pp; MS-0007: 'Melanesian dictionary'. 63 pp; MS-0009: Notebook No. 9i, 'Australian languages & South African languages', which includes notes E.M. Carr's *Australian Race* (1886), 39 pp; MS-0010: 'Dictionary of Australian and South African languages'; MS-0011: 'Maori manuscript No. 11' (concerning religion and mythology, land tenure, disputes and confiscation), c. 1870s, 84 pp; MS-0008: Notebook containing the Melanesian alphabet and Motu grammar; MS-0012: 'Maori manuscript No. 12', containing clippings and notes on the Albert Barracks Reserve, religion and mythology and a tour of Waikato, 66 pp; MS-0014: Manuscript containing Maori notes on traditions, karakia and religion; MS-0015: Manuscript containing Maori notes on mainly, genealogies, karakia and customs, c. 1880s, 160 pp+; MS-0019: Notebook containing Maori language notes; MS-0020: Notebook comprising Maketu journal and common-place book B, New Zealand, 29 November 1842–8 August 1843; MS-0021: Journal entitled 'Coromandel and Kawhia'; MS-0022: Notebook comprising a journal of a journey to Matamata, Tauranga and Waikato and common-place book A. New Zealand, 200 pp+; MS-0005: 'Hints on the study of the Maori language'; MS-0006: 'Melanesian languages'; MS-0016: Edward Shortland, Inward letterbook, Maori … Report of Speeches made at Kuiti, March 1872; MS-0017: Notebook containing Maori vocabulary and botanical notes; MS-0018: Notebook containing Maori vocabulary; MS-0023: Journal, 1843–1844. Middle Island of New Zealand; MS-0024: Journal notes kept while in the Middle Island; MS-0025: Notes on Maori vocabulary, syntax, waiata and whakatauki; MS-0034: Edward Shortland: Journal, Memoranda, Receipts and Payments; MS-0086/001-002: Outward letterbooks; MS-0013: Outward letterbook, Maori, 1853–64; MS-0385/002: Correspondence and notes; and MS-0096: Notes on Maori language, customs and traditional history, 110 pp+.
42 William Wildman to TMH, 12 December 1890. Tipped in Edward Shortland's 'Collection of papers relating to Maori and the Maori language'. MS-1166/006. HC.
43 Eugenia Shortland, to TMH, 3 November 1903. MS-0451-018/008; Eugenia Shortland, to TMH, 10 November 1903. MS-0451-018/010. HC.
44 Mary Ford to TMH, 6 July 1903. MS-0451-017/006. HC.
45 Mary Ford to TMH, 14 July 1903. MS-0451-017/007. HC.
46 Mary Ford to TMH, 18 August 1903. MS-0451-017/011. HC.
47 Note in TMH's *Selected Speeches of Sir William Molesworth* (1903). HC.
48 Note attached to letter from Mary Ford to TMH, 28 September 1903. MS-0451-017/019. HC.
49 GHD, 8 August 1903.

50 William L. Selfe to TMH, 11 August 1903. MS-0451-017/009. HC. Fifty-four correspondents and numerous letters. Webb–Selfe manuscripts. MS-Papers-0530. ATL.
51 W.L. Selfe to TMH, 30 August 1903. MS-0451-017/015. HC.
52 F&J 6: 41, 42, 44, and 46: MSS letters from Dean Henry Harper to H.S. Selfe, 13 February 1866, and 27 May 1866; Harper, Bishop of Christchurch to H.S. Selfe, 8 June 1866; MSS letters from Harper to H.S. Selfe, 4 December 1866, 4 May 1867; MS letter from Harper to H.S. Selfe, 2 July 1868. HC.
53 GHD, 4 September 1903.

Chapter 16: The CMS, the Colonial Office and Home

1 S.F. Purday to TMH, 12 August 1903. MS-0451-017/010; Letter, 1 October 1903, from W. Lang, Lay Secretary; Letter discussing an application to be submitted to the finance committee. MS-0451-018/001. HC.
2 John R. Elder (ed.), 'Preface', *The Letters and Journals of Samuel Marsden 1765–1838* (Dunedin: Coulls Somerville Wilkie and A.H. Reed for the Otago University Council, 1932), pp. 8–9.
3 TMH had three copies of Samuel Marsden's 1823 journey: his second copy was obtained through Canon J.C. Betts of Cootamundra, NSW (Marsden's grandson); the third of 141 pages was a copy of the second.
4 GHD, 12 November 1903.
5 See Trimble (1926), p. 3.
6 Alfred Lyttelton, Secretary of State for the Colonies, Colonial Office, London, to Lord Plunket, 7 September 1904. MS-0451-019/005. HC. A copy of a letter transmitting a copy of correspondence with TMH. Lyttelton wished to know if the New Zealand government should take the papers. It encloses TMH's report of 1903 (which is to be returned). The following were enclosed with the letter: H.B. Cox to TMH, 1 July 1903 (MS-0451-017/005); TMH to Under Secretary of State, Colonial Office, 11 August 1903 (MS-0451-017/008); H.B. Cox to TMH, 25 August 1903 (MS-0451-017/013); C.P. Lucas to TMH, 1 September 1903 (MS-0451-017/016); TMH to Under Secretary of State, Colonial Office, 22 October 1903 (MS-0451-018/004); H.B. Cox to TMH, 4 November 1903 (MS-0451-018/009); H.B. Cox to TMH, 18 November 1903 (MS-0451-018/012); TMH to Under Secretary of State, Colonial Office, 23 November 1903 (MS-0451-018/013); and H.B. Cox to TMH, 17 December 1903 (MS-0451-018/017). The letter and enclosures were enclosed in a letter from Pollen to TMH, 23 March 1905. See also Stuart Strachan, 'Not quite half a loaf: Dr Hocken and the "patriation" of the New Zealand Company Archives', draft paper, 2008.
7 GHD, 8 August 1903.
8 GHD, 8 August 1903 (date in error).
9 F&J 2: 9. HC.
10 Mary Alice Freeman to TMH, 20 August 1903. MS-0451-017/012. HC.
11 Ibid.
12 TMH to H.B. Cox, Under Secretary of State, Colonial Office, 11 August 1903. MS-0451-017/008. HC.
13 H.B. Cox to TMH, 25 August 1903. MS-0451-017/003; C.P. Lucas to TMH, 1 September 1903. MS-0451-017/016. HC.
14 TMH, 'The early New Zealand missions: The Rev. Samuel Marsden', *ODT*, 25 December 1905.
15 On 18 September, a box of flowers arrived, sent by TMH who was still in Devonshire. Bessie was unwell, Gladys was beginning her typewriting lessons and Robley was expected again. GHD, 11 September 1903 onwards.
16 GHD, Book II, 5 October 1903.

17 Journal of Rev. William Richard Wade, June 1834 to September 1836; Journal of John Wallis Barnicoat, February 1842 to October 1844. MS-0051, pp. 23–38. HC.
18 TMH to H.B. Cox, 22 October 1903 (copy). MS-0451-018/004. HC.
19 H.B. Cox to TMH, 4 November 1903. MS-0451-018/009. HC.
20 GHD, 12 November 1903.
21 W.P. Reeves to TMH, 16 November 1903. MS-0451-018/011. HC.
22 H.B. Cox to TMH, 18 November 1903. MS-0451-018/012. HC.
23 TMH to H.B. Cox, 23 November 1903 (copy). MS-0451-018/013. HC.
24 H.B. Cox to TMH, 17 December 1903. MS-0451-018/017. HC.
25 'Chat with Dr Hocken', *OW*, 6 January 1904, p. 26.
26 The original records remain at PRO: CO 208, England; see copy of list in TMH's collection, MS-0451-028/001, 002 and 022. HC.
27 Sketches by William Holmes, Original Pictures Collection: [A] H685; Bu H753.5. HC.
28 Gilfillan, whose family were attacked by local Wanganui Maori on 18 April 1847; cited in GHD, 13 October 1903.
29 Mrs A. Lawrence, Birmingham, to TMH, 6 October 1903. MS-0451-018/002; J.S. Ousley or Oulaf to TMH, 12 October 1903. MS-0451-018/003; K.M. Ball to TMH, 3 November 1903. MS-0451-018/007. HC.
30 TMH to Augustus Hamilton, 18 January 1906. MU000152/7/106 Folder 9. MONZ Archives.
31 See 'Variae' 31: Nos 1 and 2.
32 There was a flurry of letters from James Grice, Melbourne: 15 May, 1 June and 13 July 1906, and a cablegram, 21 June 1906, relating to J.A. Gilfillan's picture. Material pertinent to the painting is pasted in 'Variae' 31: Nos 1 and 2. HC.
33 John George Lambton, the third Earl of Durham to TMH, 19 December 1903. MS-0451-018/013. HC; Viscount Cobham to TMH, 7 December 1903. F&J 5: 181; see GHD, 13 November 1903.
34 GHD, 20 November, 17 December 1903.
35 Ibid., 19 January 1904.
36 Ibid., 23, 25 March 1904.
37 Ibid., 15 May 1904.
38 See TMH's copy of *Historical Records of New South Wales*. Vol. I. Part I Cook. 1762–1780 (Sydney: 1893), which has a tipped-in letter from Bladen, 24 September, replying to TMH's previous letter of 28 April 1896. HC.
39 Sir Samuel Way to TMH, 28 July 1903. MS-1258-003-008. HC.
40 These books arrived from Sir Samuel Way in October 1904.
41 GHD, 28 June 1904.
42 See *BiM* 422; W234.
43 11 July 1904, Royal Society of Tasmania Council minutes, pp. 72–73. Thanks to Emilia Ward, Special Collections, University of Tasmania, Hobart.
44 'Abstract of Proceedings July 11th, 1904', *Papers & Proceedings of the Royal Society of Tasmania for the years 1903–1905* (Tasmania: Printed by Davies Brothers, 1906), pp. xxxii–xxxvi; repeated in a newspaper cutting heading 'Royal Society of Tasmania'. MS-2469/001 and 002.
45 'Dr Hocken on Tour', F&J 43: July 2007, 3. See also *CW*, 27 July 1904, p. 60; Itinerary detailed in 'A three years' tour: A chat with Dr Hocken' in *OW*, 27 July 1904, p. 81.
46 GHD, 20 July 1904.
47 'A three years' tour: A chat with Dr Hocken', *OW*, 27 July 1904, p. 81.
48 Rev. Arthur Lloyd, Tokyo, to TMH, 18 February 1905. MS-0451-021/001. HC.

49 'His Excellency Admiral Heihachiro Togo, Commander in Chief of His Imperial Majesty's Combined Naval Squadron, in celebration of the victory of the Battle of Tsushima, fought on 27–28 May 1905'. MS-0451-022/001. HC.
50 TMH to John Webster, 30 November 1904. Typescript of NZMS 4/16 (7). Sir George Grey Special Collections, ACL.

Chapter 17: 'Marsden or Some Other Old Historical Subject'

1 'A Three Years' Tour. A Chat with Dr Hocken', *ODT*, 22 July 1904, p. 3; *ODT*, 25 July 1904, p. 2.
2 John Logan Campbell to TMH, 11 October 1904. MS-0451-020/001. HC.
3 Bishop William Leonard Williams to TMH, 17 October 1904. F&J 5: 181A. HC.
4 TMH, 'Travel diary' 1905. Misc-Ms-1730. HC.
5 See Parkinson, *BiM* 451, p. 229: Puckey's manuscript is now at the ATL (qMS-0330). Apparently it was not printed 'due to lack of type'.
6 Robert Mair to TMH, 5 June 1905. MS-0451-022/002. HC.
7 TMH, 'In the Far North: Ramble in search of history. Interview with Dr Hocken', *OW*, 5 April 1905, p. 15.
8 TMH to Lizzie Betts, 25 February 1904. Betts Family Papers, Vol. I. Correspondence 1827–1910. ML A2563. SLNSW.
9 R.F. Scott, St John's College, Cambridge, to TMH, 28 July 1900. MS-0451-014/005. HC.
10 S.A. Donaldson to TMH, 15 August 1904. MS-0451-019/004. HC; S.A. Donaldson to TMH, 17 January 1906. MS-0451-023/001. HC. See John R. Elder, *The Letters and Journals of Samuel Marsden 1765–1838* (Dunedin: Coulls Somerville Wilkie and A.H. Reed for the Otago University Council, 1932), p. 20 fn 3 for clarification on Marsden not attending St John's College.
11 J.E. Forty to TMH, 8 September 1905. MS-0451-022/014. HC.
12 *Notes & Queries*, 10th S.V. (19 May 1906), p. 389. R.F. Scott's 'Rev. Samuel Marsden of Paramatta' appeared in *Notes & Queries*, S9–V1 (28 July 1900), p. 66. This may have been the catalyst for TMH's enquiry.
13 Bishop Samuel E. Marsden to S. Woolly, 30 November 1905; Woolly to TMH, 1 December 1905. F&J 5: 186. HC.
14 Bishop Samuel E. Marsden to TMH, 17 May 1906. MS-0451-023/010. HC.
15 Bishop Samuel E. Marsden to TMH, 21 September 1906. MS-0451-024/009. HC.
16 'A three years' tour: A chat with Dr Hocken, *ODT*, 22 July 1904, p. 3; *ODT*, 25 July 1904, p. 2.
17 TMH to Thomas Cheeseman, 11 September 1905. Cheeseman Letters, AIM.
18 TMH, 'The early New Zealand missions: The Rev. Samual Marsden', *ODT*, 25 December 1905 and *OW*, 27 December 1905, p. 54.
19 So called by TMH in his *Bibliography*, p. 419. Vol. II of this work carried Bladen's name. Bladen and TMH knew each other and the former sent TMH information on Marsden, 1 July 1908. MS 0177/041. HC.
20 See Mr Cox, Letter to the editor, *Lyttelton Times*, 27 March 1889. Tipped in TMH's F&J 10: 149. HC.
21 Lecture 2 was read to institute members on 14 November 1905, and appeared in the *OW*, 3 January 1906, p. 23; No. 3 appeared in the *ODT*, 4 January 1906; No. 4 in *ODT*, 11 January 1906; No. 5 in *ODT*, 18 January 1906.
22 In particular: MS-0177-038 headed 'Sixth voyage'; MS-0451-022; 'Umbrella major', c. 1906. MS-0451-024. HC.
23 TMH to Percy Smith, 15 June 1906. MS-0451-023/013. HC.
24 Percy Smith to TMH, 5 December 1906. F&J 5: 187. HC.
25 Percy Smith to TMH, 28 April 1907. MS-1570-001/009. HC.

26 Percy Smith to TMH, [1907]. MS-0451-025/017. HC.
27 Percy Smith to TMH, 28 April 1907. MS-1570-001/009. HC.
28 'Answers to notes made when Hocken & I went through Marsden's Journals', [1907–09]. MS-0451-023/029. HC. It is in Smith's hand.
29 Bishop W.L. Williams to Percy Smith, 13 August 1907. MS-0451-025/011. HC.
30 Percy Smith to TMH, 21 September 1907, on letter from Williams. 13 August 1907. MS-0451-025/011. HC.
31 TMH to Percy Smith, 10 September 1908. Polynesian Society Papers, MS-Papers-1187-263-12. ATL.
32 Percy Smith to TMH, 7 September 1908. MS-0451-028/010. HC.
33 Percy Smith to TMH, 21 October 1908. MS-0451-028/016. HC.
34 TMH to Percy Smith, 10 June 1909. Polynesian Society Papers. MS-Papers 1187-263. ATL.
35 Percy Smith to TMH, 17 June 1909. MS-0451-029/012. HC.
36 TMH to Percy Smith, 23 July 1909. Polynesian Society Papers, MS-Papers 1187-263-15 and 16. ATL.
37 Percy Smith to TMH, 25 July 1909. MS-0451-029/018. HC.
38 TMH to Percy Smith, 3 August 1909. Polynesian Society Papers. MS-Papers 1187-263. ATL. Map drawn by Tuki Tahua and Ngahuruhuru, Norfolk Island, 1793. Map Collection. HC.
39 Percy Smith to TMH, 9 August 1909. MS-0451-030/008. HC.
40 TMH to Percy Smith, 27 August 1909. Polynesian Society Papers, MS-Papers-1187-263-18. ATL.
41 TMH, *Bibliography* (1909), p. 486.
42 EMH to Percy Smith, 4 June 1910. Polynesian Society Papers. MS-Papers-1187-263-5. See Elder, 'Preface', p. 8.
43 EMH to M. Betts, 3 September 1910. Betts Family Papers, Vol. I. Correspondence 1827–1910. ML A2563. SLNSW.
44 Elder, 'Preface', pp. 8–9. Elder's work is not without its inaccuracies. See Judith Binney, *Legacy of Guilt: A life of Thomas Kendall*. (Wellington: Bridget Williams Books, 2005).

Chapter 18: The Pinnacle
1 TMH, 'Catalogue of books' [1887]. MS-0044. HC.
2 'Mr Kinsey interviewed', *Star*, 7 October 1889, p. 3.
3 John Carter, cited in G. Thomas Tanselle, 'The literature of book collecting' in Jean Peters (ed.), *Book Collecting: A modern guide* (New York: R.R. Bowker Company, 1977), pp. 209–10.
4 James Davis, *Contributions towards a Bibliography of New Zealand* (Wellington: Lyon and Blair, 1887), p. [iii].
5 James Miller to TMH, 11 May 1891. MS-0451-007/006. HC.
6 See Ian McLaren, 'Book collecting and bibliography', *Bulletin* of BSANZ, No. 8 (December 1975), pp. 52–69 (56).
7 The York Gate Library is part of the Royal Geographical Society collection at the State Library of South Australia.
8 G.H. Sutherland. 'Carter, Charles Rooking', from DNZB: www.TeAra.govt.nz/en/biographies/1c8/carter-charles-rooking, Charles Rooking Carter. MS 78-149 Misc. ATL. See 'N.Z. Literature. Charles R. Carter', *Dominion*, 19 August 1933. In July 1894 the collection stood at over 333 books.
9 C.R. Carter, *Catalogue of Books on or Relating to New Zealand* (London: Printed by Bowden, Hudson & Co., 1887), p. 3.
10 Ibid., p. 7.
11 Ibid., p. 29.

12 C.R. Carter, *Second Continuation Catalogue of Books Presented by C.R. Carter, to the New Zealand Institute and Colonial Museum, Wellington, N.Z., in the Year 1893* ([London, 1893]), p. iv.
13 C.R. Carter, *Continuation Catalogue of Books Presented by C.R. Carter, J.P., to the Wellington Museum and Colonial Institute, in the Year 1892* (London: G. Norman Anderson, 1892), p. iv.
14 *Second Continuation* (1893), p. 1.
15 Grey to C.R. Carter, cited in *Second Continuation* (1893), p. 1.
16 C.R. Carter to TMH, 4 May 1896. MS-0451-010/001. HC. For the Featherston–Wakefield duel see Donald Kerr, *The Smell of Powder: A history of duelling in New Zealand* (Auckland: Random House, 2006), pp. 100–07.
17 See C.R. Carter, *Catalogue of Books* (1887). HC. Between these two publications there occurred the book sale of Christopher Beckett Denison, the British colonial administrator. Most of Denison's book collection was sold in conjunction with the *Catalogue of the Collection of Pictures, Works of Art, and Decorative Objects*, produced by Christies in 1885. According to Carter, Denison's book collection, which included a number of significant titles concerning New Zealand, was said to have cost £250,000. At sale it realised a little over £92,000. Carter himself purchased 46 books relating to New Zealand, including E.J. Wakefield's *Adventure in New Zealand* (1845), Bathgate's *New Zealand* (1880), the *Constable Miscellany* issue containing the original account of the massacre of the ship's crew of the *Boyd* (1827) and E.B. Fitton's *Condition, Prospects and Resources of New Zealand* (1856).
18 G.B. Barton, *Literature of New South Wales* (Sydney, 1866), p. [1].
19 Carole Woods, 'Henry Field Gurner (1819–1883)', *ADB*, Vol. 4 (1972), p. 309. TMH also owned the sale catalogue of books owned by Sir Alfred Stephen, George Bennett and the Rev. Daniel Draper, but not William Fairfax's *Handbook to Australasia* (1859), which lists some 86 titles under a small New Zealand section.
20 James Backhouse Walker to TMH, 28 May 1889, tipped in *List of Books Relating to Tasmania* (1884) in HPC, Vol. 63, No. 9.
21 Trimble, *Catalogue* (1912) lists 65; there are also a number of catalogues dealing with spiritualism and the occult (1908–09), and presumably these could be Bessie's.
22 James Collier to TMH, 19 July 1888. MS-0451-006/004. HC.
23 Jill Waterhouse, 'James Collier (1846–1925)', *ADB*, Vol. 8. (1981), pp. 69–70.
24 TMH to William Hall-Jones, 20 February 1906. Colonial Secretary Files, 96/1649. Cited in A.G. Bagnall, 'The rival bibliographers James Collier and TMH', *Turnbull Library Record*, Vol. 1, No. 2 (1967), pp. 22–31 (22). This is an excellent overview of the two rivals, which I have used fully.
25 TMH to William Hall-Jones, 20 February 1906. Colonial Secretary Files, 96/1649. Cited in Bagnall (1967), pp. 22–31 (22).
26 Ibid.
27 For a general account see T. Belanger, 'Descriptive bibliography' in Peters (ed.), pp. 97–115. For more detailed analysis see bibliographers Stokes, Greg, McKerrow, Bowers and Gaskell.
28 One English language edition was F.E. Raynal, *Wrecked on a Reef; Or, Twenty Months among the Auckland Isles: A true story* (London: T. Nelson & Sons, 1874). Raynal's account, first published in French in 1870 and in English in 1874, was used by Jules Verne for his book *Mysterious Island*.
29 Third Report of the Australasian Advancement of Science, Christchurch, p. xxiii. See also 'Association for the Advancement of Science', *Star*, 22 January 1891, p. 3.
30 Percy Smith to TMH, 18 December 1893. MS-0451-008/007. HC.

31 TMH to Thomas Cheeseman, 22 August 1896. Cheeseman Papers. AIM.
32 Henry Miller, preface, in Lawrence J. Shifreen and Roger Jackson, *Henry Miller: A bibliography of primary sources* (Ann Arbor, Michigan, 1993), p. [xxiii].
33 TMH to Hall-Jones, 20 February 1906. In Col. Sec. 96/1649. Cited in Bagnall (1967), pp. 22–31 (22–23). See Secretary, Royal Colonial Institute to Colonial Secretary, NZ. 7 March 1895, re: listing of NZ publications and reply on file Col. Sec. 95/1063, Col. Sec 96/1649.
34 Cited in Bagnall (1967), p. 24. Albert Pitt was attorney-general from 1903 until his death on 18 November 1906.
35 Wilson to Hall-Jones, 22 February 1906, cited in Bagnall (1967), p. 24.
36 Ibid.
37 Hall-Jones, Minute, 3 August 1906 96/1649, and Cabinet Approval, 28 June 1906. Cited in Bagnall (1967), p. 25.
38 TMH to Percy Smith, 15 June 1906. MS-0451-023/013. HC.
39 Percy Smith to TMH, 5 December 1906. F&J 5: 187. HC.
40 *Evening Post*, 4 December 1906, p. 4; 'Local and general', *OW*, 5 December 1906, p. 36.
41 See John Mackay, 'The Dominion's printing', *Star*, 14 January 1908, p. 1.
42 Ibid.
43 TMH to Augustus Hamilton, 27 October 1907. MU000152/7/106 Folder 9. MONZ Archives.
44 TMH to Percy Smith, 10 September 1908. MS-Papers-1187-263. ATL.
45 Gertrude von Tunzelmann to TMH, 21 March 1906. MS-0451-023/007. HC. The manuscript is an account of Nicholas Paul Baltazar von Tunzelmann's pioneering and discovery of a route to Lake Wakatipu with his friend William Gilbert Rees. It carries a postscript: 'I went by the name of Wakatipu in Wellington on my return from our exploring trip. NvT.' The yodelling and musical Tunzelmann (1825–1900) arrived in Wellington in 1859, was later a runholder at Fernhill on the western side of the lake and after an interim period in Australia, returned to live at Beach Bay, Walter Peak. Gertrude Hodgkinson was a daughter of Dr Samuel Hodgkinson (one of TMH's early correspondents) and Mary Hodgkinson (née Atcheson). Gertrude married W. von Tunzelmann, brother of Nicholas. See F&J 2: '1836 to 1906', 67; see also Alan de la Mare, 'Von Tunzelmann' in Jane Thomson (ed.), *Southern People* (Dunedin: Longacre/DCC, 1998), p. 528.
46 The Maori language New Zealand Church Almanac is 1845 (*BiM* S201, p. 819). Colenso's edition of the *New Testament* (1837, i.e. 1838) is *BiM* 45; *W* 20.
47 TMH to Horatio Robley, 27 November 1906. MS-0488/006. HC.
48 TMH to John Webster, 24 April 1907. Typescript of NZMS 4/16 (9). Sir George Grey Special Collections, ACL.
49 TMH to Augustus Hamilton, 25 April 1907. MU000152/7/106 Folder 9. MONZ Archives.
50 James McKerrow to TMH, 20 May 1907. F&J 2: 70. HC.
51 'Old New Zealand: Dr Hocken's researches', *Evening Post*, 18 March 1908, p. 2.
52 TMH to Justice Chapman, 19 May 1908. In Chapman, Eichelbaum and Rosenberg Family Papers MS-Papers-8670-099. ATL
53 TMH to John Webster, 10 June 1908. Typescript of NZMS 4/16. Sir George Grey Special Collections, ACL. Webster's work was registered on p. 484 of TMH's *Bibliography*.
54 Percy Smith to TMH, 21 October 1908. MS-0451-028/016. HC.
55 Advertisements, *Poverty Bay Herald*, 20 January 1909, p. 6; Advertisements, *Poverty Bay Herald*, 13 August 1909, p. 3.

56 TMH to Percy Smith, 10 June 1909. Polynesian Society Papers, MS-Papers-1187-263-13. ATL.
57 J. Mackay to TMH, 16 July 1909. MS-0451-029/014. HC.
58 TMH to Percy Smith, 23 July 1909. Polynesian Society Papers, MS-Papers-1187-263-15 and 16. ATL; Percy Smith to TMH, 28 July 1909. MS-0451-029/018. HC.
59 TMH, Introduction, *Bibliography* (1909), p. vii.
60 'An indispensable volume', *OW*, 18 August 1909, p. 66.
61 TMH, Introduction, *Bibliography* (1909), pp. v–vi.
62 'New publications', *Evening Post*, 21 August 1909, p. 13. Interestingly, R. Ramsay's *The Straw* (London: Hutchinson, 1909) is given far more copy.
63 Although a brave attempt, TMH's coverage was woefully incomplete. To realise the full number of publications, one need only examine the coverage of publications in Maori in Phillip Parkinson's *BiM*, in itself a vast improvement on Williams's early bibliography.
64 4 August 1909 entry, Augustus Hamilton's Diary. MU 000144 box 1, item 6 July 1906 to 17 December 1909. MONZ Archives.
65 'A valuable work', *Taranaki Herald*, 25 August 1909, p. 2.
66 TMH to Percy Smith, 3 August 1909. Polynesian Society Papers, MS-Papers-1187-263-18. ATL.
67 *Argus*, Friday 12 November 1909, p. 5.
68 A.H. Turnbull to W. Downie Stewart, 12 August 1909. Cited in E.H. McCormick, *Alexander Turnbull: His life his circle his collections* (Wellington: Alexander Turnbull Library, 1974), p. 224.
69 A.H. Turnbull to W. Downie Stewart, 19 August 1909. Cited in McCormick (1974), p. 224.
70 TMH to Percy Smith, 27 August 1909. Polynesian Society Papers, MS-Papers-1187-263-18. ATL.
71 Augustus Hamilton's Diary. MU 000144 box 1, item 6 July 1906 to 17 December 1909. MONZ Archives.
72 TMH to Charles Wilson, 14 September 1909. In T.M. Hocken Miscellaneous Papers, 1890–1910. MS-Papers-0380-4. ATL.
73 [A.N. Field, editor], *The Citizen*, 24 October 1909. See Bagnall's 1967 article for Field's unorthodoxies.
74 [James Collier], 'The literature of New Zealand: A criticism and a protest', *The Citizen*, 24 October 1909, pp. 485–86.
75 TMH to A.H. Turnbull, 28 February 1910. Hocken Miscellaneous Papers, 1890–1910. MS-Papers-0380. ATL.
76 Ibid.
77 J. Mackay to TMH, 16 July 1909. MS-0451-029/014. HC.
78 A.H. Turnbull to Percy Smith, 29 June 1911. MS-Papers 0057-052. ATL.
79 John Webster to TMH, 25 July 1906. MS Papers 0247-09. ATL.
80 TMH, 'A biographical sketch' in F.E. Maning's *Old New Zealand* (Christchurch: Whitcombe & Tombs, 1906), p. vii.
81 John Webster to TMH, 15 August 1906. MS Papers 0247-09. ATL. The collection now forms: Letters from Frederick Maning to John Webster, 1865–1883. MS-0050. HC. Embedded at back of the letters are various letters from Webster to TMH, dated 25 July 1906, 15 August 1906, 22 August 1906 and 25 [August] 1906, and Leys's letter to TMH, 25 August 1906. TMH added 'Of Oponini, Hokianga' under the Webster photograph.
82 John Webster to TMH, 22 August 1906. MS-Papers-0247-09. ATL. See David Colquhoun, 'Maning, Frederick Edward', from DNZB: www.TeAra.govt.nz/en/biographies/1m9/maning-frederick-edward. Colquhoun is less sure, giving 1811 or 1812. See biographical details from T. Maning, nephew of

Judge Frederick Maning, which were given to TMH, 20 February 1907. MS-0451-025/005. HC
83   Notes written in TMH's 2nd edn of Maning's *History of the War in the North of New Zealand* (1864). See HPC, Vol. 115. HC.
84   John Webster to TMH, 25 July 1906; John Webster to TMH, 22 August 1906. MS-Papers-0247-09. ATL. See David Colquhoun. 'Maning, Frederick Edward', from DNZB.
85   F. Maning to John Webster, 16 April [1874]. F&J 5: 97. HC. See also F. Maning to von Sturmer 12 June 1881, cited in John Nicholson, *White Chief: The colourful life and times of Judge F.E. Maning of Hokianga* (Penguin, 2006), p. 219.
86   F. Maning to von Sturmer 12 June 1881, cited in Nicholson, p. 219.
87   TMH, 'A biographical sketch' in Maning's *Old New Zealand* (1906), p. viii.
88   J.W. Leys to TMH, 25 August 1906. MS-Papers-0247-09. ATL.
89   'Among the books: *Old New Zealand*', *OW*, 6 March 1907, p. 79.
90   TMH to John Webster, 24 April 1907. Hocken–Webster Letters, NZ MS 4/16 (9). Sir George Grey Special Collections, ACL.
91   Ibid.
92   TMH to John Webster, 29 April 1908. Hocken–Webster Letters, NZ MS 4/16 (10). Sir George Grey Special Collections, ACL.
93   They include *Hokianga River (Upper Part)*, Admiralty Chart. 2800 (London: The Admiralty, 1861). Hocken Maps: 841 1851 aj; and *Hokianga River*, Admiralty Chart. 1091 (London: The Admiralty, 1861). Hocken Maps 841 1861 aj.
94   TMH to John Webster, 29 April 1908. Hocken–Webster Letters, NZ MS 4/16 (10). Sir George Grey Special Collections, ACL.
95   TMH to John Webster, 10 June 1908. Hocken–Webster Letters, NZ MS 4/16 (11). Sir George Grey Special Collections, ACL.
96   John Webster to TMH, 10 February 1909. MS-1570-001/011. HC.

Chapter 19: An Act of Patriotism
1   'Observance of anniversary day', *ODT*, 19 March 1897, p. 3.
2   *OW*, 8 April 1897, p. 23.
3   TMH to David Scott Mitchell, 8 March 1898. ML A1461, 130–31. Cited in Eileen Chanin, *Book Life. The life and times of David Scott Mitchell* (Melbourne: Australian Scholarly Publishing, 2011), p. 281.
4   Cited in *Dr Hocken to Mark Cohen, 1 July 1906*. A printed sheet in Robert McNab Papers, 0047-01. ATL.
5   Mary Ronnie, *Freedom to Read: A centennial history of Dunedin Public Library* (Dunedin: DCC, 2008).
6   Anderson to TMH, 25 March 1899. MS-0451-013-007. HC.
7   David Scott Mitchell to TMH, 8 April 1899. F&J 5: 165. HC.
8   See George Griffiths, 'Mark Cohen' in Jane Thomson (ed.), *Southern People* (Dunedin: Longacre/DCC, 1998), p. 98; see also Mary Ronnie, *Freedom to Read* (2008).
9   Cited in *Dr Hocken to Mark Cohen, 1 July 1906*.
10   Percy Smith to TMH, 22 June 1899. MS-0451-013/012. HC.
11   TMH to Cohen, 1 July 1906; reprinted in *ODT* under heading 'Dr Hocken's Library'. A printed sheet in Robert McNab Papers. 0047-01. ATL.
12   Ibid.
13   'Dr Hocken's gift', *OW*, 25 July 1906, p. 49.
14   Mark Cohen to Robert McNab, Saturday, [c. July 1906]. Robert McNab Papers 0047-01. ATL.
15   30 July meeting, reported in *OW*, 1 August 1906, p. 37.
16   'The Hocken Collection', compiled newspaper extracts in F&J 10: 174–81.

17 'Dr Hocken's Collection: The Premier will make no promises', *OW*, 8 August 1906, p. 12.
18 'The Hocken Collection', *ODT*, n.d., F&J 10: 174–81.
19 TMH to F.R. Chapman, 16 August 1906. MS-0451-024/003. HC.
20 'The Hocken Collection', *OW*, 22 August 1906, p. 49.
21 Cited in 'Dr Hocken's gift', *OW*, 29 August 1906, p. 49.
22 Sir Samuel Way to TMH, 20 August 1906. MS-1258-003/007. HC.
23 J. Horsfall to EMH, 17 August 1906. MS-0451-024/004. HC.
24 'The Hocken Collection: What it consists of', *ODT*, 4 August 1906, p. 9; see also compiled newspaper extracts, F&J 10: 174–81. HC.
25 'The Hocken Collection: Our final symposium', see compiled newspaper extracts, F&J 10: 174–81. HC.
26 Ibid.
27 Ibid.
28 'Dr Hocken's library and pictures', *ODT*, 29 August 1906, p. 5; see also compiled newspaper extracts, F&J 10: 174–81. HC.
29 James Allen to TMH, 11 September 1906. MS-0451-024/007. HC. See also 'The Hocken Collection', *OW*, 19 September 1906, p. 31.
30 'Dr Hocken's gift', *OW*, 19 September 1906, p. 27.
31 *Press* 25 July 1906, p. 6; 28 July 1906, p. 8. F&J 10: 174. HC.
32 'Dr. Hocken's treasures', *Press*, 28 July 1906; compiled newspaper extracts, F&J 10: 174–81. HC.
33 'The Hocken Collection', *ODT*, 25 July 1906, p. 4, F&J 10: 174. HC.
34 'Dunedin letter', *Tuapeka Times*, 6 October 1906, p. 3.
35 Mr Richards, Town Clerk, to Dr W.B. Benham, 1 February 1907. Hocken Trustees Minute book, December 1906–May 1913. MS-2847/001. Other Hocken-related purchases, minute books covered at 002-029. HC.
36 'The Hocken Collection', *OW*, 3 April 1907, p. 18.
37 W.B. Benham, to James Taine, 24 August 1907. Hocken Trustees Minute book, December 1906–May 1913, MS-2847/001, p. 3. HC.
38 'The Hocken Fund: An appeal to the people of Clutha', compiled newspaper extracts, F&J 10: 174–81. HC.
39 'Theatrical and musical notes', *OW*, 8 May 1907, p. 68.
40 Douglas MacLean to George Fenwick, 15 May 1907. Hocken Trustees Minute book, December 1906–May 1913. MS-2847/001. HC.
41 'University Council', *OW*, 12 June 1907, p. 14; W.A. Marsh, Registrar, University of Otago, to W.B. Benham, 9 August 1907. Hocken Trustees Minute book, December 1906–May 1913. MS-2847/001. HC.
42 'University Council', *OW*, 7 August 1907, p. 41.
43 'University Council', *OW*, 4 September 1907, p. 53; David Ross to George Fenwick, 11 January 1907. Hocken Trustees Minute book, December 1906–May 1913.
44 'The Deed of Trust'. Misc-MS-1566. HC.
45 William Arthur Mason, Chancellor, University of Otago, to TMH, 8 October 1907. MS-0451-025/012. HC.
46 Note by TMH, 10 January 1908. Hocken Trustees Minute book, December 1906–May 1913. MS-2847/001. HC.
47 'Otago Museum: Housing Dr Hocken's Collection', *OW*, 15 January 1908, p. 34; Specifications for Hocken Wing, 1908. Hocken Trustees Minute book, December 1906–May 1913. MS-2847/001. HC.
48 'Otago University Museum: Annual Report of the Curator', *OW*, 16 September 1908, p. 34; see also Hocken Trustees Minute book, December 1906–May 1913. MS-2847/001. HC.

49 'Otago University Museum: Annual Report of the Curator'. Ibid.
50 'The Hocken Collection: Proposals for the trustees'. Ibid.
51 W.B. Benham to J.A. Burnside, 4 November 1908 (p. 13). Ibid.
52 John Halliday Scott to Marion and Helen Scott, 24 October 1909. MS-2673/001. HC.
53 J.A. Burnside to W.B. Benham, 24 February 1909. Ibid.
54 Hocken Trustees to Scott and Wilson, 25 February 1910, p. 43; Hocken Trustees to David Scott, 25 February 1910, p. 43; Trustees to Ormand Bros, 16 April 1910, p. 56. Hocken Trustees Minute book, December 1906–May 1913. MS-2847/001. HC.
55 Hocken Trustees to A. and T. Burt, 1 May 1909, p. 31. Ibid.
56 J.A. Burnside to G. Fenwick, 26 January 1909; G. Fenwick to J.A. Burnside, 26 January 1909. Ibid.
57 W.B. Benham to J.A. Burnside, 20 October 1909, p. 34; to Orr Campbell, 24 January 1910, p. 39; J.A. Burnside to W.B. Benham, 31 December 1909. Ibid.
58 W.B. Benham to J.A. Burnside, 15 February 1910, p. 40. Ibid.
59 W.B. Benham to George Fenwick, 8 February 1909, p. 28. Ibid.
60 W.B. Benham to J.A. Burnside, 27 December 1909, p. 36. Ibid.
61 David Scott to TMH, 3 June 1909. MS-0451-029/019. HC.
62 TMH to Charles Wilson. 14 September 1909. In T.M. Hocken Miscellaneous Papers, 1890–1910. MS-Papers-0380-4. ATL.
63 TMH to George Fenwick, 24 March 1910. MS-0451-031/003. HC.1245 Trustees to Mr Burnett, 15 March 1910, p. 45. Hocken Trustees Minute book, December 1906–May 1913. MS-2847/001. HC.
64 Trustees to Mr Burnett, 15 March 1910, p. 45. MS-2469/001. HC.
65 W.B. Benham to W.H. Trimble, 15 March 1910, p. 46. Ibid.
66 'Corrections on the Echoes of the Trimbles' by Elizabeth Wyllie Smith, daughter of Dorothy Heywood Stewart. Trimble Papers. MS-2278/002. HC.
67 W.H. Trimble to W.H. Skinner, 22 September 1926. MS-0074 Trimble's New Plymouth papers. HC.
68 W.H. Trimble to TMH, 11 September 1908. MS-0451-028/030. HC.
69 Journal of Librarian. MS-0361. HC.
70 *ODT*, 1 April 1910, p. 2.
71 John Halliday Scott to his daughters Marion and Helen 3 April 1910. MS-2673/001. HC.
72 Cited in 'The Hocken Library', *ODT*, 1 April 1910.
73 TMH, cited in George Fenwick's talk on the occasion, as reported in 'The Hocken Library', 1 April 1910, *ODT*. TMH may have been hesitant on letting go his collection. In a personal note to the author, Gordon Parsonson wrote: 'Dr H.D. Skinner once told me that when it came to the bit Hocken drew back from sheer reluctance to part with his treasures.' Personal communication, February 2013.
74 'The Hocken Library', *ODT*, 1 April 1910; for the reception of TMH's Japanese and Egyptian materials about 30 May, see *Evening Star*, 30 May 1910. The Japanese material has caused much discussion over the years as there was a suggestion that some were pornographic. According to Parsonson, Benham instructed Skinner to take them to Sydney for disposal, which he prudently refused to do. They were eventually burnt. Helen Leach was also told by Skinner that this material was burnt.
75 Rogen and Clarkson to W.B. Benham, 4 March 1910. Hocken Trustees Minute book, December 1906–May 1913. MS-2847/001. HC.
76 'A glance at the books', *ODT*, 1 April 1910.
77 TMH to George Fenwick, 24 March 1910. Cited *ODT*, 1 April 1910, p. 2.

Chapter 20: The Hocken Legacy

1. Judge F.W. Pennefather to TMH, 7 June 1910. MS-1258-003/009. HC.
2. Thomas Hodgkin, Diary – Extracts on Hocken and the Museum, 1909. Micro-MS-COLL-20-1918. ATL. Hodgkin wrote *Italy and her Invaders* (1879–99), was an active member of the Quaker community, and visited New Zealand in 1909, specifically Dunedin for 10 days: 6–12 April and 24–28 April. While in Dunedin, he attended Shackleton's lecture in early April 1909, which TMH surely attended.
3. John Halliday Scott to Marion and Helen Scott, 13 February 1910. MS-2673/001. HC.
4. John Halliday Scott to Marion and Helen Scott, 15 May 1910. MS-2673/001. HC.
5. See Alfred Burton, *The Miner's Investor's Guide*, No. 3 (January 1901), pp. 234–35, and *ODT*, 24 December 1877, p. 2.
6. 'The late Dr Hocken: His will' (compiled newspaper extracts, no date); see *Sydney Daily Telegraph*, 30 May 1910; see also F&J 17, 122. HC.
7. Point 11, Dr Hocken's will, 27 April 1909.
8. Codicil 1, Dr Hocken's will, 3 April 1910.
9. Hocken Library Trustees tender notices, 20 August, 5 September 1910. Hocken Trustees Minute book, December 1906–May 1913. MS-2847/001. HC.
10. Herbert Haynes to Hocken Library Trustees, 30 May 1910; William Nees to. W.B. Benham, Secretary, Hocken Library Trustees, 28 May 1910. Hocken Trustees Minute book, December 1906–May 1913. MS-2847/001. HC.
11. *ODT*, 14 April 1910.
12. *Evening Star*, 8 April 1910.
13. W.B. Benham to the University Council, 8 April 1910. pp. 52–53. Hocken Trustees Minute book, December 1906–May 1913. MS-2847/001. HC; See James Allen to W.B. Benham, 30 August 1910. Hocken Trustees Minute book, December 1906–May 1913. MS-2847/001. HC.
14. Horatio Robley, *Moko, or Maori Tattooing* (1896). MS-0488-001. HC.
15. EMH to W.H. Trimble [24 March 1910]. MS-0488/006. HC.
16. W.H. Trimble to Hocken Trustees, 16 May 1910. Hocken Trustees Minute book, December 1906–May 1913. MS-2847/001. HC.
17. Ibid. See P. Sinclair, solicitor, to George Fenwick, 21 April 1910. Ibid. Christina was the wife of Robert Chapman. Further acquisitions were regularly printed in the *ODT* for all to read.
18. W.H. Trimble to Hocken Trustees, 16 May 1910. Hocken Trustees Minute book, December 1906–May 1913. MS-2847/001. HC.
19. W.H. Trimble to Hocken Trustees, 17 June 1910. Ibid.
20. W.H. Trimble to Hocken Trustees, 18 July 1910. Ibid.
21. W.H. Trimble to Hocken Trustees, 9 December 1910. Ibid.
22. W.H. Trimble to Hocken Trustees, 5 June 1911. Ibid.
23. W.H. Trimble to Dr W.B. Benham, 18 July 1911. Ibid.
24. See entry 25 July 1911, p. 74. Ibid. Also W.H. Trimble to Hocken Trustees, 24 October 1911. Ibid.
25. See W.H. Trimble Correspondence. MS-2293/001. HC.
26. Trustee Meeting, 24 October 1911, p. 76. Hocken Trustees Minute book, December 1906–May 1913. MS-2847/001. HC.
27. George Fenwick, Letter, 1 September 1911. Ibid.
28. W.H. Trimble to George Fenwick, 1 June 1912. Ibid.
29. W.H. Trimble to Dr W.B. Benham, Secretary, Hocken Trustees, 10 June 1912. Ibid.
30. Trimble's work on the maps stopped at No. 74. A number of other hands

continued listing the maps and plans, going through to a draft number of 123. See 'Maps and plans in the Hocken Library', MS-1458. HC.
31 W.H. Trimble to W.B. Benham, 10 June 1912. Hocken Trustees Minute book, December 1906–May 1913. MS-2847/001. HC.
32 'University Council', *CDT*, 22 June 1912. Extracted newspaper collection from 'Variae' 13: pp. 1–35.
33 W.H. Trimble, 'Journal of Librarian'. MS-0361. HC.
34 W.H. Trimble to W.B. Benham, 15 November 1912. Hocken Trustees Minute book, December 1906–May 1913. MS-2847/001. HC.
35 TMH to George Fenwick, 24 March 1910. Cited in *ODT*, 1 April 1910, p. 2.
36 Robert McNab, cited in *Evening Star*, Hocken Trustees Minute Book. MS-2847/001. HC.
37 'Dr Hocken memorial', *Evening Star*, 31 May 1910. Extracted newspaper collection from 'Variae' 13: pp. 1–35. See also W.P. Morrell, *The University of Otago: A centennial history* (Dunedin: University of Otago Press, 1969).
38 'The Hocken Collection', *Evening Star*, 3 September 1910. Extracted newspaper collection from 'Variae' 13: pp. 1–35.
39 'Hocken endowment', *ODT*, 16 July 1910. In the Hocken Collection there is a prospectus with an excerpt containing handwritten 'Promises' listing Dr Shaw 2 guineas, Messrs Malcolm 2 guineas and Adams 1 guinea.
40 Annie E. Trimble, 'Raw material of history: The Hocken Library', *Evening Star*, 5 November 1910. Compiled newspaper extracts, 'Variae' 13: pp. 1–35 (29).
41 A.H. Turnbull to W. Downie Stewart, 20 August 1910. Downie Stewart Correspondence. MS-0985-002/221. HC.
42 *Evening Star*, 9 September 1910. Extracted newspaper collection from 'Variae' 13: pp. 1–35, and also cited in F&J 4 (loose).
43 EMH to Augustus Hamilton, 24 July 1910. MU000152/005/0083. MONZ Archives. Bessie's letters to Hamilton are excellent for what went to the Dominion Museum and prices paid.
44 EMH to Augustus Hamilton, 17 July 1910. MU000152/005/0083. MONZ Archives.
45 This sum cited in Strachan's 'The Hocken Collections 1910 to 2007', in Stuart Strachan and Linda Tyler (eds), *Ka Taoka Hakena: Treasures from the Hocken Collections* (Dunedin: Otago University Press, 2007), pp. 21–26 (21). Strachan gives a very useful overview, which I have used extensively.
46 EMH to W.B. Benham, 24 July 1911. MS-0451-032. See also the Register of the Hockens' gifts to the Otago Museum, where some 451 items are recorded. Thanks to Scott Reeves, Curator, Humanities, Otago Museum.
47 EMH to W.B. Benham, [c. 1911]. MS-0451-032. The greenish-white tiki is D12.7 on the Otago Museum Register.
48 John R. Elder (ed.), 'Preface', *The Letters and Journals of Samuel Marsden 1765–1838* (Dunedin: Coulls Somerville Wilkie and A.H. Reed for the Otago University Council, 1932), p. 9.
49 EMH to W.B. Benham, 3 October 1913. MS-0451-032. HC.
50 Taiaha (D39.1552) and a paddle-shaped cultivator (D39.1551). See Otago Museum Register.
51 W.B. Benham or Trustees to Mr Allen, Chancellor of the University of Otago, 18 August 1910, pp. 63–66. Hocken Trustees Minute book, December 1906–May 1913. MS-2847/001. HC.
52 James Allen to W.B. Benham, 30 August 1910. Ibid.
53 James Allen to W.B. Benham, 23 September 1910. Ibid.
54 James Allen to W.B. Benham, 30 August 1910. Ibid.
55 Library Trustees to Council of the University, 29 October 1910, p. 72. Ibid.
56 See 'Valuable gift libraries: Their future expansion', *Evening Post*, 11 April

1919, p. 11; and 'Gift by Mr McNab', *Hawera & Normanby Star*, 10 March 1914, p. 14.
57 Annual Report (1926), p. 12. Cited by Stuart Strachan, 'The Hocken Collections 1910 to 2007', Strachan and Tyler (2007), p. 22.
58 Strachan and Tyler (2007), p. 22.
59 Cited in Dennis McEldowney (ed.), *An Absurd Ambition: Autobiographical writings E.H. McCormick* (Auckland: Auckland University Press, 1996), p. 128.
60 Ibid., p. 128.
61 Strachan, 'The Hocken Collections 1910 to 2007', Strachan and Tyler (2007), p. 23.
62 Ibid., p. 24.
63 Ibid., p. 236.
64 Ibid., p. 26.
65 Also found in *A Short History of St Philip's Church, Sydney: Jubilee 1856–1906* ([Sydney]: Published with the authority of the Rector and Parochial Council, 27 March 1906), a work that is signed by TMH and in J.R. Elder's Papers. MS-0177/031. HC.
66 George Griffiths, *Books & Pamphlets on Southern NZ: A simplified locality guide 1772 to the 21st century* (Dunedin: Otago Heritage Books, 2006), p. E5.
67 EMH, 'Notes for preface to Marsden's Journals' [1910]. MS-0451-032. HC.
68 EMH to Percy Smith, 4 June 1910. Polynesian Society Papers, MS-Papers-1187-263. ATL.
69 Cited in Michael Blain (compiler), *Clergy in the Diocese of Dunedin 1852–1919: A biographical directory of Anglican clergy who served in Otago and Southland*. First edition 2003: www.anglicanhistory.org/nz/blain_dunedin2003.pdf
70 EMH to Percy Smith, 4 June 1910. Polynesian Society Papers, MS-Papers-1187-263. ATL.
71 Interestingly, Fenwick's 'Memoir' of Hocken at the beginning of this publication is dated October 1911.
72 *ODT*, 13 February 1912. 'Variae' 13: pp. 1–35 (33).
73 Robert McNab, *From Tasman to Marsden* (Dunedin: J. Wilkie, 1914), p. 9.
74 J.R. Elder, 'Preface', *The Letters and Journals of Samual Marsden 1765–1838* (1932), pp. 8–9.
75 Downie Stewart, 'Foreword', J.R. Elder, *Marsden's Lieutenants* (Dunedin: Coulls Somerville Wilkie and A.H. Reed for the Otago University Council, 1934), p. [5].
76 Elder, 'Preface', p. 9.
77 Specifically, Elder's collection has TMH's typescript of Marsden's first voyage, some 40 closely typed pages of text, with extensive notes and instructions; the second voyage of 123 typed pages, containing notes by TMH that were incorporated into Elder's version, which is also present. E.g. footnote on Butler and Tui and Titore; the third voyage to New Zealand of 140 typed pages, with similar amendments and notes by TMH; the two versions of Marsden's fourth voyage to New Zealand – the CMS 101-page version, the other the Cootamundra one from Canon J. Betts; and the sixth voyage of 50 pages. See Elder Papers. TMH typescripts. MS-0177/006-008; 009-011, 01r4, 025, 030-031, 037-038, and 043. HC.
78 Mary Allan to J.R. Elder, 9 May [1933?]. MS-0177/035. HC.
79 Wilmarth Lewis, *Collector's Progress* (London: Constable, 1952), p. 52.
80 Information supplied by Sharon Dell, Hocken Librarian, 22 September 2014.
81 G. DCC 1956, cited in George Griffiths, *Books & Pamphlets on Southern NZ* (2006), p. 66.
82 EMH to Augustus Hamilton, Friday [August 1910]. MU000152/005/0083. MONZ Archives.

83 Cited in Carl Cannon, *American Book Collectors and Collecting from Colonial Times to the Present* (New York H.W. Wilson, 1941), p. 317.
84 George Fenwick, 'Papers relating to a memoir and bibliography of Dr Hocken'. MS-0453/012. HC.
85 W.H. Trimble, *Dr Hocken and His Historical Collection* (Dunedin, 1926), p. 2.
86 Ibid., p. 9.
87 George Griffiths, *Books & Pamphlets on Southern NZ* (2006), p. E5.

Bibliography

T.M. Hocken

PUBLICATIONS

A Holiday Trip to the Catlins District (via Willsher Bay): Being a reprint of the articles contributed to the Otago Daily Times (Dunedin: Otago Daily Times, 1892) (with George Fenwick)

Abel Tasman and His Journal: A paper read before the Otago Institute on Tuesday, 10th September, 1895 (Otago: Daily Times Print, 1895)

Contributions to the Early History of New Zealand (London: Sampson Low, Marston, 1898)

A Bibliography of the Literature Relating to New Zealand (Wellington: Government Printer, 1909)

The Early History of New Zealand: Being a series of lectures delivered before the Otago Institute; Also a lecturette on the Maoris of the South Island (Wellington: Government Printer, 1914)

PERIODICAL AND SECONDARY PUBLICATIONS

'Treatment of sea-sickness', *The Lancet*, 5 October 1861, p. 337

Great Britain Magazine and Weekly Screw, 16 March to 27 April 1861

Great Britain Gazette, 6 July, 20 July, 27 July and 3 August 1861

The Cabinet, 9 November, 8 December 1861; and twice more during voyage

The Cabinet: A repository of facts, figures, and fancies relating to the voyage of the 'Great Britain' S.S. from Liverpool to Melbourne with the Eleven of All England, and other distinguished passengers (Melbourne: J. Reid, 1862)

Wayte, G.H. (ed.), *The 'Great Britain' Miscellany* (Melbourne: Mason & Firth, 1862)

'Botany', *Otago Witness* (Town Version), 20 December 1862, p. 5

'Decrease in the number of whales', *Otago Daily Times*, 3 July 1870, p. 3

'The hot springs of New Zealand', *Saturday Advertiser*, 1 September 1877, p. 11

'The early history of New Zealand: I', *Otago Daily News*, 1 September 1880, Supplement, p. 1

'The early history of New Zealand: II', *Otago Daily News*, 18 September 1880, Supplement, p. 1

'Early pictorial illustrations of New Zealand', *New Zealand Educational and Literary Monthly Journal*, 14 June 1884, pp. 4–6

'The early history of New Zealand: III', *Otago Daily News*, 13 September 1884, Supplement, p. 1

'The early history of New Zealand: IV', *Otago Daily Times*, 26 September 1885, Supplement, p. 1

Some References and Correspondence relating to the Coronership at Dunedin, 1876–1885. Printed for private circulation, c. 1885

'The early history of New Zealand: V', *Otago Daily Times*, 18 September 1886, Supplement, p. 1

'The early history of New Zealand: VI', *Otago Daily Times*, 2 October 1886, Supplement, p. 1

'Early history of New Zealand: The Otago settlement', *Otago Daily Times*, 13 August 1887, Supplement, p. 1

'Early history of Otago', *Otago Daily Times*, 24 September 1887, Supplement, p. 1

'Notes on the derelict ship in Facile Harbour, Dusky Sound', *Transactions of the New Zealand Institute*, Vol. 22 (1887), pp. 422–28

'Some account of the earliest explorations in New Zealand, etc.', *Australasian Association for the Advancement of Science, Report of the Third Meeting: Transactions of Section E*, Vol. 3 (1891), pp. 254–70.

'Some account of the earliest literature and maps relating to New Zealand', *Transactions of the New Zealand Institute*, Vol. 27 (1894), pp. 616–34
'The etymology of the word "penguin"', *Transactions of the New Zealand Institute*, Vol. 28, 11 June 1895, p. 756
'On a piece of Aztec statuary representing the sacrifice of a human victim', *Transactions of the New Zealand Institute*, Vol. 29, 11 August 1896
'Old Maori drawings by Tui (Tooi) and Titore (Teeterree)', *New Zealand Herald*, 10 April 1897
'An account of the Fiji fire ceremony', *Transactions of the New Zealand Institute*, Vol. 31 (1898), pp. 667–72
'Relics of the old Native population on the Upper Molyneux', Otago Institute meeting, 9 August 1898, *Transactions of the New Zealand Institute*, Vol. 31 (1898), p. 738
'Notes on New Zealand earthworms' (with W.B. Benham and G.M. Thomson), Otago Institute meeting, *Transactions of the New Zealand Institute*, Vol. 31 (1898), p. 743
'A photograph of a curious nest found on the Rock and Pillar Range, *Transactions of the New Zealand Institute*, Vol. 31 (1898), p. 737
'Maori weapons and implements exhibited', Otago Institute meeting, 9 August 1898, *Transactions of the New Zealand Institute*, Vol. 31 (1898), p. 738
'Some account of the beginnings of literature in New Zealand: Part I, the Maori section', *Transactions of the New Zealand Institute*, Vol. 33 (1900), 472–90
'Some account of the beginnings of literature in New Zealand: Part II, the English newspapers', *Transactions of the New Zealand Institute*, Vol. 34 (1901), pp. 99–114
'History of the early New Zealand missions', *Otago Daily Times*, 3 October and 10 November 1905
Notes & Queries, 10th S.V. (19 May 1906), p. 389
'Early visits of the French to New Zealand', *Transactions of the New Zealand Institute*, Vol. 40 (1907), pp. 5–8
'Our early history: New Zealand Institute. Dr Hocken's address', *Otago Daily Times*, 14, 16 May 1908; reprinted *Otago Witness*, 20, 27 May 1908, pp. 17, 65
'The Fiji fire ceremony', *Japan Daily Herald*, 9 October 1909

INTRODUCTIONS
'Introductory remarks to the catalogue of the contents of the early history, Maori, and South Seas Court', *Official Catalogue of the Exhibition: New Zealand and South Seas Exhibition, Dunedin, 1889–1890* (Dunedin, 1889)
Frederick Edward Maning, *Old New Zealand* (Christchurch: Whitcombe & Tombs, 1906)
John Webster, *Reminiscences of an Old Settler in Australia and New Zealand* (Christchurch: Whitcombe & Tombs, 1908)

HOCKEN'S OWN LIBRARY
'Dr T.M. Hocken's Original Collection', printout from the Hocken Collections Pictorial Collection database
'Flotsam and Jetsam' (F&J) volumes
Hocken, T.M., 'Catalogue of books, pamphlets, maps, newspapers, prints etc. relating to New Zealand. In the Library of Dr T.M. Hocken of Dunedin, N.Z.' [1887]. MS-0044
—, 'Historical notes'. MS-0027
—, Letters to Bessie and his daughter 1883–1897 MS-1258/001; 002; 004
—, 'New Zealand notes'. MS-0037
—, Pamphlet collection (HPC)
—, Papers – 'Traditions of Maori migration to New Zealand', 1875. MS 0734

—, Papers and correspondence MS-0451
—, 'The history of our ship', typescript. Misc-MS-0516
Le François, Gladys, 'Album: Fiji, Samoa, Solomon Islands'. Album 39, 1895
—, Diary, Fish Hoek Collection (from A.G. Hocken)
—, Newspaper scrapbook and loose items. MS-2469/001 and /002
—, Papers related to the ship *Great Britain*. Misc-MS-0516
—, 'Travel diary', several volumes. Misc-MS-1730
McGill, Jean and Linda Rodda (compilers), *Catalogue of Pictures in the Hocken Library* (Dunedin: Otago University Library, 1948)
'The Deed of Trust'. Misc-MS-1566
'21 Important Letters, 1867–96'. MS 0084
'Variae' volumes

HOCKEN COLLECTIONS
Buckland, O.J., to W.H. Trimble, Hocken Librarian. MS-2547
Carew, W.S., Papers. 1874–1898. MS-0105
Cook & Allan Papers, Box 4. UN-003
Early History Society of Otago. MS-0097
Elder, J.R., Research papers and transcriptions relating to Rev. Samuel Marsden. ARC-0035 (MS-0057 and MS-0177)
Fenwick, George, Papers relating to a memoir and bibliography of Dr T.M. Hocken, October 1911. MS-0453/012
Hocken Collections: Records, Trustees Minute book, MS-2847/001; 002-029
Hocken, Joshua, Correspondence with the Methodists. Misc-MS-1300 (reproduction copies)
Letterbook containing letters from Kettle, as Principal Surveyor of the New Zealand Company, to Colonel William Wakefield and Cargill, as agents of the company, 1846–1850. MS-0083
Marsden, Samuel, Collected papers of and relating to Rev. Samuel Marsden. MS-0056
—, Correspondence, 14 June 1815 to 11 March 1816 MS-0055
Neill, Ruby, 'The Hocken family', recorded interview with. A.G. Hocken, 24 February 1960. MS-2847/62
New Zealand and South Seas Exhibition, Dunedin, Letterbook. MS-0104
—, Miscellaneous inward correspondence September 1863 to November 1865. MS-0334
New Zealand Exhibition 1889–90 (Early History, Maori & South Seas Section): MS-0335–0354
—, Directors' Minute book 1888–90. MS-0335
—, Minute book of the Early History, Maori and South Seas Committee. MS-0101
—, Letterbook regarding insurance. MS-0354
Nicholson, Sir Richard, Papers relating to Richard Nicholson – Diary, 1844. MS-0439/032
Riemenschneider, Johann Friedrich, 'On Maori habits of life'. MS-0303
Robley, Horatio, *Moko, or Maori Tattooing* (first edn, 1896), annotated and including material for a second edition. MS-0488-001
Scott, John Halliday, Papers, Letters to daughters Marion and Helen. MS-2673/001
Shortland, Edward, Papers. MS-0001-0025; MS-0086/001-002; MS-0385/002; MS-0096; MS-1166/006
Smith, Marsden, Diary, 1888–1890. Misc-MS-1255
Stewart, William Downie, Personal, political and family papers – correspondence. MS-0985-002/221
Trimble family, Papers, W.H. Trimble correspondence. MS-2293/001
Trimble, William Heywood, Log and private journal, 'Journal of Librarian'. MS-0361

—, Volume entitled 'New Plymouth letters' containing letters to Colonel William Wakefield relating to the Plymouth Company of New Zealand. MS-0074
University of Otago Medical Library Historical Collection, First Letterbook, Part II. MS-1630
Webster, John, Letters 1865–1883, from Frederick Edward Maning. MS-0050

Archives and Institutions

NEW ZEALAND
Sir George Grey Special Collections, Auckland Central Library
Auckland Library Archives (uncatalogued)
Grey, Sir George, Letters, Hocken to Grey, GL: NZ H29 (1-5); Grey to Clifford Holgate, GL: H36 (3)
Reid, John, 'Journey on SS *Great Britain*', October 1861. NZMS 763
Shillington, Edward, to Sir George Grey. GNZ MSS 124 (23)
Webster, John, Papers. NZMS 4/16

Auckland Institute and Museum Library
Cheeseman, Thomas, Papers 1890–97 and Post-1900 Correspondence Letterbook. MA 95/38/5; MA 94/40
Robley, Horatio, to Augustus Hamilton [1904], Vol. 10, Folder 11, MS 131

Cambridge Museum
Buckland Deeds Reference: IF 934 F2.17.1204

Canterbury Museum, Christchurch
Wakefield, Edward Gibbon, Papers, Vol. 1, p. 25

Dunedin City Council Archives
Rate Book Vol. 83a 1920–22, Block XV, section 6. No. 163. Dunedin Drainage & Sewerage Board Drainage Plan S 103a. Dunedin City Council Building Permit 3357, 1916

Dunedin Public Library
Petition, 29 December 1868, in Dunedin Athenaeum and Mechanics' Institute, 1858–1885, Archive 34

Otago Museum
Register of Hocken gifts to Otago Museum

Alexander Turnbull Library, Wellington
Allen, C.R., 'A few notes on Hocken' in correspondence relating to Walter Empson Burdon. Randal Matthews Papers, 1896–1965. MS-85-109-2/05
Allom Collection of Edward Gibbon Wakefield Papers, 1823–1928. qMS-0056-0059
Berggren Papers. MS-Papers 1002
Alper, G.S. to TMH, 28 December 1884. McDonnell MS-Papers-0151-27
Carter, Charles Rooking, Papers. MS 78-149 Misc.
Chapman, Eichelbaum and Rosenberg Family Papers. MS-Papers-8670-099 (MS-Group-0754)
Chapman, Henry Samuel, letter to father, 19 August 1847. Vol. 2, 1847–48. qMS
Grey, Sir George, typescript letter to TMH, 28 October 1880, bound in at front of 'Historical narrative of an attempt to form a settlement in New Zealand' by Charles, Baron de Thierry. qMS-2013

Hill Henry, T., Correspondence, 1900–02. MS 0172-005
—, Papers. 0172-004Hocken, T.M. to A.H. Turnbull, 2 May 1899. A.H. Turnbull Papers, 1868–1918. 0057-039
Hocken, T.M., Miscellaneous Papers, 1890–1910. MS-Papers-0380-4
Hodgkin, Thomas, Diary, Extracts on T.M. Hocken and the Museum, 1909. Micro-MS-COLL-20-1918
Johnstone, A.H., Papers, MS-Papers-601
Lawlor, Patrick, Papers: F.A. Brett to Pat Lawlor, 29 September 1952. MSS 77-067-2/7
Leys, J.W. to TMH, 25 August 1906. MS-Papers-0247-09
McNab, Robert, Papers, 0047-01
Phillipps, William John, Papers. MS-Papers-1222
Polynesian Society Papers. MS-Papers-1187-263-7; 1187-263-13
Sidney Scott Papers, MS-Papers-1845-1
Turnbull, Alexander H. to Percy Smith, 29 June 1911. MS-Papers 0057-052
—, Letterbooks qMS-2050-2052. Typescript and index at qMS-2053-2058
Webb-Selfe manuscripts. MS-Papers-0530
Webster, John to TMH, 25 July 1906. MS-Papers 0247-09
Wohlers, J.F.H., Collection. MS Papers 1410

Museum of New Zealand Te Papa Tongarewa
Hamilton, Augustus, Interior of Dr Hocken's house, Hamilton No. 192
—, Diary, 6 July 1906 to 17 December 1909. MU 000144, box 1
—, Papers. MU000152/005/0083; MU000152/7/106
Hocken, T.M. to W.B.D. Mantell, 14 February 1876. No. 2465/76/18/2/76, MU 000094/3/4
Hutton, F.W. to W.B.D. Mantell, 22 March 1876. No. 2497/76/ 27/3/76, MU 000094/3/4

AUSTRALIA
National Library of Australia, Canberra
Cabinet, The, No. 1 (November 1861) [2]. AJCP Reel 855
'Heathfield Harman Stephenson (1833–1896)' in Heathfield Harman Stephenson Papers and Books, Entry 437, AJCP Reel M855 AJCP Microfilm 2347
Roland, Helen, Log, journals, notes 1853–1861. MS 2758

State Library of New South Wales, Mitchell Library and Dixson Library
Anderson, Henry, 'David Scott Mitchell: Some reminiscences'. ML A 1830
Angus and Robertson Archives, 1824, 1848, 1858–1933. Z ML MSS 314 36–38
Betts Family Papers, Vol. I. Correspondence 1827–1910. ML A2563
Dixson Correspondence and Papers, and Dixson family biographical file
Hocken, T.M. to Angus and Robertson, 8 October 1899. MS-Papers-0763, from ML MSS 1116
Mitchell, David Scott to Rose Scott, 19 July 1868. ML ZA1437, pp. 79b–82
Mitchell, David Scott, Catalogues of books. ML C368-71
–, Correspondence, 1844–1907. ML A1461
Morris, Edward E., Papers. MSS 551
Scott, Rose, Papers. ML A1437

State Library of Victoria
Aspinall, Clara, 'Miss Aspinall's Diary, Melbourne to Liverpool May–August 1861', Chomley Family Papers. MS 11000, Box 3416/9
Chomley, Charles Albert, Diary. MS 11000: 2494/13

State Library of Tasmania
Clarke, George, Papers, 28/114–136

University of Tasmania, Hobart
Royal Society of Tasmania Council Minutes
'Walker's trip through New Zealand 25 February to 24 March 1898'. James Backhouse Walker Papers. W9/C3/38; W9/C1/7 (34)

BRITAIN
British Library
'Alphabetical listing of titles and authors'. Quaritch Archive. MS Add. 64,222 (of MS Add. 64,132–64, 217)
'Asia, Africa, Australia', ledger for 1899. Quaritch Archive. MS Add. 64,221
Sherborn Autographs, Vol. IX, 'Politics and Professions', MS. Add. 42,583, f.127 (Grey to Richard Owen, 3 November 1848)

Cambridge University Library
Darwin, Charles, Archive. DAR 229: 80 (ref. S 12733)

Grimsby Public Library
Circuit timetables, in Skelton Posters and Bills Collection, Reel I (30 December 1836 to 31 December 1839) and Reel II (13 January to 29 December 1836)
'Rules to be observed in the Sunday School, Great Coates', in Skelton Posters and Bills Collection, Reel I (30 December 1836 to 31 December 1839) and Reel II (13 January to 29 December 1836)

Japan Society
Japan Society catalogue, 1906
Japan Society London address book 1904–05
Minutes of the Council of the Japan Society, June 1902 to December 1908, No. 2

Lincoln Archives
Circuit records, Meth B Stamford/12/1, Circuit Steward's Account Book 1805–1836 (Meth B/Grimsby/13/1), and Quarterly Meeting Grimsby Accounts 1838–1872 (Meth B/Grimsby/13/2)

Linnean Society of London
General Minute Book No. 12, 1898–1906
Hocken, T.M. to the treasurer, Linnean Society, 20 March 1886.

Baptism and Census Records
Captain's logs, ADM 51, Reels 1762–64, 1550–71, 2900, 5712–21, 5736–78
Surgeon's logs ADM 101, Reels 3187–216; MT 32 Reel 3181
White Star log, October 1859. BT 98/6257

Royal Anthropological Institute
Council minutes of the Royal Anthropological Institute, 27 October 1903 and 10 November 1903, A10: 3 and RAI Archives: 63/1/31: Election form: Proposed 27/10/03 and elected 10/11/03, with address given: 40 Kildare Terrace, Westbourne Grove
Martindell, E.W. to W.H. Trimble, 17 January 1912. A18/*554
Proceedings of the Anthropological Institute, Vol. 3 (1903), Nos 113, 192.
RAI Archives. 63/1/31: Hocken's election form

SS Great Britain Archive, Bristol
Bill of fare, August 1861
Chomley, Charles Albert, 'Full true and particular account of the voyage of the good steam ship *Great Britain* from Melbourne to Liverpool ... 30 May–3 August, 1861'
Newspapers, SS *Great Britain*

University of Newcastle, Robinson Library
Embleton, Dennis, Papers. 16/2/1

Books and Articles

Adams, David (ed.), *Letters of Rachel Henning* (Sydney: Angus & Robertson, 1966)
Adams, Nancy M., 'Buchanan, John', from DNZB: www.TeAra.govt.nz/en/biographies/1b42/buchanan-john
Alison, Jennifer, *Doing Something for Australia: George Robertson and the early years of Angus and Robertson, publishers 1888–1900* ([Melbourne]: Bibliographical Society of Australia and New Zealand, 2009)
Allibone, S. Austin, *Critical Dictionary of English Literature and British and American Authors* (Philadelphia: Childs and Peterson, [1859–1875])
American Society of Mechanical Engineers, *An International Historic Engineering Landmark: SS Great Britain, 1843 Bristol, England* (New York, 1984)
Anderson, Atholl, 'Shortland, Edward', from DNZB: www.TeAra.govt.nz/en/biographies/1s11/shortland-edward
Annan, Lord Noel, 'The intellectual aristocracy' in J.H. Plumb (ed.), *Studies in Social History: A tribute to G.M. Trevelyan* (London: Longmans, Green, 1955), pp. 243–87
Anthropological Institute of Great Britain and Ireland, 'List of the Fellows', *Journal of the Anthropological Institute of Great Britain and Ireland*, Vol. 35 (July–December 1905), pp. 1–19
Aspinall, Clara, *Three Years in Melbourne* (London: Booth, 1862)
Auckland City Libraries, *Real Gold: Treasures of Auckland City Libraries* (Auckland: Auckland City Libraries and Auckland Library Heritage Trust by Auckland University Press, 2007)
Australian Dictionary of Biography, 2 vols (Sydney: Angus & Robertson, 1949)
Australasian Association for the Advancement of Science, *Report of the Third Meeting: Transactions of Section E*, 3 (Sydney, 1891), 254–70
Bagnall, A.G., *New Zealand National Bibliography to the Year 1960* (Wellington: Government Printer, 1969–80)
—, 'The rival bibliographers James Collier and T.M. Hocken', *Turnbull Library Record*, Vol. 1, No. 2 (1967), pp. 22–31
—, 'Sven Berggren in New Zealand', Section I', *Turnbull Library Record*, Vol. 3, No. 1 (1970), pp. 29–42
—, 'Sven Berggren in New Zealand', Section II: Tauranga and Rotorua, *Turnbull Library Record*, Vol. 3, No. 3 (1970), pp. 143–51
Bagnall, A.G. and G.C. Petersen, *William Colenso, Printer Missionary Botanist Explorer Politician: His life and journeys* (Wellington: A.H. & A.W. Reed, 1948)
Ball, Adrian, *Is Yours an SS* Great Britain *Family?* (Hampshire: Kenneth Mason, 1988)
Barton, G.B., *Literature of New South Wales* (Sydney: Thomas Richards, 1866)
Bathgate, Alexander, *Colonial Experiences, or Sketches of People and Places in the Province of Otago, New Zealand* (Glasgow: James Maclehose, 1874; Capper Press reprint, 1974)
Beaglehole, J.C. (ed.), *The Journals of Captain James Cook on his Voyage of Discovery* (Cambridge: Cambridge University Press/Hakluyt Society, 1961)

—, *The Life of Captain James Cook* (London: Adam & Charles Black, 1974)
Beattie, James, 'Natural history, conservation and Scottish-trained doctors in New Zealand, 1790–1920', in *Immigrants & Minorities*, Vol. 29, No. 2 (2011), pp. 281–307
—, 'W.L. Lindsay, Scottish Environmentalism and the "Improvement" of Nineteenth Century New Zealand', in Tony Ballantyne and Judith A. Bennett (eds), *Landscape/Community. Perspectives from New Zealand* (Dunedin: Otago University Press, 2005)
Beddie, M.K. (ed.), *Bibliography of Captain James Cook R.N., F.R.S., Circumnavigator*, 2nd edn (Sydney: Council of the Library of New South Wales, 1970)
Bedingfeld, Henry and Peter Gwynn-Jones, *Heraldry* (Leicester: Magna Books, 1993)
Beer, Eric and Alwyn Gascoigne, *Plough of the Pakeha* (Cambridge: Cambridge Independent, 1975)
Belanger, Terry, 'Descriptive bibliography' in Jean Peters (ed.), *Book Collecting: A modern guide*. (New York: R.R. Bowker, 1977), pp. 97–115
Berggren, Sven, *On New Zealand Hepaticæ* (Lund: Printed by E. Malmström, 1898)
Binney, Judith, 'Introduction', in William Yate, *An Account of New Zealand*, 2nd edn (Wellington: A.H. & A.W. Reed, 1970), pp. v–xxi
—, *Legacy of Guilt: A life of Thomas Kendall* (Wellington: Bridget Williams Books, 2005)
—, 'Kendall, Thomas', from DNZB: www.TeAra.govt.nz/en/biographies/1k9/kendall-thomas
—, 'What happened to poor Mr Yate?', *New Zealand Journal of History*, Vol. 9, No. 2 (1975), 111–25
—, 'Yate, William', from DNZB: www.TeAra.govt.nz/en/biographies/1y1/yate-william
Blair, John, *Lays of the Old Identities* (Dunedin: Wheeler, 1889)
Blake-Palmer, Geoffrey, 'Sir Frederic Truby King', in A.H. McLintock (ed.), *An Encyclopedia of New Zealand*, II (Wellington: Government Printer, 1966), pp. 221–23
Bleek, Wilhelm, *Early Printed Books, Vol. IV, Part I: England* (Cape Town: J.C. Juta, 1867)
—, *Manuscripts and Incunables Vol. III, Part I* (London: Trübner, 1862)
Booth, Robert, *The Lodge of Otago No. 844 E.C. Register of Members: 1850–1993* (Dunedin: R. Booth, 1994)
British and Foreign Medico-Chirurgical Review and Quarterly Journal of Practical Medicine and Surgery, Vol. 71 (July 1865)
British Medical Journal (28 May 1859)
Brown, Colin, Marie Peters and Jane Teal (eds), *Shaping a Colonial Church: Bishop Harper and the Anglican Diocese of Christchurch 1856–1890* (Christchurch: Canterbury University Press, 2006)
Brown, Henry, *Diary During a Tour Round the World* (Torquay: Directory Office, Fleet Street, 1874)
Brown, Robert, *Prodromus Florae Novae Hollandiae et Insulae Van Diemen* (Norimbergae, Sumtibus L. Schrag, 1827)
Brunton, Paul, 'The collector collected', in *A Grand Obsession: The D.S. Mitchell story* (Sydney: State Library of New South Wales, 2007)
Bryden, Inga (ed.), *The Pre-Raphaelites: Writings and sources*, Vol. II (London: Routledge/Thoemmes Press, 1988)
Bunting, Thomas Percival, *The Life of Jabez Bunting*, Vol. II (London: T. Woolmer, 1887)
Burmester, C.A., 'E.A. Petherick', *Australian Dictionary of Biography* (Sydney: Angus & Robertson, 1949), Vol. 2, pp. 236–37

Byrnes, Giselle M., 'Smith, Stephenson Percy', from DNZB: www.TeAra.govt.nz/en/biographies/2s33/smith-stephenson-percy

Caffyn, William, *Seventy-One Not Out: The reminiscences of William Caffyn*, edited by 'Mid-on' (Edinburgh: William Blackwood, 1889)

Callcott, Maureen, 'The governance of the Victorian city', in Robert Colls and Bill Lancaster (eds), *Newcastle upon Tyne: A modern history* (Chichester: Phillimore & Co., 2001)

Cameron, Sir Charles Alexander, *History of the Royal College of Surgeons in Ireland* (Dublin: Fannin & Co., 1886)

Cannon, Carl, *American Book Collectors and Collecting from Colonial Times to the Present* (New York: H.W. Wilson, 1941)

Carlyle, Thomas, *On Heroes, Hero-worship and the Heroic in History* (London: Routledge, [1905])

Carter, C.R., *Catalogue of Books on or Relating to New Zealand* (London: Printed by Bowden, Hudson & Co., 1887)

—, *Continuation Catalogue of Books Presented by C.R. Carter J.P., to the Wellington Museum and Colonial Institute in the Year 1892* (Covent Garden, G. Norman Anderson, 1892)

—, *Second Continuation Catalogue of Books Presented by C.R. Carter, to the New Zealand Institute and Colonial Museum, Wellington, N.Z., in the Year 1893* ([London, 1893])

Chanin, Eileen, *Book Life: The life and times of David Scott Mitchell* (Melbourne: Australian Scholarly Publishing, 2011)

Cheeseman, Thomas. F., 'On the flora of the north, Cape District', *Transactions and Proceedings of the Royal Society of New Zealand*, article XXIX, Vol. 29 (1896), pp. 333–85

Clark, John Willis and Thomas M'Kenny Hughes, *The Life and Letters of the Rev. Adam Sedgwick*. 2 vols (Cambridge: Cambridge University Press, 1890)

Clarke, George, *Notes on Early Life in New Zealand* (Hobart: J. Walch & Sons, 1903)

Coleridge, K.A., 'Revans, Samuel', from DNZB: www.TeAra.govt.nz/en/biographies/1r5/revans-samuel

[Collier, James], 'The literature of New Zealand; A criticism and a protest', *The Citizen*, 24 October 1909, pp. 485–86

—, *The Literature Relating to New Zealand: A Bibliography* (Wellington: Government Printer, 1889)

Collins, R.D.J., 'Caveat Lector: Notes on some exhibition catalogues', *Bulletin of New Zealand Art History*, 16 (1995), pp. 21–27

Colquhoun, David, 'Maning, Frederick Edward', from DNZB: www.TeAra.govt.nz/en/biographies/1m9/maning-frederick-edward

Concise Dictionary of National Biography, The, Part II, 1901–1950 (Oxford: Oxford University Press, 1964)

Cowan, James, 'Famous New Zealanders, No. 43 John Webster', *New Zealand Railways Magazine*, Vol. 11, No. 7 (1 October 1936)

Cyclopedia of New Zealand: Industrial, descriptive, historical, biographical facts, figures, illustrations. 6 vols (Wellington: Cyclopedia Co., 1897–1908), especially Vol. 4: Otago and Southland Provincial Districts

Davies, Rupert E., *Methodism* (Petersborough: Epworth Press, 1985)

Davies, Rupert E., A.R. George and Ernest Gordon Rupp (eds), *A History of the Methodist Church in Great Britain*, 4 vols (London: Epworth Press, 1965–1988)

Davis, C.O.B., *The Renowned Chief of Kawiti and other New Zealand Warriors* (Auckland: William Lambert, at the Office of the *Southern Cross*, 1855)

Davis, James, *Contributions towards a Bibliography of New Zealand* (Wellington: Lyon & Blair, 1887)

De La Mare, Alan, 'Von Tunzelmann' in Jane Thomson (ed.), *Southern People: A dictionary of Otago Southland Biography* (Dunedin: Longacre Press/Dunedin City Council, 1998), p. 528

Defoe, Daniel, *A Tour thro' the Whole Island of Great Britain*, 5th edn, Vol. III (London: Printed for S. Birt [and 11 others], 1753

Diamond, Marion, 'Henry Parkes and the strong-minded women', in *Australian Journal of Politics and History*, Vol. 138, No. 2 (August 1992), pp. 152–62

Dixson Library and Galleries, The: A brief guide (Sydney: Trustees of the Public Library of New South Wales 1959)

Dufossé, E., *Catalogues* (Paris: Dufossé, 1880–1890)

Early Historical Society of Otago, Constitution and By-laws (1884), article II. Hocken Pamphlet Collection, Vol. 166, No. 20

Eccles, Alfred, 'Address', 2 November 1869, *Transactions and Proceedings of the New Zealand Institute 1869*, Vol II, p. 429

Edge-Partington, James, *An Album of the Weapons, Tools, Ornaments, Articles of Dress of the Natives of the Pacific Islands.* [First], Second and Third series (Manchester, 1890, 1895, 1898)

Eggleton, David, *Into the Light: A history of New Zealand photography* (Nelson: Craig Potton, 2006)

Elder, J.R. (ed.), *The Letters and Journals of Samuel Marsden 1765–1838* (Dunedin: Coulls Somerville Wilkie and A.H. Reed for the Otago University Council, 1932)

—, *Marsden's Lieutenants* (Dunedin: Coulls Somerville Wilkie and A.H. Reed for the Otago University Council, 1934)

Electoral District of the City of Dunedin: Roll of persons qualified to vote, 1870–71 (Wellington, 1871)

Ellis, Elizabeth, 'David Scott Mitchell: A life and a bequest' in *A Grand Obsession: The D.S. Mitchell story* (Sydney: State Library of New South Wales, 2007)

Embleton, Dennis, *Collegium Medicum Novacastrense: The history of the Medical School, afterwards the Durham College of Medicine at Newcastle upon Tyne: for forty years from 1832 to 1872* (Newcastle upon Tyne: Reid, 1890)

Examination for a License in Medicine, Easter Term, 1856 (Durham: University of Durham, 1856)

Facer, Annette, 'Jessie Buckland' and 'Elizabeth Hocken', Charlotte Macdonald, Merimeri Penfold and Bridget Williams (eds), *The Book of New Zealand Women: Ko Kui Ma Te Kaupapa* (Wellington: Bridget Williams Books, 1991), pp. 104, 300

Fairburn, Miles, 'Wakefield, Edward Gibbon', from DNZB: www.TeAra.govt.nz/en/biographies/1w4/wakefield-edward-gibbon

[Field, A.N.,], *The Citizen*, 24 October 1909, pp. 485–86

Field, Tom and Erik Olssen, *Relics of the Goldfields: Central Otago* (Dunedin: John McIndoe, 1976)

Fife, John, *Inaugural Address Delivered at the Opening of the Newcastle-Upon-Tyne College of Practical Science, 1 October 1851* (Newcastle: M. & M.W. Lambert, 1851)

Findlay, Michael, 'Henry Frederick Hardy', in Jane Thomson (ed.), *Southern People: A dictionary of Otago Southland biography* (Dunedin: Longacre Press/Dunedin City Council, 1998), pp. 211–12

Firth, J.C., *Nation Making: A story of New Zealand savagism v. civilization* (London: Longmans, Green, & Co., 1890)

Fitzgerald, Caroline (ed.), *Letters from the Bay of Islands: The story of Marianne Williams* (Auckland: Penguin, 2004)

Fitzgerald, Michael, 'Heaphy, Charles', from DNZB: www.TeAra.govt.nz/en/biographies/1h14/heaphy-charles

Fleetwood, John F., *The History of Medicine in Ireland*, 2nd edn (Dublin: Skellig Press, 1983)

Fletcher, Brian H., *Magnificent Obsession: The story of the Mitchell Library, Sydney* (Sydney: Allen & Unwin/State Library of New South Wales, 2007)
Ford, Colin and Brian Harrison, *A Hundred Years Ago: Britain in the 1880s in words and photographs* (London: Allen Lane/Penguin, 1983)
Frame, Alex, *Grey and Iwikau: A journey into custom* (Wellington: Victoria University Press, 2002)
Frith, David, *The Trailblazers: The first English cricket tour of Australia 1861–62* (Cheshire, England: Boundary Books, 1999)
Froude, James Anthony, *Oceana, or England and her Colonies* (London: Longman, Green, 1886)
Fry, Margot, *Tom's Letters: The private world of Thomas King, Victorian gentleman* (Wellington: Victoria University Press, 2001)
Fulton, Robert Valpy, *Medical Practice in Otago and Southland in the Early Days* (Dunedin: Printed by the Otago Daily Times and Witness Newspapers Co., 1922)
Galloway, David, 'The Swedish connection in New Zealand lichenology, 1769–2004', *Symb. Bot. Upsala*, Vol. 34, No. 1 (2004), pp. 63–85
Garrett, Helen, *Te Manihera: The life and times of the pioneer missionary Robert Maunsell* (Auckland: Reed, 1991)
Gillespie, Oliver Arthur, 'Harper', in A.H. McLintock (ed.), *An Encyclopedia of New Zealand* (Wellington: Government Printer, 1966), Vol. 1, pp. 910–11
Glen, Rewa [Marguerite Maude Johnson], *The Botanical Explorers of New Zealand* (Wellington: A.H. & A.W. Reed, 1950)
Gombrich, *Art and Illusion* (London: Phaidon, 1977)
Gordon, C.M., *The Taylor and Bucklands: Early Auckland pioneer families*, 2nd edn (Auckland: Pelorus Press, 1969)
Goulding, Jeanne H., 'Cheeseman, Thomas Frederick', from DNZB: www.TeAra.govt.nz/en/biographies/3c14/cheeseman-thomas-frederick
Graham, J.M. and M.E.A Cartridge, 'Tutu poisoning in dogs', *New Zealand Veterinary Journal* (1961), p. 45
Great Britain Gazette, No. 1, Saturday 6 July 1861
Great Britain Magazine and Daily Screw, 1861
Greenwood, William, *Riemenschneider of Warea* (Wellington: A.H. & A.W. Reed, 1967)
Grey, George, *Vocabulary of the Dialects Spoken by the Aboriginal Races of S.W. Australia* (Perth: Printed by C. MacFaull, 1839), p. 1
Grey, Sir George, *Address to the Members of the New Zealand Society* (Wellington: The Spectator, 1851), pp. 8–9
—, and Wilhelm Bleek, *The Library of His Excellency Sir George Grey, K.C.B. Philology. Vol. II. Part IV New Zealand, the Chatham Islands and the Auckland Islands* (Cape Town: Saul Solomon, 1859)
Griffiths, Barbara, *Life of Henry John Chitty Harper* (Timaru, 1956)
Griffiths, George, *Books & Pamphlets on Southern NZ: A simplified locality guide 1772 to the 21st century* (Dunedin: Otago Heritage Books, 2006)
—, 'Mark Cohen' and 'Peter Thomson', in Jane Thomson (ed.), *Southern People: A dictionary of Otago Southland biography* (Dunedin: Longacre Press/Dunedin City Council, 1998), pp. 98, 511
Grove, Richard, *Green Imperialism: Colonial expansion, tropical island Edens, and the origins of environmentalism, 1600–1860* (Cambridge: Cambridge University Press, 1995)
Haast, H.V. von, *The Life and Times of Sir Julius von Haast* (Wellington: H.F. von Haast, 1948)
Haines, Robin, *Life and Death in the Age of Sail: The passage to Australia* (Sydney: University of New South Wales Press, 2006)
Hamilton, Augustus, 'Notes on some old flax mats found in Otago', *Transactions and Proceedings of the Royal Society of New Zealand*, article LXVII, Vol. 25 (1892), pp. 486–88

Harnett & Co's Dunedin Directory (Dunedin, January 1863 and 1864)

Harrop, A.J., *The Amazing Career of Edward Gibbon Wakefield* (London: Allen & Unwin, 1928)

Hastings, David, *Over the Mountains of the Sea: Life on the migrant ships 1870–1885* (Auckland: Auckland University Press, 2006)

Hastings, D. Harris, *Official Record of the New Zealand and South Seas Exhibition. Held at Dunedin, 1889–90* (Wellington: Government Printer, 1891)

Hayward, J.W. and A.E. Russell, *The Lodge of Otago No. 844, E.C. Centennial History 1860–1960* (Dunedin: The Budget Ltd, [1960])

Hocken, A.G., *Dr Hocken of Dunedin: A life* (North Otago: East Riding Press, 2008)

—, *Dr T.M. Hocken 1836–1910: A gentleman of his time* (Dunedin: Hocken Library, University of Otago, 1989)

Hocken, Joshua, *A Brief History of the Wesleyan Methodism, in the Grimsby Circuit, including References to the Horncastle, Boston, Barton, Louth, Spilsby, Alford, and Rasen Circuits* (London, 1839)

—, *Hints and Helps to Local Preachers* (London; Norwich: James Gilbert, 49 Paternoster Row; Jarrold & Sons, 1845)

Holgate, C.W., *An Account of the Chief Libraries of New Zealand* (London: Dryden Press, 1886)

Hordern House, *Captain James Cook & His Pacific Legacy Catalogue* (Sydney: Hordern House, 2007)

—, 'Captain Cook', *Catalogue* (Sydney: Hordern House, 2006)

Howe, K.R., *Singer in a Songless Land: A life of Edward Tregear 1846–1931* (Auckland: Auckland University Press, 1991)

Instructions to the Surgeons Superintendent appointed by the Court of Directors to the Emigrant Ships of the New Zealand Company, [November 1841]

Jackson, F. Arthur, 'A Fijian legend of the origin of the "Vilavilairevo" or "fire ceremony"', *Journal of the Polynesian Society*, Vol. 3, June 1894, pp. 72–75

Jackson, Ian, *The Price-codes of the Book Trade: A preliminary guide by exhumation* (Berkeley: Ian Jackson, 2010)

Jenkins, Andrew, *Stamford on Old Picture Postcards* (Nottingham: Reflections of a Bygone Age, 2002)

Kerr, Donald, *Amassing Treasures for All Times: Sir George Grey, colonial bookman and collector* (Dunedin: Otago University Press, 2006)

—, *The Smell of Powder: A history of duelling in New Zealand* (Auckland: Random House, 2006)

Kitagawa, Joseph M., *On Understanding Japanese Religion* (Princeton: Princeton University Press, 1987)

Kizu, Shigetoshi, *A 100 Years' History of the Ships Nippon Yusen Kaisha* (Tokyo: Nihon Yusen Kabushiki Kaisha, 1954)

Knight, Hardwicke and Niel Wales, *Otago News Letter*, 16 February 1867 cited in *Buildings of Dunedin: An illustrated architectural guide to New Zealand's Victorian city* (Dunedin: John McIndoe, 1988)

Lancet, The, September 1858, 2 October 1858, 4 December 1858, 7 May 1859, 21 May 1859

Lang, Andrew, *Modern Mythology* (London: Longmans, Green & Co., 1897)

Langley, S.P. and Andrew Lang, 'The fire walk ceremony in Tahiti', *Folklore*, Vol. 12, No. 4 (December 1901), pp. 446–55

[Larnach, W.J.M.], *Catalogue of Magnificent & Extensive Library … of Late Hon. W.J.M. Larnach* (Dunedin: Park, Reynolds & Co., April 1900)

Ledwich, Thomas H., *Introductory Lecture delivered in the Original School of Medicine, Peter-Street, Dublin, on Monday, 2 November 1857* (Dublin: Fannin & Co., 1857)

Lee, Mary Isabella, *The Not So Poor: An autobiography*, ed. Annabel Cooper (Auckland: Auckland University Press, 1992)

Lerner, Fred, *The Story of Libraries* (New York: Continuum, 1998), p. 99
Leslie, Margaret, Livingston Baker, Ian Church (eds), *Patea: A centennial history* (Patea: Patea Borough Council, 1981)
Lester, George, *Grimsby Methodism (1743–1889) and the Wesleys in Lincolnshire* (London: Wesleyan-Methodist Book-Room, 1890)
Lewis, Wilmarth, *Collector's Progress* (London: Constable, 1952)
Lindsay, William Lauder, *On the Toot Plant and Poison of New Zealand* (London, 1865)
Lindt, J.W., 'The fire ordeal of Beqa, Fiji Islands', *Transactions of the Royal Anthropological Society*, June 1894
Lock, John and Canon W.T. Dixon, *A Man of Sorrow: The life and times of the Rev. Patrick Brontë 1777–1861* (London: Nelson, 1965)
Lubbock, Basil, *The Colonial Clippers*, 2nd edn (Glasgow: James Brown & Son, 1921)
[McCormick, E.H.,], *An Absurd Ambition: Autobiographical writings E.H. McCormick*, ed. Dennis McEldowney (Auckland: Auckland University Press, 1996)
McCormick, E.H., *Alexander Turnbull: His life his circle his collections* (Wellington: Alexander Turnbull Library, 1974)
—, *The Fascinating Folly: Dr Hocken and his fellow collectors* (Dunedin: University of Otago Press, 1961)
—, *Letters and Art in New Zealand* (Wellington: Department of Internal Affairs, 1940)
McCready, Jim, 'Some bookplates in the Hocken Collections', *Friends of the Hocken Collection Bulletin*, No. 52 (November 2005)
Macdonald, Colin, 'FitzGerald, Sir Thomas Naghten (1838–1908)', *Australian Dictionary of Biography* (Melbourne: Melbourne University Press, 1972), Vol. 4, pp. 180–81
McGill, Jean and Linda Rodda, *Catalogue of Pictures in the Hocken Library* (Dunedin: Otago University Library, 1948)
McLaren, Ian, 'Book collecting and bibliography', *Bulletin of Bibiographical Society of Australia and New Zealand*, No. 8 (December 1975), pp. 52–69
McLean, Denis, 'Dieffenbach, Johann Karl Ernst', from DNZB: www.TeAra.govt.nz/en/biographies/1d13/dieffenbach-johann-karl-ernst
MacLeod, Angus, 'Kirk, Thomas', from DNZB: www.TeAra.govt.nz/en/biographies/2k10/kirk-thomas
McLintock, A.H., *The History of Otago: The origins and growth of a Wakefield class settlement* (Christchurch: Capper Press reprint, 1975)
—, *The Port of Otago* (Christchurch: Whitcombe & Tombs, 1951)
McNab, Robert, *From Tasman to Marsden* (Dunedin: J. Wilkie, 1914)
—, *Historical Records of New Zealand*, Vol. I. (Wellington: John Mackay, 1908)
Maning, Frederick Edward, *Old New Zealand* (Christchurch: Whitcombe & Tombs, 1906)
—, *Old New Zealand and Other Writings*, ed. Alex Calder (London: Leicester University Press, 2001)
Manion, Margaret M., Vera F. Vines and Christopher de Hamel, *Medieval and Renaissance Manuscripts in New Zealand Collections* (Melbourne: Thames & Hudson, 1989)
Markham, Edward, *New Zealand, or Recollections of It*, ed. E.H. McCormick (Wellington: Government Printer, 1963)
Martin, A.W. (ed.), *Letters from Menie: Sir Henry Parkes and his daughter* (Melbourne: Melbourne University Press, 1983)
Martin, Ged, 'Wakefield's past and future' in *Edward Gibbon Wakefield and the Colonial Dream: A reconsideration* (Wellington: Friends of the Turnbull Library/GP Publications, 1997)

Matthews, Kay Morris, 'Hill, Henry', from DNZB: www.TeAra.govt.nz/en/biographies/2h36/hill-henry
Medical Directory and General Medical Register for Ireland 1859 (London: John Churchill, 1859)
Medical Students Guide Containing the Latest Regulations of all the Licensing Medical Corporations of Great Britain and Ireland (Dublin: Fannin and Co., [1855])
Mennell, Philip, 'James Davis', *Dictionary of Australasian Biography* (London: Hutchinson & Co., 1892)
Miller, Richard Combe, *Round the World in Five Months: A diary October 1889 to March 1890*. For private circulation only. (Dartford: J. Snowden, [1891?])
Milne, James, *The Romance of a Pro-Consul: Being the personal life and memoirs of the Right Hon. Sir George Grey, K.C.B* (London: Chatto & Windus, 1899)
Minutes of Several Conversations at the … Yearly Conference, Vol. 10 (London: 1844)
Minutes of the Methodist Conferences, Vol. VII (London: 1838)
Mitchell, David, *A 'Peculiar' Place: The Adelaide Hospital, Dublin 1838–1989* (Dublin: Blackwater Press, n.d.)
Morrell, W.P., *The Dunedin Club 1858–1975: A new short history* (Dunedin: The Dunedin Club, 1976)
—, *The University of Otago: A centennial history* (Dunedin: University of Otago Press, 1969)
Morris, Edward, 'On the tracks of Captain Cook', article LXII, *Transactions and Proceedings of the New Zealand Institute*, Vol. 33 (1900), pp. 499–514
Moulton, W. Fiddian and James Hope Moulton, *William F. Moulton: A memoir* (London: Isbister & Co., 1899)
Mourot, Suzanne, with Paulette Jones, *The Great South Land: Treasures of the Mitchell and Dixson Libraries and Dixson Galleries* (Sydney: Sun, 1979)
Muensterberger, Werner, *Collecting: An unruly passion* (Princeton, NJ: Princeton University Press, 1994)
New Handbook of the Christian Year, The (England: Abingdon Press, 1992)
New Zealand Exhibition, *Official Catalogue of the New Zealand Exhibition, 1865* (Dunedin: the Commissioners, 1865)
—, *Reports and Awards of the Jurors and Appendix for the New Zealand Exhibition* (Dunedin: the Commissioners, 1865)
New Zealand Institute, *Transactions and Proceedings of the New Zealand Institute*, Vol. II (1870); Vol. III (1871); Vol. V (1873)
New Zealand Journal of Science, Vol. 1, No. 8 (March 1883), p. 391
Newcastle Upon Tyne College of Practical Science: Medical Department (Newcastle, 1855)
Newman, Charles, *The Evolution of Medical Education* (Oxford: Oxford University Press, 1957)
Nicholson, John, *White Chief: The colourful life and times of Judge F.E. Maning of Hokianga* (Auckland: Penguin, 2006)
Noble, Kaye, 'Drew, Samuel Henry', from DNZB: www.TeAra.govt.nz/en/biographies/2d18/drew-samuel-henry
Oliver, W.H., 'The Wakefield myth', *Comment*, July 1962, p. 6
Olssen, Erik, *The History of Otago* (Dunedin: John McIndoe, 1984)
Ormsby, Lambert Hepenstal, *Medical History of the Meath Hospital and County Dublin Infirmary*, 2nd edn (Dublin: Fannin & Co., 1892)
Otago Girls' High School, *Jubilee Magazine 1871–1921*
Otago Institute, *Catalogue of the Library of the Otago Institute and Museum* (Dunedin: Otago Daily Times office, 1879)
Otago Jubilee Industrial Exhibition. Official Catalogue, The (Dunedin, 1898)
Otago University Library Annual Report 2010, p. 12
Pama, C., *Die Suid-Afrikaanse Biblioteek – The South African Library: Its history, collections and librarians 1818–1968* (1968), pp. 11–12

Park Reynolds & Co., *Catalogue of Maori Relics ... Wednesday May 20, 1896.* (Dunedin: Park Reynolds & Co., 1896)

Parkin, Ray, *H.M. Bark* Endeavour: *Her place in Australian history* (Melbourne: Miegunyah Press, 2006)

Parkinson, Phillip and Penny Griffith, *Books in Maori 1815–1900: An annotated bibliography* (Auckland: Reed, 2004)

Parsonson, G.S., 'Marsden, Samuel', from DNZB: www.TeAra.govt.nz/en/biographies/1m16/marsden-samuel

Peterson, M. Jeanne, *The Medical Profession in Mid-Victorian London* (Berkeley: University of California Press, 1978)

Petherick, E.A., *Catalogue of the York Gate Geographical and Colonial Library* (London: John Murray, 1882)

—, *Catalogue of the York Gate Library formed by S. William Silver* (London: John Murray, 1886

—, Obituary of S.W. Silver, *Geographical Journal*, Vol. 25, No. 4 (April 1905), pp. 465–66

Pollard, A.W., 'Book-collecting', *Encyclopedia Britannica* (London, 1911), pp. 221–25

Poole, Alec Lindsay, 'Tutu', in A.H. McLintock (ed.), *An Encyclopaedia of New Zealand* (Wellington: Government Printer, 1966), p. 465

Porter, Frances, 'Williams, William', from DNZB: www.TeAra.govt.nz/en/biographies/1w26/williams-william

Pritchard, F.C., *The Story of Woodhouse Grove School* (Bradford, England: Woodhouse Grove School, 1978)

Quaritch, Bernard, *Contributions Towards a Dictionary of English Book Collectors* (London: Bernard Quaritch, 1892–98; New York: Burt Franklin, reprint, 1968)

Reed, Frank, 'Introduction', in Alexandre Dumas, *Captain Marion* (Christchurch: Caxton Press, 1949), pp. 12–15

Regulations to be Observed by Students Intending to Qualify themselves to Practise as Apothecaries in England and Wales 1843 (London: Gilbert & Rivington, 1843)

Reid, Gerard, 'Chapman, George Thomson', from DNZB: www.TeAra.govt.nz/en/biographies/2c16/chapman-george-thomson

Richards, Eric, 'Wakefield and Australia' in *Edward Gibbon Wakefield and the Colonial Dream: A reconsideration* (Wellington: Friends of the Turnbull Library; GP Publications, 1997)

Riseborough, Hazel, *Days of Darkness: Taranaki 1878–1884* (Wellington: Allen & Unwin, 1989)

Robertson, Anne, *Treasures of the State Library of New South Wales: The Australiana Collections* (Sydney: Collins/State Library of New South Wales, 1988)

Ronnie, Mary, *Freedom to Read: A centennial history of Dunedin Public Library* (Dunedin: Dunedin City Council, 2008)

Ross, John C., 'Alexander H. Turnbull' in *Nineteenth-Century British Book-Collectors and Bibliographers: Dictionary of literary biography*, Vol. 184 (Detroit: Bruccoli Clark Layman Book, 1997), pp. 427–34

—, 'Thomas Morland Hocken' in *Nineteenth-Century British Book-Collectors and Bibliographers*, Vol. 184 (Detroit: Bruccoli Clark Layman Book, 1997), pp. 227–34

Royal Society of Tasmania, Abstract of Proceedings, July 11th, 1904, in *Papers & Proceedings of the Royal Society of Tasmania for the years 1903–1905* (Tasmania, 1906)

'Royal visits', in A.H. McLintock (ed.), *An Encyclopedia of New Zealand* (Wellington: Government Printer, 1966), Vol. 3, p. 129

Rupke, Nicolaas, *The Great Chain of History: William Buckland and the English School of Geology* (Oxford: Clarendon Press, 1983)

Sangwan, Satpal, 'From gentleman amateurs', in Richard H. Grove, Vinita Damodaran, Satpal Sangwan (eds), *Nature and the Orient: The environmental history of South and Southeast Asia* (Delhi: Oxford University Press, 1998)

Scott, J.H. and W.M. Hodgkins, 'The Exhibition Art Gallery', in *Catalogue of the New Zealand and South Seas Exhibition* (Dunedin, 1890)
Sedgwick, Adam, *The Life and Letters of the Rev. Adam Sedgwick* (Cambridge: Cambridge University Press, 1890)
Selby, Isaac, 'Memories of Macriland', in Paul Peritas, *Hinemoa: The leap year pantomime* (Melbourne, 1925)
Serle, Percival, 'E.E. Morris', *Dictionary of Australian Biography* (Sydney: Angus & Robertson, 1949), Vol. 2, p. 161
—, 'G.B. Barton', *Dictionary of Australian Biography*, Vol. 1, pp. 56–57
Sharp, Charles Andrew, 'John Gare Butler', in A.H. McLintock (ed.), *An Encyclopedia of New Zealand* (Wellington: Government Printer, 1966), Vol. 1, pp. 280–82
Sharp, Iain, *Heaphy* (Auckland: Auckland University Press, 2008)
Shaw, Henry, *The Dublin Pictorial Guide and Directory* (1850)
Shifreen, Lawrence J. and Roger Jackson, *Henry Miller: A bibliography of primary sources* (Ann Arbor, Michigan, 1993)
Shillington, Edward, *Grey Collection* (Auckland, 1898)
Sinclair, F.R.J., 'Proudfoot, David', from DNZB: www.TeAra.govt.nz/en/biographies/2p30/proudfoot-david
Sinclair, Keith, 'Richmond, Christopher William', from DNZB: www.TeAra.govt.nz/en/biographies/1r9/richmond-christopher-william
Slugg, J.T., *Woodhouse Grove School: Memorials and reminiscences* (London, 1885)
Smith, C. Fox, *There Was a Ship: Chapters from the history of sail* (London: Methuen, 1929)
Smith, Jeff, 'The making of a diocese 1851–1882', in Robert Colls and Bill Lancaster (eds), *Newcastle upon Tyne: A modern history* (Chichester: Phillimore & Co., 2001)
Snedden, Fleur, *King of the Castle: A biography of William Larnach* (Auckland: David Bateman, 1997)
Sorrell, Paul, 'Farjeon, Benjamin Leopold', from DNZB: www.TeAra.govt.nz/en/biographies/1f1/farjeon-benjamin-leopold
—, 'Farjeon', in Jane Thomson (ed.) *Southern People: A dictionary of Otago Southland biography* (Dunedin: Longacre Press/Dunedin City Council, 1998), p. 155
Sorrenson, M.P.K., 'Mantell, Walter Baddock Durrant' from DNZB: www.TeAra.govt.nz/en/biographies/1m11/mantell-walter-baddock-durrant
Spedding, Michael, *The Turanganui River: A brief history* (Gisborne: Department of Conservation, 2006)
Spencer, A.H., *The Hill of Content: Books, art, music, people* (Sydney: Angus & Robertson, 1959)
Stack, W.J., *Through Canterbury and Otago with Bishop Harper in 1859–60* (Akaroa, 1906)
Stacpoole, John, *William Mason: The first New Zealand architect* (Auckland: Auckland University Press, 1971)
Stafford, D.M., *The Founding Years of Rotorua: A history of events to 1900* (Rotorua: Ray Richards/Rotorua District Council, 1986)
Starke, June, 'Enys, John Davies', from DNZB: www.TeAra.govt.nz/en/biographies/2e10/enys-john-davies
Starkey, H.W., *A Short History of Woodhouse Grove School 1812–1912* (1912)
State Library of New South Wales, *A Grand Obsession: The D.S. Mitchell story* (Sydney: State Library of New South Wales, 2007)
State Library of New South Wales, *Sir William Dixson: A passion for collecting* (Sydney: State Library of New South Wales, 2013)
Stephen, Alfred E., 'The late Sir William Dixson (Fellow)', *Royal Australian Historical Society Journal and Proceedings* Vol. 38, Part 6 (1952), pp. 295–96
Stevenson, Robert Louis, 'Letter to Sidney Colvin, February 1893' in *Works* (Edinburgh: Constable, 1897)

Stewart, W. Downie, 'Foreword' in *Marsden's Lieutenants* (Dunedin: Coulls Somerville Wilkie Ltd and A.H. Reed for the Otago University Council, 1934)

Strachan, Stuart and Linda Tyler (eds), *Ka Taoka Hakena: Treasures from the Hocken Collections* (Dunedin: Otago University Press, 2007)

Strachan, S.R., 'Hocken, Thomas Morland', from DNZB: www.TeAra.govt.nz/en/biographies/2h39/hocken-thomas-morland

Strathern, Gloria Margaret, 'Thomas Morland Hocken', in A.H. McLintock (ed.), *An Encyclopaedia of New Zealand*, Vol. 2 (Wellington: Government Printer, 1966), pp. 93–94

Stringer, Hugh, 'Shand, Alexander', from DNZB: www.TeAra.govt.nz/en/biographies/2s16/shand-alexander

Strong, Isobel, 'Vailima Table-talk: Robert Louis Stevenson in his home life', *Scribner's Magazine*, Vol. 19, No. 5 (May 1896)

Sutherland, G.H., ·Carter, Charles Rooking', from DNZB: www.TeAra.govt.nz/en/biographies/1c8/carter-charles-rooking

Tanselle, G. Thomas, 'The literature of book collecting', in Jean Peters (ed.), *Book Collecting: A modern guide* (New York: R.R. Bowker, 1977), pp. 209–10.

Temple, Philip, *A Sort of Conscience: The Wakefields* (Auckland: Auckland University Press, 2003)

Thom's Directory 1858 (Dublin: Alexander Thom, 1858), p. 631

Thatcher, Charles R., *Thatcher's Otago Songster* (Dunedin: Joseph Mackay, 1865)

Thomson, Arthur S., *The Story of New Zealand: Past and present, savage and civilised* (London: John Murray, 1859)

Thomson, Basil, *South Sea Yarns* (Edinburgh: William Blackwood & Sons, 1894; R. McMillan facsimile, Papakura, 1984)

Thomson, Jane (ed.), *Southern People: A dictionary of Otago Southland biography* (Dunedin: Longacre Press/Dunedin City Council, 1998)

Thomson, John Mansfield, *Farewell Colonialism: The New Zealand International Exhibition Christchurch, 1906–07* (Palmerston North: Dunmore Press 1998)

Toole, John Lawrence, *The Concise Dictionary of National Biography*, Vol. III: N–Z (Oxford: Oxford University Press, 1992), pp. 2994–95

Traue, J.E., *Committed to Print: Selected essays in praise of the common culture of the book* (Wellington: Victoria University Press, 1991)

—, *New Zealand Studies: A guide to bibliographic resources* (Wellington: Victoria University Press for the Stout Centre for the Study of New Zealand Society, History and Culture, 1985)

'Trials, Notable' in *An Encyclopedia of New Zealand*, Vol. 3 (Wellington: Government Printer, 1966), pp. 447–54

Trimble, Annie, 'A collector's sacrifice: An interview with Dr Hocken', *Evening Star*, 1 February 1908, pp. 39–41

Trimble, W.H., *Catalogue of the Hocken Library Dunedin* (Dunedin: Otago Daily Times and Witness Newspapers Co., 1912)

—, *Two Lectures on Dr Hocken and his Historical Collection* (Dunedin: Otago University/Hocken Library, 1926)

Turner, George Grey, *The Newcastle upon Tyne School of Medicine, 1834–1934* (Newcastle upon Tyne: Andrew Reid, 1934)

Twain, Mark, *Following the Equator: A journey around the world*, Vol. 1 (New Jersey: Ecco Press, 1992), ch. XXX, pp. 246–48

Tyerman, Luke, 'Life and times of the Rev. John Wesley', in Rupert Davies, A.R. George and Ernest Gordon (eds), *A History of the Methodist Church in Great Britain* (London: Epworth Press, 1978), Vol. 2, p. 98

Tyler, Linda, 'Art for Empire: Paintings in the British Art Exhibit', in John Mansfield Thomson (ed.), *Farewell Colonialism: The New Zealand International Exhibition Christchurch, 1906–07* (Palmerston North: Dunmore Press, 1998)

Tyrrell, James, *Old Books, Old Friends, Old Sydney* (Sydney: Angus & Robertson, 1952)
University of Otago, Library Annual Report 2010, p. 12
Vangioni, Peter J., (compiler), *Canterbury Society of Arts First Annual Exhibition, 18 Jan.–12 Feb. 1881* (Christchurch: Robert McDougall Art Gallery, 2000)
Walker, James Backhouse, *The Discovery of Van Diemen's Land in 1642* (Tasmania: Government Printer, 1891)
Wallace, Alfred Russel, *Protective Mimicry in Animals* (1879)
Wallace, Lewis A.R., 'On the varieties of the signatures of Tōün', *Japan Society Catalogue* (1902)
Walpole, Sarah, 'A floating museum of mankind?', *Anthropology Today*, Vol. 20, No. 4 (August 2004), p. 24
Ward, Justice, 'Inaugural address' to the Otago Institute, 24 August 1869 in *Transactions and Proceedings of the New Zealand Institute 1869*, Vol. II (April 1870), pp. 425–26
Ward, Alan, 'Davis, Charles Oliver Bond', from DNZB: www.TeAra.govt.nz/en/biographies/1d3/davis-charles-oliver-bond
Waterhouse, Jill, 'Collier, James (1846–1925)', *Australian Dictionary of Biography*, Vol. 8 (Melbourne: Melbourne University Press, 1981), pp. 69–70
Wayte, G.H. (ed.), *'Great Britain' Miscellany* (Melbourne: Mason & Firth, 1862)
Wekey, S., *New Zealand: Otago as it is, its goldmines and natural resources: Handbook* (Melbourne: F.F. Bailliere, 1862)
Welford, Richard, 'R.B. Sanderson' in *Men of Mark 'Twixt Tyne and Tweed*, Vol. III, part I (London and Newcastle upon Tyne: Walter Scott, 1895)
Wesley, John, *Plain Account of Kingswood School* in *Works* (New York: J. Emory & B. Waugh, 1831), p. 336
White, John, *Ancient History of the Maori*, Vol. II (Wellington: Government Printer, 1887–90), p. 163
—, 'Kahui-maunga at Patea', *Journal of Polynesian Society*, Vol. 16, No. 4 (1907), pp. 189–206
Whyte, Philip, 'Harris, John Williams', from DNZB: www.TeAra.govt.nz/en/biographies/1h9/harris-john-williams
Widdess, J.D.H., *The Royal College of Surgeons in Ireland and Its Medical School 1784–1984*, 3rd edn (Dublin: Royal College of Surgeons in Ireland, 1984)
Williams, Herbert W., *A Bibliography of Printed Maori to 1900* (Wellington: Dominion Museum, 1924)
Wolfe, Richard, *A Society of Gentlemen: The untold story of the first New Zealand Company* (Auckland: Penguin, 2007)
Wood, Pamela, *Dirt: Filth and decay in a New World Arcadia* (Auckland: Auckland University Press, 2005)
Woodhouse Grove School: Reminiscences, 1812–83 (Bradford: Centenary Celebration Committee, 1912)
Woods, Carole, 'Gurner, Henry Field (1819–1883)', *Australian Dictionary of Biography*, Vol. 4 (Melbourne: Melbourne University Press, 1972), p. 309
Woolcock, Helen, *Rights of Passage: Emigration to Australia in the nineteenth century* (London: Tavistock Publications, 1986)
Wright, Neil, *Lincolnshire Towns and Industry 1700–1914* (Lincoln: History of Lincolnshire Committee, 1982)
Wright-St Clair, Rex, 'Monro, David', from DNZB: www.TeAra.govt.nz/en/biographies/1m48/monro-david
Yaldwyn, John (ed.) with Juliet Hobbs, *My Dear Hector: Letters from Joseph Dalton Hooker to James Hector 1862–1893*, Museum of New Zealand Te Papa Tongarewa Technical Report 31 (Wellington: Museum of New Zealand Te Papa Tongarewa, December 1998)

Yamashita, Sinji, Joseph Bosco and J.S. Eades (eds), *The Making of Anthropology in East and Southeast Asia* (New York: Berghahn Books, 2004)
Yarwood, A.T., *Samuel Marsden: The great survivor* (Melbourne: Melbourne University Press, 1977)
Youngson, A.J., *The Scientific Revolution in Victorian Medicine* (New York: Holmes & Meier, 1979)

NEWSPAPERS
Age
Argus
Auckland Evening Star
Auckland Star
Australasian
Bookseller
Colonial and Indian News
Colonist
Daily News
Daily Southern Cross
Daily Telegraph
Evening Post
Evening Star
Freeman's Journal and Daily Commercial Advertiser (Dublin)
Inangahua Times
Leeds Mercury
London Illustrated News
Lyttelton Times
Manchester Guardian
Nelson Examiner and New Zealand Chronicle
Newcastle Courant (England)
Newcastle Journal (England)
New Zealand Herald
New Zealander
North Otago Times
Otago Daily Times
Otago News
Otago Police Gazette
Otago Provincial Gazette
Otago Witness
Pall Mall Gazette
Poverty Bay Herald
Saturday Advertiser
Scotsman
Southland Provincial Government Gazette
Star
Taranaki Herald
Tuapeka Times
Wairarapa Standard
Westminster Gazette (England)
West Coast Times

UNPUBLISHED
Buckland, Nancy M., 'The Bucklands: A continuation of C.M. Gordon's story and a revision of the Buckland and Taylor trees', typescript, Auckland, 1975
Clayton, Neil, 'The too-well-known "Toot": Encounters with the indigenous', in

'Weeds, people and contested places: Selected themes from the history of New Zealanders and their weeds, 1770-1940', PhD thesis, University of Otago, Dunedin, 2007

Fitchett, Olga, 'Dr. Hocken and his work', MA dissertation, University of Otago, Dunedin, 1928

Mee, B.R., 'The Reverend George Clarke', BA hons thesis, University of Tasmania, Hobart, 1965

Reilly, Michael, 'John White: An examination of his use of Maori oral tradition and the role of authenticity', MA thesis, Victoria University of Wellington, 1985

Strachan, Stuart, 'Not quite half a loaf: Dr Hocken and the "patriation" of the New Zealand Company archives', draft paper, October 2005

Walker, Timothy, 'Robley: Te Ropere 1840–1930', 2 vols, MA thesis, Auckland University, 1985

WEB SOURCES

The Hocken blog: https://blogs.otago.ac/thehockenblog
www.anglicanhistory.org/nz/blain_dunedin2003.pdf
www.captaincooksociety.com, formerly the Captain Cook Study Unit
www.history-nz.org/parihaka.html
www.mysite.wanadoo-members.co.uk/Farsley
www.pdavis.nl/Medical.htm
Wikipedia Lincolnshire

EMAIL CORRESPONDENCE

Captain Masaharu Akamine, NYK Maritime Museum, Yokohama, Japan, 15 August 2009
Simon Beattie, April 2008 (Quaritch)
Alison Breese and Chris Scott, Dunedin City Council, 26 October 2010
Alan Callender, Special Collections Assistant, Robinson Library, University of Newcastle upon Tyne
Ian Farquhar, Dunedin
Lydia Fraser, Textile Museum, Washington DC, 2014
David Galloway, Dunedin, 22 May 2006
Keith Giles, Sir George Grey Special Collections, Auckland Central Library
Michael Jeans, Cambridge, New Zealand
Hugh Knowles, Woodhouse Grove School historian, Yorkshire
John Montgomery, Royal United Services Institute (RUSI) Librarian, London
Jerry Morris and Michael Laird for information on Saint-Ferriol
David Murray, Hocken Library
Georgia Prince, Sir George Grey Special Collections, Auckland City Library
Michael Reilly, Dunedin, August 2006
Rev. John H. Walker and Michele Walker, Calverley Vicarage, Yorkshire

Index

Titles of books and other works, including those of Hocken, are indexed under the names of the authors and creators. Works without an identifiable author or creator are indexed under subjects or directly under titles.
Page numbers in **bold** refer to illustrations in the three sequences of plates.

A. & T. Burt 273
Abbott, Edward Immyns, *Dunedin from Little Paisley* (1849) 181
Abduction: The King v. Wakefields & Thevenot (1827) 169, 315
Abraham, C.J. 203
'Account of a fight at Matarai Gorge, 12 July 1844' 221
Adams, C.W., *A Spring in the Canterbury Settlement* (1853) 180
Adams, J.A.D. 135
Adams, William (Miura Anjin) 213
Adelaide Museum 156
Akaroa 70, 82, 85, 88, 224, 278
Album of New Zealand Views (c. 1880) 167
Aldcorn, Andrew 110
Alexander Turnbull Library, Wellington 149, 161, 165
Allan, Mary 293
Allen, C.R. 115
Allen, James 228, 262, 267, 286–87
Allom, Albert 130, 182
Allom, Thomas 130; *Part of the New Plymouth Settlement in the District of Taranaki* (lithograph, 1841) 82, 130
Anderson, Atholl 293
Anderson, Henry 171, 259, 317–18
Andersons Bay, Dunedin 64
Angas, George French 113, 250; *New Zealanders Illustrated* (1846) 108, 109, 110, 131, 265; *South Australia Illustrated* 265
Anglem, William 183
Anglo-Saxon Club 226
Angus & Robertson 18, 157, 160, 201–02, 311
Angus, Rita 290
Anzac Club, Dunedin 67
Apothecaries Act 1815 (UK) 34
Apperley Bridge, Yorkshire 28
archives: Hocken Library, University of Otago 289, 290, 295, 296; *see also* Colonial Office, British; New Zealand Company – records
Argus (Melbourne) 250, 263

Arminian Magazine (later *Methodist Magazine*) (1778–1969) 28, 32
Arney, Sir George 117
artefacts 21, 68, 69, 94, 117, 128, 140, 152, 156, 183–84, 276, 280, 302, plate **xv**
Asiatic Society, *Bulletin* 228
Aspinall, Clara 43–44, 45–46; *Three Years in Melbourne* (1862) 43
Atahapara, Dunedin 20, 67–69, 71, 115–16, 227, 296, 306, plates **viii**
Atkinson, A.S., *Notes on the Maori-Polynesian Comparative Dictionary of Mr E. Tregear* (1893) 92
Auckland 75, 100, 114, 128, 131, 150, 151, 157, 158; Government House 125, 158; Hocken's visits 77, 93, 94, 101, 102–03, 121, 129, 139, 141, 145, 146–47, 175, 188, 189, 229, 233, 254, 260
Auckland and New Ulster Agricultural and Horticultural Society (Agricultural and Pastoral Association) 114
Auckland Chronicle and New Zealand Colonist 179
Auckland Institute and Museum 124, 146, 155, 179, 204, 229; Library 69, 205
Auckland Provincial Council 114, 312
Auckland Public Library 150, 159, 163, 166, 268; catalogue 241; Hocken's gift of pamphlets and New Zealand Company reports 189; Sir George Grey Collection 150, 159, 162, 163, 166, 188, 189, 229, 241, 272, 297
Auckland Punch 169, 313
Auckland Standard 179
Auckland Star 103
Auckland Times 82, 87, 128, 179
Aumblin, J.H. 22
Australasian 284
Australasian Association for the Advancement of Science (AAAS): Anthropology Section 92, 96, 178; conference, 1891 176, 177–78, 185;

'Polynesian Bibliography with special reference to Philology' committee 92, 177, 180, 243; Report of the Third Meeting: Transactions of Section E, 3 (1891) 185

Australia: bibliographies relating to 240–41; Dixson's collecting 163, 164; *Great Britain*' voyages to 39, 48; Hocken's collecting 18, 76. 86, 201–02, 231, 232, 297; Mitchell's collecting 161–62, 163; New Zealand and South Seas Exhibition 145, 151, 152; New Zealand Exhibition, 1865 61; Petherick's intended bibliography 111, 112; Rotz's map 79, 86; Turnbull's collecting 160; *see also* New South Wales; South Australia; Tasmania; Victoria. Western Australia

Avetinus, Johannes 21–22

Baden-Powell, Robert 226
Bagnall, Graham, *New Zealand National Bibliography to the Year 1960* (1969) 253, 291
Baker, James 102
Baker, Sally 212, 213
Balclutha 269
Balfour, Henry 225
Ballance, John 92
Bampton, William 86
Bank of New Zealand, Dunedin 65
Banks, Sir Joseph 69, 79, 87, 200; diaries of voyages to Newfoundland and Labrador, 1766 112
Bannerman, William 136
Barnett, Louis E. 279
Barnicoat, John Wallis 134; 'Journal of John Wallis Barnicoat' (1842–44) 85, 125, 202, 222
Barr, James 135, 136, 137
Barraud, Charles D. 62, 140
Barton, George Burnett: *Literature of New South Wales* (1866) 240; *Poets and Prose Writers of New South Wales* (1866) 240
Batchelor, F.C. 63
Batchelor, Stanley 212, 227, 279
Bathgate, Alexander 260, 261, 277, 283, 294
Batkin, C.T. 128
Baxter, Hector 57
Baxter, James K. 290
Bay of Islands 87, 88, 102, 229–30; *see also* individual placenames

Bay of Islands Advertiser 264, 311
Bay of Plenty 93
Bayly, George, 'Journal of voyages' (1934) 288
Beal, L.O. 117; *Guide for Gold Mining Investors* (1889) 118
Beattie, James Herries 289, 293
Beckett, Mr 49
Begg, A.C. 135, 136
Bell, Francis Dillon 61, 110, 145, 188, 220
Bell, Lady 110
Bellairs, Edmund H.W. 196, 202
Benham, William Blaxland: Bessie Hocken's correspondence 117; collecting 109; and Hocken Library 262, 263, 264, 267, 268, 269, 271, 272, 274, 275, 276, 280, 284, 286, 306; Hocken's comment at Otago Institute talk 199
Bennett, George 'Farmer' 47
Bennett, George, *Wandering in New South Wales* (1834) 49
Benstead, Emily 306, 308
Berggren, Sven 75; *Fresh-water Agae collected by Dr S. Berggren in New Zealand and Australia* (1888) 75; *On New Zealand Hepaticae* (1898) 75
Bernard Quaritch, London 18
Best, Elsdon 19, 22, 109, 119, 160, 211–12; *In Ancient Maoriland* (1896) 175
Bett, Francis Arnct Blackader 23
Betts, Elizabeth (Lizzie) 111, 141, 231
Betts, Francis Matthews 141
Beverly, Arthur 72
Bible: Colenso's edition of *New Testament* (1837, i.e. 1838) 247; 'Collation of Volume of Scripture Extracts, ets. Seen through the Press by Rev. Yate & printed at Sydney, New South Wales, in 1830' 316; first complete Maori Bible (1868) 91; *Galtjindingamea-Pepa: Aranda – Wolambarinjaka* (1904) 227; Hocken's collection of books of Bible in Maori 302; *Ko te Kawenata Hou o to Tatou Ariki o te Kai Wakaora o Ihu Karaiti* (New Testament) (1842) 203; *Ko Te Kawenata Hou o to Tatou Ariki o te Kai Whakaora o Ihu Karaiti* (New Testament) (1852, W233) 120; *Ko te Rongo Pai i tuhituhia e Ruka* (1835) plates **xxvi**; *Ko te tahi wahi o te Kawenata Tawhito* (1848) 188, plates

xxvii; New Testament in Maori (1844) 91, 203; Reuther, J.G., Strehlow, Carl, *Testamenta Marra* (1897) 227; *Upoku 21* (1846) 91, 203
bibliographies: relating to Antarctica 249; relating to Australia 240–41; relating to New Zealand 237–40, 241–43, 249, 253, 293–94, 295 (*see also* Hocken, Thomas Morland: *A Bibliography of the Literature Relating to New Zealand* (1909))
Bidwill, John Carne 69; *Rambles in New Zealand* plates **xl**
Bigges, John Thomas, *Report of the Commissioner of Inquiry into the State of the Colony of New South Wales* (1822) 201
Binney, Judith 293, 296
Black, C.F. 66
Black, James G., *Chemistry for the Goldfields* (1885) 129
Blackburn, Charles, *Hints on Catalogue Titles and on Index Entries* (1884) 241
Bladen, Frank M. 226–27, 232
Blair, John, *Lays of the Old Identities* 126
Bleek, Wilhelm 158, 238
Bligh, William 275
Bluett, Thomas 82
book dealers 18, 101, 102, 108–10, 127, 138, 159–60, 162, 179, 190, 217, 226, 297; catalogues 241, 291
bookplates 19; Hocken's armorial bookplates 20, 139, 173, 295; Hocken's F.L.S. bookplates 20, 97, 113, 295; Turnbull's bookplate 160
Books and Pamphlets relating to New Zealand (dealer catalogue, 1840) 241
botanical collecting and interests of Hocken 54, 69–70, 73–74, 216, 226; *Balantiopsis Hockeni Berggr.,* liverwort named by Berggren 75; Berggren's visit 75; botanical interests 36, 49, 54, 55, 67, 68, 78, 91, 121, 215; Featon, Edward Henry and Sarah, *The Art Album of New Zealand Flora* (1889) plates **xxxiv**; flax culture publications 72; Hocken's botanical notes in books 74; Thomas Ralph's library 72–73; specimens 75
Bouvier, Louis, *Flores des Alpes* (1882) 216
Bowden, Thomas, *A Memorial Upon Colonial Education* (1868) 97
Branigan, St John 58
Brasch, Charles 289, 290
Brett, F.A. 63

Brett, Henry 103
Brett Printing and Publishing Co. 255
Britannica 96; *see also* Wellington
British and Foreign Bible Society 188
British Museum 214, 224, 229
Brodie, Walter, *New Zealand and the Constitution Act* (1861) 92
Brooke, G.V. 43
Brookes, Barbara 293
Brooking, Tom 293
Brosses, Charles de, *Histoire des navigations aux Terres Australes* (1756) 138
Brouard, Emily 160
Brown, Charles Keats 211, 212
Brown, James Elder 135, 136, plates **xxxv**
Brown, Mainwaring 136
Brown, Robert 70, 113
Brown, William (bookman, Edinburgh) 167
Brown, William (merchant, writer, politician NZ), *New Zealand and Its Aborigines* (2nd edn, 1851) 98
Brunel, Isambard Kingdom 39
Brunner, Thomas 104
Bryce, John 106
Buchanan, John 288
Buchanan, William and Allan 110
Buckland, Alfred 114, 139
Buckland, Amelia (later Matson) 127
Buckland, Elizabeth (Bessie) Mary *see* Hocken, Elizabeth (Bessie) Mary (née Buckland)
Buckland, Frank 139
Buckland, Harry, Janie and Hazel 227
Buckland, Henry 114
Buckland, James 192, 196
Buckland, Jessie 123
Buckland, John Channing 114, 123
Buckland, Marianne 115
Buckland, Susan 115
Buckland, William Thorne 114, 127
Buick, T. Lindsay, *An Old New Zealander* (1912) 291–92
Buller, Charles 82
Buller, (later Sir) Walter Lowry 92, 113, 150, 203, 261, 288
Bunting, Jabez 25, 27, 35; 'Best means of preparing missionaries for their work' 28
Bunyan, John, *Pilgrim's Progress,* Maori translation (Kemp, 1854) 109, 179, 230
Bunyan, John, *Pilgrim's Progress,* Maori translation (Puckey, 1836) 230
Burke, William 77

Burn, David 203
Burnett, William 270
Burney, James 86, 138; *Chronological History of the Voyages and Discoveries in the South Sea or Pacific Ocean* (1813) 242, 252
Burns, Agnes J. 126–27
Burns, Barnet 184–85; *A Brief Narrative of a New Zealand Chief* (1844) 184–85; broadsides advertising lectures in England 185
Burns, Thomas 64, 84, 110, 126–27, 181
Burnside, John A. 270, 271, 273, 274
Burrows, Robert ('Bob the Smasher') 230
Burton Brothers, *The Camera in the Coral Islands* [1884] 197
Burtt, Mr 102
Butler, John Gare 80, 175, 220
Butler, Samuel 170–71; 'A note on "The Tempest"'. 91

Cabinet, the 47, 48–49, 50
Caffin, James 136
Caffyn, William 'Terrible Billy', *Seventy-One Not Out* (1889) 47
Cain, Henry: *Full Report of the Trial of Thomas Hall for the Murder of Captain Henry Cain* 56–57
Calverley, near Leeds 111
Cambridge, Waikato 114
Cameron, A. 270
Campbell (binder, Dunedin) 282
Campbell, John Logan 150, 229; *The History of Maungakiekie* 229; *The Unveiling of the Statue of Sir John Logan Campbell at Cornwall Park, 24 May 1906* 247
Campbell, Orr 273
Canaday, Frank and Molly M. 290
Canterbury 82, 85, 104, 131, 180, 215, 218, 241, 265, 302; *see also* individual placenames
Canterbury Association 90, 196, 215, 219; Canterbury Association Minutes and Letterbook, June 1851–28 January 1853 215; *Plan of the Association for Founding the Settlement of Canterbury in New Zealand* (1848) plates **xxxix**
Canterbury Museum 138
Canterbury Society of Arts 104
Cantrell, R.S. 61
Cape Town, Grey Collection, National Library 159, 166, 205

Capra, Guiseppe, *L'Australia nei suoi rapporti con l'Italia* (1910) 119
Carew, Walter Sinclair 198–99
Cargill, Edward Bowes 61, 136
Cargill, Isobel 216
Cargill, John 61, 128
Cargill, W. John 128
Cargill, William 82, 84, 110, 128, 136
Carleton, Hugh 102; *The Life of Henry Williams* (1874) 93, 102
Carlyle, Thomas 26, 76
Carnegie, Andrew 247, 258, 259, 261, plates **xvii**
Carnegie Library, Dunedin 275
Carpenter, Robert Holt 98
Carrington, F.A. 105, 176; *A Synoptical Account of the Making of the Harbour at New Plymouth* 176
Carter, Charles Rooking 159, 238–40; *Catalogue of Books on or Relating to New Zealand* (1887) 239; *Continuation Catalogue of Books Presented by C.R. Carter J.P., to the Wellington Museum and Colonial Institute, in the Year 1892* (1892) 239
Carter, John 237
Cass, Thomas, *Canterbury Times* 179
Castle Donington, Yorkshire 27
Castle, Miss 250
Catlins district 96, 185–86
Cécille, Jean-Baptiste 88
Chaffers, Edward, chart of Port Nicholson (1841) 82, 128
Chambers, W. 127
Chapman, Christina 281
Chapman, Frederick Revans 136, 137, 150, 152, 225, 237, 266–67, 276, plates **xiii**; bequest to Hocken Library 288
Chapman, George 18, 101, 102; *New Zealand Almanac* 101
Chapman, Henry S. 56, 81, 82, 188, 244, 248, 263, 277, 288
Chapman's Monthly Review 277
Chaseland, Tommy 186
Chatham Islands 143, 155–56, 177, 238, 291
Cheeseman, Thomas 67, 69, 74, 124, 146, 150, 155, 179–80, 204–05, 229, 231, 243
Chomley, Charles 43, 44, 45
Choral Hall, Dunedin 84
Christchurch 63, 97–98, 104, 123, 138, 139–40, 153. 179, 181
Christchurch Orphan Asylum 90

Church, Ian, *Gaining a Foothold: Historical records of Otago's eastern coast, 1770–1839* (2008) 294
Church Missionary Society (CMS) 80, 87, 91, 142, 188, 202, 208, 220, 229, 232
Church of England 57, 90, 91–93; Anglican Book of Prayer in Maori 227; Church of England Hymns (c. 1860) 92; *He Kupu Whakamarama,* Nos 5, 6 and 9 (1898) 93; New Zealand Church Almanac (c. 1845) 92
Church of Otago Library catalogue (1861) 241
Citizen, The 251
Clapcott, Henry 61
Clarke, Cuthbert 139
Clarke, Edward Bloomfield 149
Clarke, George (1798–1875) 80, 149, 203, 207, 209, 220, 302
Clarke, George (1823–1913) 207–10, 220, 227, 230; *Notes on Early Life in New Zealand* (1903) 208
Clarke, Sarah 230, 234
Clark's sale rooms/auction house, Christchurch 104, 138, 139–40
Clayton, George Thomas, 'Kororareka in the Bay of Islands' (1845) 83, 128
Clayton, W.H. 61
Cleckheaton, Leeds area 34
Cloudy Bay 173
Clutha 270
Coates, Dandeson 91
Cobham, Viscount 226
Cockayne, Leonard 69, 249
Codfish Island 103
Cohen, Mark 258, 259, 261, 262–63, 268, 270, 306
Colenso, Elizabeth 93
Colenso, William 61, 62, 63, 69, 80, 95, 102, 170, 203, 230, 294, 302, 316; *An Account of Visits to, and Crossings Over, the Ruahine Mountain Range, Hawke's Bay, New Zealand: and of the Natural History of that Region; Performed in 1845–1847* (1884) 129; *Classification and Description of Some Newly-Discovered Ferns, Collected in the Northern Island of New Zealand in 1841–42* (1845) 70; *Ko te Rongo Pai i tuhituhia e Ruka* (1835) plates **xxvi**; *New Testament* (1837, i.e. 1838) 247
Collier, James 139, 241; *The Literature Relating to New Zealand: A Bibliography* (1889) 241–43, 244, 249, 251, 252, 253; review of Hocken's *Bibliography* 251–53, 317; *Sir George Grey* (1909) 253, 316
Collins, David, *Account of the English Colony in New South Wales* 138
Collins, Roger 296
Colombo 213
Colonial Gazette (Colonial Society) 82, 278
Colonial Museum 95–96, 109, 140
Colonial Office, British 110, 220–24, 297
Colquhoun, Daniel 157, 196, 197, 198, 216, 233, 267–68, 279, 282
Cook, James 17, 76, 79–80, 84, 86, 87, 98, 101, 131, 140, 152–53, 163, 197, 200; Andrew Kippis' first biography 138, plates **xxi**; botany 69; charts and maps 69, 163–64; copy of portrait at Trinity House, Hull 217, plates **xviii**; Hocken's search for correspondence 222; *Resolution* and *Adventure* medal 79; Silver's relics of expeditions 112; *A Voyage to the Pacific Ocean* (1784) 80, 101; *A Voyage Towards the South Pole and Round the World* (1777) 80, 243
Cook, James, Jr 24
Cook, Thomas 147
Cooper, George Sisson 104, 139; *Journal of an Overland Expedition from Auckland to Taranaki* (1851) 139, 172
Coote, Henry 62
Copeland, Joseph, *Lecture on the New Hebrides* (1866) 197
Copland, James, *The Origin and Spiritual Nature of Man* (1885) 129
Cornwall and York, Duke and Duchess of 211
Coromandel 142
Cotterill, George, *Literary Foundlings* (1864) 90–91
Cotterill, J.S. 104
Coulls Somerville Wilkie Ltd 292
Cowan, James, *The Adventures of Kimble Bent* (1912) 292
Cox, H. Bertram 221–22
Craig, William 88, 126
Crane, Walter 160, 214
Crawford, James Coutts 61
Creighton & Scales 255
Cridland, H.T., early depiction of Riccarton 124
Crozet, Julien Marie, *Nouveau voyage à la mer du sud* (1783) 79, 242

Culverwell, Evelyn 275
Cunningham, Allan 69
Cunningham, W.T., *New Zealand as a Tourist & Health Resort: A handbook to the hot lakes* [1893] 172

Dadelszen, Edward von 170
Dalrymple, Alexander 86, 252; *Historical Collection* 138; *A Letter from Mr Dalrymple to Dr Hawkesworth ...* (1773) plates **xxxvii**; *Scheme of a Voyage to Convey Conveniences of Life, Domestic Animals, Corn, Iron, etc to New Zealand* (1771) 79–80
Dance-Holland, Nathaniel, painting of Cook 80
Daniels, John 57
Darwin, Charles 69, 95, 113, 230; illuminated address from Otago Institute, and reply 107
Davie, George 155
Davies, Theo H., *Letter to His Grace the Archbishop of Canterbury* (1886) 172
Davis, Charles (Maori boy) 59
Davis, Charles Oliver Bond 93–95, 117, 178, 203; 'Lessons in Maori' (bound pamphlets by Davis and Leonard Williams) 95; *Life and Times of Patuone* (1876) 94; 'Maori etiquette' (1882) 95; *Maori Lesson Book* (3rd edn, 1874) 95; *Maori Mementos* (1855) 93; 'Maori names' (1882) 95; *A Maori Phrase Book* (1863) 95; 'Notes relating to the description of tikis, use and customs' (1885) 95; 'On the Maori word for the immortal principle in man' (1885) 95; *The Renowned Chief Kawiti* (1855) 93, 94; *Te Honae* (1885) 95, 139; *Temperance Songs in the Maori Language* (1873) 95
Davis, James Davidson, *Contributions towards a Bibliography of New Zealand* (1887) 237–38, 249
Davis, Richard 220
Davison, William 134, 182
Day, William 131
De Styrap, Jukes 34
Declaration of the Independence of New Zealand, facsimile (1877) 81, 82
Defence Forces 55
Delano, Amasa, *Narrative of Voyages* 138
Dell, Sharon 289
Desant, Alexander 66
Dick, Thomas 61
Dictionary of the New Zealand Language, A (1844) 91

Didsbury, George 104
Dieffenbach, Ernst 69
Dilke, Sir Charles Wentworth 212
Dillon, Peter, *Narrative and Successful Result of a Voyage in the South Seas* (1829) 137
Dixson, Sir William 18, 157, 163–64; Hocken's connections and interchanges 173–74
Dixson Gallery, Sydney 164
Dixson Library, State (formerly Public) Library of New South Wales 164
Docherty, William 86
Dodsley, Robert, *Annual Register* (1779) 79
Domett, Alfred 87, 188
Dominion 250
Donaldson, Robert, *Bush Lays and Rhymes* (1860) 97
Donlan, M.J.J., *Phormium Tenax, or Neptune New-Rigged* (1833) 72
Douglas, John 62
Dresden Pianoforte Company City Hall, Grand Tableaux Concert 120
Drew, Samuel 140
Drury, Byron, charts of New Zealand 256
Dublin 36–37
Dudley, Benjamin Thornton 'Journal of 4th Melanesian Voyage in the *Southern Cross*' 142
Dulau & Co. 159, 160
Dumont d'Urville, Jules 69, 79, 88, 163, 197, 235, 252; *Voyage autour du monde de la corvette "Astrolabe* (1826–29) 239; *Voyage de la corvette l'Astrolabe* (1830–35) 177
Duncan, A.M. 197
Duncan, C. 29–30
Dunedin 17, 97, 98–99, 161; clubs and associations 57–58, 67, 115–16; derivation of surrounding names 175; Fox, Sir William, *Dunedin* 124, 191; impact of gold discoveries 52–53; Kettle, Charles Henry, views of Dunedin 124, 130, 181, 191; naming of 126–27; population 52, 153; Princes Street plates **vi**; *Province of Otago in New Zealand ...* (1868) plates **xxxviii–xxxix**; Rattray Street, showing Hocken's house plates **vi**; Tuckett's *Sketch of the Rural District of New Edinburgh* ('Plan of the New Edinburgh settlement') (1844) 85, 132, 194; watercolour painting

(1851) 181; *see also* Hocken, Thomas
   Morland – Dunedin life; and names
   of suburbs, features, buildings, events
Dunedin City Council 259, 269, 284,
   286
Dunedin (Otago) Club 57–58, 212
Dunedin Diocesan Trust Board 280,
   304–05
Dunedin Free Public Library *see*
   Dunedin Public Library
Dunedin Lunatic Asylum 58
Dunedin Photographic Society 123
Dunedin Public Art Gallery 260, 268,
   280, 305
Dunedin Public Library 258, 261, 268,
   275, 288; McNab Collection 288
Dunedin Punch 63, 169, 295, 313, plates
   viii
Dunedin Sanitary Commission 53
Dunedin Volunteer Naval Brigade 55,
   107
Dunedin Young Men's Christian
   Association 54
Dunningham, Archie 288
Duperrey, Louis-Isadore 177; *Voyage
   autour du monde ... Histoire du voyage:
   Atlas* 138
Duppa, George, 'Part of the New
   Plymouth settlement in the district of
   Taranaki' (1841) 82, 125, 130
Duret, Marie 58
Durham, John George Lambton, Earl
   of 226
Duthie, John 264
Dymock, William 162

Earl, George Windsor, *The Eastern Seas*
   (1837) 119
Earle, Augustus: lithographic drawings of
   New Zealand 109; *A Narrative of a
   Nine Months' Residence in New Zealand*
   (1832) 102
Early History Society of Otago 120,
   135–37, 145
Early Settlers' and Historical Society,
   Wellington 98
Early Settlers' Association, Dunedin 260
Easton, Brian 296
Eccles, Alfred 61, 62, 70, 71
Echo, The 316
Eden, William, *The History of New
   Holland, from its First Discovery in
   1616, to the Present Time* (2nd edn
   1787) 21
Edgar, J.D. Charlton 289

Edge-Partington, James 225; *An Album
   of the Weapons, Tools, Ornaments, Articles
   of Dress of the Natives of the Pacific
   Islands* (1890) 225; *Third Series*
   (1898) 225–26
Edward, Francis 159, 162, 238, 244
Edwards, Ruth (later Hall) 66
Egypt 213–14, 226, 229
Elder, J.R.: Elder Collection, Hocken
   Library 292–93; *The Letters and
   Journals of Samuel Marsden*
   (1932) 236, 292; *Marsden's Lieutenants*
   (1934) 292
Elliott, Charles and James 87
Endeavour 79, 86, 200
England: Hockens' trip, 1882 108–13,
   114; Hockens' trip, 1901–04 211,
   212–13, 214–27, 229, 231; *see also*
   individual placenames
Enys, John Davies Gilbert 217
ephemera 21, 62, 72, 90, 110–11, 128,
   144, 154, 185, 241
Erskine, John Elphinstone, *Journal of a
   Cruise among the Islands of the Western
   Pacific* (1853) 174
Evening Post 169, 195, 215, 247, 249
Evening Star 181, 195, 258, 268, 269,
   285, 296, plates **ix**
Ewen, C.A. 160, 250, 285

Fairchild, John 86
Falwasser, Henry 82, 87, 128
Farquhar, Ian 296
Farsley, near Leeds 110–11; 'Description
   of the windows at Farsley
   Church' 110–11
Fawcett, George 58
Fawcett, Sandford and Tom 58
Featherston, Bethia (née Scott) 128
Featherston, Isaac 128, 188, 240
Featon, Edward Henry and Featon,
   Sarah, *The Art Album of New Zealand
   Flora* (1889) plates **xxxiv**
Fels, Willi 276
Fenwick, George 228, 236; *A Holiday
   Trip to the Catlins District* (1892) 96,
   185–86; and Hocken Library 268,
   269, 270, 274, 276, 283, 285;
   Hocken's connections and
   interchanges 32, 154, 190, 261, 263,
   264, 274, 276, 297; and Hocken's
   funeral 279; Hocken's letter, on
   opening of Hocken Library 301–03;
   'Memoir' of Hocken for publication
   of *The Early History of New*

Zealand 291; 'Memoir' of Hocken, for
 The Early History of New Zealand 291
Fernhill Club 211
Field, Arthur Nelson 251
Field, William H. 116
Fiji 157; Hockens' trip, 1898, and
 fire-walking ceremony 196, 197–99;
 at New Zealand and South Seas
 Exhibition 145, 149, 150–51
Filleul, W.G. 196
First Lessons in the Maori Language
 (1862) 92
Fitchett, A.R. 109
Fitchett, Olga, 'Dr Hocken and his
 work' 294
FitzGerald, Thomas Naghten 37
Fitzherbert 100
FitzRoy, Robert 265; *Remarks on New
 Zealand* (1846) 109, 166; *Voyages of
 the* Adventure *and* Beagle (1839) 239
F&J (newsletter, Friends of Hocken
 Collections) 296
Fleurieu, C.A. de 120
Flinders, Matthew 201; *Voyage to
 Australia* (1814) 169
Flotsam and Jetsam (F&J) volumes 21,
 58, 62, 99, 107, 111, 157, 206, 211,
 216, 221, 282, 295
Ford, Martha 101
Ford, Mary 217–18
Ford, Richard 217
Ford, Samuel 101, 149
Forster, Georg 69, 79, 138; *A Voyage
 Round the World* (1778) 80
Forster, Johann Reinhold 69, 79, 138; *A
 Journal of a Voyage Round the World in
 Her Majesty's Ship* Endeavour
 (1771) 80; *Observations Made During a
 Voyage Round the World* (1777) 80
Forty, James Edwin 231
Fowlds, George 160
Fowler, John Walker 211
Fox, Sir William 69, 82, 104, 123, 175;
 Dunedin 124, 191; sketchbook 124;
 W. Fox's House, Nelson (1848) plates
 xxxv
Frame, Janet 290
Frances Hodgkins Fellowship 290
Franklin, Benjamin, *Scheme of a Voyage to
 Convey Conveniences of Life, Domestic
 Animals, Corn, Iron, etc to New Zealand*
 (1771; 1882) 79–80, 112
Franklin, Lady 230
Fraser, John 180, 197
Free Church of Scotland 110, 135

Free Kindergarten Association,
 Dunedin 116
Freeman, Alice Mary 214, 221
French visits to New Zealand 79, 87–88
Friends of Hocken Collections 294, 296
Fulton, Robert: *An Account of the Fiji
 Fire-walking Ceremony or Vilavilairevo*
 (1902) 198; *Medical Practice in Otago &
 Southland* (1922) 293
Fulton, Robert Valpy 59; *Medical Practice
 in Otago and Southland in the Early
 Days* (1922) 55, 67

*Galtjindingamea-Pepa: Aranda –
 Wolambarinjaka* (1904) 227
Gardenhire, W.C., *Fiji and the Fijians and
 Travels among the Cannibals* (1871) 197
Garnett, Richard 214–15, 218, 221
Garrick, David 65
Geering, Lloyd 296
General Assembly Library of New
 Zealand 241, 244, 245, 268; catalogues
 (1885, 1897, supplement 1899) 241
Gilfillan family 99
Gilfillan, John Alexander 99, 225, 288; *A
 Native Council at War* 225; *Sketch of the
 Chief Hone Heke Pokai* (c. 1845) 124;
 *View in a Native Village in NZ (Interior
 of a Native Village or Pa in New
 Zealand)* 113, 224–25
Gillies, Robert 71
Gillies, T.B. 61
Gillies, Thomas 69
Gillies, William 196
Gilroy, Paddy 183
Gisborne 101, 184, 275
Godley, Charlotte 215–16, 217
Godley, John Robert 82, 215; *Letters from
 America* (1844) 215; *Writings and
 Speeches* (1863) 98
Godward, Bruce 290
goldfields: Otago 51, 52–53, 55; West
 Coast 90
Goring, Foster 106
Gourley, Hugh 145
Government Printer/Printing
 Office 104, 234, 242, 244, 246, 249,
 282, 291
Grand Hotel, Dunedin 227
Grant, J.G.S. 35, 63, 170, 269, 314, 316
Grants Braes (now Waverley),
 Dunedin 64
Gray, John 39, 43, 46, 47, 48–49, 50
Grear, William 29
Great Britain 53–54, 66, 226, plates **iv**;

Hocken's first voyage 39–43;
Hocken's second voyage 43–46;
Hocken's last voyage 47–51, plates **v**;
Hocken's theatrical
performances 45–46
Great Britain Gazette 44–45, 49
Great Britain Magazine and Weekly Screw 39–40, 50, plates **v**
'*Great Britain' Miscellany* 50
Greenwood, C.W. 188
Grey, Sir George 92, 93, 104, 132, 139, 145, 175, 202, 295, plates **xii**; *Address to Members of the New Zealand Society* (1851) 96; collecting 17, 18, 109, 157, 158–59, 163, 164, 168, 180, 237, 239–40, 241, 288, 297; Colllier, *Sir George Grey* (1909) 253, 317; *Early Printed Books* (Bleek's catalogue) (1867) 158; and George Clarke Jr 208, 209; gifting of collection to National Library (formerly South African Library), Cape Town 159–59, 166, 205; Governor of New Zealand 61, 64, 83, 179, 188, 208, 302; Grey Collection, Auckland Public Library 150, 159, 162, 163, 166, 188, 189, 229, 241, 272, 297; Hocken's articles for *Otago Witness* 188; Hocken's connections and interchanges 18, 106, 139, 157, 164–66, 224; Hocken's visits to Kawau Island 106–07, 165, 240; *Journal of Two Expeditions of Discovery in North-west and Western Australia* (1841) 158; *Ko nga mahinga a nga Tupuna Maori* (1854) 158; *Ko nga moteatea, me nga hakirara o nga Maori* (1853) 98, 158; *The Library of His Excellency Sir George Grey, K.C.B.. Philology. Vol. II. Part IV New Zealand, the Chatham Islands and the Auckland Islands* (with Bleek) (1859) 238; *Manuscripts and Incunables* (Bleek's catalogue) (1862) 158; *Maori Proverbs* (1857) 105; and New Zealand and South Seas Exhibition, 1889–90 145, 146–47, 149–50, 166; and New Zealand Exhibition, 1865 60–61; purchase of Kawau Island 159; and Robert Louis Stevenson 157; Shortland as assistant 207; and Turnbull 159, 166–67; *Vocabulary of the Dialects Spoken by the Aboriginal Races of S.W. Australia* (1839) 158
Greytown 98

Grice, James 225
Griffiths, David, *A Grammar of the Malagasy Language in the Ankova Dialect* (1845) 198
Griffiths, George 296
Griffiths, William: *On the Higher Cryptogamous Plants* 72, 73; *Icones Plantarum Asiaticarum* (1847–54) 72, 73; *Monocotyledonous Plants* 73
Grimsby, England 25–27
Groves, midshipman, 'Plan of Kawiti's pa at Ruapukepuke' 83, 84, 127
Gully, John 62, 104, 105; *New Zealand Scenery* (1877) 62; *The Peak of Mount Cook* 62
Gurner, Henry Field: *Books on the Colonies and Colonial Publications* (1878) 240; *Chronicle of Port Phillip* (1876) 240
Gurr, Edwin 197, 310
Guthrie, Walter 186

Haast, Julius von 61, 69, 95, 98, 138
Hadfield, Octavius 140, 206, 208, 210; *A Reply to the Question: Is a miracle opposed to reason?* (1875) 172; *The Second Year of One of England's Little Wars* (1861) 92
Haghe, Louis 131
Hakluyt publications 86, 112
Hakluyt Society 112
Hall, Mrs Brames 33
Hall, Ruth (née Edwards) 66
Hall, Thomas: *Full Report of the Trial of Thomas Hall for the Murder of Captain Henry Cain* 56–57
Hall, William 80, 220, 292, 302
Hallenstein, Bendix 258
Hall-Jones family 290
Hall-Jones, William 244, 246
Hamel, Christopher de 159
Hamilton, Augustus 22, 176, 286; Hocken's connections and interchanges 68, 147, 160, 184, 211, 224, 244, 246, 247, 250–51, 261, 262, 266; and New Zealand and South Seas Exhibition 147, 149, 150, 155, 156
Hamlin, James 209, 302
Hammond, Thomas Godfrey 180
Handcock, William, *City of Dunedin* (1864) 65
Hansard, George Albert, 'Voyage of the *Acheron*, Part 3rd (1849–51) plates **xxxi**

Hanson, Richard Davies 87
Hardwick, Jane 96
Hardy, Charles 56
Hardy, Edwin 79
Hardy, Henry Frederick 67, 131, 185
Hare, William 77
Hargreaves, Ray 296
Harper, Henry John Chitty 90–91; *[A charge delivered ... on the] Report of the Education Commissioners* (1864) 90; 'A ketch' 91; *Alms-giving: A sermon* 90
Harris, John 288–89
Harris, John Hyde 57, 58, 123, 136, 181
Harvard-Williams, Peter 289
Harwood, Octavius 146
Hastings, D.D. 156
Hatton, James Wright 111
Hawea 98
Hawke's Bay Herald 170, 316
Hawke's Bay Times 170, 316
Hawkesworth, John 86, 200; *An Account of the Voyages Undertaken by order of His Present Majesty for Making Discoveries in the Southern Hemisphere* (1773) 80, 125, 243
Hawthorne, James, *A Dark Chapter from New Zealand History* (1905) 247
Hayward, C. & W. 280
He Kupu Whakamarama, Nos 5, 6 and 9 (1898) 93
Heale, Theophilus 175
Heaphy, Charles 104; *Nelson from the Gaol* (1859) 105, 130; sketch of Port Nicholson 82; two views of Wellington (1841) 130; 'View of Nelson Haven, in Tasman's Gulf, New Zealand' (1841) 128, 130
Hearne, Tom 47
Heberley, James 182
Hector, James 61, 69, 71, 86, 95, 109, 116, 145, 212; *Phormium Tenax as a Fibrous Plant* (1872; 1889) 72
Heeres, J.E. 186
Heihachiro, Togo 228
Heke, Hone 83, 101, 117, 128, 149, 190, 203
Henning, Rachel 39
Henry, Richard 86, 123, 182
Herbert Haynes Co. Ltd 280
Herd, James 147–48, 181, 182
Héroïne 88
Hexateuch (1848) 91
Hight, James 293
Highwic, Auckland 114
Hill, Henry T. 183–84, 203, 205–06

Hill, Richard 91
Hinemoa: A love song (1881) 129
Historical Records of New South Wales 226, 232
Hitchings, Michael 289
Hobbs, John 91
Hobson, Eliza 125
Hobson, William 152, 188, 189, 207, 265
Hochstetter, Ferdinand von 69
Hocken, A.G. 296; *Dr Hocken of Dunedin: A life* (2008) 17, 55, 66, 114, 117; *Dr T.M. Hocken 1836–1910: A gentleman of his time* (1986) 17
Hocken, Andorania 25
Hocken, Anne (née Richardson) 24–25, 26, 27, 34, plates **ii**
Hocken Collections (previously Hocken Library), University of Otago 170, 171, 188–89; acquisitions, since opening 281, 282, 286, 288, 289, 290; Anzac Avenue premises 290; care and preservation of materials 271, 274, 277, 282, 286, 287; *Catalogue of the Hocken Library* (1912) 70, 217, 228, 281–83, 287, plates **xxiii**; control moved from museum to university library 288; deed of gift 270–71, 287, 294; fellowships 290, 296; Friends of Hocken Collections 294, 296; gifts and bequests 281, 282, 286, 288, 289, 290, 292–93; Hocken Picture Room 272, 273; Hocken Wing, Otago Museum 270, 271–74, 275, 276–77, 279, 280, 286–87, 290, plates **xviii, xix**; Hocken's letter to Fenwick on occasion of official opening 301–03; Hocken's provision for librarian 280; 'Journal of Librarian' (Trimble) 275, 277; *Ka Taoka Hakena: Treasures from the Hocken Collections* (Strachan and Tyler) (2007) 294; librarians and staff 280, 287–89, 294, 302–03, 305–06, 308 (*see also* Trimble, William Heywood); monetary value 282, 284; official opening 275–78; online use of collections 294; relocations 290; research and publications by users of collections 291–94; titles from Ralph library 73; use of collection 271, 272–73, 281, 283, 284, 288, 289, 294–95; visitor, to make regular inspections 271; *see also* Hocken, Thomas Morland: library; and types of materials, e.g. manuscripts

Hocken, Eliza Anne 25, 27, 34
Hocken, Elizabeth (Bessie) Mary (née Buckland) 19, 114–25, 157, 176, 181, 183, 188, 191, 192, 264, 279, plates **x**; *Arrested Attention* 123, 295, plates **xiv**; artist 122–25, 151, 224, 295; *Citadel, Cairo* plates **xvi**; close relationship with Morland 120–22, 139; copying and transcribing of works 124–25, 127, 134, 188, 222, 224, 235; and death of Morland 279, 280, 304, 306; duplicates sent to Turnbull after Morland's death 171; embroidered tablecloth in Hocken Collection 116; and Endowment Fund 285, 286; *Kowhai and Ribbonwood* 151; and Morland's 'Life of Marsden' project 235–36, 291; *Mother's Treasure Box* (1895) 123; *Mr Wohlers' Church and School House* (1896) 122, 123; *Mr Wohlers' Grave, Ringaringa Point, Stewart Island* (1896) 122, 123; musical skills 120, 136; *The Old Mission Station at Waikouaiti* (1887) (watercolour) 122, 123; *Old Mission Station, Waikouaiti* (photograph) 123; photographer 68, 123, 190, 197, 206, 216, 295; publication of lectures on the early colonisation of New Zealand 291; *Ruins of the Rev. J.F. Wohlers' House* (1896) 122, 123; season ticket to New Zealand and South Seas Exhibition plates **xi**; *Takahe (Notornis mantelli)* (1895) 122–23; translation skills 119–20, 177, 186, 228; travel to Fiji and Samoa, 1898 196, 197; travel to Japan, England and Europe, 1901–04 212, 213, 215, 216, 222, 226; and Trimble 281, 284
Hocken, Ersca 306, 308
Hocken, Gladys (later Le François) 39, 115, 116, 117, 118–19, 120, 121, 122, 175, 176, 218; *Arrested Attention*, photograph with father, by Bessie Hocken 123, 295, plates **xiv**; and Hocken Library 276, 286; and Hocken's will 304, 308; *Mother's Treasure Box*, photograph by Bessie Hocken 123; music 216, 226, 227; season ticket to New Zealand and South Seas Exhibition plates **xi**; travel diary, trip to Japan, England and Europe, 1901–04 212, 213, 215, 216, 217, 219, 220, 221, 223, 224, 226, 227;
travel to Fiji and Samoa, 1898 196, 197
Hocken, Hamilton 225
Hocken, James Richardson 24, 25, 26, 30, 34
Hocken, John Wesley 25
Hocken, Joshua (brother) 24, 25, 26, 30, 110
Hocken, Joshua (father) 24–26, 27–28, 34, 35, plates **ii**; *A Brief History of the Wesleyan Methodism, in the Grimsby Circuit* (1839) 27, plates **ii**; *Hints and Helps to Local Preachers* (1845) 28
Hocken, Julia Anne Dayke (née Simpson) 66, 107
Hocken Collections Committee 290
Hocken Endowment Memorial Fund 284–87, 290
Hocken Lecture 296
Hocken Library Trustees 268, 269, 276, 286–87, 303, 306; 'The Hocken Collection' 272
Hocken Memorial Committee 284
Hocken, Thomas Morland
 A Bibliography of the Literature Relating to New Zealand (1909) 18, 28, 92, 137, 171, 178, 234, 235, 240, 243–46, 247–49, 258, 317, plates **xxii**; Collier's review 251–53, 317; driving force for Hocken Library acquisitions 288; individual responses to 250–51; printed Maori publications component 203, 246, 251, 252, 278; reinforcement of Hocken's legacy 290–91; reviews 249–50, 251–53; Wilson's account and later review 245–46, 251
 biographies of: Fitchett, Olga, 'Dr Hocken and his work' 17, 294; Hocken, A.G., *Dr Hocken of Dunedin: A life* (2008) 17, 55, 66, 114, 117; Hocken, A.G., *Dr T.M. Hocken 1836–1910: A gentleman of his time* (1986) 17; McCormick, E.H., *The Fascinating Folly: Dr Hocken and his fellow collectors* 17, 288; Ross, John, article on Hocken in *Dictionary of Literary Biography* 17
 caricatures and lampooning of 58–59, 63, 247, 295, plates **viii, xl, xvii**
 childhood and schooling: baptism 26; family and birth 24–26; first attempt at writing 26; Sunday school 26–27; Woodhouse Grove boarding school 28, 29–33

collecting: completist approach 111; first recorded item 59–60; lifelong activity 296–98; local and indigenous 297; oldest book 70; reasons for 84, 276, 278, 296–97; *see also* Hocken, Thomas Morland: library

collecting: annotations on works collected 54, 60, 63, 64–65, 77, 91, 93, 95, 123, 125, 127, 148, 154, 172, 173, 179, 197, 214, 253, 265, 267, 281, plates **xxxv, xxxix, xxxvii**

collecting: process 17–18; advertising 102–03, plates **ix**; book dealers 18, 101, 102, 108–10, 127, 138, 159–60, 162, 179, 190 217, 226, 241, 291, 297; connections and interchanges with Grey, Turnbull, Mitchell and Dixson 157–74 (*see also* index entries for each of these collectors; and other collectors, e.g. Smith, Stephenson Percy); gifts and exchanges 18, 90, 98, 128 *see also under* types of material, e.g. manuscripts); importance of Otago Institute 18, 70–72; New Zealand Exhibition, 1865 62–63; during overseas travel 73–74; personal networking 72–73, 90, 175–83, 196, 200–05, 214, 225, 238, 240, 241–43, 246, 247, 309–18 (*see also* Hocken, Thomas Morland – travel, New Zealand; Hocken, Thomas Morland – travel, overseas); subscription copies 129; William Larnach's library sale 169–70, 173, 315

collecting: provenance markers: bookplates 20, 21, 97, 113, 139, 295; hei tiki stamp and label 20, 21, 97, 172, 295, plates **xxxvi, xxxix**; signatures 20–21, 97, 139, 168, 173, 295, plates **xxvi, xl, xxxix**

collecting: subjects: Australia 18, 76, 86, 201–02, 231, 232, 297; change from natural environment to local and national history 76–77; early settlement and colonisation 17, 69, 81–82, 90, 92, 98, 102–03, 152, 154, 181, 220–24, 267, 278; explorers, other than Cook 79–80, 137–38, 197, 278, 302; Japanese materials 226, 228, 276, 302; Otago Benevolent Institute 58; Pacific Islands 62–63, 137–38, 142, 152, 197; *see also* botanical collecting and interests of Hocken; Cook, James; Maori, Hocken's collecting; Maori language; Marsden, Samuel; missionaries; New Zealand Company; Wakefield, Edward Gibbon

collecting: types of material 17; copies or facsimiles 81, 82, 85, 91, 124–25, 127, 134, 166, 188, 202, 216, 222; presentation copies 72, 75, 91, 92, 96, 129, 154, 172, 176, 186, 201, 206, 227, 247, 254, plates **xxxvi**; *see also* artefacts; bibliographies; ephemera; manuscripts; maps, charts and plans; newspapers; oral history records; paintings and drawings; pamphlets; photographs; tokens

Contributions to the Early History of New Zealand (Settlement of Otago) (1898) 18, 75, 85, 132, 168, 181, 189–90, 309, plates **xix**; Bessie Hocken's illustrations and key plan 124; copies given to other people 207, 211, 218; dedication to Bessie Hocken 125; personal responses to 195–96, 215; publication 129, 190–95, 258; reinforcement of Hocken's legacy 290; reviews 195

death, funeral and tributes 279–80; *see also* Hocken, Thomas Morland: will

Dunedin life: arrival in Dunedin 17, 52–54; clubs and associations joined 57–58; comments and notes on 63–65; light moments 58–59; New Zealand Exhibition, 1865 61–63 return from travel to Japan and England, 1904 227–28

educator 19, 77, 83–84, 88, 129, 189, 228

fellowships: Linnean Society 20, 111, 112–13, 114 Royal Anthropological Institute 225–26

health: on board SS *Great Britain* 48; final illness (carcinoma of the oesophagus) 148, 171, 176, 212, 213, 216, 226, 235, 253, 273, 276, 277, 279, 301, 317; flu, 1897 192; reason for emigration to New Zealand 37

historian: Early History Society of Otago 135–37, 145; New Zealand and South Seas Exhibition, Dunedin, 1889–90 145–51, 152–53, 154, 156; reputation as authority on New Zealand history 88–89, 126 homes (as an adult): 40 Kildare Terrace, Westminster, London 216, 220, 223, plates **xvi**; 128 Princes Street, Dunedin 57; Atahapara, Dunedin 20, 67–69, 71, 115–16, 227, 296, 306, plates **viii**; Rattray Street, Dunedin 57, 67, plates **vi**

lectures 18, 106, plates **xiii**; *Abel Tasman and His Journal* (1895) 119–20, 186–87; on botany (17 December 1862) 54–55; on Canterbury (1891) 180; 'Decrease in the number of whales' (1870) 76–77; on early history of New Zealand (1880; 1884; 1886) 79–80, 81–84, 126, 134, 165, 166, 291; 'Early visits of the French to New Zealand' (1907) 87–88; on Fijian fire-walking ceremony (1898) 198; 'Hot springs of New Zealand' (1877) 77; 'Japan: Its people and its industries' (1904) 227; 'Maoris of the South Island' (1901) 211; on Marsden (1905–06) 80–81, 232; 'Notes on the derelict ship in Facile Harbour, Dusky Bay' (1887) 85–86, 113; 'Some account of the beginnings of literature in New Zealand: Part 1, the Maori section' (1900) 86–87, 202–03; 'Some account of the beginnings of literature in New Zealand: Part II, the English newspapers' (1901) 87, 211, 230; 'Some account of the earliest literature and maps relating to New Zealand' (1894) 86; on Southland and Otago (1877) 84–85, 88, 125, 126

library 126–27, 161; article by Mr Stephens on *Evening Post* 170; draft catalogue (1887) 137–38, 140, 237, plates **xxi**; Hocken's summation, 1906 264–65; loans from 178, 182–83; monetary value 245, 261; Wilson's account 245; *see also* Hocken Library, University of Otago

library: compilations and bound volumes 199; '21 Important Letters, 1876–96' 90, 182; Flotsam and Jetsam (F&J) volumes 21, 58, 62, 99, 107, 111, 144, 157, 206, 211, 216, 221, 282, 295; 'Maori School Books' 97; pamphlet volumes 21, 58, 72, 92, 95, 98, 113, 118, 127, 129, 142, 165–66, 169, 173, 176, 180, 201, 254, 277, 281, 282, 295; *Variae* volumes 21, 143, 176, 198, 282, 295

library, gifting of 188–89, 258–59, 297, 298; art gallery and Early Settlers' building as possible site 260, 261, 263; Cohen's proposal for new building 259–60; custody question 262, 265, 268, 269, 270, 271, 280, 284, 302–03, 305–06, 308; deed of gift 270–71; future usage 266; government contribution to housing of collection 262–63, 264, 267, 268, 271, 276, 287; 'Hocken Equipment Fund' *(Evening Star)* 270; Hudson's offer of finance 258; letter to Fenwick on occasion of Hocken Library opening 301–03; Otago Museum as possible site 260–61, 262, 263, 267–68, 269; railway site proposal 262, 263, 267, 268; subscription fund for housing of collection 261, 263–64, 267, 268, 269–70, 271, 276, 287; *see also* Hocken Library, University of Otago

marriages: Bessie 19, 114–25 (*see also* Hocken, Elizabeth (Bessie) Mary (née Buckland)); Julia 66, 107; proposal to Miss Sampson, on board *Great Britain* 44

medical career 21; coroner, Dunedin 55–57, 107, 108, plates **viii**; Dunedin practice 53–54, 59; intention to upgrade medical qualifications in England 213; Inter-Colonial Medical Congress, 1896 175; medical assessor for Otago province 77; president, Otago Medical Association 55; qualifications 37; surgeon, Dunedin Volunteer Naval Brigade, and Defence Forces 55, 107; surgeon-superintendent, *Great Britain* 39–51, 66; surgeon-superintendent, *White Star* 37–39, 66; training as apothecary 34–35; training as surgeon 35–37

memorials: *Balantiopsis Hockeni Berggr.,* liverwort named by Berggren 75; Hocken Lecture 296; Hocken Library Fellows 290, 296; Hocken

Street, Kenmure, Dunedin 295;
plaque to commemorate
Atahapara 296
names: different versions 19; Maori
version, Hakena 20, 172;
nicknames 46; noms-de-plume 40
personal characteristics: amiability 38;
authority 46; busy man 55, 60;
courage 46; courtesy 38;
energy 43, 44; enthusiasm 22, 46,
89, 117; hat wearing 63; 'intellectual
feasting' 46, 47–48;
intelligence 215; judgemental
comments 140; kindness 39, 43;
likeability 22; methodical
approach 22; outgoing
personality 90; persistence 18, 21,
22, 148–49; presence 21, 60;
self-assurance and confidence 63,
84; small stature 21, 43, 44, 46, 47,
63; social skills 90; vision 22
portraits and photographs: by Fanny
Wimperis, pastel on paper
portrait 295; by Halliday Scott,
charcoal sketch 295;
photographs 295, **ix**, plates **vii, x,
xi, xiii, xiv, xv**; *see also* Hocken,
Thomas Morland: caricatures and
lampooning of
religion: chaplain, SS *Great
Britain* 43–44, 48; Christian
faith 48, 57; church activities,
Dunedin 175; Church of
England 57, 90, 91, 175, 280,
304–05; Methodist upbringing and
schooling 26–27, 28, 29–33, 41
travel, New Zealand: Auckland,
Tauranga, Napier and Hot Springs
area, 1871 77–78, 90; Bay of Islands,
1880 87; Catlins district, 1892 96,
185–86; Christchurch, Nelson,
Wellington, Wanganui, Taranaki,
Kawau Island, 1881 104–07;
Christchurch, Wellington, Wanganui,
1888 139–41; Dunedin overland to
Bay of Islands, 1879 90, 94, 97–103;
Milford Sound, 1901 211; northern
trip, 1895 175, 183–85; northern
trip, 1897 175, 188; northern trip,
1905 229–30; northern trip,
1906 225; northern trip, 1907 233;
Oamaru and Christchurch,
1894 175, 179; Rotorua, 1909 279;
Ruapuke Island, 1896 97, plates **x**;
Stewart Island region, 1895 175,
183; Tauranga, Taupo and Hot
Springs area, 1875 78, 90, 93, 229;
Timaru, Christchurch, Wellington,
Picton, Nelson, Taranaki, Auckland,
1885 138–39; West Coast,
1876 93–94
travel, overseas: England, 1882 108–13,
114; Fiji and Samoa, 1898 157,
196–99, 258, 310; Japan, England
and Europe, 1901–04 73, 88, 119,
211–28, 229, 297; Melbourne,
1910 279
will 279–80, 285, 304–08;
beneficiaries 280, 304–06, 308; value
of estate 280
writing and editing 18, 129; *A Holiday
Trip to the Catlins District* (1892) 96,
185–86; *Abel Tasman and His Journal*
(1895) 86, 119–20, 186–87, 230;
articles for *Cabinet* 49; articles for
Great Britain Gazette 44–45, 49;
articles for *Great Britain Magazine
and Weekly Screw* 40–41, 42; articles
for '*Great Britain' Miscellany* 50;
'Collected papers' project 225; *Early
History of New Zealand, The*
(1914) 18, 83, 85, 142, 188, 200–01,
223–24, 236, 291, plates **xxii**; 'Early
pictorial illustrations of New
Zealand' (1884) 129–31; 'Early
statesmen and public men of New
Zealand' (1895) 188; experience of
writing, editing and publishing
shipboard magazines 50–51; first
appearance in print, *Lancet*
article 41; 'Historical notes' (started
1893 and 1897) 175; history of
Canterbury province 180, 202; letter
to *Otago Daily Times,* 'A Maori
house for Dunedin' 156; life of
Marsden 80, 231–36, 246, 291;
Maning, Frederick, *Old New Zealand*
new edition (1907) 254–55, 291,
plates xxxvii; 'New Zealand notes'
(between 1893 and 1897) 96, 175;
reliance on documentary sources 27;
'Some account of the beginnings of
literature in New Zealand: Part 1,
the Maori section' (1900) 86–87,
202–03; 'Some account of the
earliest explorations in New
Zealand' (1891) 185; style 27; 'The
governors of New Zealand'
(1896) 188; 'The mythology of the
Maori,' 42; translation of part of

Tasman's journal relating to New
Zealand 186–87, 211, 213; Webster,
John, *Reminiscences of an Old Settler
in Australia and New Zealand*
(1908) 255–57, 291; *see also*
Hocken, Thomas Morland:
Bibliography ... ; Hocken, Thomas
Morland: *Contributions to the Early
History of New Zealand (Settlement of
Otago)* (1898)
Hocken, William Henry 25, 30, 110
Hockin, John 20
Hockin, Thomas 20
Hodges, William 79, 164
Hodgkin, Thomas and George 279
Hodgkins, Frances 151, 229, 290
Hodgkins, Isabel Jane 116, 151
Hodgkins, William Mathew 57, 104, 151
Hodgkinson, Samuel 85, 132, 134;
Provincialism versus Centralism
(1868) 132
Hogan, P.J. 131
Hokianga 127, 148, 181, 182, 206, 230,
256; *see also* individual placenames
Hokioi, Te 170
Hokitika 90
Holgate, C.W., *An Account of the Chief
Libraries of New Zealand* 127
Holmes, William 224; *The Canterbury
Plains from the Heathcote River*
(1851) 125, 224
Hongi Hika 147, 149, 234
Hooker, Joseph Dalton 230; *Flora
Antarctica* (1847) 70; *Flora Novae-
Zelandiae* (1855) 70; *Flora Tasmaniae*
(1860) 70; *Handbook of New Zealand
Flora* (1864–67), notes by Hocken 74
Hooker, Sir William Jackson: *Companion
to the Botanical Magazine* (1835) 70;
*Directions for Collecting and Preserving
Plants in Foreign Countries* (1834) 70;
Icones Plantarum (1837) 70; *Species
Filicum, &c.* (1861) 70
Hooper, Thomas 98
Horsburgh, James 129, 190, 193
Horsfall, John Sutcliffe 117, 264
hot springs district, North Island 77, 78,
229
Hough, William 105
Houston, Margaret 56–57
Howard, Basil 293
Howes, Beatrice 287
Howorth, Henry 55, 57, 66
Hoyte, John Barr Clark,
watercolours 289

Hudson, Richard 258
Hume, Mary and Elizabeth 110
Hunter, Alexander 44, 46, 63
Huntington, Henry 297
Hursthouse, Charles Flinders 132; *The
Incorporation of Britain's Colonial with
her Home Empire* (1866) 105; *Letters
on Colonisation* (1866) 132; *The New
Zealand Handbook* (1866) 172; *New
Zealand: The Britain of the south*
(1861) 132; *New Zealandia or
Zealandia: The Britain of the south*
(1857) 98, 132
Hursthouse, Charles Wilson 176
Hutton, Frederick 96, 294

Imperial Hotel, Dunedin 108
Imperial Songs 228
Industrial Exhibition, 1862, Dunedin 57,
60, 144
Inter-Colonial Medical Congress,
1896 175

Jackson, Benjamin Daydon 111
Jackson, F. Arthur, *Fire-walking in Fiji,
Japan, India and Mauritius* (1899) 228
Jackson, Thomas 138
Jacobs, Dean 138, 203, 294
Jacobs, Henry 126
Japan 211, 212, 213, 224, 226, 227–28
Japan Daily Herald, publication of
Hocken's talk on Fijian
fire-walking 198
Japan Society 214; *Transactions* 228
Jarvey, Catherine 56
Jarvey, Elizabeth Ann 56
Jarvey, William Andrew, murder case 56,
175, 312
Jeffreys, Charles 63
Jeffreys, William 63
Jenkins, Mrs A. 149
Jenkins, William 148
Jenkins, W.N. 148
Jervois, Sir William F. Drummond 145,
188
'Jewlius Rex' 169, 313
Jobson, F.J. 148
Jobson, Rev. Dr and Mrs 33
Joel, Grace 229
Johnson, John 125
Johnstone, A.H., *Supplement to Hocken's
Bibliography of New Zealand Literature*
(1927) 290
Jones, Antonia 43, 45
Jones, Henry Festings 171

Jones, John (Wesleyan preacher, England) 26
Jones, Johnny (whaler and merchant) 103, 128; promissory notes (1855) 181
Jones, Mrs Stanley, *Handbook to the Ferns of New Zealand* 70
Jones, Sara 66
Jones, Shadrach Edward Robert 63–64
Jones, Sir Robert 296
Jordan, Henry, *Emigration to the New Colony of Australia* (1860) 172
Jose, Arthur W., *A Short History of Australasia* (1899) 202
Joubert, Jules: *Proposed New Zealand Exhibition in London* (1890) 154; *Shavings and Scrapes* (1890) 154
Journal of the Polynesian Society 142, 227, 228
Jowett, William 91
Jubilee Convalescent Fund 116
Justice Department records 289

Kahanga Club, Dunedin 115–16, 120
Karaitiana 156
Karere Maori, Te (the *Maori Messenger*) 93, 140, 203–06, 313, 316, plates **xxiii**
Karetai (Jacky White) 123, 186
Karetai, Alice 211
Kawau Island 106–07, 159
Kawiti 83, 101; 'Plan of Kawiti's Pa at Ruapekapeka' (1846) 83, 84, 127
Kelly, John L., *The South Sea Islands: Possibilities of trade with New Zealand* (1885) 197
Kemp, Henry Tacy 92, 181–82, 302
Kendall, Thomas 80, 175, 220, 225, 292, 302; *A Grammar and Vocabulary of the Language of New Zealand* (1820) 69, 109, 138, 203, plates **xxviii**; *A Korao o New Zealand* (1815) 69, 205
Kennedy, Rodney 289
Kerr, John 38
Kerry-Nicholl, J.H., *The King Country; or Explorations in New Zealand* (1884) 159
Kettle, C.C. 135, 136
Kettle, Charles Henry: Letterbook of Charles Henry Kettle, Chief Surveyor of the Settlement of Otago (1846–50) 128; *Lower Harbour at Port Chalmers* 124, 130; *Map of Suburban Lands in Settlement of Otago* (1849) 181; *View of Dunedin* (1849) 124, 130, 191; *View of part of Dunedin and Upper Harbour from Stafford Street* (1849) 181
Kidderminster Shuttle & Worcester Mercury 184
Kinder, John 142, 204, 206; collection of photographs and paintings in Hocken Library 288; *Remarks on the Report of the Commissioners on the General Synod* (1901) 206
King, Frederic Truby 228
King, James, *A Voyage to the Pacific Ocean* (1784) 80
King, John 80, 292, 302
King, Philip Gidley 234
King, Thomas 105
Kingswood School 29
Kinloch 116, 117, 122
Kinsey, Joseph 237
Kippis, Andrew, first biography of Cook 138, plates **xxi**
Kirk, Thomas 69, 113, 140
Kirk, W.H. 140
Knight, Charles 69
Knox, Frederick John 77
Knox, Robert 77
Kororareka 83, 101, 102, 221; *see also* Russell
Kupu Whakamarama, He, Nos 5, 6 and 9 (1898) 93

Labillardière, Jacques, *Voyage* 138
Laing, Robert M. 185
Lake Tarawera 78
Lanarch, Donald 66
Lancaster, G.B. (Edith Lyttleton) 251
Lancet, The 41
Landfall archive 290
Lang, Andrew 198; *Magic and Religion* (1901) 198; 'The fire walk ceremony in Tahiti' (1901) 198
Langley, S.P., 'The fire walk ceremony in Tahiti' (1901) 198
Laplace, Cyrille, *Voyage autour du monde par les mers de l'Inde et de Chine* (1833) 88
Larnach, Eliza 66
Larnach, James, *A Bibliographical History of Australia* (1855) 173
Larnach, William 66, 169–70, 173, 186, 315
Latour, H.A. de, *Education in Relation to Public Health* (1887) 129
Lawes, William George 180; *Grammar and Vocabulary of Language spoken by Motu Tribe, New Guinea* 180

Lawlor, Pat 23
Lawrence, George 261, 262
Lay Association 110
Le François, Alan plates xiv
Leach, Helen 296
Lee, John A. 68
Lee, Mary Isabella 68
Lee, Samuel, *A Grammar and Vocabulary of the Language of New Zealand* (1820) 69, 109, 138, 203, plates **xxviii**
Lesson, René Primevère 177, 252
Lewis, Wilmarth 293
Leys, J.W. 255
Lindsay, William Lauder 54, 75; *Contributions to New Zealand Botany* (1868) 54; *Observations on New Zealand Lichens* (1866) 54; 'The place and power of natural history in colonization' (1862; 1863) 54
Linnaeus, Carl 111
Linnean Society, London 111–12, 215, 216–17; Hocken's Fellowship 20, 111, 112–13, 114; Hocken's speech, 1903 217; Turnbull's Fellowship 160
Literary Foundlings (1864) 90–91, 170
Livingstone, William 192
Lloyd, Arthur 228
Lloyd, Taggart & Co. 57
Lloyd, William 57
Locke, Samuel 101
London 108–10, 111–13, 119, 159, 214–15, 216–26
Lord, William 29, 32
Lubbock, Sir John 239
Lycett, Joseph 149
Lyell, Charles 48, 95, 113; *Principles of Geology* 48
Lyttelton 104, 131
Lyttelton, Lord 90, 221; *Memorandum* (1854) 165
Lyttelton Times 98, 139–40
Lyttleton, Captain 43
Lyttleton, Edith (G.B. Lancaster) 251

Macandrew, James 135, 136; promissory notes (1853) 181
McCahon, Colin 289, 290
McCormick, E.H. (Eric) 130, 288; *The Fascinating Folly: Dr Hocken and his fellow collectors* 17, 288
MacDonald, Sir Claude 213
McDonald, David 294
McDonald, Rachel Walker 288
McDonnell, A.F. 284
Macdonnell, Thomas 99
McDonogh, Arthur Edward, *To the Inhabitants of Wellington and its Vicinity* (1843) 97
MacDougall, Donald, *The Conversion of the Maoris* (1899) 173
McEldowney, Jock 289
McGlashan, Edward 65, 72
McGlashan, John 54, 127
McGlashan, Miss 132
McIndoe, John 136
Mack, Jane 47, 48
Mackay, Alexander: *Land Purchases, Middle Island: Report* (1875) 131; *Memorandum ... on the Origin of New Zealand Company's 'Tenths' Native Reserves* (1873) 131
Mackay, John 244, 245, 247, 248, 253
McKellar, J. 176
McKenzie, Thomas (printer) 140
Mackenzie, Thomas Noble (politician) 279
McKerrow, James 247; 'On the physical geography of the lake district of Otago' 247
McLachlan, Robert 111
McLean, Donald 205
MacLean, Douglas 270
McLean, Thomas, Jr 108, 110
McLean, Thomas, Sr 108
McLintock, A.H. 52–53, 293
McMillan, James 188
Macmillan Publishers 190
McNab, Robert 109, 160, 161, 234, 251, 261, 265–66, 282, 284–85, 293; Dunedin Public Library, McNab Collection 288; fundraising lecture, 'The early history of New Zealand' 285–86; *Historical Records of New Zealand* 246, 265, 293; *From Tasman to Marsden* (1914) 292
McNichol, Elizabeth 34
McNichol, Robert 34, 35
McOwan, Peter 32
Madden, John 104
Maggs Bros Ltd 162
Magra, James, *A Journal of a Voyage Round the World in His Majesty's Ship Endeavour* 200
Main, G.M. 204
Mair, Gilbert 77, 150, 203, 209, 230
Mair, Robert 230
Maketu, Wiremu Kingi (Maketu Wharetotara) 207–08, 209
Malcolm, Margaret 308

Manawatu Gorge 100
Maning, Frederick 124, 127, 129, 154; *Hine-moa: A Maori love song* (1881) 101; *History of the War in the North of New Zealand* (1864) plates **xxxvii**; obituary plates **xxxvii**; *Old New Zealand* (1863) 101; *Old New Zealand,* new edition (1907) 254–55, 291
Mantell, Gideon 95, 140; *A Pictorial Atlas of Fossil Remains* (1850) 97
Mantell, Walter Baldock Durrant 69, 87, 95–97, 118, 129, 175, 176, 178, 183, 237; 'Lay of the disappointed' (1851) 97; *The Ostrich and Some Allied Birds Now Extinct* (1850) 97
Manukau 235
manuscripts: Hocken Library, University of Otago 275, 276, 278, 280, 282, 283, 284, 285, 288, 289, 290, 292, 294, 295
manuscripts: Hocken's collecting 17, 18, 21, 83, 126, 141, 148, 152, 153, 157, 175, 185, 193, 247, 298; annotations 60, 127, 253; botanical manuscripts 74, 91; copying 125, 133, 134; extent and descriptions of collection 21, 137, 154, 189, 265, 266, 284–85, 302; first recorded item 60; in F&J volumes 107, 157; gifts 90, 97, 100, 128, 131, 132, 133, 141–42, 176, 183, 198, 206–07; Hocken's provenance markers 20; King's papers 234; letters 90, 107 131, 132, 133, 176, 206, 209, 210, 215–16, 230, 234, 302; manuscripts on and by Maori 60, 74, 81, 181, 203 217; missionary manuscripts 69 81, 142, 220, 229, 230, 231, 232, 234, 236, 283, 292, 302; in pamphlet volumes 72, 176; purchases 18; Selfe's papers 218–19; Shortland's papers 206–07, 217; Tuckett papers 131–35, 191–92, plates **xxiv–v**; in 'Variae' volumes 21, 176, 198
Maori: Dusky Sound 182; health and disease 59–60; Hocken's article, 'The mythology of the Maori' 42; Hocken's *Bibliography,* printed Maori publications component 203, 246, 251, 252, 277; Hocken's investigations into connection with Japanese 213; Hocken's lectures 77, 86–87, 202–03; Hocken's observations while travelling 77, 78; land 92, 95, 96–97, 99, 105, 181, 207, 208; Maori Carnival, 1901 211; New Zealand and South Seas Exhibition 144, 146, 147, 148, 149, 150, 152, 153, 154, 155, 156; New Zealand Exhibition, 1865 61–62; presentation of illuminated address to Duke and Duchess of Cornwall and York 211; at Wairoa, Hocken's visit 78; *see also* New Zealand Wars; and individual books about Maori
Maori, Hocken's collecting 17, 62–63, 81, 94, 105, 302; artefacts 21, 68, 69, 94, 117, 152, 156, 183–84, 276, 280, 302, plates **xv**; manuscripts on and by Maori 60, 74, 81, 181, 203, 217; paintings and sketches 33, 68, 104, 108, 148–49, 188, 224–25, plates **xxxvi**; pamphlets 95; plans of pa 69, 83, 84, 127, 255; *see also* Maori language
Maori language 87, 91, 178–79, 180, 202–06, 209, 264, 277, 295, 302; Anglican Book of Prayer in Maori 227; Atkinson, A.S., *Notes on the Maori-Polynesian Comparative Dictionary of Mr E. Tregear* (1893) 92; Bunyan, John, *Pilgrim's Progress,* Maori translations 109, 179, 230; 'Collation of volume of scripture extracts, etc. seen through the press by Rev.Yate & printed at Sydney, New South Wales, in 1830[?]' 316; Davis, Charles Oliver Bond, *A Maori Phrase Book* (1863) 95; Davis, Charles Oliver Bond, *Maori Lesson Book* (3rd edn, 1874) 95; Davis, Charles Oliver Bond, 'Maori names' (1882) 95; Davis, Charles Oliver Bond, *Te Honae* (1885) 95, 139; Davis, Charles Oliver Bond, *Temperance Songs in the Maori Language* (1873) 95; first complete Maori Bible (1868) 91; *First Lessons in the Maori Language* (1862) 92–93; Grey, George, *Ko Nga Moteatea* (1853) 98; *He Kupu Whakamarama,* Nos 5, 6 and 9 (1898) 93; Kendall, Thomas, *A Korao o New Zealand* (1815) 69, 205; Kendall, Thomas and Lee, Samuel, *A Grammar and Vocabulary of the Language of New Zealand* (1820) 69, 109, 138, 203, plates **xxviii**; *Ko nga Katikihama e wa* (1833) 203; *Ko te Kawenata Hou o to Tatou Ariki o te Kai Wakaora o Ihu Karaiti* (New Testament) (1842) 203;

Ko te Kawenata Hou o to Tatou Ariki o te Kai Whakaora o Ihu Karaiti (New Testament) (1852, W233) 120; *Ko te Rongo Pai i tuhituhia e Ruka* (1835) plates **xxvi**; *Ko te tahi wahi o te Kawenata Tawhito* (1848) 188, plates **xxvii**; 'Lessons in Maori' (bound pamphlets by Davis and Leonard Williams) 95; *Maori Lesson Book* (3rd edn, 1874) 95; Maori version of service for ordination of priests (c. 1860) 92; *Maori-Polynesian Comparative Dictionary* (1891) 92; Maunsell, Robert, *Grammar of the New Zealand Language* (Maunsell) (1862) 141; New Testament in Maori (1844) 91, 203; Shortland, Edward, 'Collection of papers relating to Maori and the Maori language' 217; *Te Karere Maori (the Maori Messenger)* 93, 203–06, 313, 316; *Te Tangata i Mate Ai Ona Hoa Noho Tata* (The man who killed his friends with kindness; The lesson of the quilt) (1873) 93; *Upoku 21* (1846) 91, 203; Watkin, James, 'Vocabulary of Maori words compiled at Waikouaiti, 1840–1844' plates **xxx**

Maori Messenger, the *(Te Karere Maori)* 93, 140, 203–06, 313, 316, plates **xxiii**

Maori Mission Board 280, 305

Map of the Settlement of Otakou (1847) 181

maps, charts and plans: Hocken Library, University of Otago 283, 289, 290, 294, 295

maps, charts and plans: Hocken's collecting: charts 69, 79, 82, 127, 147–48, 154, 256, 261; maps 17, 18, 21, 60, 69, 79, 83, 84, 85, 86, 94, 126, 129, 133, 137, 152, 154, 176, 181, 189, 235, 261, 265, 283, plates **xxvii, xxix**; plans 69, 83, 84, 127, 178, 261, 265, plates **xxiv–v**

Marion du Fresne, Marc Joseph 79, 87–88

Markham, Edward 80, 220; 'New Zealand or recollections of it' (manuscript) 141

Marsden, J.R., *Marsden's Lieutenants* (Elder) (1934) 292

Marsden, Samuel: *An Answer to Certain Calumnies ...* (1826) plates **xxv**; discovery of Manukau 235; Dixson's letters of Marsden 163; Elder Collection, Hocken Library 292–93; in Hocken's 'Historical notes' 175; Hocken's interest in 17, 76, 79, 80–81, 84, 102, 141, 153, 173, 230–31, 236, 244, 247, 278, 286; Hocken's lectures (1905-06) 80–81, 232; Hocken's life of Marsden 80, 225, 226, 231–36, 246, 291; Hocken's visit to Marsden's birthplace 110–11; *The Letters and Journals of Samuel Marsden* (Elder) (1932) 292; letters from Josiah Pratt 288; letters to and from Wilberforce 231; lock of hair 293; manuscripts 69, 72, 81, 220, 229, 231, 234, 236, 265, 302; M[a]ori names used by 175; *Proposed Memorial to the Late Rev. Samuel Marsden, at Farsley, near Leeds* 110–11

Marsden, Samuel Edward (grandson of Samuel Marsden) 231

Marsden, William 24–25

Marshall, William B.: *N.Z. the Vocabulary of South Island words* 179; *A Personal Narrative of Two Visits to New Zealand in His Majesty's Ship* Alligator (1836) 179

Marston, Edward 194

Martin, John (pilot, Hokianga) 147, 154

Martin, Johnny (Wellington) 139

Martin, R.B. 61, 62

Martin, Robert Montgomery, *The British Colonies* 131–32

Martin, Samuel McDonald 87

Martin, Sir William 101, 158, 207, 302; *A Series of Documents on the Proposed Church Constitution in the Colonies* (1854) 92

Martin, William (Otago immigrant) 89, 196

Martin Vaz island 42

Marton 112

Mason & Firth, Melbourne 40, 50

Mason, William 61, 94, 175

Masonic Lodge of Otago No. 114 EC (later No. 844) 57

Massey, Horatio 279

Massey, W.F. 279

Masterton 99

Matson, Amelia (née Buckland) 127

Matson, Henry 127

Matson, Isabel (née Thierry) 127

Mattioli, Pietro Andrea, *Discorsi* (1621) 70

Maunsell, Robert 87, 101, 102, 139, 141–42, 158, 209–10; *Grammar of the New Zealand language* (1862) 141;

Hints on Schools Amongst the Aborigines in Five Letters to the Lord Bishop of New Zealand (1849) 92, 172; 'Journal of a winter spent on Amota Bank's Island, 24 May 1860' 142
Mayo, Henry 124
Meadon, Mr 49
Meath Hospital 37
Mechanics Institute, Auckland 268
Melbourne 37, 38, 39, 43, 47, 50–51, 226, 227
Meredith, Edwin, *Memoir of the Late George Meredith* (1897) 247
Merrett, Joseph Jenner 68; Heke, his wife Harriett and Kawiti 83; *Native feast held at Remuera, Auckland, New Zealand* (1844) 207; *Ohinemutu Pa on Lake Rotorua* 125; *Three Maoris seated in front of a whare* (1850), copy 125
Methodist church 24, 25–26, 27–28, 30, 35, 41; *see also* Wesley, John; Wesleyan Methodist Conference
Methodist Magazine (previously *Arminian Magazine*)(1778–1969) 28, 32
Methodist Overseas Mission Fund 32
microfilms of Hocken material 295, 296
Milford Sound 211
Mill, H.R. 249
Miller, Alexander 53
Miller, Henry 243
Miller, James 179
Miller, John A. 291
Miller, Richard Combe 151–52
Mills, James 197, 238
Mills, John 102
Mills, William 57
missionaries 80, 84, 87, 91, 92, 97, 207, 208, 209–10, 264, 265, 295; manuscripts 69, 81, 142, 220, 229, 230, 231, 232, 234, 236, 283, 292, 302; *see also* Church Missionary Society; and names of individual missionaries
Missionary Register 182
Mitchell, David Scott 18, 157, 161–62, 164, plates **xii**; gifting of library 161, 162–63, 259, 261, 297, 317–18; Hocken's connections and interchanges 171–73, 202, 258
Mitchell, James 173
Mitchell Library, State (formerly Public) Library of New South Wales 161, 162–63, 164, 171, 172, 259, 261, 293, 317–18
moa remains 71, 95–96, 101
Moeraki 103

Molesworth, Francis Alexander 218
Molesworth, Sir William 217–18; *Selected Speeches of Sir William Molesworth* (1903) 218
Monro, (later Sir) David 69, 134; journal 135, 207; 'Notes of a Journey through a Part of the Middle Island of New Zealand' 192; *Selection of Site of Otago Settlement* (1844) 85
Montanus, Arnoldus, *Atlas Japannensis* (1670) 226, plates **xxxii**
Moore, Frederick 224
Moran, Patrick 64
Moriori 136, 143, 177
Morrell, William Parker 293
Morris, Edward Ellis 86, 187, 200–01, 244; 'Captain Cook's first log in the Royal Navy' (article in *Cornhill Magazine*) 200; *Cook and his Companions* 200; 'Doctor John Hawkesworth' (1899) (in *Gentleman's Magazine,* 1900) 201
Mortimer, Favell Lee, *More about Jesus* (1885) 203
Morton (bookseller, Auckland) 102
Morton, Harry 293
Moss, F.C., *A Planter's Experience in Fiji* (1870) 197
Muir, Amelia 62
Müller, Frederick 186
Murder of the Rev. C.S. Volkner (1865) 91
Murison, W.D. 71
Murray, A.W., *The Bible in the Pacific* (1888) 142
Murray, F. 176
Murray, John 159, 190, 218
Museum of New Zealand Te Papa Tongarewa 185, 224
music and musical score collection, Hocken Library, University of Otago 290

Napier 77, 100, 151
Natusch, Sheila 293
Nees, William 273–74, 280
Neill, Molly 227
Neill, Ruby 117
Nelson 57, 59, 60, 82, 85, 98, 104–05, 123, 133, 134, 139, 151, 312; placard warning of outbreaks of tuberculosis and cholera 97
Nelson, Dr 57
Nelson Examiner and New Zealand Chronicle 87, 104, 105, 135, 148, 168, 179, 192, 194, 264, 310, 312

Nene, Tamati Waka 102
Nevill, Samuel Tarratt 117, 211; *A Letter Addressed to the Most Rev. The Primate of New Zealand on the Establishment of Cathedrals in Colonial Dioceses* (1886) 180
New Era dredge operation, Port of Otago 118
New Plymouth 82, 105, 124, 130, 142, 176, 275
New South Wales 163, 173, 201, 240, 260; and New Zealand and South Seas Exhibition 145, 151; *see also* Sydney
New Zealand Advertiser 316, plates **xxxiii**
New Zealand and South Seas Exhibition, Dunedin, 1889–90 18, 96, 122, 123, 144–56, 204, 237; Early History, Maori and South Seas (EHMSS) Court Committee 145, 146–48, 149–51, 152, 153, 154–55; Fine Arts Committee 151; Hocken family season tickets plates **xi**; M[a]ori whare 147, 149, 151, 156; sub-committees 150
New Zealand Association 217; *see also* New Zealand Company
New Zealand Church *Almanac* (c. 1845) 92
New Zealand Colonist and Port Nicholson Advertiser 87
New Zealand Company 17, 63, 76, 81, 82, 85, 91, 128, 129–30, 139, 173, 182, 192, 217, 295; *Instructions to the Surgeons-Superintendent on Board the Emigrant Ships of the New Zealand Company* (1841) 38; land claims 207; records 109, 110, 136, 139, 165, 189, 220–24, 241, 278, 301–02; *Supplement to the 12th Report of the New Zealand Company* ('Fat Book') (April 1844) 168; *see also* New Zealand Association
New Zealand Educational and Literary Monthly 129–31
New Zealand Examiner 314–15
New Zealand Exhibition, Dunedin, 1865 61–63, 95, 105, 140, 144; 'Decisions on points relating to the New Zealand Exhibition' (1865) 62; Hocken's spoof lecture 63; 'Notes on what sorts of exhibits are required for New Zealand Exhibition' (1865) 62
New Zealand Gazette 82, 87, 99, 128, 140, 150, 285, 311

New Zealand Gazette and Britannia Spectator 99
New Zealand Gazette and Wellington Spectator 99
New Zealand Herald and Auckland Gazette 87, 195, 311, 312
New Zealand Industrial Exhibition, Wellington, 1885 72, 138, 144
New Zealand Institute 70, 76, 95, 107; *Transactions* 186, 187, 198, 202–03, 247; *Transactions and Proceedings* 71, 85–88, 120
New Zealand International Exhibition, Christchurch, 1882 144
New Zealand International Exhibition Fine Art Section Official Catalogue (1906) 247
New Zealand Journal 82, 105, 109, 127, 128, 135, 165, 166, 240
New Zealand Journalists' Institute 175
New Zealand Jubilee and Exhibition Chronicle 154
New Zealand Magazine 277
New Zealand Mail 244
New Zealand Review 277
New Zealand Society: *Address to Members of the New Zealand Society* (1851) 96; *Rules of the New Zealand Society* (1851) 96
New Zealand Spectator and Cook's Strait Guardian 87, 168, 170, 172–73, 182, 264, 310, 312, 313, 314, 316
New Zealand Times 251, 313
New Zealand Wars 64, 83, 92, 99, 101, 102, 105, 117, 128, 149, 190, 221, 289
New Zealander 204
Newcastle 35–36, 37, 215
Newcastle Infirmary 36
Newcastle upon Tyne College of Practical Science 36, plates **iii**
newspapers: Hocken Library, University of Otago 275, 281, 282, 283, 284, 292; Hocken's lecture, 'Some account of the beginnings of literature in New Zealand: Part II, the English newspapers' (1901) 87, 211, 230; *see also* titles of individual newspapers
newspapers: Hocken's collecting 82, 128, 152, 175, 181; colony's first newspaper 82; exchanges with Cheeseman 150, 179, 204; exchanges with Mitchell 172–73; extent and descriptions of collection 264, 266, 267, 301; Hocken's interest 109, 301; letters to and from Turnbull regarding

offers of duplicates 168–69, 170, 310–13, 314–15, 316; purchase of newspapers 139–40; *Te Karere* queries 203–06
Ngahuruhuru, map of New Zealand 235, plates **xxix**
Ngai Tahu 123, 181, 294
Ngapua, Hone Heke 203
Ngati Kahungunu 100
Ngawaka, Takarei 148
Nicholas, J.L. 234; *Narrative of a Voyage to New Zealand* 138, 242
Nicholson, (later Sir) Richard 182
Nops, J.G., 'Plan of Kawiti's Pa at Ruapukepuke' 83, 84, 127
Norman, Edmund 104; *Lyttelton, Port of Victoria* (1852) 131; *Port Hill's* 131; *Town of Lyttelton* (1852) 131
Norris, Edward 188
Northern Wairoa 142
Northern War 83, 101, 102, 117, 128, 149, 190, 221
Notes & Queries 231
Nutting, Ernest 275

Oamaru 175, 181
O'Brien, George 62; *The Taieri Plains* (1867) 181
Oddfellows Hall, Dunedin 81
Ohae 230
Ohaeawai Pa 83, 117, 124
Ohinemutu 78
Oihi 234
Okaihau 230
Oliver, R.A., *A Series of Lithographic Drawings from Sketches in New Zealand* (1852) 109
Oliver, W.H. 296
Olssen, Erik 293, 296
Onslow, Earl and Countess of 116, 145
Orakei, Auckland 102
oral history records 103
Original School of Anatomy, Medicine and Surgery, Dublin 36–37, plates **iv**
Ormand Brothers 273
Otago: Anglican diocese 90; goldfields 51, 52–53, 55; Hocken's lectures 84–85, 88; jubilee celebrations 188, 189, 193, 276 (*see also* Otago Jubilee Industrial Exhibition, 1898); maps 181; New Zealand and South Seas Exhibition court 151; population 52; proposal to re-annex Southland to 58; settlement 82, 84–85, 88, 131, 132, 133, 135–37, 182, 183, 188, 189, 208, 265, 294, 302; *see also* individual placenames
Otago Acclimatisation Society 58
Otago Agricultural and Pastoral Show 123
Otago Association 136
Otago Benevolent Institute 58, 107, 136
Otago Church Settlement Group 150
Otago Daily Times 52, 53, 56, 62, 72, 135, 200; 'A glance at the books', article on Hocken Library 277; announcement of gifting of Hocken's collection 183, 258; contribution to Endowment Fund 285; Hocken's advertising of medical practice 53–54; Hocken's articles and reviews 79, 185–86; in Hocken's collection 181; Hocken's description of his collection 264; and Hocken's funeral 279; Hocken's lectures on Marsden (1905-06) 80–81, 232; Hocken's lectures: printing of, and reports on 54, 77, 79, 88, 126; Hocken's letter to Fenwick 301–03; Hocken's shares 304; Hocken's use of extracts from 193; interviews with Hocken 229, 231; New Zealand and South Seas Exhibition news 145, 156; printing of Hocken Library catalogue 283; review of Hocken's *Contributions* 194, 195; support of Hocken Library and report on opening 261, 263, 268, 269, 270, 275, 285
Otago Education Board 289
Otago Gazette see Otago Provincial Government Gazette
Otago Institute 18, 70–71, 75 76, 113, 199, 279; council 107; Hocken as president 71, 107, 248; Hocken's lectures 71, 76–77, 79–86, 119, 120, 132, 186, 198, 202–03, 211
Otago Journal 130, 168, 240, 241, 277, 312
Otago Jubilee Industrial Exhibition, 1898 156, 175, 181, 197
Otago Medical Association 55, 212
Otago Medical Board 77
Otago Museum 71, 73, 80, 95, 96, 125, 147, 156, 181, 183, 263, 288; Ethnographic Department 276, 286; Hocken Wing (*see under* Hocken Library, University of Otago); Hocken's bequest of Maori

materials 292; suggested as site for Hocken Library 260–61, 262, 263, 267–68, 269
Otago Polytechnic 294
Otago Provincial Council reports 296, 312
Otago Provincial Government Gazette 169, 284, 312, 313
Otago Punch 169, 313
Otago Society for the Prevention of Cruelty to Animals, Ladies Committee 116
Otago University Press 294
Otago Witness 94, 122, 181, 279; Hocken's articles and letter 188, 189; in Hocken's collection 168, 310; Hocken's lectures 77, 211; interviews with, and tributes to, Hocken 126, 223–24, 227–28, 230; photographs and photo-montages by Bessie Hocken 123, 216; review of Hocken's works 195, 249, 255
Otaki 188
Otokia 103
Outline History of the Gold, Coal, and Other Known Mineral Resources of New Zealand (1886) 118
Owen, G.B. 139
Owen, Richard 95, 158

Pacific Islands: Dixson's interest in exploration 163; Hocken's collecting 62–63, 137–38, 142, 152; Hocken's description, introduction to catalogue of New Zealand and South Seas Exhibition 153; Hocken's lectures 77; *see also* Fiji; Samoa; Tonga
Page, Dorothy 296
Page, W.B.G. 231
Paihia 101, 102, 209, 210
paintings and sketches: Hocken Library, University of Otago 224, 283, 288, 289, 290, 291–92, 294, 295, plates **xviii**
paintings and sketches: Hocken's collecting 17, 21, 67, 69, 82, 83, 99, 152, 154, 181, 261, 278; Bessie Hocken's works 122–23; Brown's caricatures 136, plates **xxxv**; copies and facsimiles 82, 97, 123–25; early pictorial illustrations 129–31; extent and descriptions of collection 261, 265, 283, 301; Fox's bequest 124, plates **xxxv**; gifts 85; highest individual amount paid 225; Hocken's annotations 63, 64–65, 123, 125, 148, plates **xxxv**; Hocken's views on subjects worthy of depiction 76; Holmes sketches 124–25, 224; of Maori 68, 104, 108, 148–49, 188, 224–25, plates **xxxvi**; portraits 68, 80, 85, 104, 108, 148–49, 181, 206, 207, 217, plates **xxxvi**; purchases 62, 104–05, 148, 181, 225; request to Webster 207; Williams' watercolour sketches 83, 84, 102, 117, 124, 128, 146
Pakaraka 102
Pakirikiri 184
Pakowhai Pa 100
Palmer, Edwin 103, 186
Palmer Howe, booksellers and publishers 226
Palmer, Ned 86
Palmer, William (Bill) 103
Palmerston North 100
Palsey, Captain 43, 45
pamphlets: Hocken Library, University of Otago 281, 282, 286, 287, 292
pamphlets: Hocken's collecting 54, 56, 106, 118, 127, 129, 137, 140, 154, 175, 226, 281; advertisement requesting pamphlets for purchase 102–03; Benevolent Institute 58; from Clarke 227; from Collier 241; exchange with Morris 200, 201; exchange with Shaw 180; exchanges with Cheeseman 150, 180, 204; exchanges with Grey 106, 165–66; exchanges with Mitchell 172, 173; exchanges with Turnbull 167–68, 169, 170, 171, 309; extent and description of collection 21, 166, 180, 189, 237, 245, 264, 276, 277; on flax 72; given to Mitchell 164; from Heaphy 104; from Hodgkinson 132; from Logan Campbell 229; on Maori 95; from members of Williams family 92–93, 95, 166; from Petherick 113; presented to Auckland Public Library 189; purchased from book dealers 98, 101, 102; from Smith 142, 176, 233; *see also* Hocken, Thomas Morland: library: compilations and bound volumes
Parata, Tamati 87, 211
Parihaka 105, 106, 153
Park, Reynolds & Co. 169–70, 183, 286, 315
Parker, Samuel Ebenezer 32
Parker, T. Jeffrey 190

Parkes, Henry (later Sir Henry) 43; *An Emigrant's Home Letters* (with Annie Parkes) (1896) 201
Parkinson, Phillip, *Books in Maori* (2004) 293, 295
Parkinson, Sydney 79, 86, 164, 197; *A Journal of a Voyage to the South Seas* (1773; 1784) 80, 125, 138, 200, 295
Parliamentary Library, Wellington *see* General Assembly Library of New Zealand
Parsonson, Gordon 296
Patea 105
Paterson, James 61
Patteson, John Coleridge 92
Patuone 94
Pearson, John, *The Life of William Hey* (1823) 28
Pearson, Walter 77; *The Financial Position of the Colony of NZ* (1887) 118; *In Memoriam: Sir John Richardson* (1879) 97
Pearson, W.H. 175
Peele, James, *Christchurch in 1852* 104
Pennefather, F.W. 279
Perry, Joseph 61
Perry, Matthew, *Narrative of the Expedition of an American Squadron to the China Seas and Japan* (1856) 228
Peterson, M. Jeanne 34
Petherick, Edward Augustus 11–12, 113, 136; *An Index to the Literature of Geography, Maritime and Inland Discovery, Commerce and Civilization* (1886) 112; *Catalogue of a Collection of Books Illustrative of Discovery and Colonisation in Australasia* (1890) 238, 244; *Catalogue of the York Gate Geographical and Colonial Library* (1882) 112, 238; *Catalogue of the York Gate Library Formed by S. William Silver* (1886) 238; *The Colonial Book Circular and Bibliographical Record* (1887) 113; *Library Presented to the Federated Colonies of Australia* (1896) 238; *The Torch and Colonial Book Circular* (1887; 1890) 113
Pharazyn, Robert 128
Philips, Philip, *Memories of the Past* (1888) 172
Phillpotts, George 'Toby' 207
Philosophical Institute of Canterbury 185
Philson, J.M. 129
Philson, Thomas M. 126

photographs: Hocken Library, University of Otago 288, 289, 290, 294; Hocken's collecting 17, 21, 184, 206, 228, 231
Pickersgill Harbour 123
Picton 139
pictures *see* paintings and sketches
Pihoihoi Mokemoke, Te (1863) 170
Pink and White Terraces 78
Pirates Football Club 117
Pirikawau 139
Piripi 59
Pitt Island 142
Plimmer, John 139; *A Trip Through Fairyland* (1884) 97
Plunket, Lord 275, 276–77, 279
Pogson, G.W. 117
Polack, Joel Samuel: *Manners and Customs of the New Zealanders* (1840) 98, 139; *New Zealand, being a Narrative of Travels* (1838) 79, 139
'Polynesian Bibliography with special reference to Philology' committee, AAAS 92, 177, 180, 243
Polynesian Society 19, 176–79, 197, 248, 312; *Journal* 142, 227, 228
Pomare, Hare 148
Pompallier, Jean Baptiste 88
Port Chalmers, painted view 182
Port Nicholson 76, 77, 82, 173, 209; *see also* Wellington
Port Nicholson Gazette 179
Porter, T.W.R., *Major Ropata Wahawaha, NZC, MLC: The story of his life and times* (1897) 172
Portlock, Nathaniel 201
Potatau: 'Seal of the Maori King Potatau' 94, 101, 136
Potiki, Riria 123
Potts, T.H. 140
Poverty Bay 76, 79, 92, 184
Poverty Bay Herald 248
Pratt, Josiah 288
Pratt, Thomas 117
Preservation Inlet 103
Press 98, 268, 295
Priestley, Henry 33
Proudfoot, John 124
Province of Otago in New Zealand … (1868) plates **xxxviii–xxxix**
Public Library of Victoria Catalogue (1880) 241
publishing, New Zealand 18
Puckey, William Gilbert 209, 229–30
Puketeraki 87, 211

Pungarehu 105
Purday, S.F. 220
Putiki Pa 99–100, 141
Pyke, Vincent 57, 61

Quaife, Barzillai 87
Quaritch, Bernard 109, 129, 159, 160, 162, 241
Queen Charlotte Sound 79
Queenstown 122
Quintal, Oliver 101

Rahotu 106
Ralph, Thomas Shearman 72–73; *Observations and Experiments with the Microscope on the Effects of Various Chemical Agents on the Blood* (1866) 129; *On the Occurrence of Bacteria (Bacilli) in Living Plants* [1883] 129
Rangihoua 76, 102
Raoul, Etienne, *Choix de plantes de la Nouvelle Zélande* (1846) 70, 82, 128
Rattray, James 61, 80, 136
Rayne, Septimus William 35, 37
Read, Gabriel 52
Redmayne, Thomas: 'Otago and her new doctors: A speedy cure anticipated' 63; pencil drawing of Dunedin (1864) 181; *Royal Hotel, Dunedin* (1876) 65
Redwood, Francis 98
Reed, A.H. 292, 293
Rees, William: *The Effect of Native Lands Acts Upon the Colonization of the North Island of New Zealand* (1873) 96–97; *The Life and Times of Sir George Grey* (1892) 202
Reeves, William (1825–91) 98
Reeves, William Pember (1857–1932) 215, 222, 223; *The Long White Cloud – Ao Tea Roa* (1898) 202
Regulations to be Observed by Students Intending to Qualify Themselves to Practice as Apothecaries in England and Wales (1843) 34
Reid, John 64
Reid, Stuart: 'A rare bird …' plate **xl**; *The Tickler: 100 Caricatures* (c. 1907) 247
Reischek, Andreas 141
Remuera, Auckland 102
Rennie, Alexander 136
Rennie, George 84, 125, 183
Rennie, Sir Richard 183
Returned Services Association hostel 68

Reuther, J.G., Strehlow, Carl, *Testamenta Marra* (1897) 227
Revans, Samuel 82, 87, 98–99, 140
Reynolds, Sir Joshua 62
Reynolds, W.H. 61
Rich, Francis 110
Richardson, George Rycroft 87
Richardson, J.L.C. 54
Richardson, John and Jane 24
Richardson, Mary 25
Richardson, Miss (later Grant) 35
Richmond, Christopher 56, 139
Riddiford, Edward 99
Riemenschneider, Johann Freidrich 59–60, 97, 105; 'On Maori habits of life' 60
Rigan, Mr 55
Rintoul, Robert 82
Ritchie, Thomas 155
Robert Burns Fellowship 290
Roberts, John (NZ and South Seas Exhibition president, Hocken Library Trustee) 147, 268, 270, 306
Roberts, John Mackintosh (Lieutenant-Colonel) 147
Roberts, Sherwood 294
Robertson, George 111, 157, 162, 171, 201, 259
Robertson-MacDonald, David 221
Robinson, Charles Barrington 175
Robinson, W.V. 49
Robley, Horatio Gordon 20, 95, 214, 215, 216–17, 250, 280, 286; *Moko or Maori Tattooing* (1896) 214, 281
Rochfort, John, *The Adventures of a Surveyor in New Zealand* (1853) 176
Rochon, Alexis Marie 79; *Voyages aux Indes Orientales et en Afrique* (1807) 138
Rodda, Linda: 'Calendar of Dr T.M. Hocken's personal letters and documents preserved in the Hocken Library, Otago University' 289; *Catalogue of Pictures in the Hocken Library* 289
Rogers, Frank 289
Roland, Helen 47–48, 50
Ronnie, Mary, *Freedom to Read: A centennial history of Dunedin Public Library* (2008) 258
Ross, Angus 293
Ross, David 270
Ross, John 268, 270, 306; article on Hocken in *Dictionary of Literary Biography* 17

Ross, Malcolm, *Aorangi, Or, The Heart of the Southern Alps, New Zealand* (1892) 178
Ross, Sir James 230
Roth, H. Ling 79
Rotomahana 78
Rotz, Jean 79, 86
Royal Anthropological Institute 225–26
Royal College of Surgeons of England 34, 36, 37, 215
Royal Colonial Institute 110, 112, 195, 214, 270
Royal Geographical Society 112, 215
Royal Hotel, Dunedin 64–65
Royal Princess Theatre, Dunedin 58–59
Royal Society of Tasmania 227; Library catalogue (1885) 241
royal visit, 1901 211
Ruapehu 78
Ruapekapeka Pa 83, 117, 124; 'Plan of Kawiti's Pa at Ruapekapeka' (1846) 83, 84, 127
Ruapuke Island 60, 81, 97, plates **x**
Rusden, G.W.: *Curiosities of Colonization* (1874) 173; *Lecture on the Character of Falstaff* (1870) 172
Russell 83, 101, 102, 147, 229, 230
Russell, George Frederick 127
Russell, H.R. 160
Russell, Michael, *Polynesia* (1845) 197
Russell Society 149
Russo–Japanese War 226, 228
Rutherford, John 183–84

Sala, George Augustus 117, 126
Sale, Professor and Mrs 116
Salmond, Anne 293
Salvation Army 280, 305
Samoa 157, 158, 180; Hockens' trip, 1898 196, 197, 310; at NZ and South Seas Exhibition 145, 149, 152, 154; Turnbull's letter to Gurr asking to buy publications 310
Sampson, Low, Marston & Co. 129, 190, 191–94, 196
Sampson, Miss 44
Sargood Trust 289
Saturday Advertiser 77
Saturday Review 170, 316
Saunders, William 211
Scandrett, W.B. 132
Scott and Wilson 273
Scott, David 273, 274
Scott, George 64
Scott, John Halliday 116, 118, 125, 261, 273, 279, 303, 304; charcoal on paper sketch of Hocken 295
Scott, Patrick, *The Farewell and Other Poems* (1827) 173
Seddon, Richard 215
Sedgwick, Adam 48
Seed, William 139
Selfe, Henry Selfe 90, 218–19
Selfe, Norman 163
Selfe, Sir William Lucius 218–19
Selwyn, George Augustus 91, 142, 158, 188, 203, 302
Selwyn, John Richardson 182
Sewell, Tom 47
Shamrock Hotel, Dunedin 57
Shand, Alexander 177
Shand, Lily 116
Shaw, Alexander, *Catalogue of the Different Specimens of Cloth* 138, plates **xx**
Shaw, G. Gerard 180
Shaw, George Baird, *View of Dunedin from Church Hill, 1851* 124, 181, 192
Shaw, William H. 31
Shillington, Edward 229
Shirasawa, Homi, *Iconographie des essences forestières du Japon* (1900) 226
Shogoro, Tsuboi 213
Shortland, Edward 85, 209, 294; 'Collection of papers relating to Maori and the Maori language' 217; Hocken's acquisition of papers and books 206–07, 217; 'Journal notes kept while in the Middle Island November 1843 and 4 to 21 January 1844' 207; 'Journal of an expedition through Waikato with Governor Hobson ...' 207; *Maori Religion and Mythology* (1882) 207, 217; *The Southern Districts of New Zealand* (1851) 98, 207, 217281; *Traditions and Superstitions of the New Zealanders* (1854) 207
Shortland, Eugenia 206, 217
Sibeud de Saint-Ferriol, Armand Joseph de 88
Silver, Stephen William 112, 214; *Emigrants' Guide to Australia, New Zealand, The Cape of Good Hope* (1859) 112
Simpson, James 66
Simpson, Julia Anne Dayke *see* Hocken, Julia Anne Dayke (née Simpson)
Simpson, Peter 296
Singapore 213, 226
sketches *see* paintings and sketches

Skinner, Henry Devenish 287–88
Skinner, W.H. 235
Slugg, Josiah Thomas 30
Smales, Gideon, *Whitby Authors and their Publications* (1867) 129
Smetham, James 33; *Dr Evans and Mr Allwright meeting the Maori Chiefs (The New Zealand Chiefs in Wesley's House)* (1863) 33, 104, 124, 138, 148–49, plates **xxxvi**
Smetham, Sarah 33, 148
Smith, Edmund 135
Smith, Elder & Co. 255
Smith, George 65
Smith, Maggie 46
Smith, Sir James Edward 111
Smith, Stephenson Percy: and Bessie Hocken 117, 119; *The Eruption of Tarawera* (1887) 176; *Hawaiki: The Whence of the Maori* (1898) 142, 176; *History and Traditions of the Maoris of the West Coast, North Island of New Zealand Prior to 1840* (1910) 142; and Hocken's *Bibliography* 243, 246, 248, 250; and Hocken's life of Marsden 232–35, 291; interchanges with Hocken 108, 141, 142–43, 160, 161, 176, 178, 179, 182–83, 211–12, 233, 260, 294; *The Kermadec Islands* (1887) 142, 143; *The Lore of the Whare-wananga* (1913–15) 142; Pedigree of Hursthouse (Notes) 176; *The Peopling of the North* (1898) 176; and Polynesian Society 19, 176–79, 197; *Wars of the Northern Against the Southern Tribes of New Zealand in the Nineteenth Century* (1904) 176, 182–83
Smith, William Mein 85, 314
Society for Promoting Christian Knowledge (SPCK) 291
Society for the Promotion of the Health of Women and Children 116
Society of Apothecaries 37
Solander, Daniel 69
Sorrell, Paul, *Gaining a Foothold: Historical records of Otago's eastern coast, 1770–1839* (2008) 294
Sotheby's 241
Sotheran, Henry 109–10, 159, 162
South Africa 158
South Australia 158, 180, 182, 227; and New Zealand and South Seas Exhibition 145, 151
South Australian Museum 179
South Island, proposal to separate from North 58
Southern Cross 87, 150, 168, 284, 311, 312, 316
Southland: Anglican diocese 90; Hocken's lectures 84–85; New Zealand and South Seas Exhibition court 151; proposal to re-annex to Otago 58; *see also* individual placenames
Southland Institute 109
Southland Provincial Council reports 296, 312
Spain, William 207
Sparrmann, Anders 69
Spencer, A.H. 163–64
Spencer, Herbert 241
Spencer, Seymour M. 78
St John's Church, Invercargill 114
St Kilda, Dunedin 64
St Mary's, Auckland 102
St Paul's Cathedral, Dunedin 57, 115, 120, 175, 279
St Paul's Church, Auckland 102
Stack, J.W. 176, 178, 180, 203; views of Auckland 286
Stamford, Lincolnshire 24, 27, plates **i**
Standish, H. 176
Stanley, Henry M. 118
Stanningley, Leeds area 34
Stapp, Charles 125
State Library of New South Wales 161, 201; *see also* Dixson Library, State Library of New South Wales; Mitchell Library, State Library of New South Wales
Statement of the Case of Jas. Mitchell, Esq, Late Surgeon on the Civil Establishment of New South Wales [1838] 173
Stead, C.K. 296
Stenhouse, William 58
Stephenson, Heathfield 50
Stevens, Captain 86
Stevenson, Robert Louis 157–58, 197, 310
Stewart, Captain 181, 182
Stewart, F.E. 49–50
Stewart Island 175, 181, 183
Stewart, James, *On the Establishment of a Grand Hotel and Sanatorium in the Rotorua District* (1884) 129
Stewart, John Wylie 275
Stewart, Mr (Poverty Bay) 92
Stewart, William Downie 136, 169, 196, 250, 270, 275, 279, 283, 285, 286, 292
Stirling, Edward Charles 179

Stoddart, *New Plymouth, Taranaki* (1859) 124
Stokes, John Lort, charts of New Zealand 256
Stokes, William 38
Stout, Lady 116
Stout, Sir Robert 92, 116, 145, 244, 251, 258, 279
Stowe, Leonard 104
Strachan, Stuart 76, 289, 290; *Ka Taoka Hakena: Treasures from the Hocken Collections* (2007) 294
Straubel, C.R. 293
Strelitz, Philip 57
Strode, Alfred Chetham 53, 136
Strong, Isobel 157
Stuart, Donald 58, 135, 136
Sudgen, E.G. 32
surgeons-superintendent: *Great Britain* 39–51; role and duties 37–38; *Instructions to the Surgeons-Superintendent on Board the Emigrant Ships of the New Zealand Company* (1841) 38; *White Star* 38–39
Surville, Jean François Marie de 79, 87
Swainson, William 113
Swart, Jacob 86
Switzerland 215, 216, 229
Sydney 18, 66, 108, 145, 157, 161–63, 171, 208, 212, 226–27, 301
Sydney Morning Herald 275
Symonds, Alithea 182

Takamoana, Karaitiana 100
Tancred, Thomas, *Notes on the Natural History of the Province of Canterbury* (1856) 109
Tapsell, Philip 180
Taranaki 105, 139, 142, 233; *see also* individual placenames
Taranaki Herald 249–50
Taranaki News 176
Tasman, Abel 86, 131, 152, 211, 242; Hocken's facsimile copy of journals (1898) 186–87; Hocken's lecture: *Abel Tasman and His Journal* (1895) 119–20, 186–87; Hocken's translation of part of Tasman's journal relating to New Zealand 187, 211, 213; *Journaal van de Reis naar het Onbekende Zuidland in den Jare 1642* (Jacob Swart's edn, 1860) 86, 238
Tasmania 56, 68, 86, 117, 119, 153, 181, 186, 187, 207, 208, 227, 241, 284, 301; Walker, James Backhouse, *List of Books Relating to Tasmania* (1884) 149, 240, plates **xxxvi**
Tasmanian Journal 149
Taupo 93, 120, 255
Tauranga 77, 84, 93, 101
Taylor, Caroline 99
Taylor, Joseph 25
Taylor, Richard 69, 99, 101; *Te Ika a Maui, or New Zealand and its inhabitants* (1855) 99
Taylor, William B. 183
Te Ati Haunui-a-Paparangi 99–100
Te Heuheu Iwikau 139
Te Hokioi 170
Te Kani, Hirini 184
Te Karere Maori (the Maori Messenger) 93, 140, 203–06, 313, 316, plates **xxiii**
Te Kopua 100
Te Pihoihoi Mokenoke (1863) 170
Te Puna, national union catalogue 253, 291
Te Rangi Paetahi, Mete Kingi 99–100
Te Rauparaha 207, 211, 291
Te Rauparaha, Tamihana 188
Te Tangata i Mate Ai Ona Hoa Noho Tata (The man who killed his friends with kindness; The lesson of the quilt) (1873) 92–93
Te Wana, Wiremu 148
Te Whiti o Rongomai 105, 106
Telford, John 188
Temple, E.F., *Early Settlers* 104
Temple, Philip 296
Tempsky, Gustavus Ferdinand von 105
Terra Australis Cognita (1766) 137
Terry, Charles, *New Zealand, Its Advantages and Prospects* (1842) 180
Thatcher, Charles, *Otago Songster* (1865) 63
Theomin, David 216, 228, 276
Theomin, Dorothy 216
thermal district, North Island 77, 78, 229
Thévenot, Melchisédec 250, 313; *Relations de divers voyages curieux* (1696) 138, 169, 313
Thierry, Charles Philippe Hippolyte de 81, 127, 152, 207; 'Historical narrative of an attempt to form a settlement in New Zealand' 164–65
Thompson (binder, Dunedin) 282
Thomson, Arthur S.: 'On the peculiarities in figure, the disfigurations and the customs of New Zealanders' 95; *The Story of New Zealand* (1859), including

bibliography 42, 126, 190, 238, 248, 249
Thomson, Arthur T. 71
Thomson, Basil 186
Thomson, George Craig 289
Thomson, George Malcolm 69
Thomson, J.T. 175
Thomson, Peter 74, 79
Tickler for Otago and Southland 295, plates **xvii**
Todd, Andrew 225
Tohu Kakahi 105, 106
tokens 180–81
Tokomaru 184
Tonga 158; at NZ and South Seas Exhibition 145, 149, 150
Tongariro 78
Torlesse, Charles 82
Tourist Bureau, Dunedin 261–62
Traherne, L.P. 49
Transactions and Proceedings of the New Zealand Institute 71, 85–88, 120
Transactions of the New Zealand Institute 186, 187, 198, 202–03, 247
Travels of Hildebrand Bowman (1778) 86
Travers, William 69
'Treatment of sea-sickness' (Hocken's article for *The Lancet*, 1861) 41
Treaty of Waitangi 139, 151, 152; facsimile 82, 128; Hocken's 'rescue' of 22; signing 76, 93, 181
Tregear, Edward 108, 142, 176, 178, 180, 250; *Maori-Polynesian Comparative Dictionary* (1891) 92; *Paumotuan Dictionary* (1893) 92
Trial of Captain Jarvey on a Charge of Poisoning his Wife (1865) 56
Trimble, Anna (Annie) 68–69, 120
Trimble, Annie Eliza (née Nelson) 275, 282; 'Raw material of history' 285
Trimble, Dorothy Heywood (later Stewart) 275
Trimble, Henrietta Mary Rogers (née Penn) 274–75
Trimble, William Heywood 68, 129, 201, 274–75, 281–84, 297–98; *Catalogue of the Hocken Library* (1912) 70, 217, 228, 281–83, 287, plates **xxiii**; 'Journal of Librarian' 275, 277
Trimnell, Mary Serena (née Puckey) 229–30
Trimnell, Thomas 229–30
Trinity Methodist Church 280, 305
Trollope, Anthony, *Australia and New Zealand* (1873) 180
Tsushima, Battle of 228
Tuapeka Times 268–69
Tubb, Martin 24
Tuckett, Frederick (surveyor) 60, 85, 97, 104, 181, 182; papers 131–35, 191–92; *Sketch of the Rural District of New Edinburgh* ('Plan of the New Edinburgh settlement') (1844) 85, 132, 194, plates **xxiv–v**
Tuckett, Frederick F. (nephew of surveyor) 133–34
Tuhawaiki, 'Bloody Jack' 81, 85, 186
Tuke, Arthur 105, 106
Tuki Tahua, map of New Zealand 235, plates **xxix**
Tunzelmann, Gertrude, 'Struggles of an early settler in the district around Lake Wakatipu' 247
Turanga 184
Turei, Mohi 203
Turnbull, Alexander Horsburgh 17–18, 109, 113, 159–61, 163, 185, 205, 241, 279, 286, 288, 297, plates **xii**; and Edge-Partington 225; and Hocken Library 283, 285; Hocken's connections and interchanges 18, 66–71, 157–58, 237, 309–17; response to Hocken's *Bibliography* 250, 253; *see also* Alexander Turnbull Library
Turnbull, Robert 160, 167
Turnbull, Sissy 169
Turner, Ellen 100, 315
Turton, H. Hanson, *Maori Deeds of Land Purchases in the North Island* (1877–78) 178
Tutapuiti, Hariata 148
tutu (*Coriaria arborea*) 50, 54–55
Twain, Mark 68, 117
Twopeny, R.E. 154
Twopeny, R.E.N. 145
Tylee family 100–01
Tyler, Linda, *Ka Taoka Hakena: Treasures from the Hocken Collections* (2007) 294
Tyrrell, James 162

Union Steamship Company 197
University of London 36
University of Otago 96, 184, 279, 280, 291, 294, 304, 305–06; council 269, 270, 271, 272, 273, 279, 280–81, 284, 286–87, 292, 303; *see also* Hocken Collections, University of Otago
University of Otago Capping Magazine 295
Upongongaro 99

Valpy, Arabella 183
Van der Poots, Gloria (later Strathern) 289
Vancouver, George, *Voyages* 138, 182
Varaie volumes 21, 143, 176, 198, 295
Vauxhall Pleasure Gardens, Dunedin 63–64
Ventress, Alan 162
Vestiges of Creation (1844) 48
Victoria, Australia 38, 180; and New Zealand and South Seas Exhibition 145; *Public Library of Victoria Catalogue* (1880) 241
Victoria League, Dunedin 116
Victoria, Queen 148, 151, 258
Vogel, Julius 58, 61, 63, 145; 'Jewlius Rex' 169, 313; *Official Handbook of New Zealand* (1875) 180
Volkner, C.S. 91
*Voyage de la corvette l'*Astrolabe (1830) 88

Wade, Harington E. 202
Wade, William Richard 80, 125, 202, 220; 'Journal of Rev. William Richard Wade' (1834–36) 222
Waikato (chief) 147, 149
Waikato (district) 75, 94, 100, 114, 115; see also individual placenames
Waikouaiti 103, 114, 123, 181; 'convict' bell used at mission station 128
Waimate North 149, 207, 208, 230, 234
Waitangi 102
Waitangi Falls Hotel 102
Waitara 142
Waiuku 142
Wakefield, Angela J. 221
Wakefield, C.M., *Life of Thomas Attwood* (1885) 221
Wakefield, Daniel Bell 215, 221
Wakefield, Edward Gibbon 17, 26, 76, 81–82, 99, 100, 101, 153, 173, 175, 182, 192, 196, 209, 214, 278, 315; *England and America* (1833) 252; letters 218, 221; reminiscences of Alice Freeman 221
Wakefield, Edward Jerningham 99, 175, 221, 240; *Adventure in New Zealand* 131, 251; *Illustrations to 'Adventure in New Zealand'* (1845) 265
Wakefield, William 85, 99, 128, 175, 208, 240
Walker, James Backhouse 117, 149, 186, 187, 208; *Abel Janszoon Tasman: His life and voyages* (1896) 149; *List of Books Relating to Tasmania* (1884) 149, 240, plates **xxxvi**
Wallace, Alfred Russel 113
Wallace, John Howard 140; *Manual of New Zealand* (1886) 138–39
Waller, William 172
Walsh, Philip 229, 230, 234
Wanaka (place) 121
Wanaka (ship) 108
Wanganui 99, 100, 105, 140–41, 146
Ward, C.D.R. 128
Ward, Dudley 70, 71
Ward, John, *Supplementary Information Relative to New-Zealand: Comprising despatches and journals of the company's officers of the first expedition* (1840) 173
Ward, Sir Joseph 262–63, 267, 276, 277, 279, 285
Watermeyer, E.B. 158
Watkin, James, 'Vocabulary of Maori words compiled at Waikouaiti, 1840–1844' plates **xxx**
Watt, Isaac Newton 105
Way, Sir Samuel 227, 263–64, 279
Wayte, Edward 102
Wayte, G.H. 49–50
Webber, Ernie R. 290
Webber, John 79, 101, 164; *Views in the South Seas* 138
Webster, John 127, 147, 150, 154, 206–07, 228, 230, 248, 254, 255; *The Last Cruise of the* Wanderer (1858) 206, 256; *Reminiscences of an Old Settler in Australia and New Zealand* (1908) 255–57
Webster, William 182
Weld, Frederick 104
Weller Brothers 46
Wellington 57, 76, 77, 82, 96, 98, 104, 108, 118, 123, 128, 138–39, 140, 157–58, 173, 183, 188, 209, 225
Wellington Advertiser 313
Wellington Gazette 264
Wellington Independent 87, 168, 264, 285, 310, 312, 314
Wellington Philosophical Society 105
Wellington Provincial Council reports 169, 312, 313, 314
Wellington Society 129
Wellington Spectator 105
Wentworth, W.C., *A Statistical, Historical and Political Description of the Colony of New South Wales* (1819) 20–21
Wesley, John 25, 27, 28, 29, 33, 148
Wesleyan Methodist Conference 29

Wesleyan Methodist Foreign Missionary Society 148
West Coast 90, 93–94, 151
Western Australia 152, 158
Wharetotara, Maketu (Wiremu Kingi Maketu) 207–08, 209
Whiston, F.W. 196
Whitcombe, George 255
Whitcombe & Tombs 234, 254, 256, 257; reference catalogue (1907) 247
White, Hori 184–85
White, John (Maori scholar) 177; *The Ancient History of the Maori* (1887–91) 100; *Maori Customs and Superstitions* (1861) 74; *Maori Superstitions* (1856) 74, 206; *Te Rou: or the Maori at Home* (1874) 100
White, John (suitor of Gladys Hocken) 118–19
White, Joseph Eli 267, 268, 270
White Star 38–39, 66
White, Thomas Leigh 102–03
Whitworth, R.P., *Martin's Bay Settlement West Coast of Otago* (1870) 93–94
Wicksteed, J.T. 275
Wilberforce, William 231
Wildash, Mr 43
Wildman, William 217
William Dixson Foundation 164
Williams, Arthur Edward, Taranaki war sketchbook 289
Williams family 80, 91–93, 101, 166
Williams, Henry (1792–1867) 91, 93, 102, 207, 209
Williams, Henry (1823–1904) 91
Williams, Henry Edward (Hocken Library Trustee) 268, 270, 306
Williams, Herbert 74, 92, 184; *A Bibliography of Printed Maori to 1900* (1924; and supplement by Sommerville, 1947) 293–94, 295
Williams, John (sergeant): sketch of Okaihau pa 124, 146; sketches of Ohaeawai and Pomare's pa 83, 84, 102, 117, 124, 128
Williams, John (missionary), *Narrative of Missionary Enterprises* (1867) 197
Williams, Marianne 91
Williams, Robert 72
Williams, Samuel 91, 101
Williams, William 91, 142, 150, 203, 208, 227; *A Dictionary of the New Zealand Language* (1844) 91; *Remarks upon 'Ecce Homo'* (1867) 91; *Three Letters* (1845) 91
Williams, William Leonard 92–93, 95, 182, 229, 233–34; 'Lessons in Maori' (bound pamphlets by Davis and Leonard Williams) 95; 'Maori names of plants' 74
Williamson, John 204
Wilmot, Lieutenant, *Sketch of Heke's Pah at Ohaewai* 83, 128
Wilson, Alexander 136
Wilson, Charles 160, 244–46, 251, 274; *New Rambles in Bookland* (1923) 244; *Rambles in Bookland* (1922) 244
Wilson, George Henry, *Ekino and Other Poems* (1869) 97
Wilson, J.A., *Missionary Life and Work in New Zealand* (1889) 206
Wilson, John Frederick 57
Wilson, William Scott 204
Wimperis, Fanny 295
Windle, St Helens, Lancashire 34
Wohlers, Johann Friedrich Heinrich 59, 85, 97, 131
Wood, Joan Collis 290
Wood, Joseph 109
Woodhouse Grove boarding school 28–33, plates **iii**; Hocken's 1902 visit 33; lack of library 32; little science teaching 32
Woodthorpe, Robert 236, 291, 292
Woollaston, Toss 290
Woolly, S. 231
Woon, Richard Watson 105
Worshipful Company of Apothecaries 36
Wynyard, Henry 128
Wynyard, Robert Henry 128

Yarwood, A.T. 293
Yate, William 80, 208, 210; *An Account of New Zealand* (1835) 126
York Gate Library 112; *An Index to the Literature of Geography, Maritime and Inland Discovery, Commerce and Civilization* (1886) 112; *Catalogue of the York Gate Geographical and Colonial Library* (1882) 112
Young, Nicholas 79
Young, Sir Frederick 214
Young, W.C. 65

Zoological Library, London, *Catalogue* (1887) 241